Integrative Pharmacology

Combining Modern Pharmacology with Integrative Medicine

SECOND EDITION

by Dr. Greg Sperber with Bob Flaws

Published by:
BLUE POPPY PRESS
A Division of Blue Poppy Enterprises, Inc.
4804 SE 69th Avenue
Portland, OR 97206
www.bluepoppy.com

First Edition, October 2007
Second Printing, July 2013
Third Printing, June 2014
Second Edition, October 2016
Second Printing, March 2019
Third Printing, December 2019
Fourth Printing, March 2020

ISBN 1-891845-69-1   ISBN 978-1-891845-69-7
Library of Congress Control Number: 2016953802

Cover & page design: Deborah Topping, Honora Lee Wolfe, and Eric J. Brearton

COMP Designatio n Original work

10 9 8 7 6 5 4
Printed at Frederic Printing, Aurora, CO

Acknowledgments

We are very grateful to the many people who have helped make this book a reality. To Diane Sperber, Marv Mittleman, and the late Dr. Martin Rosten and Mrs. Estelle Rosten, without whom the skills, knowledge, and education that helped create this book would not exist. To Bruce Staff, who gently kept us on track with encouragement and understanding. To Shr Fu Mike Patterson, who set the course many, many years ago. And to my wife, Ginelle, for all the support and encouragement. To the rest of our friends and families for their support. And to all those colleagues and students who gave us positive feedback and helped keep us motivated when the task seemed too large.

Contents

Introduction

INTRODUCTION TO THE SECOND EDITION

It was always the intent that the first edition of this book would not be the last. This author had asked for a six-month lead time in getting a second edition together. Three years after that lead time, it was finished. This edition is not an update to the original edition; it is an almost complete rewrite.

We were shocked at how many things had changed in just a few years. Add to that a long list of additions we wanted to make. We are very proud that we accomplished almost everything we set out to do. This addition adds:

- **Over the counter drugs**

- **A new chapter dedicated to cancer agents**

- **A new chapter devoted to illicit drugs in order to make this book a complete solution to the National Certification Commission of Acupuncture and Oriental Medicine's new outline for biomedicine**

- **Hundreds of new drugs**

- **New pregnancy risks for every drug**

- **A new section in every drug class that specifically outlines the drug-herb interaction risks**

- **An expanded section explaining the basics of drug-herb interactions**

- **Dozens of new drug-herb interactions from the research literature and, as always, classified to according to their evidence level**

- **Subcutaneous and intramuscular agents**

- **Topical agents**

Unfortunately this isn't everything. We have added intramuscular and subcutaneous agents, but still have not included intrathecal or intravenous agents. We have not included ophthalmic, nebulized, or dental-only drugs, nor those used exclusively in emergency situations.

We have also tried to make the book more useful to practitioners other than acupuncturists and Oriental medical practitioners. While we still have a long way to go with adding drug-herb interactions for Western herbs, we have started that process and hope to expand on it dramatically in future editions. Ultimately, we are simply trying to create an accessible text and reference book for pharmacology. Not an easy task, but, based on feedback from the first edition, we think we have achieved it. Please let us know one way or another and let us know how we can improve it.

While this book includes a lot of information, whether because of time or space constraints, or simply the information would not be especially useful, a lot of information is not included. Since this book is geared towards the United States market, it does not include any drugs unavailable in the US. In addition, all generic and brand names are those used in the USA and do not include names used elsewhere in the world.

HOW TO USE THIS BOOK

One of the first things the reader may notice about this book is that the authors do not skimp on the terminology. This in many ways may make for difficult reading, but as in any discipline, the terminology or jargon is important to comprehend in order to understand the subject. The authors have tried to minimize the difficulty by including handy breakout boxes with difficult terminology defined, not in the back of the book, but right where the term is used. In addition, there are lots of figures to explain concepts discussed in the text. It is hoped that these will make reading a little easier and help facilitate the internalization and learning of the terminology.

This book was designed with two purposes in mind. One purpose was to be a textbook to be used in pharmacology classes in integrative medical schools. This means it has to follow a regular progression of information and include and explain the basics of pharmacology. The second purpose was to create a reference book for integrative medical practitioners. In this role, information that needs to be quickly found should be broken down into small chunks that can be quickly and easily digested and useful in the clinic.

To make the use of this book as easy as possible, the back of the book has a list of commonly and not so commonly used abbreviations, a comprehensive glossary, and, most importantly, an extensive index.

Each drug class monograph is similar. They start with a list of the drugs based on their generic names followed by a pronunciation guide and a list of the drug's brand names. If there are no brand names, it is because the drug is sold exclusively in generic form.

PR: Pregnancy Risk. In each listing of pharmaceutical agents, this symbol indicates the drug's grade for use or contraindication during pregnancy, A through X. See the table on the following page.

This may be followed by an overview of the disease or some general information relevant to the drug class. The functions of the drug class are then illustrated followed by how each agent works and its mechanisms of action. For agents used to treat micro-organisms, there may be a section covering the spectra of organisms the agent is useful against. But most monographs continue to discuss doses of each drug. The adverse effects and any red flags for each drug are listed. In these sections, it is not the goal to be comprehensive but to demonstrate common adverse effects, those that may affect the use of the agent, those that may necessitate monitoring, and serious or life-threatening effects.

Some conventions are used throughout the book. Seeing an [O] behind a brand name means the brand name is over the counter. If there is no geriatric dosing in a given drug's dosing, the adult dosing should be considered the appropriate guideline. It is always a good idea to be at the lower end of a dosing range, if specific geriatric dosing is not given.

Off-label uses of specific drugs have generally been included in their functions and descriptions. Using a drug off label means it is being used for a purpose not approved by the Federal Drug Administration (FDA). Most of these are considered legitimate uses of the agent and may in fact have a lot of evidence supporting their use. Sometimes, the manufacturer has not gone through the FDA approval process, and other times it is an older drug without the incentive for an outside company to usher it through the very expensive process. Dosing for off-label uses is not included in this book.

After every drug entry is its pregnancy risk category (PR=). The FDA grades almost every agent for its risk if used during pregnancy, graded from "A" no risk to D and X, which is contraindicated during pregnancy. This is summarized in the table on the following page.

Interactions of each agent are listed, and these include major drug-drug interactions to be wary of and drug-herb interactions. Because of the ever-changing landscape of interactions, these sections cannot be considered comprehensive. Drug-herb interactions are a particularly rapidly changing area as more and more evidence is being accumulated almost on a daily basis.

After thought and discussion, the authors decided that a simple list of drug-herb interactions could just as easily be used against the profession as be an aid. The authors have used standard evidence-based medicine levels from the Oxford Centre for Evidence-based Medicine to grade each drug-herb interaction paper for level of evidence. These grades and what they mean are listed below:

1a Systematic Review (SR) of Random, Controlled Trials (RCTs)

1b Individual RCT with narrow Confidence Interval (CI)

2a SR of cohort studies

2b Individual cohort study including low quality RCT

2c Outcomes research–study of a cohort of patients with the same diagnosis that correlates their clinical and health outcomes to the care that they received

3a SR of case-control studies

3b Individual case-control study

4 Case-series, poor-quality cohort, and case-control studies

5 Expert opinion without explixit critical appraisal, or based on physiology bench research. Animal research falls under the category of bench research.

After an evidence level for each paper is determined, a letter grade for the overall interaction is assigned based on the level of evidence of the individual papers. For each interaction, the following criteria are employed. This assessment is in parenthesis behind the herb.

A Consistent level 1 studies

B Consistent level 2 or 3 studies or extrapolations from level 1 studies

C Level 4 studies or extrapolations from level 2 or 3 studies

D Level 5 evidence or troublingly inconsistent or inconclusive studies of any level

Of course, applying these criteria does involve a bit of subjectivity in the real world. But they have been applied as consistently as possible and should be a good guide for how serious the interaction can be. It is up to an individual practitioner how to use this information. For example one practitioner may not be comfortable prescribing herbs with any level of interaction with a drug. A bolder, hopefully more experienced, practitioner however, may be completely comfortable ignoring a Level D interaction but not an A, B, C level. It is the authors' suggestion that each interaction be assessed on its own merits and a determination made as to avoid the interaction or decide whether it is okay to proceed with the combination. In the latter case, at the bare minimum, each interaction should argue for greater surveillance in its usage. Please refer to the general discussion of how to use herbs with pharmaceutical drugs.

Finally, the last chapter is a monograph discussing how each individual drug or drug class affects the body according to Chinese medicine. By including all of these sections, it the authors' goal to make this the most comprehensive drug resource for the Oriental and integrative medical practitioner.

CATEGORY	A	B	C	D	X	N
DESCRIPTION	No human fetal risk or remote possibility of fetal harm	No controlled studies show human risk; animal studies suggest potential toxicity	Animal fetal toxicity demonstrated; human risk undefined	Human fetal risk present; but benefits outweigh risks	Human fetal risk present but does not outweigh benefits; contraindicated in pregnancy	The FDA has not assigned a risk category to these agents

Figure 1.1 Categories of drugs and their danger to a fetus.

Pharmacology Basics   2

This chapter explores basic pharmacology by looking at several areas: pharmacokinetics, common pharmaceutical interactions, and pharmacodynamics. With the information in this chapter, a basic understanding of how most drugs work and basic terminology and procedures should be accomplished. Pharmacokinetics and pharmacodynamics are the yin and yang of pharmacology and are the basis on which the whole discipline rests. Therefore a basic understanding of these areas is not only necessary but gives important insight into how drugs work in all their aspects.

Pharmacokinetics describes the action of drugs within the body, including the absorption, distribution, metabolism, and elimination of drugs in addition to the rate, or kinetics, at which a drug's actions begin and their duration. This chapter will explore each of these areas.

Pharmacodynamics looks at how drugs act in the body and the effects of different drug concentrations or doses.

Pharmaceutical interactions will explore the mechanisms that most drugs use to accomplish their therapeutic actions and will discuss common receptors upon which drugs act.

SECTION 1: PHARMACOKINETICS

▥ INTRODUCTION

The ADME scheme, which includes absorption, distribution, metabolism, and elimination combined with the kinetics or rates of a drug's actions is the basis of pharmaokinetics. The ADME scheme describes how drugs move through the body and how the body acts on the drugs. It does not describe how they act upon the body, which is the purview of pharmacodynamics. The chart below gives a general overview of ADME.

▥ ABSORPTION

Absorption is the rate and extent that the drug leaves the site of administration. For example, how long does it take for an oral drug to enter the bloodstream from the small intestine and how much of the drug makes it there? This second half is referred to as *bioavailability:* what fraction of the dose of a drug reaches its site of action or a body fluid where the drug has access to its site of action.

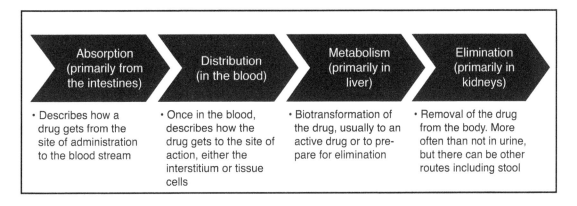

Absorption (primarily from the intestines)	Distribution (in the blood)	Metabolism (primarily in liver)	Elimination (primarily in kidneys)
• Describes how a drug gets from the site of administration to the blood stream	• Once in the blood, describes how the drug gets to the site of action, either the interstitium or tissue cells	• Biotransformation of the drug, usually to an active drug or to prepare for elimination	• Removal of the drug from the body. More often than not in urine, but there can be other routes including stool

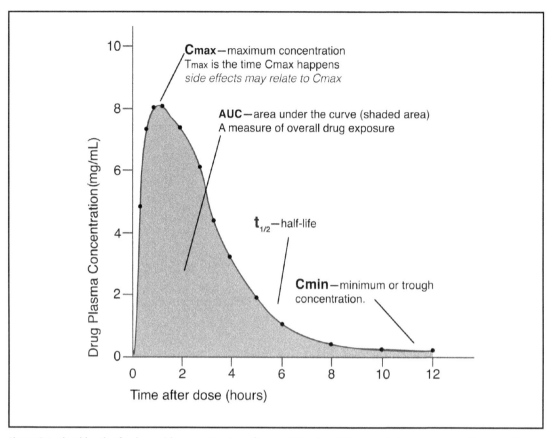

Figure 2.1: Blood levels of a drug with respect to time after an initial dose. This graphically shows several important pharmacokinetic variables including maximum concentration (Cmax), area under the curve (AUC), the drug half-life (t$_{1/2}$), and the minimum or trough concentration (Cmin).

Plasma: The fluid component of the blood

Hepatic: Pertaining to the liver

Portal system: A system that has two capillary beds rather than one. Examples include the hepatic portal system where the first capillary bed is in the intestines and the second is in the liver.

Hydrophilic: Chemicals that prefer to be in aqueous solution rather than fat- or oil-based solution

Hydrophobic: Chemicals that prefer to be in a fat- or oil based solution rather than aqueous solution

pH: A measurement of a solution's acidic or basic nature

BIOAVAILABILITY

By definition, the bioavailability of an intravenous (IV) injection is 100%. This can be plotted by having drug **plasma** concentration on the Y axis of a graph and time along the X axis (see Figure 2.1). Oral drug plasma concentrations can be plotted the same way and will always be less than IV administration. The area below each of these curves is called the *area under the curve (AUC)*. AUC is a measurement of total drug exposure over time. Bioavailability of an oral drug is computed in the following formula:

Bioavailability of oral drug = (AUC oral) / (AUC injected) X 100

Several factors can affect bioavailability:

- First-pass **hepatic** metabolism–While metabolism will be covered more in depth in Section 3 of this chapter, briefly, first-pass metabolism refers to drugs entering the hepatic **portal system** from the intestines. Hence, drugs arrive at the liver before entering the systemic circulation. Many undergo biotransformation and metabolism in the liver, and this affects the amount of active drug in the circulation. See Figure 2.2.
- Drug solubility–Very **hydrophilic** or **hydrophobic** drugs have difficulty crossing cell membranes and entering the circulation. A drug needs to be primarily hydrophobic but somewhat soluble in aqueous solutions in order to maximize drug availability.
- Chemical instability–Some drugs may be affected by the **pH** in the stomach or various degradative enzymes in the GI tract and therefore have less ability to enter the circu-

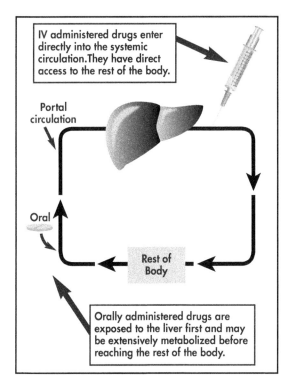

IV administered drugs enter directly into the systemic circulation. They have direct access to the rest of the body.

Portal circulation

Oral

Rest of Body

Orally administered drugs are exposed to the liver first and may be extensively metabolized before reaching the rest of the body.

Figure 2.2 First-pass hepatic metabolism. This figure shows how an oral administration of a drug must pass through the liver and have metabolism occur before going to the rest of the body. This is in contrast to an intravenous injection, which travels through the body before going to the liver.

lation as active drugs .

- Chemicophysical properties of the drug formulation–Many factors can play a role in bioavailability such as particle size, salt form, and **excipients**, among others.

Drugs can enter cells through passive diffusion, not involving a carrier protein. The physiochemical makeup of the drug helps determine how easily or difficult the drug will transverse cell membranes. This includes the concentration gradient, how lipophilic the drug is, and the surface area of the cell. This is the most common method of how a drug enters sites of action within the body.

Drugs can also enter cells through active transport, facilitated diffusion, or endo- or exocytosis (see Figure 2.3 on page 10). Facilitated diffusion is where there is a carrier protein in the cell membrane that facilitates the drug's movement to the interior. It does not require energy in order to produce this effect. Active transport is similar in that it has a protein that aids the drug's ability to enter the

cell, but it takes energy, usually in the form of **adenosine triphosphate (ATP)** to facilitate movement across the membrane. P-glycoprotein is a common example of this. Endocytosis is used by cells to engulf a large-sized drug and transport it into the cell by pinching off the cell membrane and creating a drug-filled **vesicle**. Exocytosis is the opposite of this: A cell secretes an intracellularly stored substance such as in neurotransmitter release.

Most drugs are either a weak acid or a weak base. Whether a drug is charged or neutral can affect how readily it crosses a cell membrane. Uncharged chemicals can more easily transverse membranes. Weak acids and bases can be charged or uncharged based on physiological pH. This variable is represented by pK_a. While a discussion of pK_a and the Henderson-Hasselbach equation is beyond the scope of this book, it is important to note that each drug has a different pK_a and therefore a different inherent ability to cross cell membranes.

ADMINISTRATION ROUTES

Administration routes of drugs play a large role in drug absorption. Two major methods of administration are enteral and parenteral. Enteral means through the gastrointestinal (GI) tract and parenteral means outside the GI tract and usually refers to injection.

There are also routes of administration that do not fall under either category and are considered "other" than enteral or parenteral. This includes topical, inhaled, and transcutaneous drugs. Some texts state that a rectal administration is not an enteral administration while others say it is. For the purposes of this book, it will be considered to be an enteral administration.

Enteral Administration

Oral administration, by far the most common form of enteral administration, involves swallowing a drug and having it absorbed through the gastrointestinal tract. It is the most common route of administration and is the safest, most convenient, and most economical route of administration.

Excipients: Additives to a drug formulation that affect the bulk, delivery, or availability of a drug. They are biologically inert.

Adenosine Triphosphate (ATP): The main energy storage chemical in the body

Vesicle: A storage "bubble" located in the cytoplasm of a cell, surrounded with a phospholipid bilayer

Disadvantages may include reduced drug absorption, **emesis** due to gastrointestinal irritation, destruction of some of the drug through enzymatic degradation and gastric acid, inconsistent absorption, and patient compliance issues.

Multiple factors affect absorption from the gastrointestinal tract including surface area, blood flow at the absorption site, drug state (solution, solid, or suspension), water solubility, and concentration. Oral drugs can be absorbed in the stomach or though the duodenum, which is the most common site due to its vast surface area. Most drugs absorbed in the intestine enter the hepatic portal system and enter the liver before proceeding to the rest of the body. The liver is the primary location of drug metabolism, and the drug may be significantly altered here before proceeding. This will be discussed more in depth in the metabolism section below.

A drug may be enteric coated (EC), which allows the drug to pass through the stomach without being destroyed by gastric acid. Enteric coating, however, may also limit absorption in the small intestine. Another oral drug form is the controlled-release preparation, which allows a drug to release a uniform stream to the absorption site over a relatively long period of time (8 hours, for example). Disadvantages of this form of drug include differences between patients, failure of the controlled release causing dose dumping (where the entire drug is released at once instead of over time), or reduced drug release.

Other forms of enteral administration include **sublingual** and rectal administration. Sublingual administration can be an effective method for certain drugs to enter the systemic blood stream through the mucosa of the mouth, allowing the drug to bypass the intestines and liver preventing first pass metabolism. Absorption can be very rapid as well. Few drugs, however, are chemically appropriate for this route of administration.

Rectal administration is particularly useful when oral ingestion is not possible, as when the patient is vomiting or unconscious. It is often used in young children. An advantage is that the drug bypasses the stomach and its gastric acid, which

Emesis: Vomiting

Sublingual: Below the tongue, refers to a method of administration where a drug is held under the tongue until dissolved.

could destroy some of the drug. Only about 50% of the drug enters the liver and is metabolized. Disadvantages include irregular and incomplete absorption and irritation of the rectal mucosa.

Parenteral Injection

Parenteral injections of drugs include intravenous injection, subcutaneous, intramuscular, intraarterial, and intrathecal. Intravenous (IV) injection is when an aqueous solution is injected into a vein. Subcutaneous (subcut or SubQ) injection is an injection below the skin into the subcutaneous tissues. Intramuscular (IM) injection is into a muscle. Intraarterial injection is a relatively rare administration into an artery. An intrathecal injection is an injection into the cerebrospinal fluid of the spinal subarachnoid space. Drugs, very rarely, can also be administered intraventricularly, directly into the ventricles of the brain.

Parenteral injections have many advantages over oral administration including more rapid, extensive, and predictable administration. They can be given to unconscious patients, and some drugs cannot be delivered in their active form in any other way. Disadvantages include necessity for aseptic protocols, pain, difficult self-medication, expense, and local trauma.

This book will examine many parenteral drugs but not all as many acupuncturists and integrative medical practitioners will not commonly encounter all of these agents.

Other Routes of Administration

Several other routes of administration are possible including inhalation, intranasal, topical, and transdermal. While these routes are not as common as oral and injection, many useful drugs use these routes of administration.

Medicines that are administered through inhalation are common especially in the treatment of asthma and other lung diseases. They allow for rapid delivery of the drug through the large surface area of the lung mucosa. However, only gases, very small particulates, and fine droplets of liquid can be administered this way. This route of administration can minimize systemic side effects.

A few drugs are administered intranasally, or through the nose, taking advantage of the nasal mucosa for absorption. Topical drugs can be applied to mucous membranes or to the skin and are commonly used in dermatology or when a local effect is desired. Topical drugs also include those applied to the eye. Transdermal application is related to topical administration in that it involves a patch applied to the skin that contains medication. These are becoming more common and allow for sustained drug absorption over time.

DISTRIBUTION

If drug absorption is the process where the drug enters the systemic circulation, distribution is the process through which the drug leaves the blood stream and enters the **interstitium** or tissue cells. There are four main factors that affect distribution. These are blood flow, capillary permeability, drug structure, and the degree of binding to proteins.

Blood flow to various parts of the body and specific tissues varies. This variability affects blood

Interstitium: The space between cells that is filled with fluid

Route of Administration	Advantages	Disadvantages	Notes
Enteral:			
Oral	Safe, convenient, economical	Reduced drug absorption, emesis due to gastrointestinal irritation, destruction of some of the drug through enzymatic degradation and gastric acid, inconsistent absorption, and patient compliance	Most common route of administration
Sublingual	Bypasses first pass metabolism; absorption can be very rapid.	Few drugs are chemically appropriate; erratic or incomplete absorption	Some studies have shown that many sublingual drugs are swallowed and are therefore predominantly oral.
Rectal	Bypasses the stomach and its gastric acid, which could destroy some of the drug; only about 50% of the drug enters the liver and is metabolized	Irregular and incomplete absorption, rectal mucosa irritation	
Parenteral:			
Intravenous (IV)	Rapid, extensive, and predictable administration; can be given to unconscious patients; immediate effects. Some drugs cannot be delivered in their active form in any other way.	Aseptic protocols, pain, difficult self-medication, expense, and local trauma	Considered the "gold standard," and most other forms of administration are compared to it.
Intramuscular (IM)	Similar to IV but preferable for self-administration.	Similar to IV, may affect certain lab tests such as creatinine kinase, can cause intramuscular hemorrhage, and cannot be used with anticoagulation therapy	
Subcutaneous (SC)	Similar to IV, more suitable for slow-release drugs	Similar to IV, unsuitable for drugs that need to be administered in large boluses	
Other (like intraarterial, intrathecal, intraventricular)	Each of these administrations have their own unique advantages and disadvantages, but each has a much greater inherent risk of infection and other complications.		
Other:			
Inhalation	Rapid delivery of the drug through lung mucosa, can minimize systemic side effects	Only gases, very small particulates, and fine droplets of liquid can be administered in this way.	
Topical	Act locally and avoid systemic effects		Generally only used in skin and eye conditions
Transdermal	Sustained drug absorption over time, no first pass effect, convenient, painless	Can trigger allergies and cause irritation; drugs must be very lipophilic	Good for very hydrophobic drugs that need a slow and sustained absorption and are administered in small daily doses

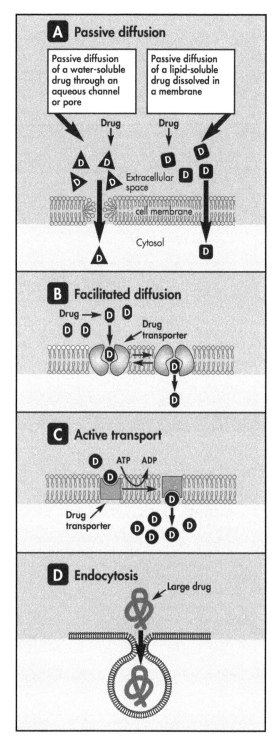

Figure 2.3 Methods of intracellular transport of extracellular compounds. A. Shows transport by passive diffusion, which does not require any energy source. B. Facilitated diffusion requires a transport protein but does not require energy. C. Active transport requires a transport protein that requires a source of energy. D. Endocytosis is a pinching off of the cell membrane.

distribution to various parts. Obviously if blood flow is decreased, there is less opportunity for a drug to move from the plasma into the area of reduced flow. The brain, liver, and kidneys have excellent blood flow, the skeletal muscles and skin less, and the adipose tissues even less.

Capillary permeability is determined by how "leaky" specific, local capillaries are. For example, due to the plasma filtration function of the spleen and liver, their capillaries are very permeable, and most drugs will be able to more easily move from the plasma. In contrast, the central nervous system (CNS) is protected by the blood-brain barrier, which is formed by tight junctions between capillary endothelial cells and is not "leaky" at all. Because of this barrier very few drugs can enter the brain; only those that are lipid soluble and without charge or polarity can enter the CNS.

As discussed previously, hydrophobic drugs can easily cross cell membranes. This affects how easily a drug can leave the circulation. Therefore, the distribution of a very hydrophobic drug is primarily determined by the amount of blood flow to a given area.

Most drugs will reversibly bind to plasma proteins. This binding slows overall distribution of the drug from the plasma and creates a reservoir of the drug within the plasma. The most common protein for drug binding is also the most common protein in the plasma: albumin. This binding is concentration dependent, meaning as plasma concentration of the drug increases, more binding occurs. Similarly, as drug concentration drops, less binding occurs. This causes the free drug concentration to be maintained as a constant fraction of the total drug in the plasma.

Plasma protein binding is affected by many factors. The first of these is the capacity of albumin to bind drugs. Can a molecule of the drug bind singly to each molecule of albumin, or can multiple drug molecules bind to each albumin? Drugs bind with varying affinities to albumin. In other words, some bind very strongly to albumin, and it is difficult for them to disassociate.

Another factor complicating plasma protein binding is competition between two or more drugs. There are two classes of drugs. Class I drugs are those where the dose is less than albumin's capacity to bind. In other words, when a class I drug is administered there will be excess albumin for further binding. Class II drugs are given in doses much greater than the ability of albumin to bind it. This causes a lot of the drug to be free and not bound to albumin. If a class I drug is administered with a class II drug, free drug levels of the class I drug will be much greater than anticipated. Remember, a bound drug is inert. In order to be active a drug must be free. Therefore combining a class I drug with a class II drug means the class I drug will have much higher concentrations of active drug than expected.

Drugs can also bind in the tissues. This can be caused by binding to lipids, proteins, or nucleic acids and creates a reservoir of a drug in the tissues. These reservoirs can serve as a major source of the drug and prolong its effects. Accumulation in the tissues can also lead to local toxicity and cause tissue damage. Any bound drug, whether in the plasma or the tissues, is an inactive drug.

VOLUME OF DISTRIBUTION

There are several different compartments of water within the body (see Figure 2.4). These can be split into an intracellular water compartment and an extracellular compartment. Based on a 70 kg person, there are 42 liters of water in the body, 28 of which are in the intracellular compartment and 14 liters in the extracellular compartment. Within the extracellular compartment, there are 10 liters in the interstitial fluids and 4 liters in the plasma. Drugs can distribute into any or all of these compartments depending on the size and hydrophobicity of the drug.

Drugs that are very large cannot escape the plasma and are almost entirely sequestered in the plasma compartment. Those drugs that are small can leave the plasma compartment. But if it is also hydrophilic, it cannot cross cell membranes and is primarily sequestered in the interstitial volume. And finally, if a drug is small and hydrophobic, it can more easily enter the cell and be distributed throughout the intracellular volume.

In pharmacokinetics, there is an artificial number that can communicate how a drug is distributed. It is called the volume of distribution or V_d. It describes how much of a drug is in the body versus the amount of drug in the plasma. The following formula shows this:

$$V_d = \text{(total amount of drug in the body)} / \text{(plasma concentration of the drug)}$$

Therefore a small V_d, less than 1, indicates that the drug is primarily sequestered in the plasma. A large V_d, greater than 1, indicates most of the drug is elsewhere.

METABOLISM

Drug metabolism refers to the biotransformation

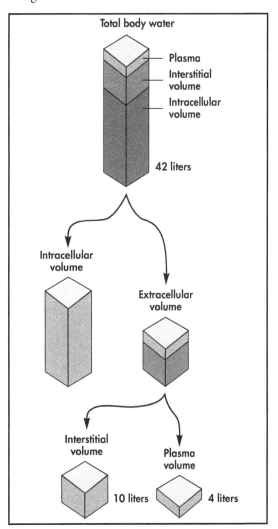

Figure 2.4: Visual representation of water within the various spaces of the body. Amounts of water are based on a 70 kg person.

of a drug into another chemical. Usually this occurs in order to facilitate elimination, as most drugs are hydrophobic, and hydrophobic chemicals are more difficult to excrete. However, some drugs are metabolized from an inactive form (called a prodrug) into an active form.

The kidney is the main organ of drug elimination. If a drug is too hydrophobic, it will simply enter the nephron and not stay within the tubule to be eliminated. In order to facilitate elimination, a drug needs to be sufficiently hydrophilic. Metabolizing the drug can accomplish this feat.

Metabolism occurs in the liver and usually involves two different phases:

Phase I reactions that do not utilize CYP450 include amine oxidation, alcohol dehydrogenation, esterases, and hydrolysis.

PHASE I: These reactions convert lipophilic drugs into more polar molecules. This may increase, decrease, or not change a drug's activity and may be enough for a drug to be eliminated by the kidney.

Many drugs are metabolized in phase I by the cytochrome P450 system. This system is involved in metabolizing **endogenous** compounds and exogenous toxins. The cytochrome P450 system is often referred to as CYP, and since there are several distinct types of CYP, this is followed by a designation denoting the specific enzyme, for example, CYP3A4 (See Figure 2.5). Specific families of CYP act on specific **substrates** and not others. Some drugs may also induce CYP and cause drugs to be metabolized more quickly. This is why patients on statin drugs (Chapter 7, Section 5) should not consume grapefruit juice, which inhibits CYP, slowing both the metabolism of the drug and its elimination, potentially increasing the drug's effective dose.

PHASE II: Phase II metabolism involves the conjugation of the drug. Conjugation involves adding a molecule to a drug. This makes the drug much more polar and hydrophilic allowing for elimination by the kidneys. Most often these drugs are inactive.

While this is the most common order of metabolism, some drugs may reverse the order with a phase II transformation occurring before phase I.

ELIMINATION

Elimination is the removal of a drug from the body. There are several methods by which a drug can be eliminated including excretion in the bile, into the intestines, the lung, or even the milk of lactating mothers. Excretion by the kidneys, however, is by far the most common route of elimination of drugs in the body.

As discussed under the metabolism section, most drugs are hydrophobic and therefore difficult to excrete by the kidneys. Therefore, drugs usually need to be metabolized into polar, hydrophilic chemicals before being eliminated.

There are three main steps to renal elimination:

1. First, as the blood enters the nephron, a portion of the blood, including a portion of the free drug, are filtered from the glomerulus into Bowman's space as glomerular filtrate.

2. In the proximal tubule of the nephron, there are relatively non-specific active transport systems that transfer anions and cations from the blood into the **lumen** of the tubule. Since there is a limited number of these transport systems, they may be overwhelmed by large drug quantities, or competition may occur between multiple drugs present at the same time.

Endogenous: Originating from within the body

Substrate: The specific chemical acted upon by an enzyme

Lumen: The opening or channel within an organ or other structure of the body; for example, the lumen of the intestines

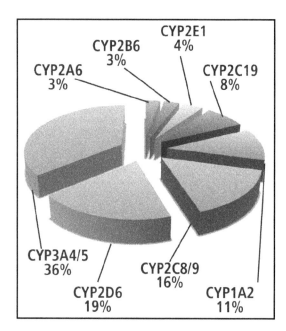

Figure 2.5: Drug metabolism. This figure shows percentages of various cytochrome P450 (CYP) isozymes within the body.

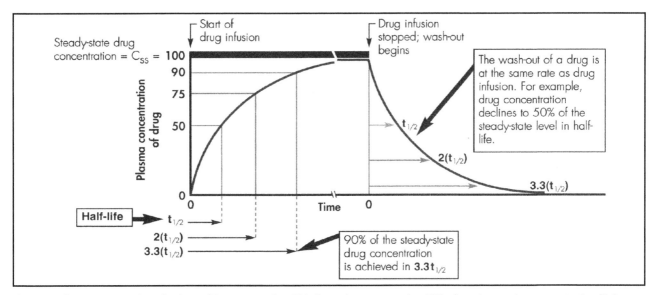

Figure 2.6: Plasma concentration of a drug with respect to time. This figure demonstrates that 90% of steady-state drug concentration (Css) occurs after 3.3 half-lives ($t_{1/2}$) when a steady infusion is initiated. The wash-out occurs at the same rate, and a drug is considered cleared after 4 half-lives.

3. Finally, in the distal tubule, reabsorption may occur. If a drug is uncharged, it may diffuse out of the tubule and back into systemic circulation. This is the main reason why drugs must undergo metabolism before excretion. Elimination of some drugs may be facilitated by manipulating the pH of urine in order to create a charged chemical that would not be there physiologically. This is called *ion trapping.*

Elimination can be described using several standardized variables. The half-life of a drug is the time required for the concentration of the drug to halve and is a function of V_d and CL or K_e, the rate constant of total body elimination of a particular drug (see Figure 2.6). CL describes the total body clearance of a drug and can be derived from adding up all the rates of elimination of a drug through every route of elimination. Therefore:

$$CL_{total} = CL_{hepatic} + CL_{renal} + CL_{pulmonary} + CL_{other}$$

It can also be computed by multiplying together K_e and V_d. These numbers can be derived through empirical investigation.

KINETICS

Kinetics are about the rates or speeds of reac-

tions. In pharmacology, kinetics are involved with everything from the speed of absorption, distribution, metabolism, and elimination as discussed above to steady-state calculations and fixed-dose, fixed-time regimens.

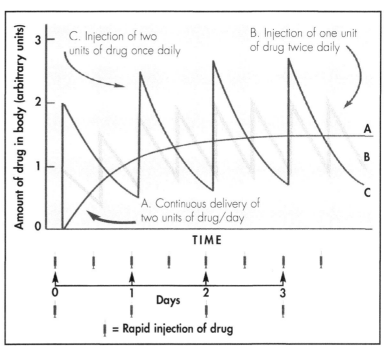

Figure 2.7: Bolus dosing. This figure shows the fluctuation around a steady-state continuous drug infusion **(A)** when using bolus dosing. Notice how the fluctuations are smaller in amplitude with smaller more frequent dosing **(B)** than larger, less frequent dosing **(C)**.

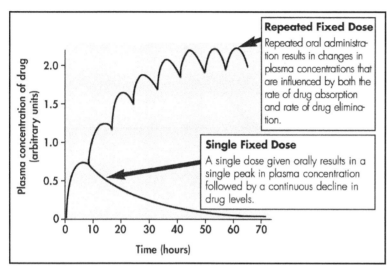

Figure 2.8: Single fixed dose versus repeated fixed dose. This figure demonstrates how a single fixed oral dose of a drug acts with respect to time as well as how repeated fixed doses will ultimately come to fluctuate around a steady state. Plasma levels of the drug are affected by the rate of absorption and the rate of elimination among other variables.

FIXED-DOSE, FIXED-TIME-INTERVAL REGIMENS

Continuous infusion of drugs can only be effectively accomplished in the hospital or under medical supervision. This makes it very inconvenient for most uses. Therefore, drugs are commonly administered in boluses (doses) either through oral administration or injection. With injections or oral dosing, the drug concentration will fluctuate around a steady state. See Figure 2.7 on page 13.

A large difference between injections and oral dosing is that injections deliver the entire drug dose immediately while oral dosing needs to take the time for absorption into account. In general, the more frequent a dose, the less fluctuation there is, though this can be modified by different drug formulations. Figure 2.8 shows the difference between a single oral drug dose and multiple doses approaching a relatively stable plasma concentration.

STEADY STATE

A steady state of a drug is reached when dosing and elimination of the drug interact to maintain a relatively stable amount in the body. A stable steady state can only be achieved through continuous IV infusion. Of the total steady-state concentration, 90% will be achieved in 3.3 half-lives. For simplicity, it is said that a drug will reach its steady state in 4 half-lives. By the same logic, a drug in steady state is said to be cleared from the body in 4 half-lives after stopping infusion of the drug. The time it takes to eliminate the drug from the body is called the wash-out period. Figure 2.6 on page 13 graphically shows the increase in plasma concentration as it approaches steady state.

To decrease the time needed to achieve steady state, a large loading dose can be given to rapidly increase the plasma concentration of the drug. Infusion is then initiated to sustain steady state.

SECTION 2: PHARMACODYNAMICS

Pharmacodynamics describes how drugs act on the body, drug receptor, and what kind of effects drug-receptor complexes create. This section will explore drug receptors, different types of actions a drug can initiate, and the therapeutic index.

▨ DRUG-RECEPTOR INTERACTIONS

Most drugs act by interacting with receptors, which are protein complexes on the cell surface or within the cell that causes changes to the cell or its functions. This causes an effect either by changing the conformation of the receptor or changing its biochemical function. In other words, a drug binds with a receptor; the drug-receptor complex then has a biological effect. This is shown in Figure 2.9 on page 16. One of the basic ideas of receptors is that they are rather specific about what binds to them. This concept is often referred to as the "lock and key." The drug or the physiological molecule is the key that fits into the "lock" of the receptor. Anything that can bind to a receptor is called a ligand. There are several terms used to describe these interactions.

REVERSIBILITY

A drug may bind reversibly or irreversibly with the receptor. A reversibly bound drug means the drug can be released from the receptor, and the receptor's biological function returns to its normal physiological state. Irreversible binding means that for the remaining life of that receptor, it will be bound to the drug and will act accordingly. Generally, drugs that irreversibly bind have much longer-term effects than those that do not.

COMPETITION

A drug may compete or not for a particular receptor. A competitive drug is one that competes with endogenous substances to be able to bind the receptor and exert an action. What binds the receptor determines its action. This may sound rather random, but really it is not. For one thing, drugs and endogenous molecules have different affinities for binding the receptor. This means that one or the other "prefers" to bind the receptor. Sometimes this is insignificant, and other times there can be huge differences in affinities. Another factor is concentrations involved. If a drug arrives at the target site in much larger concentrations than endogenous or competing substances, there will be much more binding of that drug, and affinity may have little or no impact. Non-competitive agents act at sites on the receptor that are different from and do not interfere with active sites for endogenous molecules. Another name for this is "allosteric," which means "other place or site." Therefore both can exert their effects.

RECEPTOR ACTIONS

Drugs can affect receptors in many ways. Often they are inhibitors that slow down or stop the physiological function of the receptor. Other drugs promote or increase the physiological functions of the receptors. Drugs that inhibit functions are called antagonists, while those that promote them are called agonists. Occasionally, a drug may have antagonistic effects while actually agonizing a different receptor. An example of this is epinephrine, which appears to antagonize histamine (H1) receptors but actually agonizes β_2 adrenoceptors, which have the opposite effects from the histamine receptors. This is called functional antagonism. As the actual drug effects are agonistic, their manifestations appear antagonistic. A fourth situation is that of the partial ago-

nist, which does not have the effects of a full agonist in that it may partially but not fully activate a receptor. Given different circumstances these can be considered agonistic as they promote receptor function or antagonistic as they prevent the full functioning of the drug-receptor complex.

Most drugs exert their effects on receptors, but not all. Many exceptions occur. An example of this is an antacid, which lowers acidity in the stomach, not by binding with anything but by causing a chemical reaction that raises the pH.

■ RECEPTOR FAMILIES

There are many types of receptors with which drugs can interact. The four most common are ligand-gated ion channels, G protein receptors, enzyme-linked receptors, and intracellular receptors. Each of these will be discussed below, and they are summarized in Figure 2.10 on page 17.

LIGAND-GATED ION CHANNELS

Ion channels, in general, regulate the flow of chemical ions into and out of the cell. Common ion channels control sodium (Na^+), potassium (K^+), calcium (Ca^{2+}), and chlorine (C^-). Ion channels can be controlled through several methods, the most common being voltage-gated and ligand-gated. Voltage-gated ion channels allow the flow of ions to commence when the surrounding plasma membrane reaches a certain voltage difference across its membrane. This is very useful in perpetuating an action potential in a nerve cell or in muscles as well as other physiological sites.

Ligand-gated ion channels allow the flow of ions in response to binding with a ligand (a drug or endogenous signal molecule). Ligands can activate or inhibit the flow of ions depending on whether they are agonists or antagonists. Often the flow of ions determines if a physiological effect is more or less likely. An example of this is the drug class of benzodiazepines. They act by binding the GABA receptors of neurons in the central nervous system. This is a ligand-gated chlorine channel, and the binding increases the flow of chlorine from outside the neuron to the inside. This influx reduces the chances that an action potential will occur and "dampens" the response of the neuron.

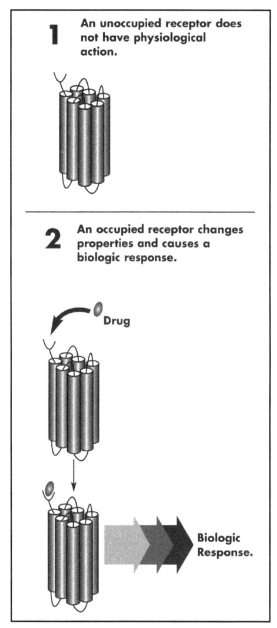

1 An unoccupied receptor does not have physiological action.

2 An occupied receptor changes properties and causes a biologic response.

Drug

Biologic Response.

Figure 2.9: How cellular receptors work. Graphic 1 shows an unoccupied and unactivated cellular receptor. **Graphic 2** shows what happens when a drug occupies the receptor and the receptor has a biologic response.

G PROTEIN-COUPLED RECEPTORS

The G protein-coupled receptors consist of a receptor that spans the plasma membrane of the cell and is attached intracellularly to a G protein that comprises three subunits: α (alpha), β (beta), and γ (gamma). A ligand binds the receptor, which causes the α subunit to bind GTP and dis-

associate into two intracellular components: the α-GTP subunit and the $\beta\gamma$ subunit. These can interact with other molecules to exert their influence on the cell. These other molecules are called second messenger systems.

SECOND MESSENGER SYSTEMS

The three most common second messenger systems are the cyclic adenosine monophosphate (cAMP) system, the inositol-1, 4, 5-triphosphate (IP^3) system, and the diacylglycerol (DAG) system. The cAMP system generally regulates protein phosphorylation (the adding of a phosphate group to a protein), which can activate or inactivate particular proteins. The IP^3 and diacylglycerol systems generally act on calcium regulation within the cell. Second messenger systems tend to magnify the effect of the initial activation as each step of the cascade acts on several other chemicals, not just one. This means one G protein activation can affect hundreds or thousands of proteins. This is called amplification. How G protein receptors work is summarized in Figure 2.11.

ENZYME-LINKED RECEPTORS

This is a transmembrane receptor with a receiving end outside the cell that binds a ligand. This activates or inhibits enzyme activity on a portion of the receptor that is on the inside (or cytosolic side) of the cell. This in turn directly exerts the effects of the receptor. While there are many types of these receptors, the most common form is that of the tyrosine kinase class. A kinase is an enzyme that adds a phosphate to another molecule, in this case, to a tyrosine (a type of amino acid) in a protein or enzyme. This may activate or deactivate the protein. It can also activate second messenger systems, such as the IP^3 system, to amplify the cascade of actions.

INTRACELLULAR RECEPTORS

These receptors remain completely within the cell in the cytosol. This means a drug needs to be lipophilic enough to pass through the cell membrane in order to bind with the receptor. Once bound, generally a small protein is displaced from the receptor that was acting as an inhibitor,

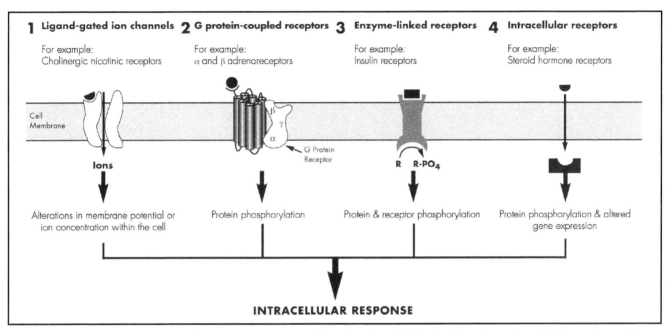

Figure 2.10: Summary of major families of cellular receptors. 1: Ligand-gated ion channels allow ion flow when activated. **2:** G protein-coupled receptors are transmembrane receptors that allow an intracellular subunit to activate enzymes and processes within the cell. **3:** Enzyme-linked receptors are another transmembrane receptor that has direct enzymatic activity when activated. **4:** Intracellular receptors respond to ligands that can pass through the cell membrane and usually activate enzymes or proteins that alter gene expression and ultimately protein production.

and the drug-receptor complex moves into the nucleus and promotes DNA transcription to mRNA and ultimately increased protein synthesis. This cascade of events can take much longer than the other receptor types, and the effects of these drugs can take hours or days to fully manifest. Steroid hormones are common ligands for these receptors. The actions of these receptors are summarized in Figure 2.12 on page 19.

RECEPTOR DESENSITIZATION

Repeated activation or inhibition of a receptor can result in changes of responsiveness. This is the cell's response to prevent long-term damage by overly strong responses. Overall, when repeated drug use results in a smaller effect, it is called tachyphylaxis. This can occur through several mechanisms. One is where the receptor actually becomes desensitized and shows a smaller effect to the drug. It can also occur through down-regulation, or less synthesis of the receptor because the DNA is not being transcribed as frequently. Another mechanism is that of endocytosis, which sequesters the membrane receptor in the cytosol where it can be either

degraded or recycled back to the cell membrane.

DOSE-RESPONSE RELATIONSHIPS

As a basic principle, the higher the concentration of a drug at the active site, the higher its pharmacological effect, up to a certain point. This is shown on a dose-response curve, which shows the effects of a drug on the y axis and the concentration of the drug on the x axis. An example of this is in Figure 2.13 on page 19. Notice that eventually, the drug has little or no additional effect even if the drug concentration increases. This is usually due to the receptors the drugs act upon being maximally utilized. From these graphs, two useful pharmacological properties can be derived: potency and efficacy.

POTENCY

Potency is the measurement of the amount of drug necessary to achieve a certain magnitude of effect. This magnitude of effect is the concentration of the drug when it has achieved 50% of the maximum effect of the drug and is referred to as EC_{50}. One of the largest contributing factors for potency is the affinity of the drug for the receptor.

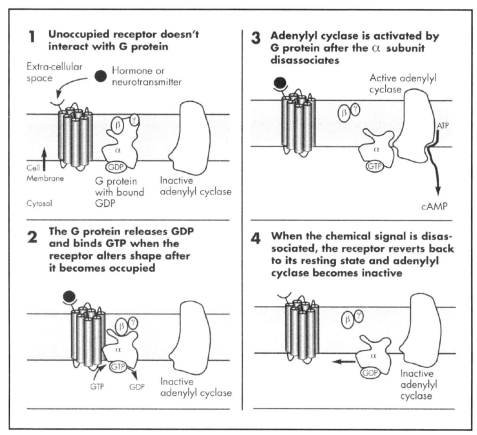

1 **Unoccupied receptor doesn't interact with G protein**

Extra-cellular space

Hormone or neurotransmitter

Cell Membrane

Cytosol

G protein with bound GDP

Inactive adenylyl cyclase

2 **The G protein releases GDP and binds GTP when the receptor alters shape after it becomes occupied**

GTP   GDP

Inactive adenylyl cyclase

3 **Adenylyl cyclase is activated by G protein after the α subunit disassociates**

Active adenylyl cyclase

ATP

cAMP

4 **When the chemical signal is disassociated, the receptor reverts back to its resting state and adenylyl cyclase becomes inactive**

Inactive adenylyl cyclase

Figure 2.11: G protein-coupled receptors activation. 1: A ligand binds and activates the transmembrane receptor. **2:** Receptor activation causes the α subunit to bind guanosine triphosphate (GTP) and displace GDP. **3:** The βγ-GTP subunit separates and activates adenylyl cyclase, which breaks down ATP into cAMP and inorganic phosphate. cAMP has various intracellular functions. **4:** The GTP is dephosphorylated to GDP, and the βγ-GDP subunit no longer activates adenylyl cyclase and disassociates reforming the G protein complex.

EFFICACY

Efficacy is a measurement of how efficiently the drug produces its effects and is dependent on the number of drug-receptor complexes formed and how efficiently these complexes create cellular responses. While potency is the concentration of a drug that produces 50% of maximal response, efficacy is not predicated on concentration at all; it simply measures the maximal effect (see Figure

2.13). This is referred to as E_{max}. Generally, while potency may have economic ramifications (i.e., the more potent the drug the less drug per dose), it is the efficacy that is more important and determines how therapeutically useful the drug is.

THERAPEUTIC INDEX

The therapeutic index (TI), also called the therapeutic margin or therapeutic window, is a measurement of how safe a drug is. It is the ratio between the toxic dose and the therapeutic dose. Since it is a ratio, the larger the number the safer the drug is. It is determined by the equation below.

Therapeutic index = TD_{50}/ED_{50}

TD_{50} is the drug dose that produces toxic effects in 50% of the population. ED_{50} is the drug dose that produces a therapeutic effect in 50% of the population.

Agents with a small therapeutic index generally need to be well monitored to avoid detrimental effects. A prime example of this is warfarin, which reduces the ability for the blood to coagulate. If not enough is given, then the blood is not anticoagulated, and the reason for prescribing the agent in the first place is more likely to occur. However, if too much is prescribed, the patient may bleed inappropriately and dangerously. To achieve the target dose and maintain its effects requires regular blood tests. Many other drugs

CATEGORY	A	B	C	D	X	N
DESCRIPTION	No human fetal risk or remote possibility of fetal harm	No controlled studies show human risk; animal studies suggest potential toxicity	Animal fetal toxicity demonstrated; human risk undefined	Human fetal risk present; but benefits outweigh risks	Human fetal risk present but does not outweigh benefits; contraindicated in pregnancy	The FDA has not assigned a risk category to these agents

Chart: FDA categories of drugs as they relate to danger of toxicity to a developing fetus.

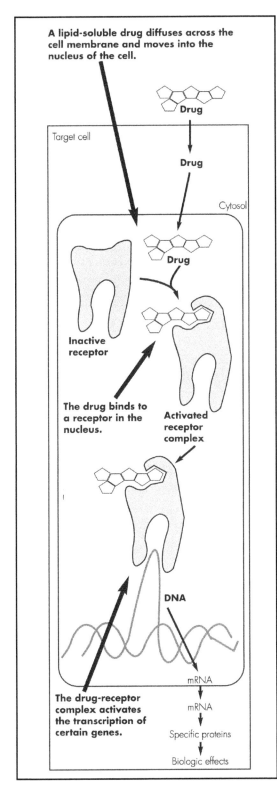

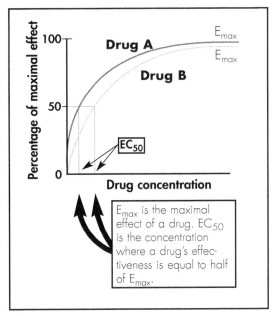

Figure 2.13: Dose-response relationships. This graph shows a percentage of maximum effect on the y axis and the drug concentration on the x axis. Each drug can be plotted with these axes. At 50% of maximal effect, the drug concentration can be determined. This is called the EC_{50}. E_{max} is defined as the maximal effect.

can push warfarin in either direction out of its therapeutic index.

An interesting comparison of the difference between the therapeutic index of warfarin on the one hand and penicillin on the other is shown in Figure 2.14 on the following page.

PREGNANCY RISKS

The Food and Drug Administration (FDA) has a risk categorization scheme showing how potentially harmful drugs are for the fetus when they are administered to a pregnant woman. They are ranked from A-D and X for absolute contraindication. A designation of N means the FDA has not assigned a risk category to a particular agent. These categories and what they mean are shown in the table on the bottom page 18. After each drug listed in the book, there is a "Pregnancy risk" **(PR=)** designation that refers to the categories in this table at the bottom of page 18 and also shown on page 3 in the previous chapter.

Figure 2.12: Intracellular receptor activation. A lipid soluble drug passes through the cell membrane and activates a receptor in the cytosol. The now activated receptor complex enters the nucleus and alters gene transcription to mRNA, which in turn alters protein translation and biologic effects.

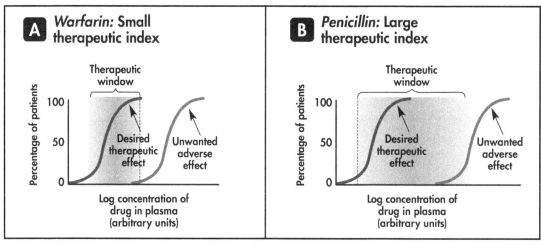

Figure 2.14: **Representations of therapeutic indices.** A. Warfarin represents a narrow therapeutic index. B. Penicillin has a large therapeutic index.

SUMMARY OF VARIABLES COMMONLY USED IN PHARMACOLOGY

AUC–Area under the curve is a measurement of bioavailability and indicates plasma drug concentration over time.

BIOAVAILABILITY–The amount of a drug that is available to act on its target site.

C–Plasma concentration of a drug.

CL–Clearance describes the removal of a drug from the body.

C_{max}–Maximum plasma concentration of a drug.

C_{ss}–Steady-state concentration of a drug. In other words, the plasma concentration where the amount of drug entering the blood equals the amount of drug removed from the blood by elimination mechanisms.

D–Total amount of drug in the body (not in the blood).

EC_{50}–The concentration of the drug when it has achieved 50% of the maximum effect of the drug; the potency of the drug.

ED_{50}–The drug dose that produces a therapeutic effect in 50% of the population.

E_{max}–The maximal effect of a drug.

HALF-LIFE–The time needed to decrease the plasma concentration of a drug by half.

K_d–Affinity of a drug for the receptor

K_e–A rate constant for drug elimination from the total body. In other words, it is a constant, different for each drug, that helps describes how fast a drug is eliminated from the body.

pH–The inverse log of the concentration of hydrogen ions. Used as a measurement of acidic and basic level: 7 is neutral, below that is acidic and above that is basic. The further away from 7 the more basic or acidic the solution is. For example, a pH of 2 is more acidic than a pH of 4.

pK_a–The inverse log of the acid constant. A measure of a drug's interaction with a proton (acid). A low pK_a indicates that the drug is more acidic, while a high pK_a indicates a more basic drug.

$T_{1/2}$–See half-life above.

TD_{50}–The drug dose that produces toxic effects in 50% of the population.

V_d–Volume of distribution. A measurement of how much drug is in the body versus how much is in the blood. A large V_d indicates wide distribution to the body, while a small V_d indicates a drug that is generally sequestered in the blood.

Drug-Herb Interactions

Drug-herb interactions are a topic of some discussion in recent years. This is for several reasons including some well-publicized case reports, the 24-hour media's need for constant news, as a possible route of attack for anti-herb activists, and because so little is known about them. Whatever the reason, the consequences for a practitioner not to be conversant in drug-herb or herb-drug interactions can be serious.

This book addresses this need in many ways. In each drug class monograph, drug-herb interactions are listed. These listings come from a wide variety of sources, but should not be considered complete. Research on interactions is constantly changing. Also, many interactions are not based on research but on case reports or expert opinions. These may or may not be valid, but are good guidelines to consider when prescribing herbs to a patient taking a pharmaceutical agent. In addition to the individual listings, this chapter discusses how a practitioner might be able to predict a drug-herb interaction even if no information is available in the scientific literature.

In the last chapter we discussed the four main aspects of pharmacokinetics: absorption, distribution, metabolism, and elimination (ADME). When combined with the therapeutic index, we then have a basis for predicting herb-drug interactions. Rather than waiting for research that may or may not occur, practitioners can make educated guesses as to whether a drug may interfere with a particular herb. The rest of this chapter will look at each of these areas and use them to predict possible interactions.

After teaching this subject for many years, this author would like to confront a myth about how to avoid drug-herb interactions. This myth says that if one separates when herbs and drugs are consumed by a few hours the potential for drug-herb interactions is reduced. This is, with an occasional exception as noted throughout this chapter, false. The interactions between administration and absorption are very complex and difficult to predict without empirical research on each and every combination of drugs and herbs, and it is just as likely that separating the administration of drugs and herbs could increase the potential for interactions, not decrease it. There has been no research, that the author knows of, showing reduced interactions from separating administration, and basic pharmacology speaks against it. Unfortunately, there are no simple answers to reducing interactions and as professionals, we should not accept easy platitudes without examining their underpinnings. The bottom line is that there is no evidence that separating administration of drugs and herbs reduces interactions and in fact, the basics of pharmacokinetics suggest that it is very hard to predict and may be just as likely to increase interactions.

To help look at these theoretical issues, there is a section towards the end of each drug class monograph titled "Interaction Issues." listing any possible concerns with drug-herb interactions.

SECTION 1: ABSORPTION

There are many factors that influence absorption and include: the pH in the stomach and small intestine, the solubility of the drugs, gastrointestinal (GI) motility, interactions with drugs, concentration, and the surface area of the absorbing organ the with which the agent is in contact.

This section will look at the most important of these areas, pH, GI motility, and binding interactions, and how they could affect the absorption of herbs or vice versa.

ACIDITY

Acidity, or pH, plays a large role in absorption for some agents. Some drugs need a very acidic environment in order to be absorbed, often in order to convert a drug into a form that is easily absorbable. This can happen when a drug is hydrophilic, but at a given pH is neutral in charge and therefore can more easily cross a membrane.

This illustrates one of the basic rules of pharmacology: passive transport of a drug requires a neutral charge. If the drug is too charged, it cannot pass through the cell membrane without assistance. The charge or neutrality, known as the ionization, of a molecule is highly dependent on the pH of the fluid it is dissolved in. Whether or not a specific pH may affect absorption is commonly determined empirically. In other words, each drug needs to be tested for these changes as they are hard to predict.

There are many drugs and herbs that can affect the pH of the stomach and intestines. Among these drug classes are antacids, proton pump inhibitors, and histamine (H2) inhibitors. From an herbal perspective, *Hai Ge Fen* (clam shell), *Hai Piao Xiao* (cuttlefish bone), and *Mu Li* (oyster shell) may have antacid effects.

GASTROINTESTINAL MOTILITY

GI motility mainly refers to intestinal peristalsis.

Increased peristalsis means a faster intestinal transit time, less contact with the wall of the intestines and therefore less ability for absorption of the substance. Of course, the opposite is also true: decreased peristalsis means slower transit time, more contact with the absorptive surfaces of the intestinal tract, and increased absorption. Either of these can have helpful or detrimental effects.

Increased motility of the GI tract may happen when using cholinergic agents and prokinetic gastrointestinal agents such as metoclopramide and cisapride. Decreased peristalsis may occur when using anti-cholinergics, narcotics, phenobarbital, and to a lesser extent some anti-depressants and antipsychotics.

BINDING

Some drugs and herbs that are cloying and sticky and can adhere to other substances consumed at the same time. While often this is due to the inherent nature of the drug or herb, sometimes that is the function of the drug as is the case of cholestyramine which is designed to sequester bile and cholesterol within the intestines and not allow them to be (re)absorbed. In general, anything taken two hours before or four hours after these substances will not be absorbed well.

Drugs that are binding include the bile acid sequestrants, sucralfate, and activated charcoal. Some herbs that may have cloying and binding properties include *E Jiao* (ass-hide glue), *Lu Jiao Jiao* (deer horn gelatin), *Bie Jia Jiao* (turtle shell gelatin), and *Gui Ban Jiao* (tortoise shell gelatin).

SECTION 2: DISTRIBUTION

Distribution, or how a drug is spread within the body, has several factors that help determine how effectively this occurs. These include protein binding almost exclusively of albumin, motility of the drug, physiological properties such as solubility, pH, and ionization, blood flow both globally, as in the form of cardiac output, and locally, as in how much blood flows to the target tissues, and reservoirs. Reservoirs include fat, particular tissues, or specific cell types. These are basically storage depots that release the drug when plasma levels drop.

Protein binding is by far the biggest factor when determining interactions. Drugs or herbs with active ingredients that are highly protein bound are very susceptible to interactions. Highly protein bound substances are over 95% bound. That means less than 5% of the agent is actually free and able to exert its effects. Therefore even a very small displacement of the bound substance could result in a dramatic increase in the amount of free agent and hence a huge difference in the agent's effects. Any interaction that can change the amount of an agent bound to albumin can have profound effects on the amount of an agent able to exert its effects.

The table below shows that if you start off with a highly protein bound drug of over 95% protein binding, a very small displacement of bound drug can lead to dramatic changes of unbound drug. Remember that an unbound drug is free to act on the body. For example, a drug that is normally 98% protein bound can, with a little displacement from another drug or herb, go to 95% protein bound. Not a dramatic shift on the bound side of the equation. But a

Percent of bound drug	Percent of unbound drug
98%	2%
95%	5%
90%	10%
80%	20%
50%	50%

huge shift on the unbound side: it went from 2% unbound to 5% unbound. This effectively means 2.5 times the "normal" amount of the drug is now free to act on the body. This could certainly cause dose related issues in a particular drug. And what if the shift is more dramatic, say from 95% bound to 80% bound. That would mean there is 4 times the "normal" amount of the drug able to act on the body. This could cause an overdose situation or at least an increase in dose-related adverse effects.

Drugs that are highly protein bound and thus open to these types of interactions include warfarin, phenytoin, oral contraceptive pills, and non-steroidal anti-inflammatory drugs (NSAIDs). While protein binding is generally specific to individual agents, these last two drug classes have many drugs that can be affected by distribution and these issues need to be taken into consideration. Unfortunately, there have not been any well-publicized studies to date examining protein binding with herbs. However, vitamin C has been shown to displace some agents from albumin.

SECTION 3: METABOLISM

Metabolism, or biotransformation of substances, has a large potential for interactions. There are many factors that affect metabolism including genetics, gender, the organ health of the liver and kidneys, organ maturity, blood pressure, diet, and whether the patient is a smoker or regular drinker of alcohol. One of the biggest targets of interactions within the realm of metabolism is the cytochrome P450 (CYP) system. As mentioned in the previous chapter, some substances may inhibit this system while others promote this system. Either can dramatically affect the actions of agents on the body. Often a substance can affect many isozymes and not just one. Also they can be weak or strong inducers or inhibitors of action. Interactions are more common with the strong inducers or inhibitors.

This book lists, under the "Interaction Issues" section of each drug class monograph, any major issues with Cytochrome P450. It will list any

strong inducers or inhibitors of CYP isozymes as well as major substrates. A major substrate is a drug that uses a significant portion of a given CYP isozyme and could theoretically affect other users of that isozyme. This could lead to reduced metabolism of multiple drugs. A strong inducer causes an increase in metabolism that could cause other drugs that utilize the isozyme to be metabolized faster. This could either make it easier to eliminate or increase the amount of active drug depending on the drug and what metabolism accomplishes. A strong inhibitor would have the opposite effect.

Many drugs can affect the CYP system. Inducers of this system include phenytoin, carbamazepine, phenobarbital, rifampin and its cousins, the sulfonylureas, and alcohol in the short term. Inhibitors of the CYP system include cimetidine, erythromycin, azole antifungals, isoniazid, sulfonamides, verapamil, propoxyphene, and alcohol in the long term. Grapefruit juice is a fairly potent inhibitor of CYP. One study (Chang, 2006) has shown strong CYP inhibition by Wu Bei Zi (Chinese nut galls), *Wu Wei Zi* (Schisandra), *Jue Ming Zi* (Cassia seed), *Shi Liu Pi* (Granatum rind), and *Tian Hua Fen* (Trichosanthes root).

SECTION 4: ELIMINATION

Elimination, which can occur through many routes, but primarily the kidney, can be affected by the health of the kidneys, organ maturity, volume of distribution, perfusion of the kidneys, and urinary pH. The most significant factor in determining interactions is how a substance affects clearance.

Patients on dialysis or who have had a kidney transplant may have significantly impaired elimination from the kidneys. Diuretics can increase clearance from the kidneys. Drugs that affect GI motility may also reduce clearance from the intestines, though this is, for most drugs, a minor route of elimination. Theoretically, herbs in the drain damp category may hasten renal clearance.

SECTION 5: THERAPEUTIC MARGIN

Since the therapeutic margin is a direct measure of the safety of a drug, any substance that has a narrow margin may have significant toxicities if thrown out of that range. What may or may not push an agent out of the safety margin is an individual response and may be predicated on many factors such as the age and gender of the patient, dietary changes, and what other drugs the patient may be taking.

There are three relatively common agents that have narrow therapeutic margins: warfarin, phenytoin, and lithium. Herbs should be used with extreme caution in patients on these agents. This is made even more worrisome given that both warfarin and phenytoin are also highly protein bound. It is the opinion of the authors that herbs should not be used in patients on these agents without permission and close monitoring by a medical doctor. Other drugs that have a narrow therapeutic margin include theophylline and many, if not most, of the tricyclic antidepressants.

SECTION 6: P-GLYCOPROTEIN

P-glycoprotein (Pgp), also known as adenosine triphosphate (ATP) binding cassette sub-family B member 1 (ABCB1), is a protein that is called an efflux transporter. This means that it transports molecules from the intracellular space to the extracellular space. It is a prime target for drug research right now as it is considered to have a large impact on drug-drug interactions and is involved with multidrug resistance, especially with anticancer chemotherapy. In fact, another name for Pgp is MDR1 which stands for multidrug resistance protein 1. As for drug-herb interactions, Pgp can interfere with several steps of the ADME (absorption, distribution, metabolism, and elimination) scheme and has the potential for many interactions.

Just like cytochrome P450 (CYP), a drug can induce, inhibit, or just be a substrate of Pgp. While inducers are not thought to have a therapeutic benefit, inhibitors are targets of active research for use to reverse multidrug resistance in cancer treatments. Increased Pgp expression has been implicated in reduced response to morphine and human immunovirus (HIV) antiretroviral drugs.

Pgp affects absorption when it is expressed in the intestines. As the drug enters the intestinal cells, Pgp causes it to be transported back out of the cell and back into the intestines. So it acts to prevent absorption and reduces the amount of the drug that enters the blood stream.

Hepatobiliary excretion may also be affected by Pgp. Pgp sits on the cellular membrane of the hepatocyte (liver cell) that is closest to the bile duct (the canalicular or apical membrane). It is thought to help facilitate excretion into the bile and intestines. Inhibition of Pgp has been shown in animals to decrease excretion, and therefore maintain serum levels, of drugs that are substrates of Pgp. In terms of drug-herb interactions, this would probably play a minor part given that most herbs and drugs are eliminated through the kidneys in urine.

Pgp is located in kidney cells and plays a role in helping excrete drugs and other xenobiotics (biological compounds from outside of the body). Because of this any interference in Pgp function may have a direct role in the elimination of drugs from the body. Therefore any induction of Pgp can lead to increased excretion of a drug and less of it in the system. By the same token, inhibition would cause decreased excretion and increased serum levels of a particular drug.

Pgp also appears to be a component of the blood-brain barrier (BBB) which protects the brain and prevents many substances from entering the central nervous system (CNS). Pgp appears to play a role in preventing substances crossing the BBB by transporting some highly lipophilic substances that normally would cross the BBB back into the blood and away from the CNS. Drugs that may be prevented from entering the brain include: ivermectin, digoxin, doxorubicin, paclitaxel, loperamide, and vinblastine. Some studies are suggesting a role in reducing concentrations of morphine and derivatives within the brain suggesting that Pgp inhibition may decrease pain when taking these agents.

Several drugs have been implicated in inhibiting Pgp in humans. These include verapamil, rifampin, quinidine, clarithromycin, traconazole, and propafenone. Digoxin, talinolol, colchicine, vincristine, doxorubicinol, tamoxifen, and daunorubicin are substrates of Pgp. St. John's Wort (*Guan Ye Lian Qiao*) has been shown in a few studies to inhibit Pgp expression.

The bottom line about P-glycoprotein is that it is actively being researched for its interactions with drugs and its potential for influencing drug-drug and drug-herb interactions. While currently these roles are not fully understood, it does appear that Pgp may have some major roles in these interactions. As such, it behooves the practitioner interested in drug-herb interactions to keep an eye on this protein.

SECTION 7: GUIDELINES FOR TREATING PATIENTS WHO ARE TAKING WESTERN DRUGS WITH CHINESE MEDICINE

The issue of combining Western drugs with herbal remedies has received attention in both public and professional media. The concern voiced by Western MDs is that such combinations may result in unknown adverse herb-drug interactions. Therefore, many Western physicians would rather their patients not take any herbal medicines and recommend against herbal remedies. While some of this concern is a valid medical issue, the authors believe that some of it is motivated by increasing competition in the health care marketplace for finite resources which were once the undisputed monopoly of Western medicine. As one will see when reading the information presented in this book, many of the specific concerns of Western practitioners are either entirely theoretical (as preceded by the words "may" or "might") or are supported by extremely small anecdotal evidence, (*i.e.*, one or two cases).

Further, when it comes to Chinese herbal medicine (中药 *zhong yao*), these concerns typically fail to take into account three important aspects of our practice. First, as professional practitioners of Chinese medicine, we do not use singles. We prescribe Chinese medicinals in complex polypharmacy formulas, not just random collections of every herbal ingredient that we know empirically treats this or that condition. Rather, these are highly synergistic combinations of medicines, intended to check and balance each other and address a condition from several different points of view. Secondly, we prescribe these formulas on the basis of each patient's personally presenting patterns (辨证论治 *bian zheng lun zhi*). This insures that the medicinals in a formula are the ones specifically needed by that individual to remedy their underlying pathology. Since we are only trying to bring the patient back to their normal balance, it is unlikely that our medicines will push the patient too far in any direction. And third, these concerns fail to take into account the many years of experience of combining Chinese and Western medicines in the People's Republic of China. In China, there are three separate health care delivery systems:

1. Pure Chinese medicine (中 医 *zhong yi*)

2. Pure Western medicine (西 医 *xi yi*)

3. Integrated Chinese-Western medicine (中 西 医 结 合 *zhong xi yi jie he*)

Hundreds of thousands of patients are treated each year in integrated Chinese-Western medical hospitals and clinics in China with simultaneously administered Western drugs and Chinese herbs. Reams of research has been published on this practice. Besides the sections on integrated Chinese-Western medicine included in most Chinese medical journals, there are also a number of Chinese journals solely devoted to integrated Chinese-Western medicine.

Unfortunately, this research is all published in Chinese; only the smallest portion has been translated into English. Thus, Western practitioners are largely unaware of this huge reservoir of clinical experience on the combination of Western drugs and Chinese medicinals. What this research routinely shows is that the combination of Western drugs and Chinese medicinals achieves:

1. Better therapeutic results than either alone

2. At lower doses of the Western drugs

3. With fewer side effects

There is virtually no discussion in the contemporary Chinese journal literature of herb-drug interactions. With so many Chinese simultaneously using Western drugs and Chinese medicinals, if such interactions were a problem in clinical practice, we would expect to see numerous discussions of this in the Chinese literature. Yet, except for the occasional single case history, there is nothing in the Chinese medical literature to suggest this is an important concern.

Therefore, when reading this book or accessing its information in clinic, we advise our readers to keep four things in mind:

1. The issue of herb-drug interactions is largely an economic battle over dwindling resources and consumer dissatisfaction.

2. The overwhelming majority of cautions and concerns are purely theoretical.

3. There is very little actual evidence of Chinese herb/Western drug interactions.

4. There is massive research proving that combining Chinese and Western medicines is clinically safe and therapeutically desirable.

In order to help allay some of the fears among practitioners of Chinese medicine about prescribing Chinese herbal medicines to patients who are also taking Western drugs, we would like to outline what we do and believe that others should do in such situations. If one has a step-by-step protocol to follow, then one has less of a sense of working in the dark and fearing the worst. Below we give our three steps in deciding if and how to prescribe Chinese herbs to patients on Western drugs. Each of these steps are composed of a number of sub-steps. Following these steps in order, one will have considered what they are doing and why in a duly diligent and thorough manner. Thus it is far less likely that a patient will experience an adverse reaction.

FIRST STEPS: LEARN THE BIOMEDICAL

1. **Find out all of the Western medicines the patient is taking and their doses.** Take a basic inventory of what Western drugs the patient is on and the doses they are taking. If one does not have all the information, it is impossible to make a good decision.

2. **Dosing is also very important.** Are the drugs prescribed at higher or less than normal doses? Why? If certain drugs, such as benzodiazepines are prescribed at much higher than normal doses, it strongly suggests tolerance and probability of addiction.

3. **Find out the purpose for each medicine.** This

means to find out why the patient has been prescribed each medication they are taking. Is a medication for its normal, labeled use or for some "off-label" purpose?

4. **Find out if the medicines are achieving their intended therapeutic effects.** In other words, are the medicines doing what the prescribing practitioner wants them to do? If they are, then that is good. At least one part of the benefit/risk equation has been met and we may not need to do anything further in terms of those therapeutic goals.

5 **Find out if the medicines are causing any side effects or adverse reactions.** Side effects (*i.e.*, risks) are the second half of the benefit/risk equation. If there are no side effects, that is also good. If the medicines are achieving their intended therapeutic effects but there are side effects, this may suggest that we focus our attention on alleviating or ameliorating these. In any case, if there are side effects, something is not entirely right. In Chinese medicine, we generally do not think that any side effects are acceptable. Since the body is one whole integrated unit, creating side effects while attempting to heal is like "paying Peter by stealing from Paul."

6. **Read up about each of these medicines.** In this book, you will find all the necessary information about commonly prescribed Western medicines, including their therapeutic effects, side effects, dosages, contraindications, and potential interactions. One can also look up Western drugs using the internet. There is no lack of easily-available information on the Western medicines our patients are taking, and we should be knowledgeable about this information.

7. **Do not say anything to the patient about these medicines.** It is very important for professional practitioners of Chinese medicine not to say anything about a patient's prescription drugs. To discuss or, more importantly, to advise our patients about their Western prescription drugs is outside our scope of practice. It is both illegal and unethical. If we believe there is a problem with one or more of a patient's Western prescription drugs, we should refer the patient back to the prescribing physician. However, we should next:

8. **Get the patient's written permission to discuss their case with the prescribing MD.** Once we have a patient's written release to discuss their case with the prescribing MD, we should voice our concerns to that physician in a collegial, professional way. We should inform the physician that the patient has sought out our care. We should explain to the physician what we intend to do and the rationale for our therapy. In closing, we should tell the physician that we would be happy to dialogue/consult with them on this case and would be happy to furnish further information about our treatment at their request.

Some Western MDs are so closed-minded that they will reject all this out of hand. However, a growing number of MDs, especially younger MDs, are open to the idea of complementary and alternative medicine (CAM). Even those who are lukewarm at best about their patients' use of CAM, know that the statistics are stacked against them. It is our experience that, as long as we approach and communicate with them in an intelligent, informed, and professional manner, many Western physicians are willing to talk and confer with us. The downside is that they will expect us to talk in their language, not ours, and we have to be ready to do so. This book should help.

SECOND STEPS: THE CHINESE MEDICINE

Steps two and three have to do with the practice of Chinese medicine. Now we are on our turf.

1. **Reframe the patient's Western medical disease diagnosis or main complaints into its/their corresponding traditional Chinese disease categories (病 *bing*).** Every Western medical disease corresponds to one of more traditional Chinese medical disease categories. For example, migraine simply corresponds to side headache (偏头痛 *pian tou tong*). Therefore, in order to know what are the commonly seen, professionally agreed upon Chinese medical

patterns of migraine, one can simply look up the disease category side headache. In this case, there is a one-to-one correspondence. However, in some diseases, such as multiple sclerosis (MS), there is not such a simple one-to-one correspondence. In that case, one lists the main clinical symptoms or features of the condition. In the case of MS, its main clinical features are loss of muscular strength and use with eventual atrophy, numbness and insensitivity, blurred vision, loss of vision, and spasticity. In Chinese medicine, loss of muscular strength and use and atrophy correspond to the disease category of wilting condition (痿 证 *wei zheng*). Numbness and insensitivity corresponds to tingling and numbness (麻 木 *ma mu*). Blurred vision corresponds to flowery vision (花 眼 *hua yan*), and loss of vision corresponds to clear-eyed blinding (清 盲 *qing mang*), while spasticity corrresponds to tetany (痉 *jing*). Therefore, we can know what patterns to look for in our MS patient by identifying which of these Chinese diseases he or she manifests and then looking under those.

This step of reframing our patient's Western disease into its corresponding Chinese medical disease/diseases is extremely important, although commonly overlooked by or unknown to Western practitioners. It helps us more quickly and accurately examine the patient for the most likely patterns they are presenting.

2. **Identify the patient's presenting patterns as they are on their Western medications.** Next, through application of the four examinations, we identify the patient's Chinese medical patterns as they exist *while on their Western medications.* Some Western practitioners have suggested we should try to figure out what the patient's patterns were or would be if they were not taking Western drugs, but nothing in the Chinese medical literature from China suggests this approach. It is, instead, unanimous that we should discriminate our patient's patterns as they are, whether the patient is taking one or more Western medi-

cines or not. These are the patterns that require remedying. Further, in an average Western patient with a chronic disease who is on one or more Western medicines, we can expect them to present not less than three patterns simultaneously and up to eight or 10. Since all these patterns typically reflect mutually engendering disease mechanisms, we must address them as one total gestalt. Such mutually engendering disease mechanisms cannot be treated one at a time but must be treated as the integrated whole that they have become.

3. **State the treatment principles** (治 则 *zhi ze*) **for each pattern in the same order as the statement of the presenting patterns.** Another step that, in our experience as teacher-mentors, is commonly omitted by Western practitioners, is the statement of treatment principles. Treatment principles are the bridge between the pattern discrimination and the treatment plan. The treatment principles tell us exactly what we need to do. For certain patterns there are professionally agreed upon standard treatment principles. The wording of these treatment principles have important technical implications. For instance, if we say that we need to enrich the kidneys, the word "enrich" tells us we need to use yin-supplementing medicinals. However, if we say we need to warm the kidneys, this means we need to use interior-warming medicinals (in contradistinction to invigorating the kidneys which means we need to use yang-supplementing medicinals). The technical precision of Chinese herbal medicine largely lies is in the technical implications of the correctly stated treatment principles.

In addition, it is important to state the treatment principles in the same order as the pattern discrimination. Remember that, in real life, patients with chronic conditions present multiple patterns simultaneously. However, the order in which we state these patterns implies a ranking of importance. The first treatment principles should correspond to the first stated pattern and so on. Treatment principles that are more important (as evidenced by their priority in statement) will be reflected by a larger number of ingredients and/or larger doses. Those treatment principles that are less important will be reflected by fewer ingredients and/or lower doses. The order of the stated treatment principles is a guide to how heavily we weight each of those principles.

4. **Add any treatment principles for acute, emergency conditions as necessary.** In Chinese medicine, there are certain emergency conditions requiring emergency treatment (急 则 治 标 *ji ze zhi biao*). Any outflow of pure substance from the body is such a condition, including great sweating, prolonged vomiting, prolonged diarrhea, polyuria, seminal emission, bleeding, and leukorrhea. In any one of these cases, we can add the treatment principles to stop vomiting, stop diarrhea, stop sweating, stop bleeding, etc. In that case, we are required to include ingredients empirically known to do just that, as necessary. Pain is likewise a tip or branch symptom that requires emergency empirical treatment to "stop pain." In other words, in these emergency conditions, we do not just treat the root patterns but definitely must also attend to branch symptoms. It is the addition of these branch treatment principles that gives us the warrant to use such condition-specific empirical treatments or ingredients.

5. **Choose the guiding formula based on the first stated treatment principle.** As stated above, the first treatment principles should be for the first stated pattern, and it is this first stated treatment principle that tells us which category in our formulas and prescriptions book we are going to find our guiding or base formula. For instance, if the first principle is to harmonize the liver and spleen, then we will find our base formula in the category of harmonizing formulas (和 剂 *he ji*), subcategory the harmonizing formulas which harmonize the liver and spleen.

6. **Make appropriate additions and subtractions based on the remaining treatment principles.**

Then we modify that formula with additions and subtractions (加 减 *jia jian*) until the ingredients in the final formula embody each of the stated treatment principles and also only those treatment principles.

7. **Be sure to do everything warranted by the treatment principles.** This means that our final formula should do everything our treatment principles have told us we should do as indicated by the patient's presenting patterns. The final formula should reflect the treatment principles exactly–containing neither more nor less than our treatment principles have warranted.

8. **Do not do anything unwarranted by the treatment principles.** This means that we should not add ingredients that do not embody, either directly or indirectly, one or more of the elements of our treatment principles. If our treatment principles do not warrant a particular ingredient, then it should not be in the formula. This step-by-step methodology is what helps keep our formulas on target for our patients. It is what insures that we do everything indicated and nothing that is not indicated.

THIRD STEPS: ADMINISTER THE CHINESE MEDICINE

If a patient is not taking any Western medicines (西 药 *xi yao*), we can directly go to the prescription and administration of our Chinese medicinals (中 药 *zhong yao*). However, if they are taking one or more prescription medications, then there are some other steps that need to be taken in order to prevent, to the best of our ability, any adverse interactions.

1. **Research each Chinese medicinal in your prescription** regarding potential interactions with the patient's Western drugs. For instance, you can look up the Western drug(s) and then see if this book suggests there are any likely interactions.

2. **If any research proves or strongly suggests a particular Chinese medicinal may cause an adverse reaction,** substitute that medicinal

with another one or simply remove it altogether. Not all the caveats contained in this book are equally supported by evidence. Many, indeed the vast majority, are only theoretical possibilities based on chemistry. However, if there really is strong evidence for a particular negative drug-herb interaction, then one should remove that medicinal from your formula. Formulas are not sacred. They have all been created by human beings and are all modifiable depending on the situation. No ingredient is so important and unique that it is absolutely indispensable. While a certain ingredient may be your preferred ingredient, all things being equal, there are always other substitutions. In some cases, one medicinal may simply be substituted by another, such as *Dang Shen* (Radix Codonopsis) or *Tai Zi Shen* (Radix Pseudostellariae) instead of *Ren Shen* (Radix Ginseng). In other cases, one may have to substitute two or more medicinals for one, as in the case of *Dan Shen* (Radix Salviae Miltiorrhizae) with *Dang Gui* (Radix Angelicae Sinensis) and *Sheng Di Huang* (uncooked Radix Rehmanniae). In yet other cases, it may simply be a matter of leaving the ingredient out of the formula altogether. In China, doctors modify formulas all the time. It may be because a particular ingredient is too expensive, it may be because an ingredient is simply out of stock, or it may be because a patient is a vegetarian and the ingredient is an animal by-product. Whatever the reason, it is not a catastrophe and Chinese doctors still get their job done. Knowing how to substitute ingredients in formulas is simply one of the working skills of a Chinese doctor.

3. **Stay within standard doses** (用 量 *yong liang*) for all medicinals and consider starting at the low end of the range. Every Chinese medicinal has a standard dose range stated in contemporary Chinese materia medicas. For instance, in Bensky *et al.*'s third edition of *Chinese Herbal Medicine: Materia Medica*, there is a standard daily dose range for each

medicinal when that medicinal is bulk-dispensed for use in a water-based decoction. The average daily dose range for Chinese medicinals is 9-10 grams per day when taken as a water-based decoction. However, the dose range of some medicinals is higher than that. For instance, *Huang Qi* (Radix Astragali) is sometimes dosed at up to 60 grams per day, and *Pu Gong Ying* (Herba Taraxaci) is often dosed at 45 grams per day. On the other hand, the standard daily dose of *Sha Ren* (Fructus Amomi) is usually given as 3-6 grams per day. As an extension of this, if prescribing Chinese medicinals to a patient on one or more prescription drugs, prudence suggests starting out with a trial dose at the low end of each ingredient's daily standard range.

4. **Also determine dosages based on the patient's age, weight, and condition.** However, one should also take into account the patient's age, weight, and the severity and nature of their condition. For instance, liver and kidney function decrease with age, and metabolites, including herbal metabolites are cleared more slowly from the body. Therefore, after 60 years of age, patients are usually dosed less than a middle-aged adult to prevent over-dosage. A dose-to-age chart is presented here.

Similarly, dose should be adjusted to weight. A person who weighs twice as much as another should typically be administered twice the amount of medicine in order to

Age-to-Dose Guidelines

0-1 month	1/18-1/14 of adult dose
1-6 months	1/14-1/7 of adult dose
6-12 months	1/7-1/5 of adult dose
1-2 years	1/5-1/4 of adult dose
2-4 years	1/4-1/3 of adult dose
4-6 years	1/3-2/5 of adult dose
6-9 years	2/5-1/2 of adult dose
9-14 years	1/2-2/3 of adult dose
14-18 years	2/3 to full adult dose
18-60 years	full adult dose
60 years +	3/4 adult dose or less

experience the same effect. A dose-to-weight chart is presented below.

Further, the nature and severity of a patient's condition should also be taken into account when determining dosages. If a patient suffers from an acute or a very severe condition, they are typically administered larger doses, while if they suffer from a chron-

Weight-to-Dose Guidelines

30-40 lbs.	20-27% of adult dose
40-50 lbs.	27-33% of adult dose
50-60 lbs.	33-40% of adult dose
60-70 lbs.	40-47% of adult dose
70-80 lbs.	47-53% of adult dose
80-100 lbs.	53-67% of adult dose
100-120 lbs.	67-80% of adult dose
120-150 lbs.	80-100% of adult dose
150-200 lbs.	100-133% of adult dose
200-250 lbs.	133-167% of adult dose
250-300 lbs.	167-200% of adult dose

ic or mild condition, they are typically administered lower doses.

5. **Administer a trial of the Chinese medicinal formula starting at a reasonably low dose (typically, 2-4 days).** If we are prescribing a decoction, no matter whether the patient is on Western drugs or not, we always only start with a two-day trial dose. However, even when prescribing ready-made Chinese medicines (such as pills, powders, and capsules) to patients concurrently on Western medications, we also suggest not exceeding a 2-4 day initial trial dose. That way, if there are any adverse reactions, one can catch them quickly and make adjustments without the patient having to throw away a several week supply of their Chinese medicinals. Therefore, after taking Chinese medicinals for 2-4 days, we always have the patient call us to give a report. Hopefully, they will have something positive to report, but we are most concerned about any seeming side effects or interactions.

6. **If no adverse reactions,** prescribe a one-week dose. If the patient does fine on their trial dose, we then prescribe for one week. At the

end of that week, we again have them call us to give a report.

7. **If still no adverse reactions, increase the dose** to the level you believe is theoretically appropriate for the patient. If we plan on mainly treating with some form of ready-made Chinese medicine, after the two-day and one-week trials, we then prescribe whatever a full bottle's worth of that medicine is. Depending on the company and the size of the bottle, that could be anything from one week to one month. If the patient is going to continue taking decoctions, we have them call us for an update once every week. In any case, we never let a patient go for more than one month without checking in with us.

8. **Monitor the patient regularly** and make adjustments as necessary. If, on any of these check-in calls, the patient says that something has significantly shifted for either better or worse, we will then typically change their Chinese medicinal formula. If the patient's situation is such that we feel we must see their tongue, feel their pulse, and ask more questions than what is efficient over the phone, then we schedule an office visit.

9. **Be available to the patient for emergencies in some manner 24/7.** The practice of medicine, including Chinese medicine, is not one to be entered lightly. Doctors have special ethical obligations that shoe salespersons do not. One obligation is to be available 24 hours per day seven days a week. Although we would prefer otherwise, most often, when patients have difficulties, these occur outside of office hours. At the very least, this means having an answering service and cell phone. In the best of all possible worlds, there would also be a 24-hour emergency Chinese medical clinic, but such things do not currently exist and are not likely to in the forseeable future. It is also very important to provide some sort of coverage during vacations and holidays. This usually means several practitioners in a given area agreeing to cover each other's practice when one is out of town. If we are going to prescribe

internal medicine, even Chinese herbal medicine, then we have to take on all the burdens and obligations of being a doctor, especially if we chose to give care to high risk patients on many Western medicines for serious diseases.

In summary of the third series of steps, we recommend "starting low and going slow." Start at a low dose and slowly increase it to therapeutic levels. This allows observation for interactions before they become serious. What is "low" depends on the patient. A patient who is generally healthy and is taking a drug or two (depending on the drugs) could be started at 1/2 to 3/4 of our desired dose. But an older patient on multiple drugs may be started at 1/4 to 1/3 of the desired dose. Ramping up to full dosage can take one-to-three weeks depending on multiple factors such as age, condition(s), constitution, chronicity, etc.

In addition, the authors recommend not trying to do too much at any one time. By this we mean, don't start a new herbal or supplement regimen at the same time a new drug is being started. Separate them so it is possible to know if the symptoms a patient is experiencing can be attributed to side effects of the new drug, interactions between the drug and the herbs, or side effects of the new herbs. If everything is thrown together, it becomes impossible to determine what is helping or not.

■ HANDLING ADVERSE REACTIONS

There are also some steps that one can follow when a patient does have what he or she thinks is an adverse reaction or herb/drug interaction.

1. **Do not panic; stay calm; stay focused; handle the problem in a step-by-step manner.** It is extremely important to keep your composure and clear head in what purports to be crisis. If you panic, this will be communicated to the patient who will respond with their own escalating fear. Instead, take a deep breath and begin by addressing the problem in a rational, step-by-step manner, assuming nothing for granted. One way to do this is to just tell yourself (not the patient) that it is not a drug-herb interaction. In this author's experience, it is almost never an interaction. So this is a pretty good assumption and allows the practitioner to keep a clear head.

2. **Determine the exact signs and symptoms of the adverse reaction, when it started, and any surrounding conditions or factors.** We are going to solve the patient's adverse reaction the same way as diagnosing their original complaint. We first need to gather enough specifics so that we can make a determination of what is really going on.

3. **Determine if, in fact, the situation was caused by your prescription, not some other factor.** One of the first things to be determined is that the problem really has been caused by the medication you have prescribed. We cannot tell how many times patients have called us saying that their Chinese herbs were causing a problem only to find out that they ate something they were not supposed to or did something which was clearly not good for them. Do not assume that the problem was caused by the Chinese medicinals you prescribed. Only accept the possibility of that after other factors have been ruled out.

4. **If you determine the situation is a reaction to your prescription, have the patient immediately stop taking the medicinals (unless it is likely the reaction is a Herxheimer reaction. More on that below.)** In many cases, the patient will already have stopped. However, if they are still taking their Chinese medicinals, they should definitely stop at this time.

5. **See the patient in the flesh as soon as possible. Try to see the patient the very next day if at all possible.** Do not just problem solve over the phone even if you otherwise could. By seeing the patient in person as soon as possible, you are conveying both professionalism and care.

6. **Review the patient's situation and your prescription.** Go over everything about the case again. Perhaps you made a wrong pattern discrimination and the herbs are wrong. It may be the patient took the medicine wrong. It may be that only a particular ingredient

caused the problem. However, in trying to determine what truly caused what, nothing should be kept off the table; everything should be looked at. According to the famous Chinese doctor Zhong Shan: "If the course of a disease is baffling without sign of improvement, you should, with trembling caution, wholeheartedly review your diagnosis and treatment."

7. **Attempt to determine what caused the reaction.**

If the patient experienced diarrhea after taking the Chinese herbs, were there any ingredients in the formula that could damage the spleen and cause loosening of the stools? If there was extreme thirst and parched throat, were there any windy, acrid, dry-natured ingredients in the formula that have damaged yin fluids? In other words, pattern discriminate the patient's adverse symptoms, then posit a disease mechanism for those symptoms. Then check the formula to see if any ingredients could have caused that disease mechanism.

8. **Remove or reduce the offending ingredient or change the prescription entirely.** If your pattern discrimination was simply wrong from the start, then the prescription as a whole is wrong. Based on your new, hopefully now correct, pattern discrimination, prescribe a new Chinese formula and start over again. However, if you can isolate what you believe to be the most likely ingredient, then take that ingredient out of the formula, either simply omitting it or substituting it with one or more other ingredients

9. **Start again slowly as before with an initial trial run at a low dose.** Begin again with a 1-2 day trial run. Be sure to stay in close contact with the patient.

10. **Monitor the patient's response and prescribe accordingly.** If everything is now ok, prescribe a larger or longer dose of the new formula. However, continue to stay in close contact with the patient until it is definitely clear that the problem has been solved.

▥ HERXHEIMER REACTIONS

Herxheimer reactions are also called "die-off reactions." A type of toxic reaction due to microbial die-off induced by correct medication, they were first identified in the early 20th century when patients treated for syphilis had toxic reactions to the massive die-off of syphylis spirochetes. When microbes die-off they leave behind cellular debris. If the body is not able to rid itself of this debris, there will be a toxic reaction, usually in the form of nausea, vomiting, diarrhea, bodily aches and pains, headache, general malaise, and possible fever. These symptoms, similar to food poisoning, last 12-24 hours and not more than 36 hours maximum. The vomiting and diarrhea are the body's attempt to detoxify itself by any means possible.

Typically, in our patients, Herxheimer reactions are due to massive, herb-caused die-off of yeast and fungi. Due to our Western diet of excessive sugars and simple carbohydrates along with iatrogenesis due to antibiotics and steroid hormone use, it is common for modern patients to have too many yeast and fungi in their bodies. While a certain population of these are necessary for our health, overgrowths of even benign yeasts and fungi can play a part in the causation and continuation of many chronic diseases. Some authors refers to this as polysystemic chronic candidiasis (PSCC), and many Chinese medicinals, especially the heat-clearing medicinals, have broad-spectrum fungicidal actions. Therefore, when a patient with a yeast overgrowth takes one or more of these broad-spectrum Chinese herbal fungicides, the result may be massive yeast die-off and a Herxheimer reaction.

If the condition truly is a Herxheimer reaction, the symptoms will be self-limiting and, after they abate, the patient will bounce back quickly. In addition, their original complaints will markedly improve. Patients with chronic spleen qi vacuity complicated by enduring, possibly deeplying damp heat are the most likely to experience Herxheimer reactions to Chinese medicinals.

HOW TO HANDLE A HERXHEIMER REACTION

1. Do not panic.

2. **Reassure the patient.** Explain to the patient what you believe is going on, that you think they are having a Herxheimer reaction. Then explain to them what a Herxheimer reaction is, that it is self-limiting and that it is actually a good thing, that they will feel much better across the board after these symptoms pass.

3. **Reduce but do not stop administration of the Chinese medicinals unless the patient simply cannot continue taking them.** The Chinese medicinals are killing off the yeast and fungal overgrowth and that is a good thing. It is something we want to happen, just not so quickly. By reducing the dosage, we slow down the die-off so that the patient's excretory systems can eliminate the toxins with fewer or no negative symptoms. We want the die-off to keep happening, but in a way the patient can comfortably bear.

4. **Promote detoxification by all means possible.** While vomiting and diarrhea are two ways of ridding the body of toxins, there are other ways that are not as uncomfortable. By drinking lots of water, we increase urination. By taking a steambath or sauna, we increase perspiration. It is also possible to take a warm bath in Epsom salts.

5. **After symptoms have abated, replace electrolytes.** After symptoms have abated, replace electrolytes lost via vomiting, diarrhea, and/or sweating. This can be done with an electrolyte-replacing sports drink like Gatorade®, or an electrolyte-replacing liquid from a pharmacy, such as Pedialyte®.

6. **Reintroduce the original prescription.** If the patient has stopped taking the original Chinese herbal formula, try reintroducing it again and see what happens.

7. **Place the patient on a "clear, bland" diet.** A Herxheimer reaction is a clear indication that a patient has a yeast and fungi problem and needs a special diet to go along with their herbs, in Chinese medicine called the clear, bland diet. It means eating lots of whole grains and little or no refined carbohydrates, lots of vegetables and some regular lean animal protein. It also means cutting out, or severely limiting, sugars and sweets, including sweet fruits and fruit juices. In also means avoiding food made through fermentation, such as alcohol, vinegar, cheese, and breads or anything that goes easily moldy. Such a clear, bland diet does two things. First, it starves yeasts and fungi of the simple sugars they need for reproduction. Secondly, it eliminates or minimizes the intake of dead yeast bodies that may cause allergic reactions.

8. **Stress the importance of diet in the patient's overall treatment plan.** While many patients think that acupuncture or Chinese herbs alone can cure their disease, rarely is it the case. According to the great Tang dynasty doctor Sun Si-miao, the superior practitioner first adjusts the patient's diet and lifestyle. Only if that is not adequate, should they then administer acupuncture or prescribe herbs. While not realistic in our patient population, this does point to the importance of diet in the cause and cure of so much disease. In particular, if a patient has had a Herxheimer reaction after taking Chinese herbs, diet is simply going to have to be accepted as part of the treatment plan.

OPENING LINES OF COMMUNICATION

When treating patients who are also under the care of a Western physician and taking one or more prescription drugs, it is going to be important to open meaningful lines of communication with that physician. Here are the steps we suggest when attempting such communication with one of your patient's Western physicians.

1. Send the prescribing physician(s) an introduction packet containing the following:

   A. Professional-looking folder to hold all the information in the packet

   B. Introductory letter

C. Business card

D. Prescription pad

E. Curriculum vitae

F. General brochure about Chinese medicine

G. Possible brochure or article(s) about Chinese medicine and the patient's personal condition

H. Abstracts of any research on the patient's condition and Chinese medicine

2. **Follow up with a phone call several days to one week later. In that case:**

A. Speak professionally.

B. Speak their lingo.

C. Offer to provide any follow-up information the doctor may request, including personal references, further reading materials on Chinese medicine, statistics, etc.

D. Be courteous and polite, but do not be cowed or intimidated.

3. **Consider taking the doctor to lunch or making a face-to-face appointment. In that case:**

A. Dress and groom they way you think they will dress and groom.

B. Speak professionally.

C. Speak their lingo.

THE FACTS ON INTEGRATED CHINESE-WESTERN MEDICINE

A huge number of patients have been treated with integrated Chinese-Western medicine in China over the past 50 years. In 1981, the Ministry of Health and Chinese Association of Science & Technology founded the Chinese Association of Integrated Chinese-Western Medicine to support systematic research on the integration of these two medicines. Since then large numbers of clinical trials, cohort studies, and laboratory experiments have been conducted into all aspects of integrated Chinese-Western medicine. During the early years of this research, there were many criticisms about failings in research design and statistical analysis. However, year by year, there is a steady improvement to the point that we now see randomly assigned, placebo-controlled, double-blind studies being conducted in China on this subject. In October 1997, the First World Conference on Integrated Chinese-Western Medicine was held in Beijing, and over 1,300 representatives attended from all over the world.

A huge body of literature documenting these outcomes exists. This consists of:

A. Textbooks

B. Journals

C. Clinical trials and cohort studies

D. Case histories

The only reason that this body of literature is not better known is because it is written in Chinese, and very few Westerners are able to read Chinese. However, in their attempts to get the results of this research more widely disseminated, more and more Chinese medical journals are including English language abstracts and are submitting their contents to such online databases as PubMed. In point of fact, the refusal of Western practitioners to give serious credence to this body of literature is pure ignorance and smacks of both parochialism and racism.

Western practitioners of Chinese medicine should have no doubt about the benefits of combining Chinese and Western medicines. The facts show that such a combination achieves:

A. Better therapeutic effects

B. At lower doses of Western drugs

C. With fewer or no side effects

We introduced these three facts previously, but we believe they should be a mantra memorized and repeated by every Western practitioner of Chinese medicine, both to instill confidence in what we do and to counter the arguments of the many naysayers who would cast suspicion on our medicine.

FINAL ADVICE

1. **Do not be afraid to prescribe Chinese medicinals to patients on Western medicines.** Except for a very few Western drugs, there is very little true potential for adverse Chinese herb-Western drug interactions. This bugaboo only exists in the Western mind due to profound ignorance of 50 years of integrated Chinese-Western medicine in China.

2. **Speak up and out against our competitors'**

scare tactics. **Do not be passive.** Western practitioners of Chinese medicine have so far bought into and been scared by this specter of herb-drug interactions promoted by our competitors in the health care marketplace. However, once we know the facts, we need to speak up and out against these detractors with their unsupported "mays" and "mights." If we fail to rebut these arguments, they have free sway within our society, and our very silence condemns us to our seeming acquiescence.

3. **While reading over a thousand studies about drug-herb interactions,** this author sees one problem over and over: the lack of discussion about dosing. While a title of a scientific article may be something like "this drug when combined with this herb causes death or hospitalization" in almost every case, somewhere buried deep in the article (never in the abstract), they mention the dose of the herb and it is 10, 20, or even 50 times higher than we use. Everything, including water, is poison at a high enough dose. And that is not a drug-herb interaction, it is an over dosage. Do not let our competitors be inexact or even shady about this information.

4. **Do be careful when prescribing Chinese medicinals to patients on Western medications.** While there is no real proof that the routine use of Chinese medicinals in patients con-

comitantly taking Western drugs is harmful, we still must be careful. And we will have to be careful for a long time. There is no way to rule out every potential Chinese medicinal combination with every potential Western medical combination. We are going to be working in an environment of trial and error for a long, long time, and, therefore, we are going to have to be careful and duly diligent. This means:

A. Do your research.

B. Start off cautiously.

C. Do not attempt to treat conditions you have not been trained to treat.

D. Stick within professional standards of care (SOC).

5. **Open lines of communication with your patients' prescribing physicians as discussed above.**

6. **In everything you do as a professional, foster the knowledge that integrated Chinese-Western medicine is not only safe but more effective than either medicine alone.**

7. **Foster confidence in your patients and in their other caregivers:**

A. By speech, demeanor, dress, and grooming

B. By written information

C. By public speaking

D. By networking

E. By constant continuing education

Drugs Affecting The Autonomic Nervous System

The nervous system is broken down into two major divisions: the central nervous system (CNS) and the peripheral nervous system (PNS) (Figure 4.1). The CNS includes the brain and spinal cord; the PNS includes everything outside of these structures (with the possible exception of the enteric nervous system). The PNS can be broken down in two different ways. One way is to discuss efferent and afferent signals. Efferent signals are those going toward the effector organs (viscera, muscles, glands). One way to remember this is to think of *e*fferent nerves *e*xit the brain (both words begin with "e"). Afferent nerves carry impulses from sensors towards the brain and spinal cord. The afferent nerves tell us what is going on in the body or environment, while efferent nerves allow us to act on that information.

The second way the PNS can be broken down is into the autonomic nervous system (ANS) versus the somatic system. The somatic system, also called the voluntary system, generally involves efferent nerves that affect muscles and afferent nerves that involve conscious sensation. In contrast, the autonomic nervous system is generally unconscious. It controls most of the organs and regulatory apparatus of the body and with a few exceptions (such as breathing), is not affected by conscious effort.

The efferent ANS can be further broken down into the sympathetic and parasympathetic divisions. The sympathetic division is involved in the fight or flight response and generally prepares the body for action. The parasympathetic division is geared toward relaxation and rumination and allows the body to recuperate and digest food and

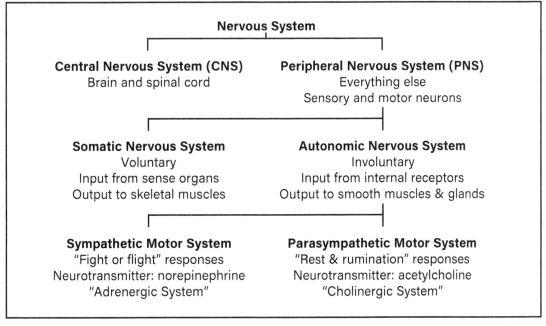

Figure 4.1: The human nervous system. This figure shows how the nervous system in humans can be broken down into several subsystems. These include several pairs of systems: the central nervous system vs. the peripheral nervous system, which can be broken down into the somatic and autonomic nervous systems, which can be further broken down into the sympathetic and parasympathetic nervous systems.

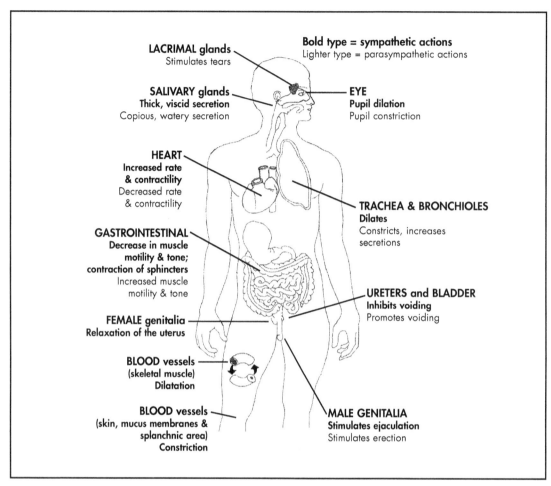

Figure 4.2: Sympathetic and parasympathetic organ innervation. This figure shows the actions of the sympathetic nervous (in bold) and parasympathetic nervous systems on various organs.

drink most efficiently. The sympathetic and parasympathetic divisions tend to balance each other, and most target organs are innervated by both divisions as shown in Figure 4.2.

The efferent pathways in the efferent ANS consist of two neurons, one that begins near the spinal cord and travels to a **ganglion** where it **synapses** with another neuron and ultimately affects a target organ. The neuron from the spinal cord to the ganglion is called the preganglionic neuron, while the neuron from the ganglion to the target organ is called the ganglionic or postganglionic neuron. The cell body of the preganglionic neuron is located within the CNS, while the cell body of the postganglionic neuron is located in the ganglion itself.

Sympathetic neurons emerge from the CNS in the thoracic and lumbar regions of the spinal cord and most immediately synapse in the **paravertebral** or chain ganglia located just lateral to the spinal column. The postganglionic neurons travel from these ganglia to their target organ. This means they have a short preganglionic neuron and a long postganglionic one. Generally, the preganglionic neuron uses acetylcholine as a neurotransmitter, while the postganglionic neuron uses norepinephrine (previously called noradrenaline).

The parasympathetic division emerges from the CNS from the cranial and sacral areas of the spinal cord. This division generally has long preganglionic neurons that extend to ganglia near or

---

Ganglion: A collection of nerve cells outside of the CNS

Synapse: A junction between two nerves or a nerve and an effector organ

---

Paravertebral: Near the vertebral column

on their effector organs where they synapse with the postganglionic neurons. These neurons are very short and extend to the effector organs. Preganglionic parasympathetic neurons, just like preganglionic sympathetic neurons, use acetylcholine as a neurotransmitter. The postganglionic neuron also uses acetylcholine as a neurotransmitter. There is a difference, however. In ganglionic synapses (between the pre- and postganglionic neurons), a specific receptor called a nicotinic receptor receives the acetylcholine (ACh). In the synapse between the postganglionic neuron and the effector organ, muscarinic receptors are prominent. While they both accept acetylcholine, there are enough differences between these two types of receptors to be pharmacologically useful, as will be demonstrated by some of the drugs in this chapter. These differences are seen in Figure 4.3.

There are over 300 identified neurotransmitters in the nervous system. Neurotransmitters are chemicals that allow a signal to pass from one neuron to another. In the ANS, there are three major types of neurotransmitters that interact with cell membrane receptors. Acetylcholine is one of these transmitters. Neurons that utilize this chemical are called cholinergic. Two other types, mainly used in the sympathetic division, are norepinephrine and epinephrine. If a neuron uses either of these transmitters it is called adrenergic. Neurotransmitters will bind with a cell membrane receptor, which can activate a second messenger system to act on the interior of the cell.

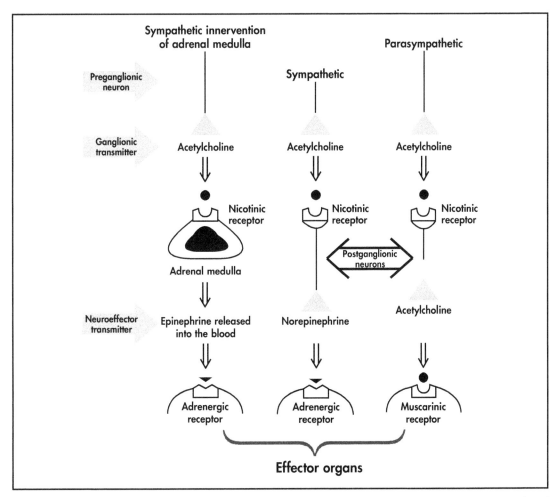

Figure 4.3: Sympathetic and parasympathetic innervation of effector organs. This shows all preganglionic and preadrenal neurons use acetylcholine as a neurotransmitter, which is received by nicotinic receptors. The postganglionic neurons of the sympathetic system, however, use norepinephrine as a primary neurotransmitter, while the postganglionic neurons of the parasympathetic system primarily use acetylcholine and activate muscarinic receptors.

SECTION 1: CHOLINERGIC AGONISTS

AMBENONIUM (am be NOE nee um) PR=C
(Mytelase®)

BETHANECHOL (be THAN e kole) PR=C
(Urecholine®)

CEVIMELINE (se vi ME leen) PR=C *(Evoxac®)*

GUANIDINE (GWAHN i deen) PR=N

PILOCARPINE (pye loe KAR peen) PR=C
(Isopto®Carpine, Pilopine HS®, Salagen®)

Cholinergic agonists act to increase the postsynaptic stimulation of a cholinergic neuron, which could be a preganglionic para- or sympathetic neuron, a postganglionic parasympathetic neuron, or a neuron that synapses with the adrenal medulla. While all cholinergic neurons employ acetylcholine as a neurotransmitter, acetylcholine is not often used therapeutically except in the eye. There are several analogues of acetylcholine that are used therapeutically. They act like acetylcholine but have longer durations of action. These are called direct cholinergic agonists. The life cycle of acetylcholine is shown in Figure 4.4.

FUNCTION

Bethanechol and Pilocarpine primarily stimulate muscarinic receptors. Bethanechol is used primarily to stimulate an atonic bladder especially in cases of nonobstructive urinary retention postpartum or postoperatively. An off-label use is to increase intestinal motility and tone in cases of reflux esophagitis.

Pilocarpine is used topically to the cornea in cases of glaucoma. It is orally used to stimulate salivation in cases of xerostomia due to radiation therapy and Sjögren's syndrome.

Ambenonium is used in the treatment of myasthenia gravis. Cevimeline is used to treat the symptom of dry mouth in Sjögren's syndrome. Guanidine is for treatment of **Eaton-Lambert syndrome** and should not be used for myasthenia gravis.

MECHANISM OF ACTION

Direct cholinergic agonists act by stimulating the postsynaptic membrane receptor just as acetylcholine would. However, since none of the agents in this category are readily broken down by acetylcholinesterases, they have a much longer duration of effect than acetylcholine.

DOSAGES

AMBENONIUM, for *adults*, 5-25 mg 3-4 times/d. Some patients may have a dose as high as 50-75 mg.

BETHANECHOL, *for children*, 0.3-0.6 mg/kg/d divided 3-4 times/d. *For adults*, for urinary retention, **neurogenic** bladder, and/or bladder atony, initiate at 10-50 mg 3-4 times/d. Some patients may require dosages of 50-100 mg qid. *For the elderly*, use the lowest effective dose. This should be taken 1 hour before meals or 2 hours after.

CEVIMELINE, for *adults*, 30 mg 3 tid.

GUANIDINE, for *adults*, for Eaton-Lambert syndrome, initiate at 10-15 mg/kg/d in 3-4 divided doses, gradually increase to 35 mg/kg/d or more until side effects occur.

PILOCARPINE, in *adults*, for xerostomia, following head and neck cancer, 5 mg 3 tid, 10 mg 3 tid for Sjögren's syndrome, 5 mg 4 qid.

ADVERSE EFFECTS

Side effects of these agents include: general stimulation of cholinergic neurons such as headache, urinary urgency, nausea, **miosis**, **diaphoresis**, hypotension, salivation, flushing, abdominal pain and cramps, **bronchospasm**, and diarrhea. Together, these effects are often referred to as cholinergic or muscarinic side effects.

RED FLAGS

Any shortness of breath may be an indication of

Eaton-Lambert syndrome: A form of muscle weakness that tends to be associated with lung cancer

---

Neurogenic: Stemming from or caused by the nervous system

Miosis: Constriction of the pupil

Diaphoresis: The act of perspiring or sweating

Bronchospasm: A muscle spasm causing narrowing of the airways of the lung, usually accompanied by a cough and wheeze

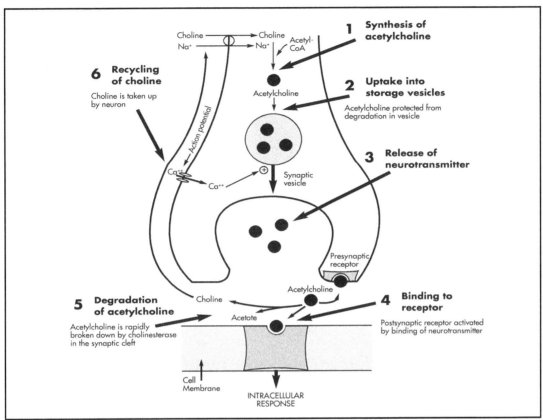

Figure 4.4: The life cycle of acetylcholine. 1. Acetylcholine (ACh) is produced in the neuron's cell body and transported down the axon into the axonal terminal. **2.** In the terminal, ACh is stored until needed in synaptic vesicles. **3.** When an action potential initiates release of ACh, the vesicle blends into the presynaptic cell membrane and releases ACh into the synaptic cleft. **4.** ACh diffuses across the cleft and activates the postsynaptic membrane receptor. **5.** Cholinesterase in the synaptic cleft breaks down ACh into acetate and choline. **6.** Choline is reabsorbed by the presynaptic neuron and remade into acetylcholine.

bronchospasm and may rapidly progress to an inability to breathe and should be treated as soon as possible.

Patients with asthma should not take these agents as they can precipitate an attack. Hyperthyroid patients may develop atrial **fibrillation** and should avoid these agents. In patients with coronary insufficiency, because of the hypotensive effects of these agents, they may cause a cardiac event.

■ INTERACTIONS

HERB

PILOCARPINE
- *Gan Cao* (Licorice) (Indeterminate)—may treat overdoses by increasing the metabolism of certain drugs such as barbituates, chloral hydrate,

urethane, cocaine, picrotoxin, pilocarpine, nicotine, and caffeine (Chinese language article cited in Chen & Chen, 2004) Indeterminate level of evidence.

■ INTERACTION ISSUES

A: Cholinergic effects may increase GI motility and therefore decrease absorption.

D:

M:

E: Cholinergic effects may increase GI motility and therefore affect elimination of drugs or herbs that excrete from the intestines.

TI: There is a narrow margin between the appearance of adverse effects with Ambenonium and serious toxic effects.

> Fibrillation: Recurrent, abnormal muscle contraction that is not physiologically useful

SECTION 2: ANTICHOLINESTERASES (REVERSIBLE)

DONEPEZIL (doh NEP e zil) PR=C *(Aricept®, Aricept ODT®)*

GALANTAMINE (ga LAN ta mene) PR=B *(Razadyne®, Razadyne® ER)*

NEOSTIGMINE (nee oh STIG mene) PR=B *(Prostigmin®)*

PYRIDOSTIGMINE (peer id doe STIG mene) PR=C *(Mestinon®, Mestinon Timespan®, Regonol®)*

RIVASTIGMINE (ri va STIG mene) PR=B *(Exelon®)*

Anticholinesterases act by preventing the breakdown of acetylcholine in the synaptic cleft. This causes acetylcholine to remain in the cleft for a longer period of time and prolongs activation of the postsynaptic membrane receptor as seen in Figure 4.4. These anticholinesterases can be reversible or irreversible. The reversible anticholinesterases can be used therapeutically. The irreversible types are used as insecticides and possibly nerve agents in chemical warfare.

FUNCTION

Neostigmine and pyridostigmine are used in the diagnosis and treatment of myasthenia gravis, a disease characterized by skeletal muscle weakness and fatigability. It is caused by an autoimmune reaction to postsynaptic ACh membrane receptors. They are also used as prophylaxis to biochemical weapons such as cholinesterase inhibitor poisons.

Donepezil, galantamine, and rivastigmine are used in the treatment of Alzheimer's disease to improve cognition and global function, and delay or slow progression of the disease.

Donepezil is occasionally used off-label for children with attention deficit hyperactivity disorder (ADHD).

MECHANISM OF ACTION

Anticholinesterases act by binding and reversibly inactivating acetylcholinesterase (AChE) in the synaptic cleft between neurons. AChE breaks down acetylcholine (ACh) in the synaptic cleft so that it can be recycled by the presynaptic neuron. Inhibiting AChE causes ACh to remain in the cleft for longer causing increased activation and action of the postsynaptic membrane receptors.

In other words, it makes it seem as if there is more ACh than there actually is.

DOSAGES

DONEPEZIL, for *adults*, for dementia of Alzheimer's type, initiate at 5 mg/day nocte; may increase to 10 mg/day after 4-6 weeks. In moderate to severe cases may be increased further to 23 mg once daily after 3 months. All dosing should occur at bedtime.

GALANTAMINE, for *adults*, using immediate release tablets or solution, for mild to moderate Alzheimer's dementia, initiate at 4 mg bid for 4 weeks. If well tolerated, increase to 8 mg bid. After 4 or more weeks increase to 12 mg bid. Normal therapeutic range is 16-24 mg/d in two doses taken with breakfast and dinner. If using extended-release capsules, initiate at 8 mg once daily for 4 weeks; if well tolerated, increase to 16 mg once daily for 4 or more weeks, increase to 24 mg once daily; normal therapeutic range is 16-24 mg once daily, taken with breakfast.

NEOSTIGMINE, for myasthenia gravis: for *children*, 2 mg/kg/d divided every 3-4 hours; IM or subcutaneous is used for treatment at a dose of .01-.04 mg/kg every 2-4 hours and IM can be used for diagnosing at a .04 mg/kg dose. For *adults*, 15 mg every 3-4 hours up to a maximum of 375 mg/d. Can be used IM for diagnosis with a single dose of .02 mg/kg, IM, subcutaneous as treatment of myasthenia gravis with a dose of .5-2.5 mg every 1-3 hours up to 10 mg daily and in bladder atony: to prevent at .25 mg every 4-6 hours for 2-3 days or treatment at .5-1 mg every 3 hours for five doses.

PYRIDOSTIGMINE, for myasthenia gravis: for *children*, 7 mg/kg/d divided into 5–6 doses; IM: .05-.15 mg/kg/dose. For *adults*, this agent is highly individualized with normal dosing ranges of 60-1500 mg/d, usually 600 mg/d divided into 5-6 doses for sustained release formulation, use dosing ranges between 180-540 mg once or twice daily. For pretreatment for Soman nerve gas exposure by the military, for adults, 30 mg every 8 hours beginning several hours prior to exposure, discontinue at first sign of nerve agent exposure, then begin atropine and pralidoxime. IM dose is approximately 1/30 of oral dose.

RIVASTIGMINE, for mild to moderate Alzheimer's dementia, initiate at 1.5 mg bid; may increase by 3 mg/d (1.5 mg/dose) every 2 weeks based on toleration up to a maximum recommended dose of 6 mg bid; for mild to moderate Parkinson's-related dementia, initiate at 1.5 mg bid; may increase by 3 mg/d (1.5 mg/dose) every 4 weeks based on toleration up to a maximum recommended dose of 6 mg bid. For transdermal patch: initiate at 4.6 mg/d; if tolerated, may be increased, after 4 or more weeks, to 9.5 mg per day.

ADVERSE EFFECTS

Side effects of these agents include: general stimulation of cholinergic neurons such as headache, urinary urgency, nausea, miosis, diaphoresis, hypotension, salivation, flushing, abdominal pain and cramps, bronchospasm, and diarrhea.

RED FLAGS

Any shortness of breath may be an indication of bronchospasm and may rapidly progress to an inability to breath and should be treated as soon as possible.

INTERACTIONS

No major interactions are noted. However:

INTERACTION ISSUES

A: Cholinergic effects may increase GI motility and therefore decrease absorption.

D: Donepezil is 96% protein bound.

M:

E: Cholinergic effects may increase GI motility and therefore affect elimination of drugs or herbs that excrete from the intestines.

TI:

SECTION 3: ANTIMUSCARINIC AGENTS

ATROPINE (A troe peen) PR=B/C *(Atropen®, Atropine Care™, Bonnatal®,[1] Donnatal Extentabs®,[1] Lomotil®,[2] Lonox®,[2] Motofen®[3])*

BENZTROPINE (BENZ troe peen) PR=C *(Cogentin®)*

BIPERIDEN (bye PER i den) PR=C *(Akineton®)*

DARIFENACIN (dar i FEN a sin) PR=C *(Enablex®)*

DICYCLOMINE (dye SYE kloe meen) PR=B *(Bentyl®)*

FESOTERODINE (fes oh TER oh deen) PR=C *(Toviaz™)*

GLYCOPYRROLATE (glye koe PYE roe late) PR=B (injection)/C (oral) *(Curposa™, Robinul®, Robinul® Forte)*

HYOSCYAMINE (hye oh SYE a meen) PR=C *(Anaspaz®, Cystospaz®, Donnatal®,[1] Donnatal Extentabs®,[1] HyoMax®SR, HyoMax®SL, HyoMax™DT, HyoMax™FT, Hyonatol,[1] Hyosine, Levbid®, Levsin®/SL, Levsin®, Symax® DuoTab, Symax®FasTab, Symax®SL, Symax®SR, Urelle®,[6] Urimar-T[6])*

IPRATROPIUM (eye pra TRO peum) PR=B *(Atrovent®, Atrovent®HFA, Combivent®,[50] DuoNeb®,[50] Duovent® UDV)*

MEPENZOLATE (me PEN zoe late) PR=B *(Cantil®)*

METHSCOPOLAMINE (meth skoe POL a meen) PR=C *(aeroKid™,[9] Dry Max,[9] Duradyl®,[9] Pamine Forte®, Pamine®, PCM,[9] Rescon X®[9])*

...continued on the following page

OXYBUTYNIN (ocks ee BYOOT i nene) PR=C
(Gelnique®, Oxytrol®)

PROCYCLIDINE (proe SYE kli deen) PR=C
(Kemadrin®)

PROPANTHELINE (proe PAN the leen) PR=C

SCOPOLAMINE (skoe POL a meen) PR=C
*(Donnatal®, Donnatal Extentabs®,[1]
Hyonatol,[1] Isopto® Hyoscine, Murocoll-2®,[22]
Transderm Scōp®)*

SOLIFENACIN (sol i FEN a sin) *(VESIcare®)* PR=C

TIOTROPIUM (ty oh TRO pee um) PR=C
(Spiriva® HandiHaler®)

TOLTERODINE (tole TER oh deen) PR=C
(Detrol®, Detrol® LA)

TRIHEXYPHENIDYL (trye heks ee FEN i dil) PR=C

TRIMETHOBENZAMIDE (trye meth oh BEN za mide) PR=C *(Tigan®)*

TROSPIUM (TROSE pee um) PR=C *(Sanctura™, Sanctura®XR)*

Muscarinic receptors are primarily located on the effector organ post synaptic membrane in the parasympathetic division of the autonomic nervous system. There are several subtypes of muscarinic receptors, designated M1-M5, each acting on different areas of the body. These subtypes of receptors allow for different agents to act on different parts of the body. For example, some agents work on the bladder almost exclusively.

FUNCTION

Atropine is used as an antispasmodic agent as it relaxes the gastrointestinal tract and the bladder. It is used topically in the eye for diagnostic procedures. It is also used to decrease respiratory secretions prior to surgery.

Benztropine, biperiden, procyclidine, and trihexyphenidyl are used to treat Parkinson's in an adjunctive role and to treat extrapyramidal symptoms (EPS) induced by other drugs.

Dicyclomine is used as an antispasmodic in treating irritable bowel syndrome (IBS).

Glycopyrrolate is used to inhibit salivation and secretions in the respiratory tract preoperatively, and as an adjunct treatment of peptic ulcers. A new preparation of this agent is also used to prevent drooling in neurologic conditions such as cerebral palsy.

Hyoscyamine is used as adjunctive therapy for peptic ulcers, in irritable bowel syndrome, for neurogenic bladder/ bowel, spasmodic GI tract disorders, parkinsonism, and dry acute rhinitis.

Detrussor: Pertaining to the detrussor urinae muscle, which forms the external muscle layer of the bladder

---

Antiemetic: An agent that suppresses nausea and vomiting

Ipratropium and tiotropium are bronchodilators used as inhalers with acute asthma, chronic obstructive pulmonary disease (COPD), bronchitis, and emphysema. More information on these conditions is found in Chapter 8. Ipratropium can be used nasally to help treat colds and rhinitis whether allergic or nonallergic in origin.

Mepenzolate is used as adjunctive treatment for peptic ulcer disease. More information about peptic ulcer disease is in Chapter 9, Section 1.

Methscopolamine is used, in combination with other drugs, in cases of allergic reactions such as rhinitis and skin reactions, lung congestion, and vasomotor rhinitis.

Propantheline is used as an antispasmodic and antisecretory agent in the treatment of peptic ulcers, IBS, pancreatitis, and urinary bladder spasm.

Darifenacin, fesoterodine, oxybutynin, solifenacin, tolterodine, and trospium act on the bladder to treat overactive bladder and urinary incontinence. Oxybutynin is also used in patients over 6 years old in treating neurogenic **detrussor** overactivity.

Trimethobenzamide is used as an **antiemetic** to prevent postoperative nausea and vomiting and nausea from gastroenteritis. Scopolamine is used to prevent nausea and vomiting from motion sickness or recovery from anesthesia and surgery. Can be injected preoperatively to create amnesia, sedation, and tranquilization and to prevent nausea and vomiting and decrease salivary and respiratory secretions. It can also be used to treat symptoms of parkinsonian spastic states and spasms of the gastrointestinal tract (such as in irritable bowel syndrome).

MECHANISM OF ACTION

Antimuscarinic agents, also known as muscarinic receptor antagonists, act by binding to post-synaptic receptor sites and preventing binding of ACh to these receptors.

DOSAGES

ATROPINE, for *children* under 5 kg, 0.02 mg/kg/dose 30-60 minutes preop, then every 4-6 hours as needed. For *children* over 5 kg, 0.01-0.02 mg/kg up to a maximum 0.4 mg/dose 30-60 minutes preop with a minimum dose of 0.1 mg. For *adults*, 0.4 mg, may repeat in 4 hours if necessary; IM or subcutaneous: 0.4-0.6 mg 30-60 minutes preop and repeat every 4-6 hours as needed.

BENZTROPINE, for *children* under 3 years, oral or IM, for drug-induced extrapyramidal symptoms, 0.02-0.05 mg/kg/dose 1-2 times/d. For *adults*, for drug-induced extrapyramidal symptoms, oral or IM, 1-4 mg 1-2 times/d; for parkinsonism, oral or IM, 0.5-6 mg/d in 1-2 divided doses. For acute dystonia, IM 1-2 mg.

BIPERIDEN, for *adults*, for parkinsonism, 2 mg 3-4 times/d, for extrapyramidal symptoms, 2 mg 1-3 times/d. For the *elderly*, initiate at 2 mg 1-2 times/d.

DARIFENACIN, for *adults*, initiate at 7.5 mg once daily; may be increased to 15 mg once daily.

DICYCLOMINE, for *adults*, initiate at 20 mg, qid, then increase up to 160 mg/d. IM 20 mg qid. For the *elderly*, initiate at 10-20 mg qid and increase as necessary to 160 mg per day.

FESOTERODINE, for adults, 4 mg once daily; can be increased to 8 mg.

GLYCOPYRROLATE, for *children*, 40-100 mcg/kg/dose 3-4 times/d. For chronic drooling in children 3-16, .02 mg/kg tid increasing by .02 mg/kg every 5-7 days as tolerated to a maximimum of .1 mg/kg, or 1.5-3 mg/dose, tid. IM, <2 years, 4-9 mcg/kg 30-60 mins preoperatively, >2 years 4 mcg/kg 30-60 mins preoperatively. For *adults*, IM 4 mcg/kg 30-60 mins preoperative.

HYOSCYAMINE, for *children*, for GI disorders, for *children* <2 years: 3.4 kg, 4 drops up to a maximum of 24 drops/d; 5 kg, 5 drops, up to a maximum of 30 drops/d; 7 kg, 6 drops up to a maximum of 36 drops/d; 10 kg, 8 drops up to a maximum of 48 drops/d. For *children* 2-12 years: 10 kg, 0.031-0.033 mg up to a maximum of 0.75 mg/d; 20 kg, 0.0625 mg up to a maximum of 0.75 mg/d; 40 kg, 0.0938 mg up to a maximum of 0.75 mg/d; 50 kg, 0.125 mg up to a maximum of 0.75 mg/24 hours. For *adults*: 0.125-0.25 mg every 4 hours or prn ac up to a maximum of 1.5 mg/d; for timed release, 0.375-0.75 mg every 12 hours up to a maximum 1.5 mg/d. IM or subQ, .25-.5 mg; may repeat up to 4 times/d.

IPRATROPIUM, for *children* 12 and under, for an acute asthma exacerbation, using a metered dose inhaler, 4-8 inhalations every 20 mins prn for up to 3 hours. For *children* 5-11, intranasal use for colds, 2 sprays in each nostril tid. Children over 5 for rhinitis or 4 for seasonal allergic rhinitis can use adult dosing. For *adults* with an acute asthma exacerbation using a metered dose inhaler, 8 inhalations every 20 mins prn up to 3 hours; for bronchospasm associated with COPD, 2 inhalations qid up to 12 inhalations/d. Intranasal use for colds: 2 sprays in each nostril 2-3 times/d, for allergic or nonallergic rhinitis, 2 sprays in each nostril 2-3 times/d; for seasonal allergic rhinitis, 2 sprays in each nostril qid. For colds, safety and effectiveness has not been established for use longer than 4 days.

MEPENZOLATE, for *adults*, for peptic ulcer disease, 25-50 mg qid with meals.

METHSCOPOLAMINE, for *adults*, 2.5 mg 30 minutes ac and 2.5-5 mg nocte; may increase dose to 5 mg bid.

OXYBUTYNIN, for *adults*, 5 mg 2-3 times/d up to a maximum of 5 mg qid; extended release, initiate at 5-10 mg once daily, up to a maximum of 30 mg/d. Topical gel: 1 100mg/g satchet once a day; transdermal: one 3.9 mg/d patch twice a week. For the *elderly*, 2.5-5 mg 2-3 times/d.

PROCYCLIDINE, for *adults*, 2.5 mg tid pc; can increase up to a maximum of 20 mg/d if necessary.

PROPANTHELINE, for *children*, as an antisecretory, 1-2 mg/kg/d in 3-4 doses; as an antispasmodic, 2-3 mg/kg/d in doses every 4-6 hours and at bedtime. For *adults*, 15 mg tid ac and 30 mg nocte. For the *elderly*, 7.5 mg tid ac and at bedtime. Can increase to maximum 30 mg tid.

SCOPOLAMINE, for *children*, as an antiemetic, subcutaneous .006 mg/kg, perioperative. For *children* 6 months to 3 years, IM and subQ, .1-.15 mg; for *children* 3-6 years, .2-.3 mg. For *adults*, transdermal patch can be used preoperatively (1 patch behind ear the night before surgery or 1 hour prior to cesarean section and remove 24 hours after surgery); for motion sickness (1 patch behind the ear at least 4 hours prior to exposure and every 3 days prn, effective if applied 2-3 hours before anticipated need, optimal 12 hours before); or for chemotherapy-induced nausea and vomiting (1 patch every 72 hours). Scopolamine hydrobromide can be used as an antiemetic (subQ .6-1 mg), preoperative (IM or subQ, 0.3-0.65 mg) sedation, or tranquilization (IM or subQ, .6 mg 3-4 times/d), parkinsonism, spasticity (oral, 0.4-0.8 mg, may repeat every 8-12 hours prn; may be cautiously increased), or motion sickness (oral, 0.4-0.8 mg; may repeat every 8-12 hours prn starting at least 1 hour before exposure is recommended).

SOLIFENACIN, for *adults*, 5 mg/d; may increase to 10 mg/d.

TIOTROPIUM, for adults, in COPD, oral inhalation of an 18 mcg capsule once daily.

TOLTERODINE, for *adults*, immediate release tablet, 2 mg bid, which may be lowered to 1 mg bid; extended release capsule, 4 mg once a day, which may be lowered to 2 mg daily.

TRIHEXYPHENIDYL, for *adults*, initiate at 1 mg/d, increase 2 mg every 3-5 days up to a usual dose of 6-10 mg/d in 3-4 divided doses; 12-15 mg/d may be required.

TRIMETHOBENZAMIDE, for *children*, over 40 kg, same as adult. For *adults*, 300 mg 3-4 times/d. IM 200 mg 3-4 times/d; for postoperative nausea and vomiting, IM 200 mg and another 200 mg an hour later.

Mydriasis: Dilation of the pupil

Supraventricular tachycardia: A heart rate of over 100 bpm caused above the ventricle, either at the atria, SA node, or AV junction

TROSPIUM, for *adults*, 20 mg bid, extended release dose at 60 mg once daily. For the *elderly* 75 years or over, consider initial dose of 20 mg once daily (based on tolerability) nocte.

ADVERSE EFFECTS

Common side effects of these agents include: blurred vision, confusion, drowsiness, **mydriasis**, constipation, dry mouth, tachycardia, restlessness, headache, and urinary retention.

Atropine is contraindicated for use with narrow-angle glaucoma patients.

RED FLAGS

Tachycardia can progress to **supraventricular tachycardia** or atrial fibrillation, both of which need immediate medical care.

INTERACTIONS

HERB

SCOPOLAMINE may have the following herb interactions:

- *Fu Ling* (Poria) (D)—in combination with *Ren Shen, Yuan Zhi*, and *Shi Chang Pu* was shown to decrease impairment of memory registration due to scopalamine in mice (Nishiyama, Zhou, Takashina & Saito, 1994) Level 5 evidence.
- *Dang Gui* (D)—was found to relieve amnesia in rats caused by scopalamine and cycloheximide (Hsieh, Lin, Lin & Wu, 2000) Level 5 evidence.
- *Ren Shen* (Ginseng) (D)—in combination with *Fu Ling, Yuan Zhi*, and *Shi Chang Pu* was shown to decrease impairment of memory registration due to scopalamine in mice (Nishiyama, Zhou, Takashina & Saito, 1994) Level 5 evidence.
- *Shi Chang Pu* (Acorus) (D)—in combination with *Ren Shen, Yuan Zhi*, and *Fu Ling* was shown to decrease impairment of memory registration due to scopalamine in mice (Nishiyama, Zhou, Takashina, Saito, 1994) Level 5 evidence.
- *Yuan Zhi* (Polygala) (D)—in combination with *Ren Shen, Fu Ling*, and *Shi Chang Pu* was shown to decrease impairment of memory

registration due to scopolamine in mice (Nishiyama, Zhou, Takashina & Saito, 1994) Level 5 evidence.

INTERACTION ISSUES

A: Anticholinergic effects may decrease GI motility and therefore increase absorption.
D: Darifenacin is 98% protein bound; tolterodine is greater than 96% protein bound
M: Darifenacin is a major substrate of CYP3A4

and a moderate inhibitor of CYP2D6. Fesoterodine and solifenacin are a major substrate of CYP3A4; tolterodine is a major substrate of both CYP2D6 and CYP3A4.
E: Anticholinergic effects may decrease GI motility and therefore affect elimination of drugs or herbs that excrete from the intestines.
TI:

SECTION 4: DIRECT-ACTING ADRENERGIC AGONISTS

β_2-SELECTIVE ADRENERGIC AGONISTS:

ALBUTEROL (al BYOO ter ole) PR=C
(AccuNeb®, Combivent®[50], DuoNeb®[50], ProAir®HFA, Proventil® HFA, Ventolin®HFA, VoSpire ER®)

FORMOTEROL (for MOH te rol) PR=C
(Foradil®, Aerolizer®, Dulera®[9], Percoromist®, Symbacort®[67])

INDACATEROL (in da KA ter ol) PR=C

LEVALBUTEROL (leve al BYOO ter ol) PR=C
(Xopenex®, Xopenex HFA™)

METAPROTERENOL (met a proe TER e nol) PR=C

PIRBUTEROL (peer BYOO ter ole) PR=C
(Maxair®, Autohaler®)

SALMETEROL (sal ME te role) PR=C *(Advair Diskus®,[8] Serevent® Diskus®)*

TERBUTALINE (ter BYOO ta leen) PR=B

VILANTEROL (VYE lan ter ol) PR=C *(Breo® Ellipta®[5])*

α_1-SELECTIVE ADRENERGIC AGONISTS:

MIDODRINE (MI doe dreen) PR=C

NAPHAZOLINE (naf AZ oh lene) *(Privine®)*

OXYMETAZOLINE (oks ee mee TAZ oh leen) PR=N

(12 Hour Nasal Relief [O], 4-Way® 12 Hour [O], Afrin® Extra Moisturizing [O], Afrin® Original [O], Afrin® Severe Congestion [O], Afrin® Sinus [O], Dristan® [O], Duramist Plus [O], Neo-

Synephrine® Nighttime12-Hour [O], Nostrilla® [O], NRS® [O], Vicks®, Sinex® VapoSpray 12-Hour [O], Vicks® Sinex® VapoSpray 12-Hour UltraFine Mist [O], Vicks® Sinex® VapoSpray Moisturizing 12-Hour UltraFine Mist [O])

PHENYLEPHRINE (fen il EF rin) PR=C *(4-Way®, 4-Way® Fast Acting [O], 4-Way® Menthol [O], AK-Dilate®, Aldex®CT, Aldex®DM, Alka-Seltzer Plus® Day Cold [O], AllanVan-DM,[12] Altafrin, Ambi 10PEH/400GFN [O],[10] Anu-Med [O], Benadryl® Maximum Strength Severe Allergy and Sinus Headache [O],[53] Benadryl® Allergy and Cold [O],[53] Benadryl® Allergy and Sinus Headache [O],[53] Benadryl-D® Allergy & Sinus [O],[55] Benadryl-D® Children's Allergy & Sinus [O],[55] BPM PE,[54] Bromfed®,[54] Bromfed®-PD,[54] C-Tan D,[54] C-Tan D Plus,[54] Carbaphen 12®,[15] Cetafen Cold® [O],[13] Codal-DM[12] [O], Cold Control PE [O],[53] Coldcough PD,[14] Comtrex® Maximum Strength, Non-Drowsy Cold & Cough [O],[56] Contac® Cold + Flu Maximum Strength Non-Drowsy [O],[13] Corfen DM,[16] Dallergy-JR®,[11] DiHydro-PE [O],[14] Dimaphen Cold & Allergy [O],[54] Dimetapp® Children's Cold & Allergy [O],[54] Dimetapp® Children's Nighttime Cold & Congestion [O],[55] Ed-A-Hist™ [O],[11] Ed ChlorPed D [O],[11] EndaCof [O],[16] Excedrin® Sinus Headache [O],[13] Father John's® Plus [O],[16] Fenesin PE IR,[10] FormulationR™ [O], J-Max [O],[10] Liquibid® D-R [O],[10] Liquibid® PD-R [O],[10] Little Noses®, Little Noses® Decongestant [O], LoHist [O],[11] LoHist Peb [O],[54] Mapap® Multi-Symptom Cold [O],[56] Mapap® Sinus PE [O],[13] Maxichlor*

...continued on the following page

PEH [O],[11] Maxiphen DM,[58] Maxiphen DMX,[58] Medent®-PEI [O],[10] Medicone®, Medicone® Suppositories [O], MediPhenyl®, Medi-First®, Medi-First® Sinus Decongestant [O], Medi-Phenyl [O], Mucinex® Children's Multi-Symptom Cold [O],[58] Mucinex® Cold [O],[10] Mucus Relief Sinus [O],[10] Murocoll-2®, Mydfrin®, MyHist-DM, Nalex®-A,[17] Nasohist™ [O],[11] Neo DM,[16] Neofrin®, Neo-Synephrine®[Mild, Regular, and Extra-Strength], NoHist [O],[11] NoHist DM [O],[16] NoHist LQ [O],[11] Norel® SR,[52] Novahistine DH,[14] Nu-COPD [O],[10] One Tab™ Allergy & Sinus [O],[53] One Tab™ Cold & Flu [O],53 OneTab™ Congestion & Cold [O],[10] PE-Hist-DM [O],[16] PediaCare®, PediaCare® Children's Decongestant [O], PediaCare® Children's Multi-Symptom Cold [O],[57] PE-Poly-Hist DM,[12] Preparation H® [O], Promethazine VC,[59] Rectacaine® [O], Refenesen™ PE [O],[10] Rescon GG [O],[10] Rhinall® [O], Rinal®, Robafen CF Cough & Cold [O],[58] Robitussin® Children's Cough & Cold CF [O],[58] Robitussin® Peak Cold Maximum Strength Multi-Symptom Cold [O],[58] Robitussin® Peak Cold Multi-Symptom Cold [O],[58] Robitussin® Peak Cold Nasal Relief [O],[13] Robitussin® Peak Cold Nighttime Multi-Symptom Cold [O],[53] Ru-Hist-D,[23] Safetussin® CD [O],[57] Sinex®, Sudafed PE®, Sudafed PE® Children's [O], Sudafed PE® Children's Cold & Cough [O],[57] Sudafed PE® Congestion [O], Sudafed PE™ Nasal Decongestant [O], Sudafed PE® Nighttime Cold [O],[53] Sudafed PE® Non-Drying Sinus [O],[10] Sudafed PE® Pressure + Pain [O],[13] Sudafed PE® Severe Cold [O],[53] Sudafed PE® Sinus + Allergy [O],[11] Sudagest™ PE, Theraflu® Daytime Severe Cold & Cough [O],[56] Theraflu® Nighttime Severe Cold & Cough [O],[53] Theraflu® Sugar-Free Nighttime Severe Cold & Cough [O],[53] Theraflu Warming Relief® Daytime Multi-Symptom Cold [O],[56] Theraflu Warming Relief® Daytime Severe Cold & Cough [O],[56] Theraflu® Warming Relief™ Flu & Sore Throat [O],[53] Theraflu® Warming Relief™ Nighttime Severe Cold & Cough [O],[53] Triaminic® Children's Chest & Nasal Congestion [O],[10] Triaminic® Children's Cold & Allergy [O],[11] Triaminic® Children's Night Time Cold & Cough [O],[55] Triaminic® Children's Thin Strips® Night Time Cold & Cough [O],[55] Triaminic® Day Time Cold & Cough [O],[57] Triaminic Thin Strips® Children's Cold with Stuffy Nose [O], Triaminic Thin Strips®, Triaminic Thin Strips® Children's Day Time Cold & Cough [O],[57] Tronolare®, Tronolane® Suppository [O], Tusscough DHC™,[14] Tylenol® Allergy Multi-Symptom Nighttime [O],[53] Tylenol® Children's Plus Cold and Allergy Sinus Pain & Pressure[O],[13] Tylenol® Cold Head Congestion Daytime [O],[56] Tylenol® Cold Multi-Symptom Daytime [O],[56] Tylenol® Sinus Congestion & Pain Daytime [O],[13] VapoSpray™, Vicks®, Vicks® DayQuil® Cold & Flu Multi-Symptom [O],[56] Vicks® DayQuil® Sinex® Daytime Sinus [O],[13] Vicks® Nature Fusion™ Cold & Flu Multi-Symptom Relief [O],[56] Vicks® VapoSpray™ 4-Hour Decongestant [O], Virdec [O][11])

PROPYLHEXEDRINE (proe pil HEKS e drene) PR=C *(Benzedrex® [O])*

TETRAHYDROZOLINE (tet ra hie DROZ a lene) PR=C *(Tyzine®; Tyzine® Pediatric)*

α₂-SELECTIVE ADRENERGIC AGONISTS:

CLONIDINE (KLON i deen) PR=C *(Catapres-TTS®-1, Catapres-TTS®-2, Catapres-TTS®-3, Catapres®, Clorpres®,[60] Duraclon®, Kapvay™, Nexiclon™ XR)*

GUANABENZ (GWAHN a benz) PR=C

GUANFACINE (GWAHN fa seen) PR=B *(Intuniv™, Tenex®)*

METHYLDOPA (meth il DOE pa) PR=B

TIZANIDINE (tye ZAN i deen) PR=C *(Zanaflex®)*

Many of these agents are used to treat asthma and are inhaled for maximum effect.

Adrenergic neurons are similar in function to cholinergic neurons in that they both have mechanisms of releasing a neurotransmitter, breaking down that neurochemical in the synaptic cleft, and reabsorbing and recycling the chemicals. This process is shown in Figure 4.5 on page 50. In the synaptic cleft, it is catecholo-methyltransferase (COMT) that breaks down norepinephrine. In addition, monoamine oxidase (MAO) also helps metabolize norepinephrine and other **catecholamines.**

There are 2 major families of adrenergic receptors: α (alpha) and β (beta). Each family has subtypes. α_1 receptors are located on the postsynaptic membrane of effector organs and generally cause constriction of smooth muscle. α_2 receptors are located on the presynaptic membrane of adrenergic neurons and on specific pancreas cells. When norepinephrine is released into the synaptic cleft, some diffuses across the cleft and activates postsynaptic receptors. Some, however, activates receptors on the presynaptic membrane. These α_2 receptors cause **feedback inhibition** and **down regulate** the release of further norepinephrine from the presynaptic neuron. In other words, α_1 receptors cause many of the classic functions of the sympathetic system, while α_2 receptors lower or prevent such functions.

β receptors also come in two major types. Rather than being separated by whether the receptor is on the post- or presynaptic membrane, β receptors are separated by their affinity for norepinephrine versus epinephrine. β_1 receptors have an equal affinity for norepinephrine and epinephrine while β_2 receptors have a much higher affinity for epinephrine. Norepinephrine is a neurotransmitter released into the synaptic cleft between neurons and effector organs, while epinephrine is a hormone that is circulated in the blood stream to cause more global effects. See a summary of the effects of adrenoceptors in Figure 4.6, page 51.

FUNCTION

β_2-selective adrenergic agonists are primarily used in the treatment of asthma and COPD because they cause **bronchodilation.** While some are available for oral use, most are inhaled.

α_1-selective adrenergic agonists are used primarily in the treatment of hypotension or as a nasal decongestant. Phenylephrine can be used topically or as suppositories in the treatment of hemorrhoids.

α_2-selective adrenergic agonists are used primarily in the treatment of systemic hypertension.

Tizanidine is primarily used as a muscle relaxant to treat skeletal muscle spasms.

MECHANISM OF ACTION

Each of these agents works by binding with adrenergic membrane receptors and initiating physiological actions. Most of the β_2-selective adrenergic agonists work on pulmonary receptors because the agent is inhaled.

α_1-selective adrenergic agonists primarily activate receptors in vascular smooth muscle causing contraction and an increase in peripheral vascular resistance, a primary affector of blood pressure, which is discussed more in depth in Chapter 6.

α_2-selective adrenergic agonists act somewhat paradoxically. Theoretically, activation of these receptors would cause **vasoconstriction** and an increase in hypertension. However, in vivo, these agents primarily work on the cardiovascular control centers in the CNS causing a systemic decrease in sympathetic activity from the brain due to physiological feedback inhibition. This causes a generalized lowering of blood pressure. Localized vasoconstriction explains using these agents as a nasal decongestant.

DOSAGES

ALBUTEROL, for *children*, 2-6 years, 0.1-0.2 mg/kg/dose tid up to a maximum of 12 mg/d; 6-12 years, 2 mg/dose 3-4 times/d up to a maximum 24 mg/d; for extended release, 4 mg every 12 hours up to a maximum 24 mg/d, for metered-dose inhaler (90 mcg/puff), 4 years or over, 2 puffs every 4-6 hours prn; 5-11 years, 2 puffs every 4-6 hours prn; in severe exacerbations of asthma in children under 12, 4-8 puffs every 20 minutes for 3 doses, then every 1-4 hours prn; as prevention of exercise-induced bronchospasm in children 4 years or under, 1-2 puffs 5 minutes prior to exercise; over 4 years, 2 puffs 5-30 minutes prior to exercise. For *children* over 12 years and *adults*, 2-4 mg/dose 3-4

Catecholamines: Sympathomimetic neurotransmitter family that includes epinephrine, norepinephrine, and dopamine

Feedback inhibition: Where an intermediate or final product of a biological pathway stops or slows down one of the initiating steps and eventually reduces the end results of that pathway

Down regulation: The inhibition of a particular biological function

Bronchodilation: A widening of the lumen of the bronchi, allowing increased airflow to and from the lungs

Vasoconstriction: A decrease in the diameter of a blood vessel

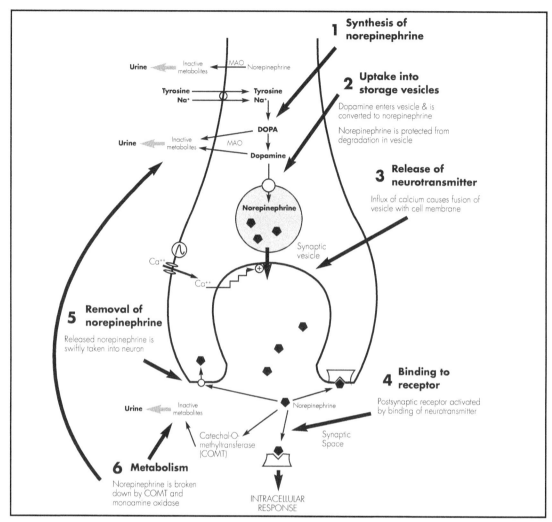

Figure 4.5: The life cycle of norepinephrine in an adrenergic synapse. 1: Dopamine is produced in the neural cell body and transported to the synaptic terminal or is locally produced from local metabolites. **2:** The dopamine is stored in synaptic vesicles where it is metabolized to norepinephrine. **3:** Norepinephrine is released into the synaptic cleft when stimulated by calcium influx due to an action potential. **4:** Norepinephrine binds to a postsynaptic membrane receptor. **5:** Norepinephrine is reuptaken into the synaptic terminal. **6:** Norepinephrine can also be broken down by catechol-o-methyltransferase (COMT) or monoamine oxidase (MAO).

times/d up to a maximum 32 mg/d; extended release, 8 mg every 12 hours up to a maximum of 32 mg/d; metered-dose inhaler, 2 puffs every 4-6 hours prn; in severe exacerbations of asthma, 4-8 puffs every 20 minutes for up to 4 hours, then every 1-4 hours prn; as prevention of exercise-induced bronchospasm, 2 puffs 5-30 minutes prior to exercise. For the *elderly*, 2 mg 3-4 times/d, up to a maximum 8 mg qid.

CLONIDINE, for *children*, for ADHD, extended release, 6 or older initiate at 0.1 mg nocte, increase .1 mg/d every week until desired result, should be dosed bid up to a maximum of 0.4 mg/d. For *adults*, for hypertension, initiate at .1 mg bid increase to effective dose usually .1-.8 mg/d up to a maximum recommended 2.4 mg/d. For extended release, initiate at .17 mg at bedtime and increase .09mg/d every week to a usual dose range of .17-.52 mg/d up to a maximum of .52 mg/d. For transdermal initiate at .1 mg/d applied every week and increase .1 mg/d every 1-2 weeks to a usual dose range of .1-.3 mg/d. For the *elderly*, .1 mg nocte and gradually increase as necessary.

FORMOTEROL, Foradil®: for asthma or COPD maintenance, 12 mcg capsule inhaled every 12 hours up to 24 mcg/d, for exercise-induced bronchospasm, 12 mcg capsule at least 15 minutes before exercise prn; Performist®: COPD maintenance, 20 mcg bid up to a maximum of 40 mcg/d.

GUANABENZ, for *adults*, initiate at 4 mg bid, increase 4-8 mg/d every 1-2 weeks up to a maximum of 32 mg bid. For *elderly*, initiate at 4 mg once daily; increase every 1-2 weeks.

GUANFACINE, for *adults* or *children* over 12, for hypertension, 1 mg usually at bedtime, may increase at 3-to-4-week intervals up to a usual dose of 0.5-2 mg once daily. For *children* 6 or over and *adolescents*, for ADHD, initiate at 1 mg once daily; may add 1 mg per week as tolerated up to a maximum dose of 4 mg/d.

INDACATEROL, for *adults*, one inhalation of 75 mcg once daily.

LEVALBUTEROL, for *children* 4 and older, using a metered-dose inhaler, for bronchospasm, 2 puffs every 4-6 hours prn, for exacerbation of asthma, 4-8 puffs every 20 minutes for 3 doses, then every 1-4 hours prn. For *adults*, using a metered-dose inhaler, for bronchospasm, 2 puffs every 4-6 hours, for exacerbation of asth-

ma, 4-8 puffs every 20 minutes for up to 4 hrs, then every 1-4 hours prn.

METAPROTERENOL, for *children* under 6, 1.3-2.6 mg/kg/d divided every 6-8 hours; for children 6-9 (or under 27 kg), 10 mg/dose 3-4 times/d; for *children* over 9 (or above 27 kg) and *adults*, 20 mg 3-4 times/d.

METHYLDOPA, for *children*, initiate at 10 mg/kg/d in 2-4 doses, increase every 2 days prn up to a maximum of 65 mg/kg/d not to exceed 3 g/d. For *adults*, initiate at 250 mg 2-3 times may increase every 2 days prn up to a maximum of 3 g/d, with a usual dose range of 250-1000 mg/d in 2 doses.

MIDODRINE, for *adults*, 10 mg tid during daytime hours (every 3-4 hours) when patient is upright, up to a maximum of 40 mg/d.

NAPHAZOLINE, for *adults*, intranasal: 1-2 drops or sprays every 6 hours prn; should not use for more than 3 days.

OXYMETAZOLINE, for nasal congestion, for *adults* and *children* 6 or older, 2-3 sprays into each nostril bid for no more than 3 days.

PHENYLEPHRINE, for *children* 4-6, 2.5 mg every 4 hours prn for no longer than 7 days (maximum dose of 15 mg/d), intranasal: 1 drop (.125% solution) in each nostril every 2-4 hrs

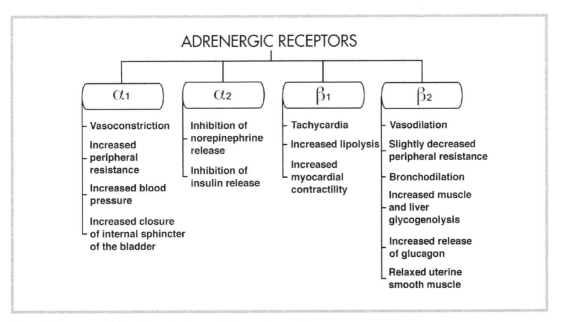

Figure 4.6: Summary of the different subtypes of adrenergic receptors.

prn for a maximum of 3 days; for children 6-12, 5 mg every 4 hours prn for no longer than 7 days (maximum dose of 30 mg/d), intranasal: 2-3 sprays (.25% solution) in each nostril every 4 hrs prn for a maximum of 3 days; for *children* over 12, intranasal: 2-3 sprays or 2-3 drops (.25% to .5% solution) in each nostril every 4 hrs prn for a maximum of 3 days; for *adults* and children over 12, 10 mg every 4 hours prn for no longer than 7 days (maximum dose of 60 mg/d); for hemorrhoids, apply ointment or 1 suppository up to 4 times per day; for *adults*, intranasal: 2-3 sprays or 2-3 drops (.25% to 1% solution) in each nostril every 4 hrs prn for a maximum of 3 days.

PIRBUTEROL, for *children* 12 and older and adults, for prevention, 2 inhalations every 4-6 hours, for treating bronchospasm, 2 inhalations with 1-3 minutes in between, followed by a third inhalation, not to exceed 12 inhalations per day.

PROPYLHEXEDRINE, for nasal congestion, for *adults* and *children* 6 or older, 2 inhalations with a minimum of two hours in between each application.

SALMETEROL, for *children* 4 and over and *adults*, for asthma or COPD maintenance and prevention, 1 inhalation bid, for exercise-induced asthma prevention, 1 inhalation prior to exercise.

TERBUTALINE, for *children* under 12, oral, initiate at .05 mg/kg/dose tid, can increase to a maximum of .15 mg/kg/dose 3-4 times per day or 5 mg per day, subQ, .005-.01 mg/kg/dose up to a maximum of .4 mg/dose every 15-20 minutes for 3 doses; may repeat every 2-6 hours prn; for *children* 12-15, oral, 2.5 mg every 6 hrs tid up to a maximum of 7.5 mg per day; for children over 15, 5 mg every 6 hrs tid up to a maximum of 15 mg/d. For *adults*, for asthma or bronchoconstriction, oral, 5 mg every 6 hrs tid up to a maximum of 15 mg per day, for adults and children 12 and over, SubQ, .25 mg may repeat every 15-30 mins up to a maximum of .5 mg per 4-hour period.

TETRAHYDROZOLINE, for nasal congestion, for *children* 2-6, 2-3 drops .05% solution in each nostril every 4-6 hrs prn, should not be used more than every 3 hours; for *adults* and *children* 6 or older, 2-4 drops or 3-4 sprays of .1% solution in each nostril, should not be used more frequently than every 3 hours.

TIZANIDINE, for *adults*, 2-4 mg tid, usual initial dose is 4 mg; may increase 2-4 mg prn every 6-8 hours to maximum three doses in any 24-hour period and maximum 36 mg/d.

VILANTEROL, this drug is used only in combination with other drugs and therefore its individual dosing is not covered here.

ADVERSE EFFECTS

Common side effects of most of these agents include: cardiac arrhythmias, hyperactivity, headache, insomnia, nausea, tachycardia, and tremors. In some diabetic patients, β_2 agonists may cause **hyperglycemia**.

α_2-selective adrenergic agonists have different adverse effects including dry mouth and sedation in at least 50% of patients. Other effects include sexual dysfunction, **bradycardia**, and contact dermatitis with the use of patches for drug delivery. Withdrawal reactions may occur after abrupt discontinuation of clonidine in some hypertensive patients.

RED FLAGS

β_2 agonists may initiate significant arrhythmias and cardiac **infarction** in susceptible patients.

The FDA has issued a warning regarding the use of long-acting β_2 agonists (LABA), including salmeterol and formoterol. Recent studies have shown that there has been more asthma-related deaths in patients who use regular asthma treatments when combined with LABAs than with regular treatment alone. The warning emphasizes that LABAs should not be used for the acute treatment of asthma attacks.

INTERACTIONS

HERB

α₁-SELECTIVE ADRENERGIC AGONISTS

• *Gan Cao* (Licorice) (D)–theoretically may reduce the effects of antihypertensive agents such as alpha-1 adrenergic blockers, ACEI, α_2 receptor antagonists, beta-adrenergic blockers, calcium channel blockers, clonidine, guanabenz, guanadrel, guanethidine, guanfacine, hydralazine, methyldopa, minoxidil, and reserpine, and concurrent use should be undertaken with caution (Kowalak & Mills, 2001) Level 5 evidence.

CLONIDINE

- *Gan Cao* (Licorice) (D)–theoretically may reduce the effects of antihypertensive agents such as alpha-1 adrenergic blockers, ACEI, α_2 receptor antagonists, beta-adrenergic blockers, calcium channel blockers, clonidine, guanabenz, guanadrel, guanethidine, guanfacine, hydralazine, methyldopa, minoxidil, and reserpine, and concurrent use should be undertaken with caution (Kowalak & Mills, 2001) Level 5 evidence.
- *Ma Huang* (Ephedra) (B-)–based on ephedrine content, clonidine may potentiate the pressor effects of ephedrine in a human study of IV ephedrine (Nishikawa, Kimura, Taguchi & Dohi, 1991) Level 2b evidence.

MIDODRINE

- *Ma Huang* (Ephedrine) (D)–based on ephedrine content, may potentiate midodrine's pressor effects, expert opinion (Gruenwald, Brendler & Jaenicke, 2004) Level 5 evidence.

PHENYLEPHRINE

- *San Qi* (Notoginseng) (D)–may interact with phenylephrine-induced contraction as mentioned in an in vitro review article (Kwan, 1995) Level 5 evidence.
- *Xi Yang Shen* (American ginseng) (D)–was shown to enhance the vasoconstrictive effects of phenylephrine in an in vitro review article (Kwan, 1995) Level 5 evidence.

SYMPATHOMIMETIC DRUGS

- *Chen Pi* (Tangerine peel) (Indeterminate)–contains constituents that stimulate the sympathetic nervous system and should be used with caution in those taking antihypertensive, antidiabetic, antihyperthyroid, and/or antiseizure medications (Chinese language article cited in Chen & Chen, 2004).
- *Ma Huang* (Ephedra) (D)–ephedrine content,

may increase sympathomimetic activity of sympathomimetic drugs such as furazolidone and procarbazine, expert opinion (Gruenwald, Brendler & Jaenicke, 2004) Level 5 evidence.
- *Ma Huang* (Ephedra) (D)–may potentiate sympathomimetic drugs and induce hypertension, expert opinon (Mills & Bone, 2000) Level 5 evidence.
- *Qing Pi* (Citrus Viride) (Indeterminate)–contains constituents that stimulate the sympathetic nervous system and should be used with caution in those taking antihypertensive, antidiabetic, antihyperthyroid, and/or antiseizure medications (Chinese language article cited in Chen & Chen, 2004).
- *Rou Cong Rong* (Cistanche) (Indeterminate)–may interact with sympathomimetics, monoamine oxidase inhibitors, selective serotonin inhibitors, and tricyclic antidepressants by increasing the activities of neurotransmitters such as norepinephrine, dopamine, and serotonin (Chinese language article cited in Chen & Chen, 2004).
- *Zhi Ke* (Aurantium fruit, bitter orange) (Indeterminate)–contains constituents that stimulate the sympathetic nervous system and should be used with caution in those taking antihypertensive, antidiabetic, antihyperthyroid, and/or antiseizure medications (Chinese language article cited in Chen & Chen, 2004) Indeterminate level of evidence.
- *Zhi Shi* (Aurantium immaturus) (Indeterminate)–contains constituents that stimulate the sympathetic nervous system and should be used with caution in those taking antihypertensive, antidiabetic, antihyperthyroid, and/or antiseizure medications (Chinese language article cited in Chen & Chen, 2004).

Hyperglycemia: Too much glucose in the blood

Bradycardia: A heart rate that is too slow, defined as less than 60 bpm

Infarction: A sudden stoppage of blood flow that causes tissue death

▪ INTERACTION ISSUES

A:

D: Indacaterol is approximately 95% protein bound, salmeterol 96%

M: Salmeterol and guanfacine are major substrates of CYP3A4; tizanidine is a major substrate of CYP1A2

E:

TI:

Pgp: Indacaterol interacts with Pgp.

SECTION 5: MIXED–ACTION ADRENERGIC AGONISTS

EPHEDRINE (e FED rin) PR=C

EPINEPHRINE (ep i NEF rin) PR=C *(EpiPen 2-Pak®, EpiPen Jr 2-Pak®, Twinject®)*

PSEUDOEPHEDRINE (soo doe e FED rin) PR=C *(Advil® Allergy Sinus,[33] Advil® Cold & Sinus [O],[63] Advil® Multi-Symptom Cold,[33] Alavert™ Allergy and Sinus [O],[24] Aleve®-D Sinus & Cold [O],[20] Aleve®-D Sinus & Headache [O],[20] Allegra-D® 12 Hour,[43] Allegra-D® 24 Hour,[43] Allerfrim [O],[19] Ambifed DM,[42] Ambifed-G [O],[32] Ambifed-G DM,[42] Anaplex® DM,[31] Aprodine [O],[19] Bromaline® DM [O],[31] Bromdex D,[31] Bromfed® DM,[31] Bromphe-nex™ DM [O],[31] Brotapp [O],[65] Brotapp-DM,[31] Cheratussin® DAC,[35] Children's Nasal Decongestant [O], Clarinex-D® 12 Hour,[47] Clarinex-D® 24-Hour,[47] Claritin-D® 12 Hour Allergy & Congestion [O],[24] Claritin-D® 24-Hour Allergy & Congestion [O],[24] CoActifed®,[18] Codar® D,[30] Congestac® [O],[32] Contac® Cold + Flu Maximum Strength Non-Drowsy [O], Covan®,[18] Dicel® Chewable [O],[37] Dicel®DM Chewables [O],[38] DiHydro-CP,[40] EndaCof-DC,[30] ExeFen-DMX,[42] ExeFen-IR,[32] J-Tan D-PD [O],[65] Kidkare Children's Cough/Cold [O],[38] Lodrane® D [O],[65] LoHist-D [O],[37] LoHist PSB [O],[65] LoHist PSB DM [O],[31] Loratadine-D 12-Hour [O],[24] M-END DM [O],[38] Maxichlor PSE [O],[37] Maxichlor PSE DM [O],[38] Maxifed [O],[32] Maxifed DM,[42] Maxifed DMX,[42] Maxifed-G [O],[32] Mucinex® D Maximum Strength [O],[32] Mucinex® D [O],[32] Mytussin® DAC,[35] Neo DM,[31] Neutrahist PDX [O],[38] Neutrahist Pediatric [O],[37] Notuss®-DC,[30] Oranyl [O], Ornex® [O],[64] Ornex® Maximum Strength [O],[64] Pedia Relief™ Cough-Cold [O],[38] Pedia Relief Cough and Cold [O],[62] PediaHist DM,[31] Pediatex® TD,[19] Pediatric Cough & Cold [O],[38] Phenylhistine DH [O],[39] Proprinal® Cold and Sinus [O],[63] Q-Tapp [O],[65] RAtio-Cotridin,[18] Refenesen Plus [O],[32] Rescon DM [O],[38] Resperal-DM,[31] Rezira™,[41] Semprex®-D[44] Silafed [O],[19] Silfedrine Children's [O], Sudafed® 12-Hour [O], Sudafed® 12-Hour Pressure + Pain [O],[20] Sudafed® 24-Hour [O], Sudafed® Children's [O], Sudafed® Children's Cold & Cough [O],[62] Sudafed® Maximum Strength Nasal Decongestant [O], SudaTex-G [O],[32] Sudo-Tab® [O], SudoGest [O], SudoGest 12-Hour [O], SudoGest Children's [O], SudoGest™ Sinus & Allergy [O],[37] Tricode® AR,[39] Tricode® GF,[35] Tripohist™ D,[19] Zutripro™,[36] ZyrTEC-D® Allergy & Congestion [O][66])*

■ FUNCTION

Ephedrine can be used as a **bronchodilator** in asthmatic patients, though less and less for this purpose with the advent of β_2-selective adrenergic agonists. It was used in the past for treating complete heart block, narcolepsy, and depressive states, but other agents have supplanted it. It is used for urinary incontinence though evidence of effectiveness is unclear. It may also be used to treat hypotension due to spinal anesthesia.

Epinephrine is used as an inhaled agent in the treatment of asthma, commonly acute, and other conditions of bronchospasms. It is also available over the counter as an inhaled agent to treat nasal congestion. In IV, IM, or subcutaneous injection form, it is used in the acute treatment of hypersensitivity reactions.

Pseudoephedrine is used in a wide variety of over-the-counter and prescription mixtures as a nasal decongestant.

MECHANISM OF ACTION

These agents are called mixed-action because they have several effects. Primarily they have both direct and indirect agonist effect in that they promote the release of norepinephrine from the presynaptic neuron as well as direct effects on the postsynaptic membrane receptors. Both α and β receptors are stimulated (see Section 4 above).

DOSAGES

EPHEDRINE is only used in an oral or injectable form for unlabeled uses. It is still used intravenously for certain conditions such as hypotension.

EPINEPHRINE, for *infants* and *children*, as a bronchodilator, subcutaneous: .01 mg/kg up to a maximum dose of .5 mg every 20 min for 3 doses; for *children* under 4, nebulized: .05 ml/kg up to a maximum dose of 3 ml over 15 minutes; for *children* 4 or older, look at adult dosing; for hypersensitivity reactions, subcutaneous or IM (preferred) .01 mg/kg up to a maximum dose of .3 mg every 5-15 mins, for self-administration: subcutaneous in *children* 15-29 kg, .15 mg may be repeated in 5-15 mins; for *children* 30 kg or over, .3 mg may be repeated in 5-15 mins, IM: for *children* 10-25 kg, .15 mg, for *children* 25 kg or over, .3 mg. For *children* 6 or over and *adults*, as a decongestant, intranasal: 1 mg/ml locally. For *adults*, as a bronchodilator, subcutaneous: .3-.5 mg every 20 mins for 3 doses, nebulized: .5 ml, for hypersensitivity reactions, IM (preferred) or subcutaneous: .2-.5 mg every 5-15 mins, self-administration: .3 mg, may repeat in 5-15 mins.

PSEUDOEPHEDRINE, for *children* 4-5, 15 mg every 4-6 hrs up to maximum 60 mg/d; for *children* 6-12, 30 mg every 4-6 hrs up to a maximum 120 mg/day; for *children* over 12 and *adults*, immediate release: 60 mg every 4-6 hrs; extended release: 120 mg every 12 hrs or 240 mg/d up to a maximum 240 mg/d. For the *elderly*, use cautiously, 30-60 mg every 6 hrs prn.

ADVERSE EFFECTS

Common side effects of ephedrine include insomnia and potentially hypertension. Headache, insomnia, nausea, and dry mouth are common side effects of pseudoephedrine.

RED FLAGS

Tachyphylaxis may occur with chronic use. Cardiovascular patients should always use sympathomimetic agents with caution.

INTERACTIONS

These agents should be used with caution in patients with cardiovascular disease, hypertension, or hyperthyroidism.

DRUG

Sympathomimetic amines, such as ephedrine and pseudoephedrine, may reduce the antihypertensive effects of reserpine, veratrum alkaloids, methyldopa and mecamylamine. Effects of these agents may be increased with MAOI and adrenergic blockers.

HERB

EPHEDRINE

- *Lu Cha* (Green tea) (D)–based on ephedrine content, may increase adrenergic stimulation of caffeine as present in *lu cha*, expert opinion (Gruenwald, Brendler & Jaenicke, 2004) Level 5 evidence.
- *Lu Cha* (Green tea) (A)–may increase thermogenesis and weight loss when combined with methylxanthines such as caffeine, as in *lu cha* in both mice (Dulloo & Miller, 1986a) Level 5 evidence; and human studies (Dulloo & Miller, 1986b) Level 2b evidence; (Malchow-Moller, Larsen, Hey, Stokholm, Juhl & Quaade, 1981) Level 2b evidence; (Boozer, Daly, Homel, Solomon, Blanchard, Nasser *et al.*, 2002) Level 1b evidence, (Greenway, de Jonge, Blanchard, Frisard & Smith, 2004) Level 2b

---

Bronchodilation: Relaxation and an increase in the diameter of the lung's bronchi allowing more airflow

---

Tachyphylaxis: When repeated drug use results in a smaller effect

---

Sympathomimetic: Either mimicking or stimulating the sympathetic nervous system

---

Amines: Any molecule that includes the element nitrogen

evidence;(Astrup, Breum, Toubro, Hein & Quaade, 1992) Level 1b evidence.

- *Ma Huang* (Ephedra) (D)–based on ephedrine content; may potentiate the sympathomimetic effects of ephedrine and pseudoephedrine, expert opinion (Gruenwald, Brendler & Jaenicke, 2004) Level 5 evidence.

PSEUDOEPHEDRINE

- *Ma Huang* (Ephedra) (D)–based on ephedrine content; may potentiate the sympathomimetic effects of ephedrine and pseudoephedrine, expert opinion (Gruenwald, Brendler & Jaenicke, 2004) Level 5 evidence.

SYMPATHOMIMETIC DRUGS

- *Chen Pi* (Tangerine peel), *Qing Pi* (Citrus Viride), *Zhi Ke* (Aurantium fruit, bitter orange), *Zhi Shi* (Aurantium immaturus) (Indeterminate)–contains constituents that stimulate the sympathetic nervous system and should be used with caution in those taking antihypertensives, antidiabetic, antihyperthyroid, and antiseizure medications (Chinese language article cited in Chen & Chen, 2004) Indeterminate level of evidence.

- *Ma Huang* (Ephedra) (D)–based on ephedrine content; may increase sympathomimietic activity of sympathomimietic drugs such as furazolidone and procarbazine, expert opinion (Gruenwald, Brendler & Jaenicke, 2004) Level 5 evidence.

- *Ma Huang* (Ephedra) (D)–may potentiate sympathomimetic drugs and induce hypertension, expert opinon (Mills & Bone, 2000) Level 5 evidence.

- *Rou Cong Rong* (Cistanche) (Indeterminate)–may interact with sympathomimetics, monoamine oxidase inhibitors, selective serotonin inhibitors, and tricyclic antidepressants by increasing the activities of neurotransmitters such as norepinephrine, dopamine, and serotonin (Chinese language article cited in Chen & Chen, 2004) Indeterminate level of evidence.

SECTION 6: ALPHA-ADRENERGIC BLOCKING AGENTS

ALFUZOSIN (al FYOO zoe sin) PR=B (*Uroxatral®*)

DOXAZOSIN (doks AY zoe sin) PR=C (*Cardura®, Cardura® XL*)

PHENOXYBENZAMINE (fen oks ee BEN za mene) PR=C (*Dibenzyline®*)

PHENTOLAMINE (fen TOLE a mene) PR=C (*OraVerse™*)

PRAZOSIN (PRA zoe sin) PR=C (*Minipress®*)

SILODOSIN (SI lo doe sin) PR=B (*Rapaflo®*)

TAMSULOSIN (tam SOO loe sin) PR=B (*Flomax®, Jalyn®61}*)

TERAZOSIN (ter AY zoe sin) PR=C (*Hytrin®*)

TETRABENAZINE (tet ra BEN a zene) PR=C (*Xenazine®*)

▦ FUNCTION

These agents are primarily used to treat benign prostatic hyperplasia (BPH).

Phenoxybenzamine is used to treat intractable hypertension and excessive sweating. Currently its main use is in the treatment of pheochromocytoma. In the past, phenoxybenzamine has been used in the treatment of benign prostatic hyperplasia. However, newer agents are safer and more effective, supplanting this use.

Doxazosin, prazosin, tamsulosin, and terazosin are used in the treatment of hypertension, commonly in the treatment of benign prostatic hyperplasia, and occasionally, congestive heart failure.

Phentolamine is used in the diagnosis of and to treat hypertension from pheochromocytoma. In addition, it is used to treat necrosis due to extravasation of drugs that have alpha adrenergic effects. It also reverses soft tissue anesthesia from local dental anesthetic containing a vasoconstrictor.

Tetrabenazine is used in the treatment of **chorea** associated with Huntington's disease.

Chorea: An abnormal involuntary movement disorder usually like quick movements of the hands and feet that resemble dancing

MECHANISM OF ACTION

Alpha adrenergic receptors have many functions (see section 4 of this chapter) including vasoconstriction, increased peripheral vascular resistance, increased blood pressure, and increased closure of the bladder's internal sphincter. Alpha blockers prevent these effects by binding, either reversibly or irreversibly, to the postsynaptic membrane α receptors. Both α_1 and α_2 receptors are blocked to varying degrees by these agents, but most of the therapeutic effects are caused by α_1 inhibition. This receptor blockage prevents receptor activation by norepinephrine and other catecholamines. Phenoxybenzamine irreversibly binds to α receptors.

Reduction in hypertension is caused by reducing total peripheral resistance, one of the major constituents of blood pressure (see Chapter 6). It achieves this by causing peripheral vascular dilation.

Relief of BPH symptoms is accomplished by relaxing the smooth muscles of the neck of the bladder and prostate allowing less constricted flow of urine.

DOSAGES

ALFUZOSIN, for *adults*, 10 mg once daily.

DOXAZOSIN, for *adults*, immediate release: 1 mg once daily; for maximum benefit may increase to 2 mg once daily. For the *elderly*, initiate at 0.5 mg once daily. For hypertension, maximum dose is 16 mg/d; for BPH, usual dose range is 4-8 mg/d up to a maximum 8 mg/d. Extended release: for BPH, 4 mg once daily with breakfast; may increase based on response and tolerability every 3-4 weeks to a maximum recommended dose of 8 mg/d.

PHENOXYBENZAMINE, for *children*, initiate at .25-1 mg/kg/d up to a maximum of 10 mg. For *adults*, initiate at 10 mg bid; dosage should be increased by 10 mg every other day, usually to 20-40 mg 2 or 3 times a day.

PHENTOLAMINE, for *children*, for a diagnosis of pheochromocytoma, IM: 0.05-0.1 mg/kg/dose, up to a maximum 5 mg; for surgery for pheochromocytoma hypertension, IM: 0.05-0.1 mg/kg/dose given 1-2 hrs before procedure; repeat prn every 2-4 hrs, maximum of 5 mg; for reversal of soft tissue anesthesia, submucosal oral injection: for *children* 15-30 kg, 0.2 mg maximum; over 30 kg and under 12 years of age, 0.4 mg maximum. For *adults*, for pheochromocytoma, IM: 5 mg; for pheochromocytoma hypertension surgery, IM: 5 mg given 1-2 hrs before procedure and repeated prn every 2-4 hrs; for reversal of soft tissue anesthesia, submucosal oral injection: .2 mg if one-half cartridge of anesthesia was administered, .4 mg if 1 cartridge was administered, .8 mg if 2 cartridges were administered.

PRAZOSIN, for *adults*, for hypertension, initiate at 1 mg/dose 2-3 times/d, the usual maintenance dose is 1-10 mg/d bid up to a maximum daily dose of 20 mg.

SILODOSIN, for *adults*, for BPH, 8 mg once per day with a meal.

TAMSULOSIN, for *adults*, 0.4 mg once daily administered approximately 30 mins. following the same meal each day. For patients who fail to respond after 2–4 wks of dosing, the dose can be increased to 0.8 mg once daily.

TERAZOSIN, for *adults*, for hypertension, initiate at 1 mg nocte; slowly increase dose to achieve desired blood pressure, up to 20 mg/d; usual dose range is 1-20 mg once daily for benign prostatic hyperplasia; initiate at 1 mg nocte, increasing as needed; most patients require 10 mg/d; if no response after 4-6 weeks, may increase to 20 mg/d.

TETRABENAZINE, for *adults*, for Huntington's disease, initiate at 12.5 mg once daily; may increase to 12.5 mg bid after 1 wk; may be increased by 12.5 mg/d weekly. Use greater than 37.5 mg/d should be divided into 3 doses, up to a maximum single dose of 25 mg.

ADVERSE EFFECTS

Phenoxybenzamine can cause postural hypotension, nausea and vomiting, nasal stuffiness, ejaculation inhibition, and tachycardia.

A major adverse effect of doxazosin, prazosin, tamsulosin, and terazosin is called a "first-dose" effect and can cause an exaggerated hypotensive effect upon first dosage that can precipitate **syncope**. Other adverse effects include dizziness, orthostatic hypotension, nasal congestion, fatigue, headache, and drowsiness. These agents can also cause sodium and fluid retention and are frequently used with a diuretic.

Syncope: Momentary loss of consciousness, a faint

▨ RED FLAGS

Tachycardia in severely compromised cardiac patients may be life threatening.

▨ INTERACTIONS

DRUG

Caution should be observed when terazosin is administered concomitantly with other antihypertensive agents, especially the calcium channel blocker verapamil, to avoid possible significant hypotension. When using terazosin and other antihypertensive agents concomitantly, dose reduction and retitration of either agent may be necessary.

HERB

ALPHA RECEPTOR ANTAGONISTS

• *Gan Cao* (Licorice) (D)–theoretically may reduce effects of antihypertensive agents such as alpha-1 adrenergic blockers, ACEI, α_2 receptor antagonists, beta-adrenergic blockers, calcium channel blockers, clonidine, guanabenz, guanfacine, hydralazine, methyldopa, minoxidil, and reserpine. Undertake concurrent use with caution, expert opinion (Kowalak & Mills, 2001) Level 5 evidence.

INTERACTION ISSUES

A:

D: Doxazosin is approximately 98% protein bound, prazosin 92-97% protein bound, silodosin approximately 97% bound, tamsulosin 94-97% bound, terazosin 90-95% bound.

M: Alfuzosin, silodosin, and tamsulosin are major substrates of CYP3A4. Tetrabenazine is a major substrate of CYP2D6.

E:

TI:

Pgp: Prazosin induces Pgp; silodosin is a substrate

SECTION 7: BETA-ADRENERGIC BLOCKING AGENTS

ALPHA AND BETA ANTAGONISTS:

CARVEDILOL (KAR ve di lole) PR=C *(Coreg®, Coreg CR®)*

LABETALOL (la BET a lole) PR=C *(Trandate®)*

NON-SELECTIVE ANTAGONISTS:

NADOLOL (nay DOE lole) PR=C *(Corguard®, Corzide®45)*

PENBUTOLOL (pen BYOO toe lole) PR=C *(Levatol®)*

PINDOLOL (PIN doe lole) PR=B

PROPRANOLOL (proe PRAN oh lole) PR=C *(Inderal® LA, InnoPran XL™)*

SOTALOL (SOE ta lole) PR=B *(Betapace®, Betapace AF®, Sorine®)*

TIMOLOL (TIM oh lole) PR=C

β_1-SELECTIVE ANTAGONISTS:

ACEBUTOLOL (a se BYOO toe lole) PR=B *(Sectral®)*

ATENOLOL (a TEN oh lole) PR=D *(Tenormin®, Tenoretic®)*

BETAXOLOL (be TAKS oh lole) PR=C *(Betoptic® S, Kerlone®)*

BISOPROLOL (bis OH proe lole) PR=C *(Dutoprol™,49 Zebeta®, Ziac®15)*

METOPROLOL (me toe PROE lole) PR=C *(Lopressor®, Lopressor HCT®,49 Toprol-XL®)*

NEBIVOLOL (ne BIV oh lole) PR=C *(Bystolic®)*

*Please note: all beta-adrenergic blocking agents end with the suffix –lol.

FUNCTION

Beta-adrenergic blocking agents, also known as beta antagonists or simply beta blockers, have numerous effects on the human body. The most common function of these agents is in the cardiovascular system though they are used in a variety of other areas. There are two general types of beta blockers that are readily prescribed orally. These are the non-selective beta antagonists and the β_1-selective antagonists.

Non-selective antagonists block both β_1 and β_2 receptors. They are used in various capacities including treatment of hypertension, migraines, hyperthyroidism, angina pectoris, myocardial infarction, and glaucoma (in ocular preparations).

β_1-selective antagonists, also called cardioselective, are used in treating hypertension in specialized situations such as previous intolerance to side effects of other beta blockers or diabetic hypertensive patients.

Carvedilol and Labetalol, while classified as non-selective beta-adrenergic blockers, also antagonize alpha adrenoceptors, especially in the periphery. This causes peripheral vasodilation and further reduction in blood pressure due to decreased peripheral vascular resistance. This is opposed to other beta blockers that cause peripheral vasoconstriction. They are particularly useful in patients who cannot have increased peripheral vascular resistance (such as peripheral vascular disease) and heart failure.

MECHANISMS OF ACTION

Beta-adrenergic blocking agents work by competitively binding with postsynaptic adrenergic membrane receptors and preventing their normal activation by adrenergic neurotransmitters. There are two main types of beta receptors: β_1 and β_2.

β_1 receptors are located primarily in the heart and normally increase the heart rate, increase the contractility of the heart muscle, and can speed **atrioventricular node** conduction. Each of these can increase the work of the heart and therefore the oxygen required by the heart. In patients with heart disease, the coronary arteries are narrowed restricting the amount of blood and therefore oxygen getting to the heart. β_1 blockers work by blocking these normal functions of β_1 receptors and reducing the amount of oxygen required by the heart and therefore protecting it from **hypoxia** and infarction. In addition, decreased heart rate and contractility reduces cardiac output and lowers blood pressure. β_1 receptors are also found in the kidneys where they stimulate **renin** release and in adipose tissues where they stimulate **lipolysis**. The effects in these areas are relatively small, and they play little or no clinical role.

Non-selective beta antagonists also block the normal function of β_2 receptors. These receptors are found in the vascular smooth muscle of the arterioles (except in the skin and brain) and normally cause vasodilation. Blocking β_2 receptors therefore will vasoconstrict and increase peripheral resistance (please see Chapter 6 for a more thorough discussion of this). Rather than counteracting the β_1-induced reduction of blood pressure, it mediates it causing a gradual reduction in blood pressure rather than a dramatic decrease. β_2 blockers also cause **bronchoconstriction** and reduce **glycogenolysis** in the liver. Bronchoconstriction is particularly an issue and explains some of the side effects and red flags for non-selective antagonists.

Reduced blood pressure can induce a compensatory mechanism in the kidneys due to decreased renal perfusion. This results in increased sodium retention and increased blood plasma volume. Occasionally, this can cause a rise in blood pressure rather than a decrease. In these cases, a diuretic may be added to the drug regimen to prevent sodium retention.

Non-selective β antagonists are also used in the treatment of migraines, glaucoma, and hyperthyroidism. It is believed that these agents prevent migraine onset by reducing catecholamine-induced vasodilation. In glaucoma, beta blockers

---

Atrioventricular node: Part of the electrical conducting system of the heart, considered the "gateway" between the atrial conducting system and the ventricular conducting system

Hypoxia: A state where oxygen levels are below normal

Renin: An enzyme that converts angiotensinogen to angiotensin I

Lipolysis: The splitting of a fat molecule

Bronchoconstriction: A decrease in the diameter of the lungs' bronchi allowing for less airflow

Glycogenolysis: Splitting of glycogen to release glucose

Intraocular: Within the eye

can be applied locally and decrease secretion of aqueous humor and thus reduce **intraocular** pressure. These agents help hyperthyroidism by counteracting the widespread sympathetic stimulation normally seen in this condition.

Sotalol has **antiarrhythmic** effects in addition to its beta-blocking effects.

Antiarrhythmic: An agent that counteracts an arrhythmia or abnormal heartbeat rhythm

▦ DOSAGES

ACEBUTOLOL, for *adults*, for hypertension, 400-800 mg/d, up to a maximum of 1200 mg/d;usual dose range is 100-400 mg/d bid; for angina or ventricular arrhythmias, 400-800 mg/d, up to a maximum of 1200 mg/d. For the *elderly*, consider smaller doses; do not exceed 800 mg/d.

ATENOLOL, for *children*, for hypertension, 0.5-1 mg/kg per dose daily; usual dose range of 0.5-1.5 mg/kg/d, up to a maximum 2 mg/kg/d up to 100 mg/d. For *adults*, for hypertension, 25-50 mg once daily; may increase to 100 mg/d; for angina pectoris, 50 mg once daily; may increase to 100 mg/d, some patients may require 200 mg/d; for postmyocardial infarction, 100 mg/d or 50 mg bid for 6-9 days.

BETAXOLOL, for *adults*, for hypertension, 5-10 mg/d; may increase dose to 20 mg/d after 7-14 days. For the *elderly*, initiate at 5 mg/d.

BISOPROLOL, for *adults*, for hypertension, initiate at 2.5-5 mg once daily; may be increased to 10 mg and then up to 20 mg once daily; usual dose is 2.5-10 mg once daily.

CARVEDILOL, for *adults*, for congestive heart failure, immediate release: initiate at 3.125 mg bid for two weeks. If tolerated, may double dose every two weeks up to a maximum 25 mg bid for those with severe failure or under 85 kg and 50 mg bid for those over 85 kg with mild to moderate failure; for extended release: 10 mg once daily. If tolerated, can be doubled every two weeks; for left ventricular dysfunction following myocardial infarction, immediate release: initiate at 3.125-6.25 mg bid and increase to double every 3 to 10 days, based on tolerability, to target of 25 mg bid; for extended release: initiate at 10-20 mg once daily and

increase if tolerated every 3-10 days to a target of 80 mg/d; for hypertension, for immediate release: initiate at 6.25 mg bid, can be doubled every 1-2 weeks up to a maximum of 25 mg bid, for extended release: initiate at 20 mg once daily; can be doubled every 1-2 weeks up to a maximum 80 mg/d.

LABETALOL, for *adults*, initiate at 100 mg bid; may increase as needed every 2-3 days by 100 mg to usual dose of 100-400 mg bid; may require up to 2.4 g/d.

METOPROLOL, for hypertension, immediate release: for *children* 1-17 years old, initiate at 1-2 mg/kg/d up to a maximum of 6 mg/kg/day or 200 mg/d, administer in 2 divided doses; extended release: for *children* 6 years or older, initiate at 1 mg/kg once daily up to a maximum initial dose of 50 mg/d. For *adults*, for hypertension, initiate at 50 mg bid; increase to a usual dose of 50-100 mg/d; may increase dose at weekly intervals to a maximum 450 mg/d; for extended release: initiate at 25-100 mg once daily; may increase weekly to maximum 400 mg/d; usual dose is 50-100 mg/d; for angina, initiate at 50 mg bid; usual dose range is 50-200 mg bid; maximum dose is 200 mg bid; extended release: initiate at 100 mg/d; maximum dose is 400 mg/d; for heart failure, extended release: initiate at 25 mg once daily; may double dose every 2 weeks to a target dose of 200 mg/d.

NADOLOL, for *adults*, initiate at 40 mg/d;increase by 40-80 mg every 3-7 days until optimum clinical response is obtained; doses up to 160-240 mg/d in angina and 240-320 mg/d in hypertension may be necessary; for hypertension, usual dosage range is 40-120 mg once daily. For the *elderly*, consider initiating at a lower dose.

NEBIVOLOL, for *adults*, for hypertension, initiate at 5 mg once daily; may be increased every 2 weeks to maximum dose of 40 mg once daily.

PENBUTOLOL, for *adults*, initiate at 20 mg once daily; usual dose range is 10-40 mg once daily.

PINDOLOL, for *adults*, for hypertension, initiate at 5 mg bid; increase prn by 10 mg/d every 3-4 weeks up to a maximum daily dose of 60 mg; usual dose range is 10-40 mg bid; for antidepressant augmentation, 2.5 mg tid. For the *elderly*, initiate at 5 mg once daily; increase as necessary by 5 mg/d every 3-4 weeks.

PROPRANOLOL, for *adults*, for stable angina, 80-320 mg/d in doses divided 2-4 times/d, long-acting formulation, initiate at 80 mg once daily up to a maximum 320 mg once daily; for essential tremor, initiate at 40 mg bid initially; usual range is 120-320 mg/d; for hypertension, initiate at 40 mg bid; increase dosage every 3-7 days; usual range is 120-240 mg/d in 2-3 doses, maximum dose is 640 mg. Usual dose range is 20-80 mg bid for extended release formulations: *Inderal® LA,* initiate at 80 mg once daily; usual dose is 120-160 mg once daily up to a maximum dose of 640 mg; *InnoPran XL®,* initiate at 80 mg nocte; may be increased every 2-3 weeks to a maximum of 120 mg; for hypertrophic subaortic stenosis, 20-40 mg 3-4 times/d, *Inderal® LA,* 80-160 mg once daily; for migraine headache prophylaxis, initiate at 80 mg/d divided every 6-8 hours; increase by 20-40 mg/dose every 3-4 weeks up to a maximum of 160-240 mg/d given in divided doses every 6-8 hours; *Inderal® LA,* initiate at 80 mg once daily; usual range is 160-240 mg once daily; for myocardial infarction prophylaxis, 180-240 mg/d in 3-4 divided doses; for pheochromocytoma, 30-60 mg/d in divided doses; for tachyarrhythmias, 10-30 mg/dose every 6-8 hours. For the *elderly*, refer to adult except for the following: for hypertension, consider lower initial doses and increase to response; for tachyarrhythmias, initiate at 10 mg bid; increase every 3-7 days to a usual dose of 10-320 mg/d in 1-2 divided doses.

SOTALOL, for *adults*, for ventricular arrhythmias (*Betapace®, Sorine®*), initiate at 80 mg bid; may be increased to 240-320 mg/d; allow 3 days between dose increases; usual daily dose of 160-320 mg/d in 2-3 divided doses; some patients, with life-threatening refractory ventricular arrhythmias, may require doses as high as 480-640 mg/day; for atrial fibrillation or atrial flutter (Betapace AF®), initiate at 80 mg bid; the dose may be increased to 120 mg bid; this may be further increased to 160 mg bid if response is inadequate.

TIMOLOL, for *adults*, for hypertension, initiate at 10 mg bid; may be increased weekly to a usual dose of 10-20 mg bid up to a maximum of 60 mg per day; to prevent myocardial infarction, use is 10 mg bid. For migraine prophylaxis, initiate at 10 mg bid; may increase to a maximum of 30 mg/d.

ADVERSE EFFECTS

In general these agents can cause arrhythmias if suddenly stopped, along with sexual impairment and metabolic disturbances such as reduced glycogenolysis and **glucagon** secretion, which can cause fasting hypoglycemia. Cold extremities, fatigue, insomnia, nightmares, and depression may also occur. Beta-blockers may increase the symptoms of peripheral vascular disease or cause Raynaud's phenomenon and, due to their decreasing blood pressure and therefore kidney perfusion, may increase sodium retention.

RED FLAGS

Beta-blockers should not be discontinued abruptly as they can exacerbate angina pectoralis and increase the risk of sudden death.

Since these agents can cause bronchoconstriction, they can be life threatening if given to patients with chronic obstructive pulmonary disease or asthma.

Beta-blockers can induce congestive heart failure in susceptible patients with impaired myocardial function such as compensated heart failure, acute myocardial infarction, and **cardiomegaly**. However, several studies have indicated that beta-blocker treatment is beneficial in mild to moderate cases of congestive heart failure.

Beta-blockers can decrease glycogenolysis and glucagon secretion. This can cause insulin-dependent diabetics to have severe hypoglycemia after insulin injection. In addition, beta-blockers may increase the normal response to hypoglycemia.

> Glucagon: A pancreatic hormone that causes the breakdown of glycogen and elevates serum glucose levels

> Cardiomegaly: An enlarged heart

Because of these effects, while beta-blockers may still be used in insulin-dependent diabetics, caution and close monitoring are necessary.

While bradycardia is a normal effect of these drugs, they can cause life-threatening brady-arrhythmias in patients with atrioventricular conduction defects and on drugs that may reduce AV node conduction such as verapamil.

■ INTERACTIONS

DRUG

Life-threatening bradyarrhythmias may occur in patients who are also taking drugs that may reduce AV node conduction (such as digoxin, verapamil, and diltiazem), alpha-blockers (prazosin, terazosin), and alpha-adrenergic stimulants (epinephrine and phenylephrine).

Propranolol and possibly other beta-blockers can interact with cimetidine, furosemide, and chlorpromazine potentiating antihypertensive effects. This is due to interference with the enzymes of metabolism.

Metoprolol and propranolol's effects can be mitigated by drugs that increase metabolism such as barbiturates, phenytoin, and rifampin.

HERB

ANTIHYPERTENSIVES

- *Chen Pi* (Tangerine peel) (Indeterminate)– contains constituents that stimulate the sympathetic nervous system and should be used with caution in those taking antihypertensives, antidiabetic, antihyperthyroid, and/or antiseizure medications (Chinese language article cited in Chen & Chen, 2004) Indeterminate level of evidence.
- *Gan Cao* (Licorice) (D)–theoretically may reduce effects of antihypertensive agents such as alpha-1 adrenergic blockers, ACEI, α_2 recepor antagonists, beta-adrenergic blockers, calcium channel blockers, clonidine, guanethidine, hydralazine, methyldopa, minoxidil, and reserpine, and concurrent use should be undertaken with caution (Kowalak & Mills, 2001) Level 5 evidence.
- *Ma Huang* (Ephedra) (C)–based on ephedrine content, antagonizes the effects of antihyperten-

sives (White, Gardner, Gurley, Marx, Wang, & Estes, 1997) Level 3b evidence. Antihypertensives including ACE inhibitors and beta-blockers may be antagonized by *Ma Huang*, and severe hypertension may result. This is speculative (Mills & Bone, 2000) Level 5 evidence.
- *Qing Pi* (Citrus Viride) (Indeterminate)– contains constituents that stimulate the sympathetic nervous system and should be used with caution in those taking antihypertensives, antidiabetic, antihyperthyroid, and/or antiseizure medications (Chinese language article cited in Chen & Chen, 2004) Indeterminate level of evidence.
- *Sheng Ma* (Cimicifuga) (D)–may potentiate the effect of antihypertensive agents, and concurrent use should be undertaken with caution. Expert opinion (Gruenwald, Brendler & Jaenicke, 2004) Level 5 evidence.
- *Zhi Ke* (Aurantium fruit) (Indeterminate)– contains constituents that stimulate the sympathetic nervous system and should be used with caution in those taking antihypertensives, antidiabetic, antihyperthyroid, and/or antiseizure medications (Chinese language article cited in Chen & Chen, 2004) Indeterminate level of evidence.
- *Zhi Shi* (Aurantium immaturus) (Indeterminate)–contains constituents that stimulate the sympathetic nervous system and should be used with caution in those taking antihypertensives, antidiabetic, antihyperthyroid, and/or antiseizure medications (Chinese language article cited in Chen & Chen, 2004) Indeterminate level of evidence.

BETA-ADRENERGIC BLOCKERS

- *Gan Cao* (Licorice) (D)–theoretically may reduce the effects of antihypertensive agents such as alpha-1 adrenergic blockers, ACEI, α_2 receptor antagonists, beta-adrenergic blockers, calcium channel blockers, clonidine, hydralazine, methyldopa, minoxidil, and reserpine, and concurrent use should be undertaken with caution (Kowalak & Mills, 2001) Level 5 evidence.
- *Ma Huang* (D)–antihypertensives including ACE inhibitors and beta-blockers may be

antagonized by *Ma Huang,* and severe hypertension may result. This is speculative (Mills & Bone, 2000) Level 5 evidence.

PROPRANOLOL

• *Hei Hu Jiao* (Black pepper) (B-)–increased absorption kinetics of propranolol, the amount of theophylline, and increased maximum concentrations of both in a small human crossover study (Bano, Raina, Zutshi, Bedi, Johri & Sharma, 1991) Level 3b evidence.

INTERACTION ISSUES

A:

D: Carvedilol is greater than 98% protein bound, nebivolol approximately 98% bound, penbutolol 80-98% protein bound

M: Betaxolol is a major substrate of CYP1A2. Bisoprolol is a major substrate of CYP3A4. Carvedilol, metoprolol, and timolol are major substrates of CYP2D6. Propranolol is a major substrate of CYP1A2 and CYP2D6.

E:

TI:

Pgp: Carvedilol and propranolol inhibit Pgp, nadolol is a substrate of Pgp

ENDNOTES

[1] Combination of Atropine, Hyoscyamine, Scopalamine, and Phenobarbital.

[2] Combination of Atropine and Diphenoxylate.

[3] Motofen contains Difenoxin in addition to Atropine and is used in treating diarrhea.

[4] Prosed/DS and Prosed/EC are a combination of Methenamine, Phenyl Salicylate, Methylene Blue, Benzoic Acid, Atropine Sulfate, and Hyoscymine Sulfate used in treating lower urinary tract inflammation and urination.

[5] Combination of Vilanterol and Fluticsone.

[6] Combination of Hyoscyamine, Methenamine, Sodium Biphosphate, Phenyl Salicylate, and Methylene Blue.

[7] Combination of Atropine, Hyoscyamine, Scopolamine, and Phenobarbital.

[8] Advair Diskus comes in three varieties: 100/50, 250/50, and 500/50. The first number is the dosage of Fluticasone in mcg, and the second number is the dosage of almeterol, which is a constant 50 mcg.

[9] Combination of Mometasone and Formoterol.

[10] Combination of Guaifenesin and Phenylephrine.

[11] Combination of Chlorpheniramine and Phenylephrine.

[12] Combination of Dextromethorphan, Phenylephrine, and Pyrilamine.

[13] Combination of Acetomaminophen and Phenylephrine.

[14] Combination of Chlorpheniramine, Dihydrocodeine, and Phenylephrine.

[15] Combination of Bisoprolol and Hydrochlorothiozide.

[16] Combination of Dextromethorphan, Chlorpheniramine, and Phenylephrine.

[17] Combination of Chlorpheniramine, Phenylephrine, and Phenyltoloxamine.

[18] Combination of Pseudoephedrine, Triprolodine, and Codeine.

[19] Combination of Pseudoephedrine and Triprolodine.

[20] Combination of Pseudoephedrine and Naproxen.

[21] Combination of Acetaminophen, Caffeine, Hydrocodone, Chlorpheniramine, and Phenylephrine.

[22] Combination of Phenylephrine and Scopalamine.

[23] Combination of Pyrilamine and Phenylephrine.

[24] Combination of Pseudoephedrine and Loratadine.

[25] Combination of Chlorthalidone and Clonidine.

[26] Aldoclor combines Methyldopa 250 mg and Chlorthiazide 250 mg.

[27] Aldoril combines Methyldopa and Hydrochlorothiazide in various dosages.

[28] Combination of Amphetamine and Dextroamphetamine.

[29] Combination of Ephedrine and Guaifenesin.

[30] Combination of Pseudoephedrine and Codeine.

[31] Combination of Brompheniramine, Pseudoephedrine, and Dextromethorphan.

[32] Combination of Guaifenesin and Pseudoephedrine.

[33] Combination of Pseudoephedrine, Ibuprofen, and Chlorpheniramine.

[34] Combination of Phenylephrine, Chlorpheniramine, and Dihydrocodeine.

[35] Combination of Codeine, Guaifenesin, and Pseudoephedrine.

[36] Combination of Chlorpheniramine, Pseudoephedrine, and Hydrocodone.

[37] Combination of Pseudoephedrine and Chlorpheniramine.

[38] Combination of Chlorpheniramine, Pseudoephedrine, and Dextromethorphan.

[39] Combination of Codeine, Chlorpheniramine, and Pseudoephedrine.

[40] Combination of Chlorpheniramine, Pseudoephedrine, and Dihydrocodeine.

[41] Combination of Pseudoephedrine and Hydrocodone.

[42] Combination of Pseudoephedrine, Guaifenesin, and Dextromethorphan.

[43] Combination of Pseudoephedrine and Fexofenadine.

[44] Combination of Pseudoephedrine and Acrivastine.

[45] Combination of Nadolol and Bendroflumethiazide.

[46] Combination of Dorzolamide and Timolol.

[47] Combination of Pseudoephedrine and Desloratadine.

[48] Combination of Atenolol and Chlorthalidone.

[49] Combination of Metoprolol and Hydrochlorothiazide.

[50] Combination of Ipratropium and Albuterol.

[51] Combination of Ipratropium and Fenoterol.

[52] Combination of Acetaminophen, Chlorpheniramine, Phenylephrine, and Phenyltoloxamine.

[53] Combination of Acetaminophen, Diphenhydramine, and Phenylephrine.

[54] Combination of Brompheniramine, and Phenylephrine.

[55] Combination of Diphenhydramine and Phenylephrine.

[56] Combination of Acetaminophen, Dextromorphine, and Phenylephrine.

[57] Combination of Dextromorphine and Phenylephrine.

[58] Combination of Guaifenesin, Dextromethorphan, and Phenylephrine.

[59] Combination of Promethazine and Phenylephrine.

[60] Combination of Clonidine and Chlorthalidone.

[61] Combination of Dutasteride and Tamsulosin.

[62] Combination of Pseudoephedrine and Dextromethorphan.

[63] Combination of Pseudoephedrine and Ibuprofen.

[64] Combination of Pseudoephedrine and Acetaminophen.

[65] Combination of Pseudoephedrine and Brompheniramine.

[66] Combination of Pseudoephedrine and Cetrizine.

[67] Combination of Budesonide and Formoterol.

■ CHINESE MEDICAL DESCRIPTIONS

The Chinese medical explanation of the drug categories in this chapter may be found in Chapter 15 on pages 385–417.

Drugs Affecting the Central Nervous System

The central nervous system (CNS) includes the brain and spinal cord and provides the integration and command functions of the nervous system. Impulse propagation is very similar to that of the autonomic nervous system (ANS) in how an action potential is transferred from one neuron to another: there is a presynaptic neuron that releases a neurotransmitter into the **synaptic cleft,** which activates a postsynaptic membrane receptor that causes voltage changes in the postsynaptic neuron. The major differences between the ANS and the CNS are that there are many more neurotransmitters used in the CNS, the neurons in the CNS have many more connections with other neurons, and neurotransmitters can inhibit as well as excite the postsynaptic neuron.

In other words, it can make an action potential more possible or less possible.

This occurs because neurochemicals can bind to receptors with ion channels that allow various ions to flow with their gradient pressure. Different ion channels can cause **hyperpolarization** or **depolarization** in the postsynaptic neural membrane. When a depolarization occurs, it is called an excitatory postsynaptic potential (EPSP) and increases the likelihood of a nerve impulse. This is caused by an influx of Na^+ ions. With enough EPSPs, depolarization can surpass a threshold, and an action potential is created.

Synaptic cleft: The space between the two neurons of a synapse; the space into which the neurotransmitters are released

Hyperpolarization: The state where a neuron's membrane is more electrically negative than normal, and therefore it is more difficult to initiate an action potential

Depolarization: The state where a neuron's membrane is more electrically positive than normal and therefore closer to initiating an action potential

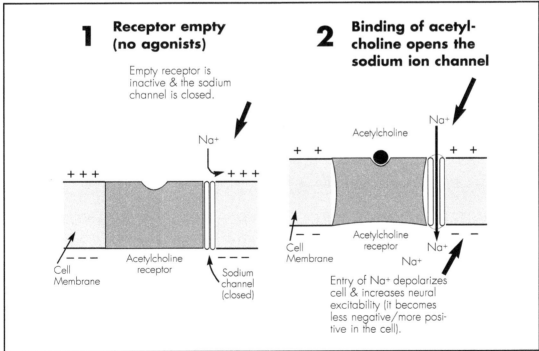

Figure 5.1: Acetylcholine transmits an excitatory postsynaptic potential (EPSP). 1: No acetylcholine binding the postsynaptic receptor maintains the closed ion channel. 2: When acetylcholine binds the receptor, it opens the sodium channel and allows influx of sodium ions (Na^+) and increases excitability and brings the membrane closer to threshold and depolarization.

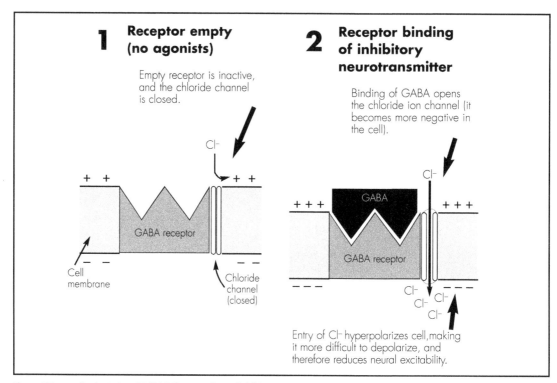

Figure 5.2: γ-aminobutyric acid (GABA) transmits an inhibitory postsynaptic potential (IPSP). **1:** No GABA binding the postsynaptic receptor maintains the closed ion channel. **2:** When GABA binds the receptor, it opens the chlorine channel and allows influx of chlorine ions (Cl⁻) and decreases excitability and brings the membrane farther from threshold and depolarization.

Norepinephrine and acetylcholine are common EPSP neurotransmitters. An excitatory neurochemical reaction is shown in Figure 5.1 (previous page).

Inhibitory postsynaptic potentials or IPSPs are the result of hyperpolarization of the postsynaptic membrane making it less likely that an action potential will be generated. They are usually caused by an influx of chlorine ions (Cl-) and/or an efflux of K^+ ions causing the resting membrane potential to be lowered making it more difficult for threshold to be achieved. Gamma aminobutyric acid (GABA) and glycine are common IPSP neurotransmitters. Figure 5.2 shows an IPSP.

Most CNS neurons receive both EPSP and IPSP inputs. It is only when the summation of these inputs allows the postsynaptic membrane potential to increase past the threshold is an action potential initiated.

SECTION 1: DRUGS FOR PARKINSON'S DISEASE

AMANTADINE (a MAN ta dene) PR=C

BENZTROPINE *(See Chapter 4, Section 3)*

TRIHEXYPHENIDYL *(See Chapter 4, Section 3)*

ANTIMUSCARINIC AGENTS: *(See Chapter 4, Section 3)*

COMT INHIBITORS:

ENTACAPONE (en TA ka pone) PR=C
(Comtan®, Stalevo™²¹)

TOLCAPONE (TOLE ka pone) PR=C *(Tasmar®)*

DOPAMINE RECEPTOR AGONISTS:

APOMORPHINE (a poe MOR fene) PR=C
(Apokyn®)

BROMOCRIPTINE (broe moe KRIP tene) PR=B
(Cycloset®, Parlodel®, SnapTabs®)

CABERGOLINE (ca BER goe lene) PR=B
(Dostinex®)

PRAMIPEXOLE (pra mi PEKS ole) PR=C
(Mirapex®, Mirapex® ER®)

ROPINIROLE (roe PIN i role) PR=C *(Requip®, Requip® XL™)*

ROTIGOTINE (roe TIG oh tene) PR=C

LEVODOPA:

CARBIDOPA (kar bi DOE pa) PR=C *(Lodosyn®, Parcopa™,[1] Sinemet®,[1] Sinemet® CR,[1] Stalevo™[21])*

LEVODOPA (lee voe DOE pa) *(Parcopa™, Sinemet®,[1] Sinemet® CR,[1] Stalevo™[2])*

MONOAMINE OXIDASE B INHIBITORS:

RASAGILINE (ra SA ji lene) PR=C *(Azilect®)*

SELEGILINE (se LE ji lene) PR=C *(Eldepryl®, Emsam®, Zelapar®)*

Primary Parkinson's disease is caused by an unexplained degeneration of dopamine-producing cells primarily in the subsantia nigra, other areas of the brain stem, and the basal nuclei. The basal nuclei (previously called basal ganglia), located in the center of the brain, aid in movement, specifically starting, stopping, and monitoring intensity of movements, especially slow or stereotyped movements.

Common symptoms of Parkinson's disease are a pill-rolling tremor of one hand, muscle rigidity (cogwheel rigidity), slow movement (bradykinesia), decreased movement (hypokinesia), and difficulty in initiating movement (akinesia), aches, fatigue, masklike face, shuffling gait with small steps, **festination**, a tendency to fall when the center of gravity is displaced, **micrographia**, and difficulty with activities of daily living (ADLs).

Normally the substantia nigra projects neuronal axons into the striatum, which release dopamine that inhibits neurons in the striatum where normal gross intentional movements of the body are processed on the way from the cortex and the thalamus. The substantia nigra neurons fire tonically, meaning they are a relatively constant inhibitory influence on the striatum neurons. In primary Parkinson's disease, this constant negative tone is reduced or absent, causing degeneration and loss of muscular control (see Figure 5.3 on the next page).

Secondary Parkinson's disease has similar signs and symptoms but is caused by another idiopathic degenerative disease, drugs, or exogenous toxins. The most common cause of secondary parkinsonism is the use of antipsychotic drugs or reserpine, which block dopamine receptors.

FUNCTION

Treatment strategies for Parkinson's disease include increasing the availability of dopamine in the striatum. These strategies include direct supplementation of a dopamine precursor (levodopa), reduction of peripheral metabolism of levodopa (carbidopa), dopamine receptor agonists (ropinirole and pramipexole), reducing dopamine metabolism within the CNS (rasgiline and selegiline), as well as symptom control with amantadine and antimuscarinic agents (see Chapter 4, Section 3).

Pramipexole, ropinirole, and rotigotine are also used in the treatment of moderate to severe restless legs syndrome (RLS).

Cabergoline is a dopamine receptor agonist; however, it is not used for the treatment of Parkinson's disease. Rather, it is used for the treatment of hyperprolactinemia. It will be discussed further in the chapter discussing hormones.

Amantadine is also used to treat and prevent influenza A viral infections and **extrapyramidal symptoms** induced by other drugs.

Bromocriptine is also used in the treatment of hyperprolactinemia, acromegaly, neuroleptic malignant syndrome, and type 2 diabetes mellitus.

MECHANISM OF ACTION

Levodopa is a precursor of dopamine. When it enters the brain it helps supplant the lowered dopamine levels and offset the effects of Parkinson's disease. Carbidopa is an inhibitor of L-amino acid decarboxylase in the periphery, which allows more absorption of levodopa into the brain. Without carbidopa only about 1% of orally administered levodopa will enter the brain while the peripheral metabolites would cause many side effects. In modern practice levodopa is almost always administered with carbidopa. Please see Figure 5.4 on page 69.

Festination: Overly hasty movement

Micrographia: Very small writing

Extrapyramidal symptoms: Exhibiting movement disorders, especially postural and locomotor, resembling Parkinson's disease

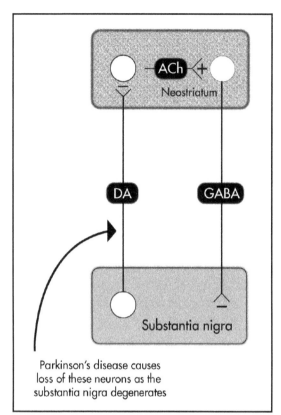

Figure 5.3: Relationship of neurotransmitters in the corpus striatum and substantia nigra. Dopamine (DA) released from a substantia nigra neuron normally provides a constant negative tone on neostriatum neurons, which releases acetylcholine (ACh) that in turn positively effects a neuron to release γ-aminobutyric acid (GABA) in the substantia nigra, which causes reduced secretion of dopamine.

Amantadine, originally developed as an antiviral agent, has been shown to have antiparkinsonism effects due to an unknown mechanism possibly by increasing synthesis, release, or reuptake of dopamine. As for its antiviral action, it prevents the uncoating of influenza A virus and prevents viral penetration into the host.

COMT inhibitors: Catechol-o-methyltransferase (COMT) is an enzyme that **catabolizes** levodopa and dopamine. The COMT inhibitors inhibit the action of this enzyme reducing the degradation of levodopa in the periphery and allowing more administered levodopa to enter the brain where it can be metabolized to dopamine. Tolcapone acts both peripherally and centrally, while entacapone acts primarily

Catabolism: Biological processes that primarily break down large storage and other chemicals, often releasing energy in the process

Isoenzymes: Subtypes of a specific enzyme

in the periphery. This is shown graphically in Figure 5.5 on page 70.

Dopamine-receptor agonists: These agents are direct agonists of striatal dopamine receptors meaning that they bind with postsynaptic membrane receptors and activate them in similar ways as dopamine would.

Monoamine oxidase B inhibitors: There are two **isoenzymes** of monoamine oxidase (MAO). MAO B is the predominant form in the striatum and helps break down dopamine in the synaptic cleft. MAO B inhibitors reduce this breakdown allowing more dopamine to stay in the synaptic cleft longer to help reduce the effects of the lowered dopamine in Parkinson's disease. For more information on MAO inhibitors, see Section 6 on page 97.

DOSAGES

AMANTADINE, for *children*, for influenza A, 1-9 years, 2.5 mg/kg/d bid, up to a maximum dose of 150 mg/d; 10 and over and under 40 kg, 2.5 mg/kg/d bid; 10 or over and over 40 kg, 100 mg bid; initiate within 24-48 hours after onset of symptoms. For *adults*, for drug-induced extrapyramidal symptoms, 100 mg bid; may increase to 300 mg/d; for Parkinson's disease, 100 mg bid as sole therapy; may increase to 400 mg/d if needed with close monitoring;initial dose is 100 mg/d if with other serious illness or with high doses of other anti-Parkinson drugs; for influenza A viral infection, 200 mg once daily or 100 mg bid; initiate within 24-48 hours after onset of symptoms and continue until 24-48 hours after symptoms disappear; for influenza A prophylaxis, 200 mg once daily or 100 mg bid.

APOMORPHINE for *adults*, for Parkinson's disease "off" episode, subcutaneous injection: a test dose must be physician-administered, initial test of 2 mg: if patient tolerates and respond start at 2 mg; may increase by 1 mg every few days to a maximum 6 mg; if patient tolerates 2 mg test but does not respond, do a second test dose of 4 mg.

BROMOCRIPTINE, for *children* and adolescents 11-15, for hyperprolactinemia, initiate at 1.25-2.5

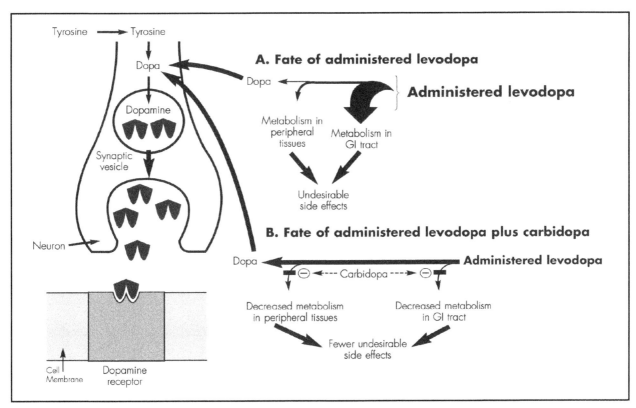

Figure 5.4: Metabolism of levodopa when released. A: Levodopa alone causes lots of adverse effects due to its widespread metabolism. **B:** Levodopa administered with carbidop,a which prevents peripheral metabolism and allows more levodopa to be present in the brain and adds greatly to its efficacy.

mg daily; usual range is 2.5-10 mg/d. For 16 years and over and *adults*, for hyperprolactinemia, 1.25 mg bid, increased by 2.5 mg/d every 2-7 days to a usual dose range of 2.5-30 mg/d; for neuroleptic malignant syndrome, 2.5-5 mg every 8-12 hours to a maximum of 45 mg/d; for acromegaly, initiate at 1.25-2.5 mg daily, increasing by 1.25-2.5 mg daily as necessary every 3-7 days to a usual dose of 20-30 mg/d and a maximum of 100 mg/d; for parkinsonism, initiate at 1.25 mg bid; may be increased by 2.5 mg/d every 2-4 weeks prn to a maximum dose of 100 mg/d. For type 2 diabetes mellitus, initiate at 0.8 mg once daily; may increase weekly by 0.8 mg as tolerated; usual dose range is 1.6-4.8 mg daily up to a maximum of 4.8 mg daily.

CARBIDOPA, for *adults*, 75-100 mg/d.

ENTACAPONE, for *adults*, 200 mg with each dose of levodopa/carbidopa, up to a maximum of 8 times/d; maximum daily dose is 1600 mg/d.

LEVODOPA is always used in combination with other agents in this class of drugs and usually includes doses of 100 mg to 250 mg bid to tid.

PRAMIPEXOLE, for *adults*, for Parkinson's disease, immediate release: initiate at 0.5 mg/d tid;increase gradually every 5-7 days to a range of 1.5-4.5 mg/d; extended release formulation: initiate at 0.375 mg once daily; increase gradually to 0.75 mg once daily; may increase by 0.75 mg/dose every 5-7 days or longer to a maximum recommended dose of 4.5 mg/d; for restless legs syndrome, initiate at 0.125 mg once daily 2-3 hours before bedtime; may be doubled every 4-7 days up to 0.5 mg/d.

RASAGILINE, for *adults*, for Parkinson's disease (monotherapy), 1 mg once daily; for adjunctive therapy with levodopa, initiate at 0.5 mg once daily; may increase to 1 mg once daily.

ROPINIROLE, for *adults*, for Parkinson's disease, immediate release: starting dose is 0.25 mg tid;based on patient response, the dose should be increased in weekly increments: week 1, 0.25 mg tid, week 2, 0.5 mg tid, week 3, 0.75 mg tid,

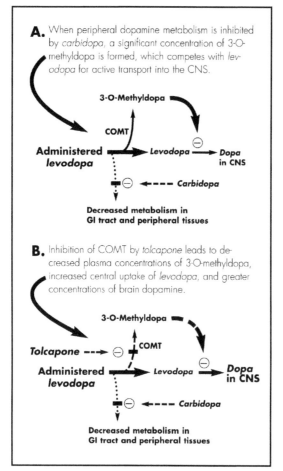

A. When peripheral dopamine metabolism is inhibited by *carbidopa*, a significant concentration of 3-O-methyldopa is formed, which competes with *levodopa* for active transport into the CNS.

B. Inhibition of COMT by *tolcapone* leads to decreased plasma concentrations of 3-O-methyldopa, increased central uptake of *levodopa*, and greater concentrations of brain dopamine.

Figure 5.5: How coadminstration of COMT inhibitors and carbidopa can affect levodopa metabolism. A: Adding carbidopa to administered levodopa decreases metabolism of levodopa in the GI tract and periphery sparing it for the brain. **B:** COMT inhibition prevents formation of 3-O-methyldopa, which increases CNS uptake of levodopa and more dopa in the brain.

week 4, 1 mg tid; after week 4, if necessary, daily dose may be increased by 1.5 mg/d on a weekly basis up to a dose of 9 mg/d, and then by up to 3 mg/d weekly to a total of 24 mg/d; for Parkinson's disease discontinuation taper, should be gradually tapered over 7 days as follows: reduce frequency of administration from tid to bid for 4 days, then reduce to once daily for remaining 3 days; for extended release: initiate at 2 mg once daily; may increase 2 mg/d with at least a week between increases up to a maximum of 24 mg/d. For restless legs syndrome, initiate at 0.25 mg once daily 1-3 hours nocte;may increase after 2 days to 0.5 mg/d, and

after 7 days to 1 mg/d and upward in 0.5 mg increments every week after that until reaching 3 mg/d during week 6. If symptoms persist or reappear, daily dose may be increased to a maximum of 4 mg beginning week 7.

ROTIGOTINE, for *adults*, for Parkinson's disease, topical/transdermal: for early stage, initially apply 2 mg/d patch once daily; may increase by 2 mg/d weekly; lowest effective dose is 4 mg/d; can use up to a maximum dose of 6 img/d; for advanced-stage, initially apply 4 mg/d patch once daily; may increase by 2 mg/d weekly up to a maximum dose of 8 mg/d; for restless legs syndrome (RLS), topical/transdermal: initially apply 1 mg/d patch once daily, may increase by 1 mg/d weekly up to a maximum dose of 3 mg/d.

SELEGILINE, for *adults*, Parkinson's disease, 5 mg bid with breakfast and lunch or 10 mg in the morning. For the *elderly*, for Parkinson's disease, initiate at 5 mg in the morning. For orally disintegrating tablet (Zelapar®), for *adults*, for Parkinson's disease, initiate at 1.25 mg daily for at least 6 weeks; may increase to 2.5 mg daily. For depression, transdermal (Emsam®): initiate at 6 mg once daily; may increase by 3 mg/d every 2 weeks up to a maximum 12 mg/d.

TOLCAPONE, for *adults*, initiate at 100 mg tid;may increase to 200 mg tid.

▧ ADVERSE EFFECTS

In general, adverse effects are caused by having too much activation of central nervous system dopamine receptors by these agents. These include visual and auscultatory hallucinations, and **dyskinesia**.

AMANTIDINE: Restlessness, dizziness, agitation, confusion, hallucinations, orthostatic hypotension, urinary retention, peripheral edema, dry mouth, and at high doses, acute toxic **psychosis** may occur.

ANTIMUSCARINIC AGENTS: (see Chapter 4, Section 3).

COMT INHIBITORS: The adverse effects of these agents are similar to those of levodopa/carbidopa; however, tolcapone is **hepatotoxic,** and liver enzymes must be closely monitored during its use.

DOPAMINE RECEPTOR AGONISTS: Pergolide can cause profound hypertension upon initiation; therefore it must be initiated at low doses and slowly increased. Pramipexole and ropinirole can cause nausea; fatigue; and, rarely, sudden attacks of sleep during ordinary daily activities. Because of having fewer adverse effects, these two agents are becoming the initial treatment of Parkinson's disease displacing levodopa.

LEVODOPA: In the periphery, too much dopamine stimulation can cause **anorexia**, nausea, and vomiting due to stimulation of the **emetic** center. In the heart it can lead to **tachycardia**, hypotension, and **ventricular extrasystoles.** In the iris, the **adrenergic** effects of dopamine may cause **mydriasis. Blood dyscrasias** and a positive reaction to the **Coomb's test** may occur. Saliva and urine may become brownish due to **catecholamine oxidation** forming melanin pigment. Beside the effects noted above, levodopa may cause mood changes, anxiety, and depression.

MONOAMINE OXIDASE B INHIBITORS: In advanced Parkinson's disease, selegiline may exacerbate the adverse motor and cognitive effects of levodopa. Other adverse effects include anxiety and insomnia.

INTERACTIONS

Levodopa may cause an increase in intraocular pressure and should be used with caution in glaucoma patients. It may also exacerbate symptoms in psychotic patients.

DRUG

MAO inhibitors (other than selegiline, due to its selectivity) can induce a hypertensive crisis from too much catecholamine production when used with levodopa. Antipsychotic drugs are contraindicated with levodopa as they block dopamine receptors and can cause parkinsonian syndrome on their own. Exceptions to this are the newer "atypical" antipsychotic agents such as clozapine. Apomorphine requires an antiemetic

before dosing. However, serotonin antagonists should not be used in this capacity as they may cause severe hypotension when combined.

Selegiline may cause stupor, rigidity, agitation, and hyperthermia when used with meperidine. Other interactions with selegiline have been reported with tricyclic antidepressants and serotonin-reuptake inhibitors.

HERB

BROMOCRIPTINE

- *Ma Huang* (Ephedra) (D)–may increase toxicity due to **sympathomimetic** effects. Speculative (Mills & Bone, 2000) Level 5 evidence.

MONOAMINE OXIDASE INHIBITORS (MAOI)

- *Gan Cao* (Licorice) (D)–may increase toxicity of MAOIs due to constituents that noncompetitively inhibit MAO, bench research (Hatano, Fukuda, Miyase, Noro, & Okuda, 1991) Level 5 evidence.
- *Ma Huang* (Ephedra) (B)–ephedrine content may cause hypertension with MAOI use, expert opinion (Blumenthal, 1998) Level 5 evidence. One case report: patient who stopped an MAOI (phenelzine) and ingested a combination pill of ephedrine, caffeine, and theophylline 24 hours later, developed encephalopathy, neuromuscular irritability, sinus tachycardia, hypotension, rhabdomyolysis, and hyperthermia (Dawson, Earnshaw & Graham, 1995) Level 4 evidence. Other possible effects include **arrhythmias**, chest pain, **hyperpyrexia**, and death (Gruenwald, Brendler & Jaenicke, 2004). One human study showed an increase in cardiovascular symptoms (Dingemanse, 1993) Level 2c evidence. Avoid *Ma Huang* for at least 2 weeks after stopping MAOIs (Brinker, 2001).

Dyskinesia: Impairment or inability to execute voluntary movements

Psychosis: A severe emotional and behavioral disorder that includes symptoms of gross distortion of a person's mental capacity, ability to recognize reality, inability to relate to others, or perform ADLs

Hepatotoxic: Toxic to the liver

Anorexia: Lack or loss of appetite

Emetic: an agent to cause vomiting

Tachycardia: A rapid heart rate defined as over 100 bpm

Ventricular extrasystoles: An extra contraction started in a ventricle

Adrenergic: Pertaining to nerve fibers in the SNS that react to epinephrine, norepinephrine, or dopamine neurotransmitters

Mydriasis: Dilation of the pupil

Blood dyscrasia: Abnormal condition of the blood

Coomb's test: A test for antibodies damaging red blood cells; may indicate many blood diseases

Catecholamines: Sympathomimetic neurotransmitter family that includes epinephrine, norepinephrine, and dopamine

Oxidation: A chemical reaction that either increases the oxygen of a molecule or loses an electron from a molecule

Sympathomimetic: Either mimicking or stimulating the sympathetic nervous system

Arrhythmia: Irregular heartbeat

Hyperpyrexia: Very high fever

- *Ren Shen* (Ginseng) (D)–rare cases of manic-like symptoms documented with concurrent use of phenelzine. Use caution with *Ren Shen* and phenelzine and similar antidepressants, expert opinion (Fugh-Berman, 2000) Level 5 evidence.
- *Rou Cong Rong* (Cistanche) (Indeterminate)–may interact with sympathomimetics, monoamine oxidase inhibitors, selective serotonin inhibitors, and tricyclic antidepressants by increasing the activities of neurotransmitters such as norepinephrine, dopamine, and serotonin (Chinese language article cited in Chen & Chen, 2004) Indeterminate level of evidence.
- *Yin Guo Ye* (Gingko leaf) (B/C against potentiation)–theoretically may potentiate effects of MAOI. Animal studies substantiate this effect (Sloley, Urichuk, Morley, Durkin, Shan *et al.*, 2000) Level 5 evidence, (White, Scates & Cooper, 1996) Level 5 evidence; however, a human study did not (Fowler, Wang, Volkow *et al.*, 2000) Level 2c evidence.
- *Ying Su Ke* (Opium husks) (D)–phenoth-iazines, monoamine oxidase inhibitors, and tricyclic antidepressants may exacerbate the depressant and CNS suppressive effects of *ying su ke*, expert opinion (Chen & Chen, 2004) Level 5 evidence.

VITAMIN

Vitamin B_6 (pyridoxine) increases peripheral metabolism of levodopa, reducing its effectiveness.

OTHER

Levadopa may cause false positives or negatives for glucose and ketones on some urinary dipstick tests.

INTERACTION ISSUES

A:

D: Entacapone is 98% protein bound; tolcapone is over 99% bound

M: Rasagiline is a major substrate of CYP1A2; selegiline is a major substrate of CYP2B6

E:

TI:

Pgp:

SECTION 2: DRUGS FOR OTHER NEURODEGENERATIVE DISEASES

ANTI-ALZHEIMERS DRUGS:

ANTICHOLINESTERASES *(See Chapter 4, Section 2)*

MEMANTINE (me MAN tene) PR=B *(Namenda®)*

DRUGS FOR MULTIPLE SCLEROSIS:

CORTICOSTEROIDS *(See Chapter 7, Section 4)*

IMMUNOSUPPRESSIVE DRUGS *(See Chapter 10, Section 10)*

DALFAMPRIDINE (dal FAM pri dene) PR=C *(Ampyra™)*

FINGOLIMOD (fin GOL i mod) PR=C *(Gilenya®)*

GLATIRAMER (gluh TEER a mer) PR=B *(Copaxone®)*

DRUGS FOR AMYOTROPHIC LATERAL SCLEROSIS:

RILUZOLE (RIL you zole) PR=B *(Rilutek®)*

There are many neurodegenerative diseases characterized by progressive deterioration of specific neurons. We have already discussed Parkinsons disease in the first section of this chapter. Multiple sclerosis (MS), Alzheimer's disease, and amyotrophic lateral sclerosis (ALS) are other relatively common neurodegenerative diseases. The deterioration of the neurons happens in different parts of the central nervous system in these diseases and can affect movement, cognition, or both.

Alzheimer's disease is said to affect 5.1 million people. It is characterized by the progressive loss of cholinergic neurons in a specific area of the brain, called nucleus basilis of Maynert. It causes a progressive dementia. Drugs used to treat this condition are palliative and can cause short-term positive effects, but do not do anything to reverse the underlying neurodegeneration.

Multiple sclerosis is an autoimmune inflammatory disease that causes demyelination of CNS neurons. It can have an erratic progression and cause anything from an acute neurologic episode to chronic, debilitating, progressive disease over 10-20 years. Treatment involves attempts to prevent the autoimmune inflammation and includes corticosteroids and immunosuppressive drugs. Chemotherapeutic drugs and some newer MS-specific drugs may also be used.

Amyotrophic lateral sclerosis, also known as Lou Gehrig's Disease, is a progressive degeneration of motor neurons that eventually causes paralysis and death.

FUNCTION

Dalfampridine, fingolimod, and glatiramer are used to treat MS, generally in the alleviation of signs and symptoms, and while they may have some effect on progression of the disease, it is a rather small effect.

Memantine is often used with acetyl cholinesterase inhibitors and has been shown to slow memory loss in both Alzheimer's and vascular dementia.

Riluzole, while similar to drugs used to treat Alzheimer's disease, is used exclusively to treat ALS. It can improve life span and postpone the need for ventilation in ALS sufferers.

MECHANISMS OF ACTION

Dalfampridine is a potassium channel blocker that allows prolongation of action potentials and hence stronger nerve conduction.

Fingolimod is a sphingosine 1-phosphate (S1P) receptor modulator. It ultimately acts by reducing the number of lymphocytes in the CNS and therefore reduces inflammation.

Glatiramer is a synthetic polypeptide that resembles the proteins in the myelin sheath. It is proposed this may cause one or more of the following effects. It can activate T-lymphocyte sup-

pressor cells that would lower T-cell attack, or it may actually be a direct decoy to the T-cell attack.

Memantine is a NMDA-receptor, a type of glutamate receptor, antagonist. Overstimulation of NMDA receptors can initiate apoptosis, or programmed cell death, which can lead to the neurodegeneration. This drug partially blocks the NMDA receptor ion channels, slowing calcium influx and preventing overstimulation and apoptosis of the neurons.

Riluzole is also an NMDA-receptor antagonist that blocks glutamate, sodium channels, and calcium channels.

DOSAGES

DALFAMPRIDINE, for *adults*, for MS, 10 mg bid; for *adults*, .5 mg once a day.

GLATIRAMER, for *adults*, for MS, SubQ: 20 mg daily.

MEMANTINE, for *adults*, for Alzheimer's disease, immediate release: initiate at 5 mg/d, increase by 5 mg/d to a target dose of 20 mg/d, and wait 1 week or more between dose changes;doses over 5 mg/d should be given in 2 doses, extended release: initiate at 7 mg once daily, increase by 7 mg/d to a maximum 28 mg/d, wait 1 week or more between dose changes.

RILUZOLE, for *adults*, for ALS, 50 mg every 12 hours.

ADVERSE EFFECTS

Dalfampridine affects the CNS and can cause insomnia, dizziness, headache, and seizures.

Fingolimod can cause headaches, hepatic enzyme changes, depression, dizziness, and migraines.

Glatiramer has a wide array of ADRs including pain, anxiety, rash, weakness, infection, and fever.

Memantine causes adverse effects that are difficult to separate from those of the disease itself: confusion, agitation, and restlessness.

Riluzole can cause CNS depression, including dizziness, sleepiness, motor weakness, and hepatic and renal impairment.

RED FLAGS

Riluzole may cause neutropenia within the first 2 months of treatment.

INTERACTIONS

INTERACTION ISSUES

A:

D: Fingolimod is more than 99.7% protein bound; riluzole is 96% bound.

M: Riluzole is a major substrate of CYP1A2.

E:

TI:

Pgp:

SECTION 3: NEUROLEPTIC OR ANTIPSYCHOTIC DRUGS

Neuroleptic drugs, also called antischizophrenic drugs, antipsychotic drugs, or sometimes major tranquilizers are primarily used in treating schizophrenia and other psychotic states but can also be used to treat delirium and manic states. In general, the drugs in this category work by blocking dopamine and serotonin receptors. In addition, most drugs in this category have many and serious side effects. They are not curative and do not treat the underlying causes of psychosis but allow the patient to function in a supportive environment. Because of the side effects, it can be difficult for patients to maintain antipsychotic use indefinitely. Patient compliance is a major issue with this class of drugs.

According to the *DSM-IV-TR* (American Psychiatric Association, 2000), psychosis can be defined as a condition with delusions and hallucinations, with or without insight to the pathological nature of the hallucinations. Definitions may also include "positive" schizophrenic signs and symptoms such as disorganized speech and grossly disorganized or catatonic behavior. Major disorders that have psychotic features include schizophrenia, schizophreniform disorder, schizoaffective disorder, delusional disorder, brief psychotic disorder, shared psychotic disorder, psychotic disorder due to a general medical condition, substance-induced psychotic disorder, and psychotic disorder not otherwise specified. Psychotic features may also be present in other disorders but are not considered main features in the condition. Examples of this include dementia and major depressive disorder with psychotic features.

Schizophrenia is a relatively common and

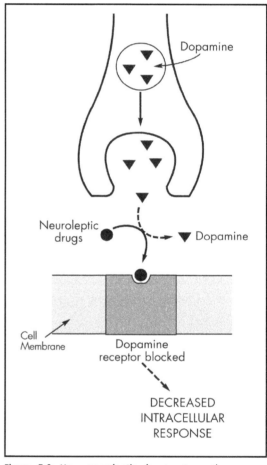

Figure 5.6: How neuroleptic drugs act on the neuron. Neuroleptic drugs engage dopamine receptors and prevent the physiological binding and effects of dopamine.

quite debilitating disorder that may have a prevalence as high as 2% of the population. It affects males more frequently than females, and, for an unknown reason, the patient population has a much higher IQ than the general population. Age of onset is usually late teens through mid-20s. While there is a genetic component to this disease,

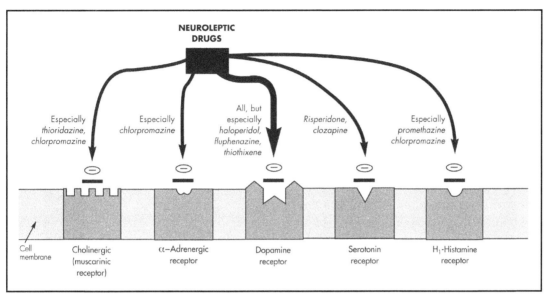

Figure 5.7: The effects of various neuroleptic drugs on specific neural receptors.

it is not clear-cut and does not explain the majority of cases. The actual cause of most cases is unknown, but many theories have been posited.

The classes of drugs vary primarily in their chemical structure. This can cause differences in potencies and factors. However, all the drugs in this section block dopamine receptors in the brain preventing activation of these receptors (see Figure 5.6 on previous page). In this regard they are opposites of antiparkinsonian drugs such as L-dopa. It appears that most of the dopamine-blocking activity is in the mesolimbic system of the brain. This area of the brain is associated with the pleasure feelings from recreational drugs and may play roles in emotions, goal-driven activities, and the ability to learn. Another primary area of action for these drugs is in the basal nuclei, which plays a role in control of posture and **extrapyramidal movements**.

Clinically, neuroleptics are broken down into two classes: typical, or traditional, and atypical. Typical neuroleptics have been used clinically for much longer than atypicals. They tend to have more and more serious side effects especially in regard to extrapyramidal effects. Generally newer, "atypical" antipsychotics also or primarily inhibit serotonin receptors. This may account for the lower incidence of side effects and extrapyramidal effects when compared with the typical neuroleptics. Also most of these drugs will affect other receptors such as cholinergic, α-adrenergic, and H1-histamine receptors. See Figure 5.7 above.

> Extrapyramidal movements: Those movements generally used to maintain posture and other involuntary movements

CLASS 1: FIRST GENERATION, OR TYPICAL, NEUROLEPTICS

CHLORPROMAZINE (klor PROE ma zene) PR=N

DROPERIDOL (droe PER i dole) PR=C

FLUPHENAZINE (floo FEN a zene) PR=N

HALOPERIDOL (ha loe PER i dole) PR=C (Haldol®, Haldol® Decanoate)

LOXAPINE (LOKS a pene) PR=N (Loxitane®)

PERPHENAZINE (per FEN a zene) PR=N

PIMOZIDE (PI moe zide) PR=C (Orap®)

PROCHLORPERAZINE (proe klor PER a zene) (Compro®)

THIORIDAZINE (thye oh RID a zene) PR=C

THIOTHIXENE (thye oh THIKS ene) PR=N

TRIFLUOPERAZINE (trye floo oh PER a zene) PR=N

◼ FUNCTION

This class of drugs is most commonly used for treatment of schizophrenia and psychosis. In IV and IM form, they can be used for the acute treatment of mania. Chlorpromazine, droperidol, perphenazine, and prochlorperazine are used in treating nausea and vomiting. Prochlorperazine and trifluoperazine can be used in anxiety.

Chlorpromazine is also used for treating intractable hiccups. Behavioral symptoms associated with dementia can be treated with thioridazine or trifluoperazine. Pimozide is indicated for the treatment of the motor and phonic tics of Tourette's disorder.

It should be noted that promethazine belongs in this chemical class of drugs; however, it is used primarily for its antihistaminic action and has no therapeutic value as an antipsychotic.

◼ MECHANISMS OF ACTION

This class of agents works primarily by blocking dopamine receptors in the brain preventing activation of these receptors. In this regard they are the opposite of antiparkinsonian drugs such as L-dopa. It appears that most of the dopamine-blocking activity is in the mesolimbic system of the brain. This area of the brain is associated with the pleasure feelings from recreational drugs and may play roles in emotions, goal-driven activities, and the ability to learn. Another primary area of action for these drugs is in the basal nucleus,i which play a role in control of posture and extrapyramidal movements. In addition, these drugs may affect other receptors such as cholinergic, α-adrenergic, and H1-histamine receptors.

Some agents in this class have antiemetic effects; that is they prevent nausea and vomiting. These effects are caused by dopamine blockage within the chemoreceptor trigger zone of the medulla oblongata, which is a vomit center of the brain.

◼ DOSAGES

CHLORPROMAZINE, for *children* 6 months or older, for schizophrenia/psychoses, 0.5-1 mg/kg/dose every 4-6 hours; older children may require 200 mg/d or higher; IM: 0.5-1 mg/kg/dose every 6-8 hours, up to a maximum 40 mg/d for children under 5 years or 22.7 kg or 75 mg/d for 5-12 years or 22.7-45.5 kg; for nausea and vomiting, 0.5-1 mg/kg/ dose every 4-6 hours prn; IM: 0.5-1 mg/kg/dose every 6-8 hours, up to a maximum 40 mg/d for children under 5 years or 22.7 kg or 75 mg/d for 5-12 years or 22.7-45.5 kg. For *adults*, for schizophrenia/psychoses, 30-800 mg/d in 1-4 divided doses; usual dose is 200-600 mg/d, though some patients may need as much as 1-2 g/d; IM: initiate at 25 mg; may repeat 25-50 mg in 1-4 hours; increase to a maximum of 400 mg/dose every 4-6 hours; usual dose range is 300-800 mg/d; for hiccups, oral or IM: use 25-50 mg tid or qid; for nausea and vomiting, 10-25 mg every 4-6 hours; IM: 25-50 mg every 4-6 hours.

DROPERIDOL, for *children* 2-12 years, for prevention of postoperative nausea and vomiting (PONV), IM: 0.1 mg/kg; additional doses may be used with caution to achieve desired effect. For *adults*, for prevention of PONV, IM: initiate at 2.5 mg; additional doses of 1.25 mg may be cautiously administered to achieve desired effect.

FLUPHENAZINE, for *adults*, initiate at 2.5-10 mg/d in divided doses every 6-8 hours, maintain at 1-5 mg/d; for acute therapy, 6-20 mg/d for up to 6 weeks, maintain at 6-12 mg/d; IM: initiate at 1.25 mg; may need 2.5-10 mg/d in divided doses at 6-8 hour intervals; once stabilized, transition to oral maintenance. In the *elderly*, initiate at 1-2.5 mg/d.

HALOPERIDOL, for *children* 3-12 years (15-40 kg), initiate at 0.5 mg/d in 2-3 divided doses, increase by 0.5 mg every 5-7 days up to a maximum of 0.15 mg/kg/d; usual maintenance is 0.05-0.075 mg/kg/d in 2-3 divided doses for nonpsychotic or Tourette's disorder, or 0.05-0.15 mg/kg/d in 2-3 divided doses for psychotic disorders. For *children* 6-12 years, for sedation or psychotic disorders, IM (lactate): 1-3 mg/dose every 4-8 hours up to a maximum of 0.15 mg/kg/d; convert to oral therapy as soon as possible. For *adults*, for psychosis, 0.5-5 mg 2 or 3 times/d, up to a usual maximum of 30 mg/d; IM (lactate): 2-5 mg every 4-8 hours prn; IM (decanoate): initiate at 10-20 times the daily oral dose every 4 weeks, maintenance dose is 10-15 times initial oral dose.

LOXAPINE, for *adults*, 10 mg bid initially; increase dose until psychotic symptoms are controlled within a usual dose range of 20-100 mg/d in 2-4 divided doses, maximum dose is 250 mg/d.

PERPHENAZINE, for *adults*, for schizophrenia, initiate at 4-8 mg tid; reduce to minimum effective dose; maximum dose is 24 mg/d; in hospitalized patients, 8-16 mg 2-4 times per day up to a maximum of 64 mg/d; for nausea and vomiting, 8-16 mg/d in divided doses; reduce to minimum effective dose; maximum dose is 24 mg/d.

PIMOZIDE, for *children* 2-12, for Tourette's disorder, initiate at .05 mg/kg nocte; may increase every 3 days to a usual effective range of 2-4 mg/d; maximum is .2 mg/kg/d or 10 mg/day. For *adults*, for Tourette's disorder, initiate at 1-2 mg/d and increase as needed every other day; maximum dose is 10 mg/d or .2 mg/kg/d. In the *elderly* initiate at 1 mg/d.

PROCHLORPERAZINE, for *children*, as an antiemetic, (therapy >1 day usually not required), not recommended for use in *children* <9 kg or <2 years, 0.4 mg/kg/24 hours in 3-4 divided doses; 9-13 kg, 2.5 mg every 12-24 hours as needed up to a maximum of 7.5 mg/d, 13.1-17 kg, 2.5 mg every 8-12 hours prn up to a maximum of 10 mg/d; 17.1-37 kg, 2.5 mg every 8 hours or 5 mg every 12 hours prn up to a maximum of 15 mg/d; as an antipsychotic (not recommended in *children* <9 kg or <2 years), 2.5 mg 2-3 times/d, do not give more than 10 mg the first day; increase dosage as needed to maximum daily dose of 20 mg for 2-5 years and 25 mg for 6-12 years. For *adults*, 5-10 mg; 3-4 times/d; may require doses as high as 150 mg/d for effectiveness; as an antiemetic, 5-10 mg tid or qid up to a usual maximum of 40 mg/d; for non-psychotic anx-

iety, 15-20 mg/d in divided doses, not to exceed 20 mg/d for longer than 12 weeks.

THIORIDAZINE, for *adults*, for schizophrenic psychosis, initiate at 50-100 mg tid, gradually increasing as tolerated up to a maximum dose of 800 mg/d in 2-4 divided doses.

THIOTHIXENE, for *adults*, for mild-moderate psychosis use 2 mg tid up to 20-30 mg/day; for severe psychosis, initiate at 5 mg bid and increase gradually up to a maximum dose of 60 mg; for rapid tranquilization of an agitated patient, 5-10 mg administered every 30-60 minutes; average total dose for tranquilization is 15-30 mg.

TRIFLUOPERAZINE, for *children* 6-12 years, for schizophrenia/psychoses, in hospitalized or well-supervised patients, initiate at 1 mg 1-2 times/d; gradually increase until symptoms are controlled or adverse effects become troublesome; maximum dose is 15 mg. For *adults*, for schizophrenic psychoses, 1-2 mg bid; for non-psychotic anxiety, 1-2 mg bid with a 6 mg/d maximum; treatment should not exceed 12 weeks.

ADVERSE EFFECTS

Antipsychotic agents have numerous and severe adverse effects that are induced primarily by their numerous effects on non-dopamine receptors or in non-therapeutic areas of the brain. Different agents in this class have different side effect profiles, with some agents more likely to cause certain effects, while others are more likely to cause others. These effects can be broken down as follows:

- Parkinsonian effects–Because this class of drugs is designed to decrease the effects of dopamine, they may induce Parkinson's-like effects including loss of balance, tremors, and other extrapyramidal motor effects. These effects can be reduced with the use of anticholinergic drugs such as benztropine or by using antipsychotic agents with anti-cholinergic action including thioridazine and chlorpromazine. Fluphenazine has low anticholinergic effects and can cause more extrapyramidal motor effects than other drugs in this class.

• Tardive dyskinesia–This motor disorder includes involuntary movements such as lateral jaw movements and "fly-catching" movements of the tongue. Usually occurring after extended use of neuroleptic agents, it can be very disconcerting for the patient. While it can diminish or disappear within 3 months when a patient is taken off of neuroleptic agents, it is often irreversible. Permanence is thought to occur because there is an increased number of dopamine receptors synthesized making the patient hypersensitive to dopamine.

• Anticholinergic effects–Antipsychotics with strong anticholinergic effects such as thioridazine and chlorpromazine may cause such effects as blurred vision, dry mouth, sedation, confusion, constipation, and urinary retention due to inhibition of gastrointestinal and urinary smooth muscle.

• Other effects may include drowsiness especially in early stage administration, lowered blood pressure, orthostatic hypotension, amenorrhea, galactorrhea, infertility, and impotence. Significant weight gain is common.

▨ RED FLAGS

Neuroleptic malignant syndrome can occur with the use of any neuroleptic drugs and may be fatal. Symptoms include muscle rigidity, fever, stupor, unstable blood pressure, and myoglobinemia. Discontinuation of the neuroleptic and possible administration of dantrolene or bromocriptine may be necessary.

▨ INTERACTIONS

DRUG

Chlorpromazine is contraindicated in patients with seizure disorders as it can lower the threshold for seizures. All neuroleptics may aggravate epilepsy.

HERB

ANTIPSYCHOTICS

• *Bing Lang* (Betel nut) (C)–two cases have been reported where concurrent use of *Bing Lang* (in heavy doses and over the long term) and antipsychotic medication has exacerbated extrapyramidal symptoms (Deahl, 1989) Level 4 evidence.

• *Da Fu Pi* (Betel nut peel) (C)–two cases have been reported where concurrent use of *Da Fu Pi* (in heavy doses and over the long term) and antipsychotic medication has exacerbated extrapyramidal symptoms (Deahl, 1989) Level 4 evidence.

DOPAMINE ANTAGONISTS

• *Man Jing Zi* (Vitex, chastetree fruit) (D)– dopamine antagonists may be weakened due to its dopaminergic effects, expert opinions (Blumenthal, 1998; Mills & Bone, 2000) Level 5 evidence.

PHENOTHIAZINES, which include: acetophenazine, chlorpromazine, fluphenazine, mesoridazine, perphenazine, prochlorperazine, thioridazine, and trifluoperazine.

• *Bing Lang* (Betel nut) (D)–may exacerbate cholinergic extrapyrimidal side effects of phenothiazine, expert opinion (Stockley, 1996) Level 5 evidence.

• *Ying Su Ke* (Opium husks) (D)–phenothiazines, monoamine oxidase inhibitors, and tricyclic antidepressants may exacerbate the depressant and CNS suppressive effects of *Ying Su Ke*, expert opinion (Chen & Chen, 2004) Level 5 evidence.

INTERACTION ISSUES

A:

D: Chlorpromazine is 92-97% protein bound; pimozide is 99% bound

M: Chlorpromazine is a major substrate and a moderate inhibitor of CYP2D6; fluphenazine and perphenazine are major substrates of CYP2D6; haloperidol is major substrate and moderate inhibitor of both CYP2D6 and 3A4, pimozide is a major substrate of CYP1A2 and 3A4; thioridazine is a major substrate and a strong inhibitor of CYP2D6; thiothixene and trifluoperazine are major substrates of CYP1A2.

E:

TI:

Pgp:

CLASS 2: SECOND GENERATION, OR ATYPICAL, NEUROLEPTICS

ARIPIPRAZOLE (ay ri PIP ray zole) PR=C
(Abilify®, Abilify Discmelt®)

ASENAPINE (a SEN a pene) PR=C *(Saphris®)*

CLOZAPINE (KLOE za pene) PR=B *(Clozaril®, FazaClo®)*

ILOPERIDONE (eye loe PEAR i done) PR=C *(Fanapt®)*

LURASIDONE (loo RAS i done) PR=B *(Latuda®)*

OLANZAPINE (oh LAN za pene) PR=C
(Symbyax®,[19] Zyprexa®, Zydis®)

PALIPERIDONE (pal ee PER i done) PR=C
(Invega®, Sustenna®)

QUETIAPINE (kwe TYE a pene) PR=C
(Seroquel®, Seroquel XR®)

RISPERIDONE (ris PER i done) PR=C
(Risperadal®, Risperdal® Consta®, Risperdal® M-Tab®)

ZIPRASIDONE (zi PRAY si done) PR=C *(Geodon®)*

FUNCTION

This class of drugs is most commonly used for treatment of schizophrenia and psychosis. In comparison to the "typical" neuroleptics of the previous subclass, these agents tend to have fewer (though still significant) side effects and tend to be more effective in those that have not responded well to the typical agents. Clozapine is generally used only when a patient is unresponsive to other neuroleptic agents because its use is associated with blood dyscrasias. Some of the atypical neuroleptics may be helpful in treating the "negative" symptoms of schizophrenia unlike the typical agents, which primarily work on the positive symptoms and do not alleviate the negative.

Several of the drugs in this class are used for controlling mania in bipolar disorder. Many have off-label uses in treating such diseases as Tourette's syndrome and autism in pediatric cases.

Risperidone was recently approved by the FDA to treat irritability associated with autism in children and adolescents. Behaviors included under the heading of irritability include temper tantrums, deliberate self-harm, and aggression.

MECHANISMS OF ACTION

While the previous class of agents works primarily by blocking dopamine receptors in the brain preventing activation of these receptors, these agents also have significant action to inhibit serotonin receptors. They also have a different profile of inhibiting dopamine receptor subtypes than the typical agents. For example, clozapine has rel-

atively equal affinity for D1 and D2 receptors, while most typical agents work primarily on D2 receptors. In addition, these drugs may affect other receptors such as cholinergic, α-adrenergic, and H1-histamine receptors.

DOSAGES

ARIPIPRAZOLE, for *children,* for bipolar I disorder with acute manic or mixed episodes, for children 10 years or older, to stabilize: initiate at 2 mg once daily for 2 days, then 5 mg once daily for 2 days, then increase to target of 10 mg once daily as monotherapy or as adjunct to lithium or valproic acid; dose increases may be made in 5 mg increments up to a maximum of 30 mg/d; for irritability associated with autistic disorder, for *children* 6 years or older, initiate at 2 mg once daily for 7 days; increase to 5 mg once daily; can increase in 5 mg increments at intervals of 1 week or longer prn; maximum dose is 15 mg/d; for schizophrenia, for *adolescents* 13 years or older, initiate at 2 mg once daily for 2 days, then 5 mg once daily for 2 days, then increase to 10 mg once daily; may increase in 5 mg increments to a maximum dose of 30 mg/d. For *adults,* for acute agitation from schizophrenia or bipolar mania, IM: 9.75 mg as a single dose; typical range is 5.25-15 mg; may repeat at 2-hour or more intervals up to a maximum of 30 mg/d; for bipolar I disorder with acute manic or mixed episodes, to stabilize: for monotherapy, initiate at 15 mg once daily, may increase to 30 mg once daily; as an adjunct to lithium or valproic acid, initiate at 10-15 mg once daily; may increase to 30 mg once daily; for depression (adjunctive with antidepressants), initiate at 2-5 mg/d; typical range is 2-15 mg/d, may increase dose up to 5 mg/d at 1 week or longer intervals; for schizophrenia, 10-15 mg once daily; may increase to a maximum of 30 mg once daily.

ASENAPINE, for *adults*, for schizophrenia, sublingual: initiate at 5 mg bid; may increase to 10 mg bid if tolerated after 1 week; for bipolar disorder, sublingual: for monotherapy, initiate at 10 mg bid; decrease to 5 mg bid if not tolerated; for combination therapy with lithium or valproate, 5 mg bid; may increase to 10 mg bid, if tolerated.

CLOZAPINE, for *adults*, for schizophrenia, initiate at 12.5 mg once or twice daily; increase in increments of 25-50 mg/d as tolerated to a target range of 300-450 mg/d after 2 weeks; may be increased to 600-900 mg/d. For suicidal behavior in schizophrenia or schizoaffective disorder, initiate at 12.5 mg once or twice daily; increase as tolerated in 25-50 mg/d increments to a target range of 300-450 mg/d after 2 weeks; mean dose is approximately 300 mg/d; typical range is 12.5-900 mg. Terminate cautiously; if dosing is interrupted for 48 hours or more, must be restarted at 12.5-25 mg/d; may increase more rapidly than initially; for planned termination, gradual reduction over a 1-2 week period is recommended. For the *elderly*, for schizophrenia, experience is limited; initiate at 12.5-25 mg/d, increase as tolerated by 25 mg/d to desired response; may require slower titration; daily increases may not be tolerated.

ILOPERIDONE, for *adults*, for schizophrenia, initiate at 1 mg bid; recommended range is 6-12 mg bid; increase in 2 mg increments every 24 hours on days 2-7.

LURASIDONE, for *adults*, for schizophrenia, initiate at 40 mg once daily; maximum recommended dose is 160 mg daily.

OLANZAPINE, for *children*, initiate at 2.5 mg/d and increase to maximum 20 mg/d (.12-.29 mg/kg/d). For *adults*, initiate at 5-10 mg once daily, increase to 10 mg daily within 5-7 days and increase 5 mg/d at 1-week intervals to maximum 20 mg/d; maintenance dose ranges from 10-20 mg/d, and while doses of up to 50 mg/d have been used, efficacy and safety have not been established; for acute mania associated with bipolar disorder, initiate at 10-15 mg once daily; may increase 5 mg/d not less than every 24 hours until a maintenance dose of 5-20 mg/d. For the *elderly*, may choose to initiate at a lower dose of 2.5-5 mg/d.

PALIPERIDONE, for *adolescents* 12-17, for schizophrenia, initiate at 3 mg once daily. For *adults*, for schizoaffective disorder, usual dose is 6 mg mane, usual range is 3-12 mg daily; for schizophrenia, usual dose is 6 mg mane, range is 3-12 mg daily; IM: initiate at 234 mg on treatment day 1 followed by 156 mg 1 week later (though can be 3-11 days after), both administered in the deltoid muscle; maintain at 117 mg every month administered in either the deltoid or gluteal muscle; monthly maintenance range is 39-234 mg; the monthly dose may be administered 7 days before or after the 1-month point.

QUETIAPINE, for *children*, for children 10 years and older, for mania in bipolar disorder, immediate release tablet: initiate at 25 mg bid on day 1, increase to 50 mg bid on day 2, and increase by 100 mg/d each day until target of 400 mg/d is reached on day 5; may increase up to 600 mg/d at increments of 100 mg/d or less; usual dose range is 400-600 mg/d; maintain at lowest therapeutic dose and occasionally reassess; for *adolescents* 13 years or older, for schizophrenia, immediate release tablet: initiate at 25 mg bid on day 1, increase to 50 mg bid on day 2, increase 100 mg/d each day until target of 400 mg/d is reached on day 5; may increase up to 800 mg/d at increments 100 mg/d or less, usual range is 400-800 mg/d. For *adults*, for depression of bipolar disorder, for immediate or extended release tablet: initiate at 50 mg once daily the first day, increase to 100 mg once daily on day 2, increase by 100 mg/d each day until a target of 300 mg once daily is reached by day 4; for mania of bipolar disorder, immediate release tablet: initiate at 50 mg bid on day 1, increase by 100 mg/d to 200 mg bid on day 4; may increase to a target of 800 mg/d by day 6 in increments of 200 mg/d or less; usual range is 400-800 mg/d; extended release tablet: initiate at 300 mg on day 1; increase to 600 mg on day 2, and adjust dose to 400-800 mg once daily on day 3; for schizophrenia/psychoses, immediate release tablet: initiate at 25 mg bid, increase total daily dose on the second and third day of 25-50 mg increments divided 2-3 times/d; if tolerated, increase to 300-400 mg/d in 2-3 divided doses by day 4; usual maintenance dose range is 300-800 mg/d; extended-release tablet: initiate at 300 mg once daily, increase by 300 mg/d or less in at least 1-day intervals;usual maintenance range is 400-800 mg/d; for ICU delirium, initiate at 50 mg bid;may increase in increments of 50 mg bid twice daily every day up to a maximum of 400 mg/d. For the *elderly* over 65, usually require 50-200 mg/d of immediate release tablets or 50 mg/d of extended release tablets with a slower titration schedule than adults; increase immediate release dose by 25-50 mg/d or extended release dose by 50 mg/d to effective dose.

RISPERIDONE, for *children* 5 years or older and *adolescents*, 15 to 20 kg, for autism, initiate at 0.25 mg daily; may increase to 0.5 mg daily after at least 4 days; maintain 14 or more days;may increase further by 0.25 mg daily every 2 or more weeks; clinical trials show larger than 1 mg/d doses do not increase therapeutic effect; may be given once a day or divided into two daily doses; 20 kg or over, initiate at 0.5 mg daily; may increase dose to 1 mg after 4 or more days; maintain for at least 14 days; may increase by 0.5 mg daily every 2 or more weeks; clinical trials show that larger than 2.5 mg/d doses (3 mg/d in children over 45 kg) do not increase therapeutic effect; may be given once a day or divided into 2 daily doses. For *children* and *adolescents* 10-17 years, for bipolar mania, initiate at 0.5 mg once daily; may be adjusted by 0.5-1 mg daily every 24 hours or longer to a dose of 1-2.5 mg daily.

For *adolescents* 13-17 years, for schizophrenia, initiate at 0.5 mg once daily; may be increased by 0.5-1 mg daily every 24 or more hours to 3 mg daily. For *adults*, for bipolar mania, recommended starting dose is 2-3 mg once daily; increase by 1 mg daily in every 24 or more hours, if necessary; usual dose range is 1-6 mg daily; for bipolar I maintenance, IM: 25 mg every 2 weeks; some may benefit from doses of 37.5-50 mg; dose changes should not be made more frequently than every 4 weeks; for schizophrenia, initiate at 2 mg daily in 1-2 divided doses; may be increased by 1-2 mg daily every 24 or more hours; recommended dose range is 4-8 mg daily; IM: initiate at 25 mg every 2 weeks; some may benefit from doses of 37.5-50 mg. For *elderly*, initiate at 0.5 mg bid; may increase to 1.5 mg bid in increments of no more than 0.5 mg bid; increases above 1.5 mg bid should occur in at least 1 week intervals; IM: 25 mg every 2 weeks; a lower initial dose of 12.5 mg may be appropriate.

ZIPRASIDONE, for *adults*, for acute bipolar mania, initiate at 40 mg bid; may increase to 60 mg or 80 mg bid on second day of treatment; for schizophrenia, initiate at 20 mg bid; may increase every 2 days or more to a maintenance range of 20-100 mg bid; for acute agitation in schizophrenia, IM: 10 mg every 2 hours or 20 mg every 4 hours up to a maximum of 40 mg/d; oral therapy should replace IM as soon as possible.

ADVERSE EFFECTS

Antipsychotic agents have numerous and severe adverse effects that are induced primarily by their numerous effects on non-dopamine receptors or in non-therapeutic areas of the brain. Different agents in this class have different side effect profiles, with some agents more likely to cause certain effects; others are more likely to cause others. These effects can be broken down as follows:

• Pakinsonian effects–Because this class of drugs is designed to decrease the effects of dopamine, they may induce Parkinson's-like effects including loss of balance, tremors, and other extrapyramidal motor effects. The atypical neuroleptics generally have a lower potential for causing extrapyramidal effects.

- Tardive dyskinesia–This is a motor disorder that includes involuntary movements such as lateral jaw movements and "fly-catching" movements of the tongue. It can be very disconcerting for the patient. It usually occurs after extended use of neuroleptic agents. While it can diminish or disappear within 3 months when a patient is taken off of neuroleptic agents, it is often irreversible. The permanence is thought to occur because of an increased number of dopamine receptors synthesized making the patient hypersensitive to dopamine. Clozapine and risperidone have a lower risk for causing tardive dyskinesia.
- Anticholinergic effects–Antipsychotics with strong anticholinergic effects such as clozapine and olanzapine may cause such effects as blurred vision, dry mouth, sedation, confusion, constipation, and urinary retention due to inhibition of gastrointestinal and urinary smooth muscle.
- Other effects may include drowsiness especially early in administration, lowered blood pressure, orthostatic hypotension, amenorrhea, **galactorrhea**, infertility, and impotence. Significant weight gain is common.

Galactorrhea: Abnormal production and secretion of milk from the breasts or any white discharge from the nipple

Clozapine is contraindicated in patients with seizure disorders as it can lower the threshold for seizures.

▨ RED FLAGS

Neuroleptic malignant syndrome can occur with the use of any neuroleptic drug and may be fatal. Symptoms include muscle rigidity, fever, stupor, unstable blood pressure, and myoglobinemia. Discontinuation of the neuroleptic and possible administration of dantrolene or bromocriptine may be necessary.

An FDA Boxed Warning indicates that patients taking atypical antipsychotics for treating dementia-related behavioral disorders resulted in an increased risk of death when compared with a placebo, and they should not be used for this purpose.

According to an FDA Dear Healthcare Provider letter, monitoring of WBCs is necessary when taking clozapine.

▨ INTERACTIONS

All neuroleptics may aggravate epilepsy.

DRUG

Should not be used with citalopram.

HERB

ANTIPSYCHOTICS

- *Bing Lang* (Betel nut) (C)–two cases have been reported where concurrent use of *Bing Lang* (in heavy doses and over the long term) and antipsychotic medication has exacerbated extrapyramidal symptoms (Deahl, 1989) Level 4 evidence.
- *Da Fu Pi* (Betel nut peel) (C)–two cases have been reported where concurrent use of *Da Fu Pi* (in heavy doses and over the long term) and antipsychotic medication has exacerbated extrapyramidal symptoms (Deahl, 1989) Level 4 evidence.

DOPAMINE ANTAGONISTS

- *Man Jing Zi* (Vitex, chastetree fruit) (D)–dopamine antagonists may be weakened due to its dopaminergic effects, expert opinions (Blumenthal, 1998; Mills & Bone, 2000) Level 5 evidence.

CLOZAPINE, OLANZEPINE, QUETIAPINE

- *Chai Hu* (Bupleurum), *Che Qian Zi* (Plantago seed), *Shu/Sheng Di Huang* (Rehmannia), *Wu Wei Zi* (Schisandra), *Zhi Zi* (Gardenia), *Mu Tong* (Akebia) (B)–a large epidemiological study (n=1795) showed increased adverse effects in patients taking *chai hu, zhi zi, wu wei zi, shu/sheng di huang, mu tong*, and *che qian zi* with clozapine, quetiapine, or olanzapine (Zhang, Tan *et al.*, 2011) Level 2c evidence.
- *Guan Ye Lian Qiao* (St. John's wort) (C)–a single case of a schizophrenic woman stabilized on clozapine displayed deterioration in her condition after self-administering St. John's wort (Van Strater & Bogers, 2012) Level 3b evidence.

RISPERIDONE

- *Yin Guo Ye* (Gingko) (D)–clinical cases indicate interactions of ginkgo with antiepileptics, aspirin (acetylsalicylic acid), diuretics, ibuprofen, risperidone, rofecoxib, trazodone, and warfarin (Izzo & Ernst, 2009) Level 4 evidence.

INTERACTION ISSUES

A:

D: Aripiprazole is 99% or greater protein bound; asenapine is 95% bound; clozapine is 97% bound; iloperidone is approximately 95% bound; lurasidone is approximately 99% bound; ziprasidone is over 99% bound.

M: aripiprazole is a major substrate of CYP2D6 and 3A4; asenapine is a major substrate of CYP1A2; clozapine is a major substrate of CYP1A2 and a moderate inhibitor of 2D6; iloperidone is a major substrate of CYP2D6; lurasidone and quetiapine are major substrates of CYP3A4; risperidone is a major substrate of CYP2D6.

E:

TI:

Pgp: Paliperidone and risperidone are substrates of Pgp.

SECTION 4: ANXIOLYTIC AND HYPNOTIC DRUGS

BARBITURATES:

AMOBARBITAL (am oh BAR bi tal) PR=D
 (Amytal®)

BUTABARBITAL (byoo ta BAR bi tal) PR=D
 (Butisol Sodium®)

BUTALBITAL (byoo TAL bi tal) PR=C *(Alagesic LQ,[3] Anolor 300,[3] Ascomp® with Codeine, Dolgic® Plus,[3] Esgic®,[3] Esgic-Plus™,[3] Fioricet®,[3] Fioricet® with Codeine,[12] Fiorinal®, Fiorinal® with Codeine, Margesic,[3] Orbivan™,[3] Orviban® CF,[4] Phrenilin® Forte,[4] Promacet,[4] Repan®,[3] Sedapap®,[4] Zebutal®[3])*

PHENOBARBITAL (fe no BAR bi tal) PR=B or D *(Pregnancy rating depends on manufacturer*

PRIMIDONE (PRI mi done) PR=D *(Mysoline®)*

SECOBARBITAL (see koe BAR bi tal) PR=D
 (Seconal®)

BENZODIAZEPINES:

ALPRAZOLAM (al PRAY zoe lam) PR=D
 (Alprazolam Intensol™, Niravam™, Xanax®, Xanax XR®)

CHLORDIAZEPOXIDE (klor dye az e POKS ide) PR=D *(Limbrax®[5])*

CLOBAZAM (KLOE ba zam) *(Onfi™)*

CLONAZEPAM (kloe NA ze pam) PR=D
 (Klonopin®)

CLORAZEPATE (klor AZ e pate) PR=D
 (Tranxene® T-Tab®)

DIAZEPAM (dye AZ e pam) PR=D *(Diastat®, Diastat® AcuDial®, Diazepam Intensol®, Valium®)*

ESTAZOLAM (es TA zoe lam) PR=X

FLURAZEPAM (flure AZ e pam)

LORAZEPAM (lor A ze pam) PR=D *(Ativan®, Lorazepam Intensol™)*

MIDAZOLAM (MID aye zoe lam) PR=D

OXAZEPAM (oks A ze pam) PR=C or D*

QUAZEPAM (KWAY ze pam) PR=X *(Doral®)*

TEMAZEPAM (te MAZ e pam) PR=X *(Restoril®)*

TRIAZOLAM (trye AY zoe lam) PR=X *(Halcion®)*

OTHER ANXIOLYTIC AND HYPNOTIC AGENTS:

ANTIHISTAMINES *(See Chapter 8, Section 2)*

BUSPIRONE (byoo SPYE rone) PR=B

CHLORAL HYDRATE PR=C *(Somnote®)*

ESZOPICLONE (es zoe PIK lone) PR=C
 (Lunesta®)

MEPROBAMATE (me proe BA mate) PR=N

RAMELTEON (ra MEL tee on) PR=C *(Rozerem®)*

ZALEPLON (ZAL e plon) PR=C *(Sonata®)*

ZOLPIDEM (zole PI dem) PR=C *(Ambien®, Ambien CR®, Edluar™, Intermezzo®, Zolpimist®)*

*Depending on the source, Oxazepam is given a pregnancy rating of C or D or none. In the author's opinion, it should be considered category D as are most benzodiazepines.

Anxiety is an unpleasant state of fear, apprehension, uneasiness, or tension that may come from an unknown source or have a known trigger. It usually involves some sympathetic activation and may have symptoms such as tachycardia, palpitations, sweating, and trembling. This category of pharmaceutical agents helps to counteract anxiety as well as insomnia.

Anxiety disorders include panic attacks, phobias, obsessive-compulsive disorder, post-traumatic stress disorder, acute stress disorder, generalized anxiety disorder, anxiety due to a medical condition, and substance-induced anxiety disorder.

FUNCTION

The word anxiolytic means "splitting anxiety," and most of the agents in this category have this effect of breaking down anxiety. Hypnotics as a class of drugs help people sleep. Another name for hypnotic is sedative. Most hypnotics have anxiolytic effect,s and most anxiolytics can cause drowsiness. In the case of benzodiazepines, each agent has a similar mechanism of action but based on its strength and length of duration can fall into either category. Benzodiazepines can be used to induce relaxation of muscles and are used as anticonvulsants. In summary, benzodiazepines can be effective in treating anxiety disorders, muscular disorders, seizures, and sleep disorders.

Another use of benzodiazepines is in causing anterograde amnesia. Important before anxiety-producing or unpleasant procedures, this causes a form of conscious sedation where the patient can still respond to instructions during the procedure but does not remember the procedure.

Barbiturates are predominantly hypnotic and for the most part, due to their induction of physical dependence and severe **withdrawal** symptoms, have been supplanted by the benzodiazepines. Here we only discuss oral barbiturates, but they are also available in injectable form. Thiopental is an injectable barbiturate that is commonly used as an **anesthetic**.

Eszopiclone, ramelteon, zaleplon, and zolpidem are often used as hypnotics,

Withdrawal: The psychological and/or physical syndrome caused by abrupt cessation of the use of a drug in a habituated individual

Anesthetic: A drug that reversibly decreases nerve function and causes loss of ability to perceive pain and/or other sensations

while buspirone is an anxiolytic. Chloral hydrate and antihistamines such as diphenhydramine and doxylamine are sedative in nature. The antihistamines will be covered more thoroughly in Chapter 8.

Clobazam is used as adjunctive treatment for seizures associated with Lennox-Gastaut syndrome, a severe form of epilepsy.

MECHANISMS OF ACTION

BENZODIAZEPINES

GABA is a neurotransmitter that induces hyperpolarization by opening a Cl- channe, which in turn causes an inhibitory postsynaptic potential (IPSP), and is primarily found in the CNS. Benzodiazepines bind to a specific benzodiazepine receptor that is adjacent to the postsynaptic GABA membrane receptors and increases the affinity of GABA for its receptors. This increased affinity causes more GABA action, increased Cl- ion influx, enhanced IPSP, and more neuronal inhibition than GABA alone. This is shown in Figure 5.8.

BARBITURATES

Barbiturates work similarly to benzodiazepines in that they enhance GABA binding to its receptors. They do not, however, do so by binding to benzodiazepine receptors as they actually make benzodiazepine binding easier rather than displacing them. They work by prolonging the length of time that Cl- channels are open rather than increasing the frequency of their opening as benzodiazepines do. In lower concentrations, barbiturates appear to reduce the excitatory effects of the neurotransmitter glutamate. At anesthetic concentrations, they suppress the opening of Na^+ channels, and at higher concentrations, K^+ channel conductance is reduced.

OTHER ANXIOLYTIC AND HYPNOTIC AGENTS

Buspirone has a completely different mechanism than benzodiazepines or barbiturates. It is a partial serotonin receptor agonist, does not have anticonvulsant activity, and does not cause **tolerance** or **dependence**. It is also not effective for panic attacks or OCD. Eszopiclone, ramelteon, zaleplon, and zolpidem are benzodiazepine receptor agonists. Although they do not resemble benzodiazepines, they do act on their receptors but show more sedative than anxiolytic effects. They have only weak anticonvulsant effects and do not appear to cause tolerance or withdrawal symptoms.

Chloral hydrate probably works by having barbiturate-like effects from one of its metabolites, trichloroethanol.

DOSAGES

ALPRAZOLAM, for *adults*, for anxiety, immediate release: initiate at .25-.5 mg tid; may increase every 3-4 days up to a usual maximum of 4 mg/d; for panic disorder, immediate release: initiate at .5 mg tid; may increase every 3-4 days by less than or equal to 1 mg/d; mean effective dose is 5-6 mg/d, though some patients may need as much as 10 mg/d; extended release: .5-1 mg once daily; may increase every 3 to 4 days by less than or equal to 1 mg per day up to a usual dose range of 3-6 mg/d. For the *elderly*, immediate release: initiate at .25 mg bid or tid;extended release: initiate at .5 mg once daily.

AMOBARBITAL, for *children* 6-12, IM: 65-500 mg. For *adults*, as a hypnotic, IM: 65-200 mg nocte, up to a maximum single dose of 1000 mg; as a sedative, IM: 30-50 mg bid or tid up to a maximum single dose of 1000 mg.

BUSPIRONE, for *children* over 6 and *adolescents*, for GAD, initiate at 5 mg bid; increase 5 mg/d

> **Tolerance:** The need for increasing doses of a substance in order to maintain the same effect or to avoid negative symptoms

> **Dependence:** The psychological and physical need for a substance

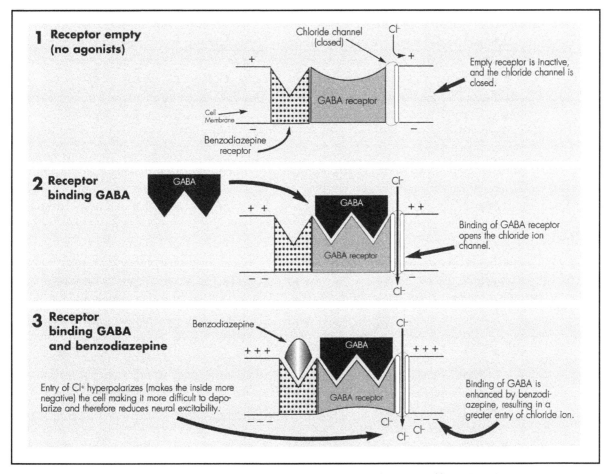

Figure 5.8: GABA receptor attenuation due to the presence of a benzodiazepine. 1: The GABA and benzodiazepine receptors are empty, and the adjacent chlorine ion channel is closed. **2:** GABA binding to its receptor causes the chlorine ion channel to open and an influx of chlorine ions. **3:** When the benzodiazepine receptor is bound to a benzodiazepine in addition to GABA binding, the chlorine ion channel allows an even greater influx of chlorine ions (and consequent hyperpolarization) than the GABA-GABA receptor complex alone.

every 2-3 days prn; up to 20-30 mg/d and maximum 60 mg/d divided into 2-3 doses. For *adults*, for GAD, 7.5 mg bid; may increase 5 mg per day every 2-3 days to a maximum of 60 mg per day; target dose for most people is 10-15 mg bid. For the *elderly*, initiate at 5 mg bid; increase by 5 mg/d every 2-3 days prn up to target dose of 20-30 mg/d and a maximum daily dose of 60 mg/d.

BUTABARBITAL, for *children*, for preoperative sedation, 2-6 mg/kg/dose up to a maximum of 100 mg. For *adults*, as a sedative, 15-30 mg tid or qid; as a hypnotic, 50-100 mg nocte; for preop, 50-100 mg 1-1.5 hours before surgery.

BUTALBITAL is used in combination with other drugs and therefore does not have an individual dosing regimen.

CHLORAL HYDRATE, for *children*, for sedation or anxiety, 5-15 mg/kg/dose every 8 hours up to a maximum of 500 mg per dose; prior to an EEG, 20-25 mg/kg/dose, 30-60 minutes prior to EEG; may repeat in 30 minutes up to a maximum of 100 mg/kg or 2 g total; as a hypnotic, 20-40 mg/kg/dose up to a maximum of 50 mg/kg/d or 1 g or 2 g dose per day; for conscious sedation, 50-75 mg/kg/dose 30-60 minutes before procedure; may repeat in 30 minutes prn up to a total maximum dose of 120 mg/kg or 1 g total. For *adults*, for sedation or anxiety, 250 mg tid; as a hypnotic, 500-1000 mg nocte or 30 minutes prior to procedure, not to exceed 2 g per day. For the *elderly*, as a hypnotic 250 mg nocte.

CHLORDIAZEPOXIDE, for *children*, under 6 years, not recommended; over 6 years, for anxiety, 5 mg 2-4 times/d; may be increased to 10 mg bid or tid in some patients. For *adults*, for mild to moderate anxiety, usual dose of 5-10 mg tid or qid; for severe anxiety, 20-25 mg tid or qid; for preoperative anxiety, 5-10 mg tid or qid on the days preceding surgery; for ethanol withdrawal symptoms, initiate at 50-100 mg; may be repeated in 2-4 hours as necessary up to a maximum of 300 mg per day. For the *elderly*, 5 mg 2-4 times per day; avoid use if possible due to long-acting metabolite.

CLOBAZAM, for *adults* and *children* 2 and older, for adjunctive treatment of Lennox-Gastaut syndrome, for patients 30 kg and smaller, initiate at 5 mg once daily for at least 1 week, increase to 5 mg bid for at least 1 week, and then to 10 mg bid; for patients over 30 kg, initiate at 5 mg bid for at least 1 week, increase to 10 mg bid for at least 1 week, then to 20 mg bid. For the *elderly*, for adjunctive treatment of Lennox-Gastaut syndrome, for patients 30 kg and smaller, initiate at 5 mg once daily for at least 2 weeks, increase to 5 mg bid for at least 1 week; may increase to 10 mg bid; for patients over 30 kg, initiate at 5 mg once daily for at least 1 week, increase to 5 mg bid for at least 1 week, and then to 10 mg bid; after at least 1 week, may increase to 20 mg bid.

CLONAZEPAM, for *children* under 10 years or 30 kg, for seizure disorders, initiate at 0.01-0.03 mg/kg/d up to a maximum 0.05 mg/kg/d given in 2-3 divided doses; increase by no more than 0.5 mg every third day until seizures are controlled or adverse effects seen; usual maintenance dose is 0.1-0.2 mg/kg/d divided 3 times/d, not to exceed 0.2 mg/kg/d. For *adults* and *children* over 10 or >30 kg, for seizure disorders, initiate at .5 mg tid, may increase by 0.5-1 mg every third day until seizures are controlled or adverse effects seen up to a maximum of 20 mg/d; usual maintenance dose is 0.05-0.2 mg/kg; for panic disorder, 0.25 mg bid; increase in increments of 0.125-0.25 mg bid every 3 days to a target dose of 1 mg/d with a maximum of 4 mg/d.

CLORAZEPATE, for *children* 9-12 years, as an anticonvulsant, initiate at 3.75-7.5 mg/dose bid; increase dose by 3.75 mg weekly, not to exceed 60 mg/d in 2-3 divided doses. For *children* >12 years and *adults*, as an anticonvulsant, initiate at 7.5 mg/dose 2-3 times/d;increase dose by 7.5 mg weekly, not to exceed 90 mg/d. For *adults*, for anxiety, 7.5-15 mg 2-4 times per day; for ethanol withdrawal, initiate at 30 mg, then 15 mg 2-4 times per day on first day; maximum daily dose is 90 mg;gradually decrease dose.

DIAZEPAM, for *children*, for conscious sedation for procedures, 0.2-0.3 mg/kg up to a maximum of 10 mg, 45-60 minutes prior to procedure; for sedation/muscle relaxation/anxiety, 0.12-0.8 mg/kg/d in divided doses every 6-8 hours; IM: .04-0.3 mg/kg every 2-4 hours up to maximum of 0.6 mg/kg within an 8-hour period; for febrile seizure prophylaxis, 1 mg/kg/d divided every 8 hours; initiate at first sign of fever and continue for 24 hours after fever resolution; for muscle spasms associated with tetanus, IM: for *infants* over 30 days and *children* under 5, 1-2 mg every 3-4 hours prn; for *children* 5 years or over, 5-10 mg every 3-4 hours prn. For *adolescents*, conscious sedation for procedures, 10 mg. For *adults*, for acute ethanol withdrawal, 10 mg tid or qid during first 24 hours, then decrease to 5 mg tid or qid prn; for anxiety, oral or IM: 2-10 mg 2-4 times per day; for muscle spasms, IM: initiate at 5-10 mg, then 5-10 mg in 3-4 hours prn; larger doses may be required if associated with tetanus; as adjunct therapy as a skeletal muscle relaxant, 2-10 mg tid or qid; for rapid tranquilization of agitated patient, 5-10 mg given every 30-60 minutes; average total dose is 20-60 mg. For the *elderly*, initiate at 2-2.5 mg 1-2 times/d, may increase gradually as needed and tolerated.

ESTAZOLAM, for *adults*, 1 mg nocte; some patients may require 2 mg; start at doses of 0.5 mg in debilitated or small *elderly* patients.

ESZOPICLONE, for *adults*, for insomnia, initiate at 2 mg nocte up to a maximum dose of 3 mg. For the *elderly*, for difficulty falling asleep, initiate at 1 mg nocte up to a maximum dose of 2 mg; for difficulty staying asleep, 2 mg nocte.

FLURAZEPAM, for *children* >15 years, 15 mg nocte. For *adults*, 15-30 mg nocte. For the *elderly*, 15 mg nocte.

LORAZEPAM, for *children* over 12, for anxiety, sedation, and procedural amnesia usual dose is 0.05 mg/kg with a range of 0.02-0.09 mg/kg every 4-8 hours. For *adults*, as an antiemetic, 0.5-2 mg every 4-6 hours prn; for anxiety, sedation, and procedural amnesia, 1-10 mg

per day in 2-3 divided doses; usual dose is 2-6 mg per day or 1-2 mg 1 hr before procedure; for insomnia, 2-4 mg nocte. For the *elderly*, for anxiety, sedation, and procedural amnesia, 1-2 mg per day in divided doses.

MEPHOBARBITAL, for *children*, for epilepsy, 6-12 mg/kg/d in 2-4 divided doses; for sedation, <5 years, 16-32 mg 3-4 times/d; >5 years, 32-64 mg 3-4 times/d. For *adults*, for epilepsy, 200-600 mg/d in 2-4 divided doses; for sedation, 32-100 mg 3-4 times/d.

MEPROBAMATE, for *children*, 6-12 years, for anxiety, 200-600 mg per day in 2-3 doses.

MIDAZOLAM, for *children*, for preoperative or preprocedural sedation, 0.25-0.5 mg/kg as a single dose preprocedure, up to maximum 20 mg, administered 20-30 minutes prior to procedure; *children* under 6 may require as much as 1 mg/kg as a single dose while in *children* 6-16 years of age 0.25 mg/kg may suffice; IM: 0.1-0.15 mg/kg 30-60 minutes before procedure; usual range is 0.05-0.15 mg/kg; maximum dose is 10 mg. For *adults*, for preoperative or preprocedural sedation, IM: 0.07-0.08 mg/kg 30-60 minutes prior to procedure; usual dose is 5 mg. For the *elderly*, for preoperative or preprocedural sedation, IM: 2-3 mg or 0.02-0.05 mg/kg 30-60 minutes prior to procedure.

OXAZEPAM, for *adults*, for anxiety, 10-30 mg tid or qid; for ethanol withdrawal, 15-30 mg tid or qid; as a hypnotic, 15-30 mg. For the *elderly*, for anxiety, 10 mg bid or tid; increase gradually as needed to a total of 30-45 mg/d.

PENTOBARBITAL, for *children*, as a hypnotic or sedative, 100 mg IM. For *adults*, as a hypnotic or sedative, 150-200 mg IM.

PHENOBARBITAL, for *children*, for sedation, 2 mg/kg tid; for preoperative sedation, oral or IM: 1-3 mg/kg 1-1.5 hours before operation; for anticonvulsant maintenance, for *infants*, 5-8mg/kg/d in 1-2 doses; for *children* 1-5, 6-8 mg/kg/d in 1-2 doses; for *children* 5-12, 4-6 mg/kg/d in 1-2 doses; for *children* over 12, 1-3 mg/kg/d in divided doses or 50-100 mg bid or tid. For *adults*, for sedation, oral or IM: 30-120 mg/d in 2-3 doses; for preoperative sedation, IM: 100-200 mg 1-1.5 hours before operation; as an anticonvulsant or for **status epilepticus,** after an IV loading dose, the maintenance oral dose is 1-3 mg/kg/d in divided doses or 50-100 mg bid or tid.

PRIMIDONE, for seizure disorders, for *children* under 8, initiate at 50 mg nocte days 1-3; for days 4-6, 50 mg bid; for days 7-9, 100 mg bid; usual dose is 375-750 mg/d in 3-4 divided doses. For seizure disorders, for *children* over 8 and *adults*, 100-125 mg/d nocte days 1-3; 100-125 bid days 4-6; 100-125 mg tid days 7-9; usual dose is 750-1500 mg/d in divided doses 3-4 times/d with maximum 2 g/d.

QUAZEPAM, for *adults*, initiate at 15 mg nocte; may be reduced to 7.5 mg after a few nights.

RAMELTEON, for *adults*, as a hypnotic, one 8 mg tablet within 30 minutes of bedtime.

SECOBARBITAL, for *children*, for preoperative sedation, 2-6 mg/kg up to a maximum dose of 100 mg/dose, 1-2 hours before operation; for sedation, 6 mg/kg/d divided every 8 hours. For *adults*, as a hypnotic, usual dose range 100 mg nocte, usual range of 100-200 mg/d.

TEMAZEPAM, for *adults*, 15-30 mg nocte. For *elderly* or debilitated patients, initiate at 7.5 mg nocte.

TRIAZOLAM, for *adults*, as a hypnotic, 0.125-0.25 mg nocte; maximum dose 0.5 mg per day; for the *elderly*, for short-term use for insomnia, 0.125 mg nocte; maximum dose 0.25 mg per day.

ZALEPLON, for *adults*, for insomnia, 10 mg nocte; usual range is 5-20 mg. For *elderly*, 5 mg nocte; maximum dose 10 mg/d.

ZOLPIDEM, for *adults*, for insomnia, 10 mg nocte, extended release: 12.5 mg nocte; sublingual: women, 1.75 mg nocte prn; men, 3.5 mg nocte prn. For *elderly*, 5 mg nocte; extended release: 6.25 mg nocte; sublingual: 1.75 mg nocte prn.

■ ADVERSE EFFECTS

The biggest adverse effects in this category are those of psychological and physical dependence, tolerance, and withdrawal. In addition, rebound insomnia, where insomnia becomes worse upon termination, can result after using these agents. Drowsiness and confusion are also common side effects of these agents.

Benzodiazepines can cause decreased long-term recall and acquisition of new knowledge, weakness, headache, blurred vision, vertigo, nausea and vomiting, epigastric distress, diarrhea, joint pains, chest pains, and incontinence. At high doses, they can cause **ataxia**.

Barbiturates have varied and profound adverse effects, which is the main reason benzodiazepines have largely replaced them in common use. These effects include the common adverse effects above as well as fine motor impairment, vertigo, nausea and vomiting, diarrhea, irritability, and "drug hangover," a feeling of tiredness after the patient awakes with possible nausea and dizziness. They can cause addiction and withdrawal that can be life threatening and includes tremors, nausea and vomiting, seizures, delirium, and cardiac arrest. Overdosage has been the leading cause of death among drug overdoses for decades and can cause severe depression of respiration and the cardiovascular system.

Chloral hydrate is a gastrointestinal irritant and can cause epigastric distress, nausea and vomiting, and an unpleasant taste. In addition, it can cause light-headedness, malaise, ataxia, and nightmares. While less likely than when using barbiturates, a drug hangover may occur. Rapid withdrawal may cause delirium, seizures, and death.

Eszopiclone can cause headache, digestive complaints, abnormal dreams, itching, and unpleasant taste. Tolerance has not been ruled out.

Zolpidem can cause nightmares, gastrointestinal upset, agitation, headache, dizziness, and daytime drowsiness. Late-night administration may result in morning sedation, delayed reaction time, and **anterograde amnesia**.

Zaleplon has similar side effects as placebos. As a relatively new drug, however, it may develop a more comprehensive adverse effect profile may develop over time.

Buspirone can cause headaches, dizziness, nervousness, and light-headedness. Sedation and cognitive dysfunction are minimal, and dependence is uncommon.

Status epilepticus: A potentially fatal state where seizures follow one another without any refractory period in between

Ataxia: Incoordination of voluntary muscles resulting in jerky movements that may affect the limbs, head, or trunk

Anterograde amnesia: Loss of memory of events after a trauma, disease, or agent is consumed

RED FLAGS

The biggest red flag in this category of drugs is that of dependence. It is important to reduce dosage of these agents slowly.

While overdosage of barbiturates is a common cause of death, overdosage of benzodiazepines very rarely results in death unless alcohol or other sedatives are involved.

Barbiturates can cause allergic reactions and tend to be more common in those patients who have asthma, **urticaria**, and **angioedema**. In addition, barbiturates may cause serious respiratory difficulty in patients with pulmonary insufficiency.

Rarely, patients who chronically use chloral hydrate may exhibit sudden, acute intoxification from an overdose or hepatic damage. This can be fatal. Renal injury may also occur.

INTERACTIONS

Many of these agents have additive effects to one another and to alcohol and should not be taken together except under physician supervision.

DRUG

The use of benzodiazepines and valproate may cause psychotic episodes.

The use of barbiturates with isoniazid, methylphenidate, and MAOIs may increase CNS depressant effects.

Due to increased hepatic enzyme induction, oral contraceptives may be more rapidly metabolized and therefore their effects reduced when co-administered with phenobarbital.

HERB

ALPRAZOLAM
• *Guan Ye Lian Qiao* (St. John's wort) (C)–decreases blood concentrations (Izzo & Ernst, 2009) Level 2b evidence.

ANTICONVULSANTS
• *Yin Guo Ye* (Gingko leaf) (D)–may precipitate epileptic seizures (Gruenwald, Brendler & Jaenicke, 2004) Level 5 evidence.

ANTISEIZURE DRUGS
• *Chen Pi* (Tangerine peel), *Qing Pi* (Citrus Viride), *Zhi Ke* (Aurantium fruit), *Zhi Shi* (Aurantium immaturus) (Indeterminate)–

contains constituents that stimulate the sympathetic nervous system and should be used with caution in those taking antihypertensives, antidiabetic, antihyperthyroid, and/or antiseizure medications (Chinese language article cited in Chen & Chen, 2004) Indeterminate level of evidence.

BARBITURATES
• *Bai He* (Lily bulb) (Indeterminate)–shown to increase sleeping time induced by barbiturates (Chinese language article cited in Chen & Chen, 2004) Indeterminate level of evidence.
• *Bai Jiang Cao* (Dahurian patrinia herb) (Indeterminate)–has a sedative effect and may increase sedative effects of drugs (Chinese language article cited in Chen & Chen, 2004) Indeterminate level of evidence.
• *Bai Shao* (White peony root) (Indeter-minate)–has a sedative and analgesic effect and may increase sedative effects of drugs (Chinese language article cited in Chen & Chen, 2004) Indeterminate level of evidence.
• *Chan Tui* (Cicada moulting) (Indeterminate)–has an inhibitory effect on the CNS potentiating sedative drugs (Chinese language article cited in Chen & Chen, 2004) Indeterminate level of evidence.
• *Gan Cao* (Licorice) (Indeterminate)–may treat overdoses by increasing the metabolism of certain drugs such as barbiturates, chloral hydrate, urethane, cocaine, picrotoxin, pilocarpine, nicotine, and caffeine (Chinese language article cited in Chen & Chen, 2004) Indeterminate level of evidence.
• *Hu Po* (Amber) (Indeterminate)–potentiates barbiturate's sedative effect (Chinese language article cited in Chen & Chen, 2004) Indeterminate level of evidence.
• *Jiao Gu Lan* (Gynostemma) (Indeterminate)–has sedative, hypnotic, and analgesic effects and may increase sedative effects of drugs (Chinese language article cited in Chen & Chen, 2004) Indeterminate level of evidence.
• *Lang Dan Cao* (Gentiana) (Indeterminate)–

Urticaria: Skin condition consisting of wheals, usually the result of hypersensitivity; commonly called hives

Angioedema: Large circumscribed area of subcutaneous edema of sudden onset frequently caused by an allergic reaction

has a sedative effect and may increase sedative effects of drugs (Chinese language article cited in Chen & Chen, 2004) Indeterminate level of evidence.

- *Niu Huang* (Cow gallstone) (Indeterminate)–has a mild sedative effect and may increase sedative effects of drugs (Chinese language article cited in Chen & Chen, 2004) Indeterminate level of evidence.
- *Qin Jiao* (Gentiana macrophylla root) (Indeterminate)–has an inhibitory effect on the CNS potentiating sedative drugs (Chinese language article cited in Chen & Chen, 2004) Indeterminate level of evidence.
- *Shen*-calming medicinals (D)–may have marked sedative and tranquilizing effects and may increase sedative effects of drugs, expert opinion (Chen & Chen, 2004) Level 5 evidence.
- *Suan Zao Ren* (Zizyphus) (Indeterminate)–has sedative and hypnotic effects and may increase sedative effects of barbiturates (Chinese language article cited in Chen & Chen, 2004) Indeterminate level of evidence.
- *Tian Ma* (Gastrodia) (Indeterminate)–potentiates barbiturates' sedative effect (Chinese language article cited in Chen & Chen, 2004) Indeterminate level of evidence.
- *Tian Nan Xing* (Arisaema) (Indeterminate)–has a marked sedative and analgesic effect and may increase sedative effects of drugs (Chinese language article cited in Chen & Chen, 2004) Indeterminate level of evidence.
- *Wu Jia Pi* (Acanthopanax) (Indeterminate)–has a mild sedative effect and may increase sedative effects of drugs (Chinese language article cited in Chen & Chen, 2004) Indeterminate level of evidence.
- *Xi Jiao* (Rhinoceros horn) (Indeterminate)–has a sedative effect and may increase sedative effects of drugs (Chinese language article cited in Chen & Chen, 2004) Indeterminate level of evidence.
- *Xie Cao* (Valerian root) (Indeterminate)–potentiates barbiturates' sedative effect (Chinese language article cited in Chen & Chen, 2004) Indeterminate level of evidence.

- *Zhi Zi* (Gardenia, cape jasmine fruit) (Indeterminate)–has a sedative effect and may increase sedative effects of drugs (Chinese language article cited in Chen & Chen, 2004) Indeterminate level of evidence.

BENZODIAZEPINES

- *Bai Jiang Cao* (Dahurian patrinia herb) (Indeterminate)–has a sedative effect and may increase sedative effects of drugs (Chinese language article cited in Chen & Chen, 2004) Indeterminate level of evidence.
- *Bai Shao* (White peony root) (Indeterminate)–has a sedative and analgesic effect and may increase sedative effects of drugs (Chinese language article cited in Chen & Chen, 2004) Indeterminate level of evidence.
- *Chan Tui* (Cicada moulting) (Indeterminate)–has an inhibitory effect on the CNS potentiating sedative drugs (Chinese language article cited in Chen & Chen, 2004) Indeterminate level of evidence.
- *Dan Shen* (Salvia root) (D)–high-dose extracts of a single constituent strongly inhibited benzodiazepine receptor binding by flunitazepam in vitro; highest dose reversed some effects of diazepam in mice (Lee, Wong, Chui, Choang, Hon & Chang, 1991) Level 5 evidence.
- *Jiao Gu Lan* (Gynostemma) (Indeterminate)–has a sedative, hypnotic, and analgesic effects and may increase sedative effects of drugs (Chinese language article cited in Chen & Chen, 2004) Indeterminate level of evidence.
- *Lang Dan Cao* (Gentiana) (Indeterminate)–has a sedative effect and may increase sedative effects of drugs (Chinese language article cited in Chen & Chen, 2004) Indeterminate level of evidence.
- *Niu Huang* (Cow gallstone) (Indeterminate)–has a mild sedative effect and may increase sedative effects of drugs (Chinese language article cited in Chen & Chen, 2004) Indeterminate level of evidence.
- *Qin Jiao* (Gentiana macrophylla root) (Indeterminate)–has an inhibitory effect on the CNS potentiating sedative drugs (Chinese

language article cited in Chen & Chen, 2004) Indeterminate level of evidence.

- *Shen*-calming herbs (D)–may have marked sedative and tranquilizing effects and may increase sedative effects of drugs, expert opinion (Chen & Chen, 2004) Level 5 evidence.
- *Tian Ma* (Gastrodia) (Indeterminate)–potentiates barbiturates' sedative effect (Chinese language article cited in Chen & Chen, 2004) Indeterminate level of evidence.
- *Tian Nan Xing* (Arisaema) (Indeterminate)–has a marked sedative and analgesic effect and may increase sedative effects of drugs (Chinese language article cited in Chen & Chen, 2004) Indeterminate level of evidence.
- *Wu Jia Pi* (Acanthopanax) (Indeterminate)–has a mild sedative effect and may increase sedative effects of drugs (Chinese language article cited in Chen & Chen, 2004) Indeterminate level of evidence.
- *Xi Jiao* (Rhinoceros horn) (Indeterminate)–has a sedative effect and may increase sedative effects of drugs (Chinese language article cited in Chen & Chen, 2004) Indeterminate level of evidence.
- *Zhi Zi* (Gardenia, cape jasmine fruit) (Indeterminate)–has a sedative effect and may increase sedative effects of drugs (Chinese language article cited in Chen & Chen, 2004) Indeterminate level of evidence.

BUSPIRONE

- *Guan Ye Lian Qiao* (St. John's wort) (C) and *Yin Guo Ye* (Ginkgo leaf)–were concurrently used with buspirone and fluoxetine. One case report noted a hypomanic episode occurred in a patient, which ended with cessation of herbs (Spinella & Eaton, 2002) Level 4 evidence (Izzo & Ernst, 2009) Level 4 evidence.
- *Yin Guo Ye* (Gingko leaf) (C-) and St. John's wort–were concurrently used with buspirone and fluoxetine. One case report noted that a hypomanic episode occurred in a patient, which ended with cessation of herbs (Spinella & Eaton, 2002) Level 4 evidence.

CHLORAL HYDRATE

- *Gan Cao* (Licorice) (Indeterminate)–may

treat overdoses by increasing the metabolism of certain drugs such as barbiturates, chloral hydrate, urethane, cocaine, picrotoxin, pilocarpine, nicotine, and caffeine (Chinese language article cited in Chen & Chen, 2004) Indeterminate level of evidence.

DIAZEPAM

- *Bai Zhi* (D)–has an inhibitory effect on cytochrome P 450 in rats, which can lead to increased plasma concentration of testosterone, diazepam, tolbutamide, nifedipine, and bufuralol and potentially other drugs (Ishihara, Kushida, Yuzurihara, Wakui, Yanagisawa *et al.*, 2000) Level 5 evidence.
- *Dan Shen* (Salvia root) (D)–high-dose extracts of a single constituent strongly inhibited benzodiazepine receptor binding by flunitazepam in vitro and at the highest dose reversed some effects of diazepam in mice (Lee, Wong, Chui, Choang, *et al.*, 1991) Level 5 evidence.

MIDAZOLAM

- *Guan Ye Lian Qiao* (St. John's Wort) (C) – Decreases blood concentrations (Izzo & Ernst, 2009) Level 2b evidence.
- *Yin Guo Ye* (Gingko) (C) – In vivo use of Gingko biloba extract in a small cohort showed a decrease in midazolam (Robertson, Davey, Voell, Formentini, *et al.*, 2008) Level 4 evidence.

QUAZEPAM

- *Guan Ye Lian Qiao* (St. John's wort) (C) – decreases blood concentrations (Izzo & Ernst, 2009) Level 2b evidence.

SEDATIVES

- *Bai Jiang Cao* (Dahurian patrinia herb) (Indeterminate)–has a sedative effect and may increase sedative effects of drugs (Chinese language article cited in Chen & Chen, 2004) Indeterminate level of evidence.
- *Bai Shao* (White peony root) (Indeterminate)–has a sedative and analgesic effect and may increase sedative effects of drugs (Chinese language article cited in Chen & Chen, 2004) Indeterminate level of evidence.
- *Chan Tui* (Cicada moulting) (Indeterminate)–has an inhibitory effect on the CNS potentiating sedative drugs (Chinese language article

cited in Chen & Chen, 2004) Indeterminate level of evidence.

- *Lang Dan Cao* (Gentiana) (Indeterminate)– may increase sedative effects of drugs (Chinese language article cited in Chen & Chen, 2004) Indeterminate level of evidence.
- *Niu Huang* (Cow gallstone) (Indeterminate)– has a mild sedative effect and may increase sedative effects of drugs (Chinese language article cited in Chen & Chen, 2004) Indeterminate level of evidence.
- *Qin Jiao* (Gentiana macrophylla root) (Indeterminate)–has an inhibitory effect on the CNS potentiating sedative drugs (Chinese language article cited in Chen & Chen, 2004) Indeterminate level of evidence.
- *Shen*-calming herbs (D)–may have marked sedative and tranquilizing effects and may increase sedative effects of drugs, expert opinion (Chen & Chen, 2004) Level 5 evidence.
- *Tian Nan Xing* (Arisaema) (Indeterminate)– has a marked sedative and analgesic effect and may increase sedative effects of drugs (Chinese language article cited in Chen & Chen, 2004) Indeterminate level of evidence.
- *Xi Jiao* (Rhinoceros horn) (Indeterminate)– sedative effect may increase sedative effects of drugs (Chinese language article cited in Chen & Chen, 2004) Indeterminate level of evidence.
- *Zhi Zi* (Gardenia, cape jasmine fruit) (Indeterminate)–has a sedative effect and may increase sedative effects of drugs (Chinese language article cited in Chen & Chen, 2004) Indeterminate level of evidence.

Vitamins

- Due to increased hepatic enzyme induction, vitamins D and K may be more rapidly metabolized and therefore their effects reduced when coadministered with phenobarbital.

INTERACTION ISSUES

A:

D: Buspirone is 86-95% protein bound; chlordiazepoxide is 90-98% bound; the metabolite (nordiazepam) of clorazepate is 97-98% bound; diazepam is 98% bound; flurazepam and midazolam are approximately 97% bound; oxazepam is 86-99% bound; quazepam is greater than 95% bound; temazepam is 96% bound.

M: Alprazolam, buspirone, chlordiazepoxide, clonazepam, clorazepate, eszopiclone, flurazepam, midazolam, triazolam, and zolpidem are major substrates of CYP3A4; amobarbital is a strong inducer of CYP2A6; clobazam is a major substrate of CYP2C19, moderate inhibitor of CYP2D6, and weak to moderate inducer of CYP3A4; diazepam is a major substrate of both CYP2C19 and 3A4; pentobarbital is a strong inducer of both CYP2A6 and CYP3A4; phenobarbital is a major substrate of CYP2C19 and strong inducer of CYP1A2, 2A6, 2B6, 2C8, 2C9, and 3A4; primidone is a strong inducer of CYP1A2, 2B6, 2C8, 2C9, and 3A4; quazepam is a moderate inhibitor of CYP2B6; ramelteon is a major substrate of CYP1A2; secobarbital is a strong inducer of CYP2A6, 2C8, and 2C9.

E:

TI:

Pgp: Clobazam is a substrate of Pgp.

SECTION 5: CENTRAL NERVOUS SYSTEM STIMULANTS

PSYCHOMOTOR STIMULANTS:

AMPHETAMINE (am FET a mene) PR=C (Adderall®,[12] Adderall XR®[12])

DEXMETHYLPHENIDATE (dex meth il FEN i date) PR=C (Focalin® XR, Focalin®)

DEXTROAMPHETAMINE (deks troe am FET a mene) PR=C (Adderall®,[12] Adderall XR®,[12] Dexedrin®, Dextrostat®, Spansule®, Procentra®)

LISDEXAMFETAMINE (lis dex am FET a mene) PR=C (Vynase®)

METHAMPHETAMINE (meth am FET a mene) PR=C (Desoxyn®)

METHYLPHENIDATE (meth il FEN i date) PR=C (Concerta®, Daytrana®, Metadate® CD, Metadate® ER, Methylin®, Ritalin-SR®, Ritalin®, Ritalin® LA)

METHYLXANTHINES:

CAFFEINE (KAF EEN) PR=N (Anacin® Advanced Headache Formula,[43] [O], Cafcit®, Cafergot®,[6] Enerjets [O], Excedrin® Extra Strength [O], Excedrin® Migraine,[43] [O], Fem-Prin®,[43] [O], Fioricet® with Codeine,[3] Goody's® Extra Strength Headache Powder,[43]

[O], Goody's® Extra Strength Pain Relief,[43] [O], Migergot®,[6] No Doz® Maximum Strength [O], Pain-Off,[43] [O], Trezix™,[17] Vanquish® Extra Strength Pain Reliever,[43] [O], Vivarin® [O])

THEOPHYLLINE DERIVATIVES (See Chapter 8, Section 1)

OTHER STIMULANTS:

ARMODAFINIL (ar moe DAF i nil) PR=C (Nuvigil®)

MODAFINIL (moe DAF i nil) PR=C (Alertec®, Provigil®)

This category covers CNS stimulants. While some of the compounds in this category have beneficial effects, many of the most common addictions in our population belong here. This category of drugs can be broken down into two major sections. The first is psychomotor stimulants, which include the pharmaceuticals listed above as well as nicotine from cigarettes and over-the-counter (OTC) smoking cessation products; caffeine from coffee, OTC stimulants and pain relieving compounds; amphetamines;and cocaine.

The second division in this category is that of psychotomimetic or hallucinogenic drugs, which includs lysergic acid diethylamide (LSD), phenclidine (PCP), and tetrahydrocannabinol (THC), the main active ingredient in marijuana. In other words, a large number of illicit and not so illicit drugs fall under this category of drugs. We will look at only those drugs that have clinical value and are prescribed.

FUNCTION

Amphetamine is used primarily as an antiobesity drug though its effectiveness is questionable. It is also used illegally as a recreational drug.

Dextroamphetamine is used to treat obesity, narcolepsy, and attention-deficit hyperactivity disorder (ADHD).

Methamphetamine is used to treat obesity and ADHD. It is also used illegally as a recreational drug.

Dexmethylphenidate and methylphenidate are used in treating ADHD and narcolepsy.

Methylphenidate is used in treating ADHD and narcolepsy. It is also one of the most prescribed medications for children, with an estimated 4-6 million children using it daily.

Modafinil is used to treat narcolepsy and obstructive sleep **apnea** (OSA) and off label for ADHD and fatigue associated with MS and other disorders.

Apnea: Absence of breathing

Methylxanthines are primarily used to relax the smooth muscle of bronchioles in the treatment of asthma. Caffeine, while used for this purpose in the past, is currently the most widely consumed stimulant in the world. It is also used for short-term treatment of apnea in premature infants.

MECHANISM OF ACTION

AMPHETAMINES

These agents work by causing the presynaptic neuron to release norepinephrine and other catecholamines into the synaptic cleft and physiological activation of the postsynaptic membrane receptors. Higher doses may cause release of another catecholamine, dopamine. Lisdexamfetamine is a pro-drug that is converted into dextroamphetamine in the body.

METHYLXANTHINES

These drugs work by inhibiting phosphodiesterase enzymes (PDEs), which break down the **intracellular** signal chemicals of cyclic AMP (cAMP) and cyclic GMP (cGMP). By inhibiting PDEs, more cAMP and cGMP remain in the intracellular space causing increased signal transduction and enhanced activity of select endogenous **autocoids**, hormones, and neurotransmitters. Ultimately, the medulla's respiratory center becomes more sensitive to carbon dioxide and stimulates breathing by increasing the central drive.

Intracellular: Within the cell

Autocoid: Chemical substance produced by one type of cell that affects different cells in the same region; a local hormone or messenger

Bronchoconstriction: A decrease in the diameter of the lung's bronchi allowing for more airflow

Theophylline also acts as a competitive adenosine receptor antagonist. While this can have wide-ranging and variable effects, it is most relevant to note that adenosine can cause **bronchoconstriction** in asthmatics and potentiate the immune response from mast cells. So by antagonizing adenosine, theophylline allows bronchodilation and reduction in the immune response, which is also a component of asthma.

Modafinil's mechanism of action is unknown.

▓ DOSAGES

AMPHETAMINE, for narcolepsy, for children 6-12, initiate at 5 mg/d mane; may be increased 5 mg weekly up to 60 mg/d; for children 12 and over and *adults*, initiate at 10 mg mane; may be increased 10 mg weekly up to 60 mg/d. For ADD, tablets: for children 3-5, initiate at 2.5 mg mane; may be increased 2.5 mg weekly up to 40 mg/d in 2-3 divided doses; for children 6 and over, initiate at 5 mg mane;may be increased 5 mg weekly up to 40 mg/d in 2-3 divided doses; extended release capsules: for children 6-12, initiate at 5-10 mg mane; may be increased 5-10 mg weekly up to 30 mg/d; for children 13-17 initiate at 10 mg mane; may be increased 20 mg after one week; for adults, initiate at 20 mg/d.

ARMODAFINIL, for *adults*, for narcolepsy or obstructive sleep apnea/hypopnea syndrome (OSAHS), for shift work sleep disorder (SWSD), 150 mg once daily 1 hour prior to work shift.

CAFFEINE, for *children*, as a stimulant, IM, SubQ: 8 mg/kg every 4 hours prn; for *children* over 12 years and *adults*, as a stimulant, 100-200 mg every 3-4 hours prn. For *adults*, for respiratory depression, IM: 250 mg as a single dose; may repeat prn; maximum single dose should be limited to 500 mg; maximum amount per day should be limited to 2500 mg.

DEXMETHYLPHENIDATE, for *children* 6 years or over, immediate release, initiate at 2.5 mg bid; may be adjusted by 2.5-5 mg weekly up to a maximum dose of 20 mg/d; doses should be taken at least 4 hours apart; extended release, initiate at 5 mg/d, may be adjusted by 5 mg/d weekly up to a maximum of 30 mg/day. For *adults*, immediate release, initiate at 2.5 mg bid; may be adjusted to 2.5-5 mg weekly up to a maximum 20 mg/d; doses should be taken at least 4 hours apart; extended release, initiate at 10 mg/d; dose may be adjusted 10 mg/d weekly up to a maximum dose of 40 mg/d.

DEXTROAMPHETAMINE, for *children*, for narcolepsy, 6-12 years, initiate at 5 mg/d; may increase 5 mg weekly until side effects appear up to a maximum dose of 60 mg/d; for ADHD in *children* 3-5 years old, initiate at 2.5 mg/d; increase by 2.5 mg/d in weekly intervals until optimal response is obtained, usual dose range is 0.1-0.5 mg/kg/dose up to a maximum of 40 mg/d; in *children* 6 years or older, 5 mg once or twice daily; increase 5 mg/d weekly until optimal response is obtained; usual dose range is 0.1-0.5 mg/kg/dose every morning up to a maximum of 40 mg/d. For *adults*, for narcolepsy, initiate at 10 mg/d; increase at 10 mg/day weekly until side effects appear up to a maximum dose of 60 mg/d.

LISDEXAMFETAMINE, for *children* 6 or over and *adults*, for ADHD, initiate at 30 mg once daily mane; may increase 10 or 20 mg daily every week until an optimal response is achieved up to a maximum dose of 70 mg/d.

METHAMPHETAMINE, for *children* 6 years or older and *adults*, for ADHD, 5 mg 1-2 times/d;

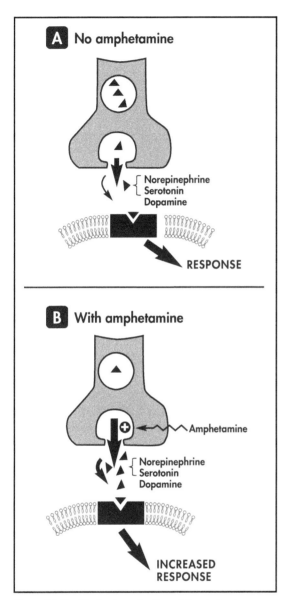

Figure 5.9 The Mechanism of action of Amphetamines.

may increase 5 mg per day weekly until optimum response is achieved, usually 20-25 mg/d. For *children* 12 years or older and *adults*, for exogenous obesity, 5 mg 30 minutes ac; treatment should not exceed a few weeks.

METHYLPHENIDATE, for ADHD, immediate release and Metadate® ER, Methylin® ER, Ritalin® SR for *children* 6 years and older and *adults*, initiate at 5 mg bid before breakfast and lunch; increase by 5-10 mg/d weekly up to a maximum dose of 60 mg/d; extended release products Metadate® CD and Ritalin® LA, ini-

tiate at 20 mg daily; may be increased 10-20 mg weekly up to a maximum of 60 mg/d; Concerta®: for *children* 6-17, initiate at 18 mg once mane; may increase dose 18 mg weekly up to a maximum dose of 54 mg/d in *children* 6-12 years or 72 mg/d in *adolescents* 13-17 years. For *adults*, for narcolepsy, 10 mg bid or tid, up to 60 mg/d.

MODAFINIL, for narcolepsy or OSAHS,[45] initiate at 200 mg mane; for SWSD, initiate at 200 mg taken 1 hour prior to start of work shift.

ADVERSE EFFECTS

Common side effects of most of these agents include: headache, chilliness, palpitations, fatigue, depression, arrhythmias, angina, hyper- or hypotension, excessive sweating, dry mouth, metallic taste, nausea and vomiting, anorexia, diarrhea, and abdominal cramping.

Overdosage can cause restlessness, irritability, insomnia, dizziness, tremor, hyperactive reflexes, talkativeness, tension, weakness, and fever. Other side effects include anxiety, confusion, libido changes, delirium, paranoid hallucinations, panic, aggressiveness, and suicidal or homicidal thoughts and tendencies, especially in mental health patients.

Dependence and **tolerance** often occur with chronic use of amphetamine, methamphetamine, and dextroamphetamine.

Moderate doses of methylxanthines can result in insomnia, anxiety, and agitation. High-dose toxicity can cause tachycardia, palpitations, hypotension, **emesis**, and convulsions. Lethal doses can cause cardiac arrhythmias. Stopping use can induce lethargy, irritability, and headache.

Dependence: The psychological and physical need for a substance

Tolerance: The need for increasing doses of a substance in order achieve similar effects or to avoid negative symptoms

Emesis: Vomiting

RED FLAGS

Cardiac collapse can occur with amphetamine, methamphetamine, and dextroamphetamine. Overdosage can cause convulsions, coma, cerebral hemorrhaging, and death. These agents have been associated with precipitating an initial psychotic break in schizophrenics.

The FDA has issued a warning for using

dextroamphetamine for the treatment of attention-deficit hyperactivity disorder and narcolepsy. There have been reports of sudden death in association with CNS stimulant treatment at usual doses in children and adolescents with structural cardiac abnormalities or other serious heart problems.

Cardiac arrhythmias can result from very high doses of methylxanthines. Addiction, overdosage, and death (improbable in methylxanthine use, though more common in theophylline than caffeine) can result from abuse of any of the drugs in this category.

INTERACTIONS

These agents are contraindicated in patients with glaucoma, advanced arteriosclerosis, symptomatic cardiovascular disease, moderate to severe hypertension, and hyperthyroidism. These should not be given to patients who are in an agitated state or who have a history of drug abuse.

DRUG

Should not be used within the first 14 days of initiating monoamine oxidase inhibitor (MAOI) therapy as it can cause a **hypertensive crisis**. Interactions may occur with concurrent use of anticonvulsant medications.

Hypertensive crisis: A sudden, severe, life-threatening increase in blood pressure

Methylphenidate may inhibit the metabolism of coumarin anticoagulants, anticonvulsants (*e.g.*, phenobarbital, phenytoin, primidone), and some antidepressants (tricyclics and selective serotonin reuptake inhibitors). Dose adjustment of these drugs may be required when given with methylphenidate.

Cardiac arrhythmias can result from very high doses of methylxanthines. Addiction, overdosage, and death (improbable in methylxanthine use, though more common in theophylline than caffeine) can result from abuse of any drugs in this category.

Phenytoin and barbiturates increase clearance of theophylline twofold, while oral contraceptive pills (OCP), rifampin, and cigarette smoking increase clearance to a lesser degree. Cimetidine and erythromycin slow clearance.

HERB

CAFFEINE

• *Chan Tui* (Cicada moulting) (Indeterminate)–has an inhibitory effect on the CNS reducing the stimulant effect of caffeine (Chinese language article cited in Chen & Chen, 2004) Indeterminate level of evidence.

• *Gan Cao* (Licorice) (Indeterminate)–may treat overdoses by increasing the metabolism of certain drugs such as barbiturates, chloral hydrate, urethane, cocaine, picrotoxin, pilocarpine, nicotine, and caffeine (Chinese language article cited in Chen & Chen, 2004) Indeterminate level of evidence.

• *Gou Teng* (Gambir) (Indeterminate)–reverses caffeine's stimulating effects without affecting the use of barbiturates (Chinese language article cited in Chen & Chen, 2004) Indeterminate level of evidence.

• *Ma Huang* (Ephedra) (D)–based on ephedrine content, may increase adrenergic stimulation of caffeine, expert opinion (Gruenwald, Brendler & Jaenicke, 2004) Level 5 evidence.

• *Ma Huang* (Ephedra) (A)–may increase thermogenesis and weight loss when combined with methylxanthines such as theophylline and caffeine in both mice (Dulloo & Miller, 1986a) Level 5 evidence; and human studies (Dulloo & Miller, 1986b) Level 2b evidence; (Malchow-Moller, Larsen, Hey, Stokholm, Juhl & Quaade, 1981) Level 2b evidence; (Boozer, Daly, Homel, Solomon, Blanchard *et al.*, 2002) Level 1b evidence; (Greenway, de Jonge, Blanchard, Frisard & Smith, 2004) Level 2b evidence; (Astrup, Breum, Toubro, Hein & Quaade, 1992) Level 1b evidence.

• *Ma Huang* (Ephedra) (B)–ephedrine, a chief component of Ma Huang increases the incidences of side effects such as agitation, tremors, and insomnia and raises blood pressure and heart rate in higher doses and plasma glucose, insulin, and C-peptide in all doses in human subjects (Astrup, Toubro, Cannon, Hein & Madsen, 1991) Level 2c evidence; (as cited in Brinker, 2001, p. 88). Another study confirmed these effects but noted the transient nature of the side effects (Astrup & Toubro, 1993) Level 2c evidence. A well-constructed RCT showed that these negative effects were transient and equaled placebo levels after 8 weeks (Astrup, Breum, Toubro, *et al.*, 1992) Level 1b evidence.

• *Niu Huang* (Cow gallstone), *Suan Zao Ren* (Zizyphus) (Indeterminate)–has a mild sedative effect and may decrease the effects of caffeine (Chinese language article cited in Chen & Chen, '04) Indeterminate level of evidence.

METHYLXANTHINES

• *Ma Huang* (Ephedra) (A)–may increase thermogenesis and weight loss when combined with methylxanthines such as theophylline and caffeine in both mice (Dulloo & Miller, 1986a) Level 5 evidence; and human studies (Dulloo & Miller, 1986b) Level 2b evidence; (Malchow-Moller, Larsen, Hey, Stokholm, Juhl & Quaade, 1981) Level 2b evidence; (Boozer, Daly, Homel, Solomon, Blanchard, & Nasser, *et al.*, 2002) Level 1b evidence; (Greenway, de Jonge, Blanchard, Frisard & Smith, 2004) Level 2b evidence; (Astrup, Breum, *et al.*, 1992) Level 1b evidence.

SYMPATHOMIMETIC DRUGS

• *Chen Pi* (Tangerine peel) (Indeterminate)–contains constituents that stimulate the sympathetic nervous system and should be used with caution in those taking antihypertensives, antidiabetic, antihyperthyroid, and antiseizure medications (Chinese language article cited in Chen & Chen, 2004) Indeterminant level of evidence.

• *Ma Huang* (Ephedra) (D)–based on ephedrine content, may increase sympathomimetic activity of drugs such as furazolidone and procarbazine, expert opinion (Gruenwald, Brendler & Jaenicke, 2004) Level 5 evidence.

• *Ma Huang* (Ephedra) (D)–may potentiate sympathomimetic drugs and induce hypertension, expert opinon (Mills & Bone, 2000) Level 5 evidence.

• *Qing Pi* (Citrus Viride), *Zhi Ke* (Aurantium fruit, bitter orange), *Zhi Shi* (Aurantium immaturus) (Indeterminate)–contains constituents that stimulate the sympathetic nervous system and should be used with caution in those taking antihypertensive, antidiabetic, antihyperthyroid, and/or antiseizure medications (Chinese language article cited in Chen & Chen, 2004) Indeterminate level of evidence.

• *Rou Cong Rong* (Cistanche) (Indeterminate)–may interact with sympathomimetics, monoamine oxidase inhibitors, selective serotonin reuptake inhibitors, and tricyclic antidepressants by increasing the activities of neurotransmitters such as norepinephrine, dopamine, and serotonin (Chinese language article cited in Chen & Chen, 2004) Indeterminate level of evidence.

INTERACTION ISSUES

A:

D:

M: Armodafinil is a major substrate of CYP3A4, a moderate inhibitor of CYP2C19, and a weak to moderate inducer of CYP3A4; caffeine is a major substrate of CYP1A2. Methamphetamine is a major substrate of CYP2D6; modafinil is a major substrate of CYP3A4, a strong inhibitor of CYP2C19, and a weak/moderate inducer of CYP1A2, CYP2B6, and CYP3A4.

E:

TI: Theophylline has a narrow therapeutic index.

SECTION 6: ANTIDEPRESSANTS

Depression is a collection of mood disorders that include symptoms of depressed, irritable, and/or anxious mood. Other signs and symptoms may include slumped posture, poor eye contact, monosyllabic or absent speech, guilt, self-denigration, lessened ability to concentrate, indecisiveness, diminished interest in usual activities, social withdrawal, hopelessness, helplessness,

Anhedonia: Inability to feel pleasure or happiness from activities that would normally provide such feelings

recurrent thoughts of death and suicide, **anhedonia**, loss of libido, and changes of appetite, either reduced or increased.

Mood disorders that may employ the following therapeutic agents include: major depressive disorder, dysthymic disorder, depressive disorder not otherwise specified, bipolar I and II disorders, cyclothymic disorder, bipolar disorder not otherwise specified, mood disorder due to a gen-

eral medical condition, substance-induced mood disorder, and mood disorder not otherwise specified.

All effective antidepressants potentiate, either directly or indirectly, the effects of serotonin (5-HT), dopamine (DA), and/or norepinephrine (NE). This fact has led to the monoamine theory of depression which states that deficiency of monoamines such as 5-HT and NE in certain areas of the brain cause depression.

CLASS 1:
TRICYCLIC/POLYCYCLIC ANTIDEPRESSANTS

AMITRIPTYLINE (a mee TRIP ti lene) PR=C

AMOXAPINE (a MOKS a pene)

CLOMIPRAMINE (kloe MI pra mene) PR=C *(Anafranil®)*

DESIPRAMINE (des IP ra mene) PR=N *(Norpramin®)*

DOXEPIN (DOKS e pin) PR=C *(Silenor®)*

IMIPRAMINE (im IP ra mene) PR=N *(Tofranil®, Tofranil-PM®)*

MAPROTILINE (ma PROE ti lene) PR=B *(Ludiomil)*

NORTRIPTYLINE (nor TRIP ti lene) PR=N *(Pamelor®)*

PROTRIPTYLINE (proe TRIP ti lene) PR=N *(Vivactil®)*

TRIMIPRAMINE (trye MI pra mene) PR=C *(Surmontil®)*

The name of this class of antidepressants refers to the carbon rings in their chemical structure. Though some may have more than three carbon rings in their structure, the main molecular backbone contains three of these rings, and generally this class is referred to by the name tricyclic antidepressants even if they do have more carbon rings than three. They are generally broken down into older tricyclic antidepressants (TCAs) and second-generation TCAs. While each generation of TCAs works similarly, they do have different pharmacokinetics, and their side effect profiles may be less onerous in the second-generation TCAs.

FUNCTION

This class of drugs is obviously used to treat depression. In addition, imipramine has been used for bedwetting in children over 6 because it can cause contraction of the internal sphincter of the bladder. Some of these drugs are also used in treating obsessive-compulsive disorder and pain.

MECHANISMS OF ACTION

A controversy exists as to the mechanism of action of TCAs. They definitely prevent reuptake of norepinephrine (NE) and serotonin (5-HT) into the presynaptic neuron terminals. This causes more NE and 5-HT to remain in the synaptic cleft and increased activation of the postsynaptic receptors (see Figure 5.10). However, the amount of the reuptake inhibition does not correlate with the effectiveness of the agent. In addition, full antidepressant effects are not apparent for at least 2-3 weeks after drug initiation, while the reuptake inhibition is immediate.

Because of these discrepancies, other theories have been posited that explain their effectiveness as antidepressants. One leading theory is that other adaptations occur in the brain in the presence of these agents. These changes are not completely understood but may include increased postsynaptic receptor formation. There may be an effect of desensitizing dopamine **autoreceptors**, which may cause extra dopamine to remain in the synaptic cleft and may contribute to their antidepressant effects.

Autoreceptors: A receptor located on a neuron that binds a neurotransmitter from the same neuron which then regulates that neuron

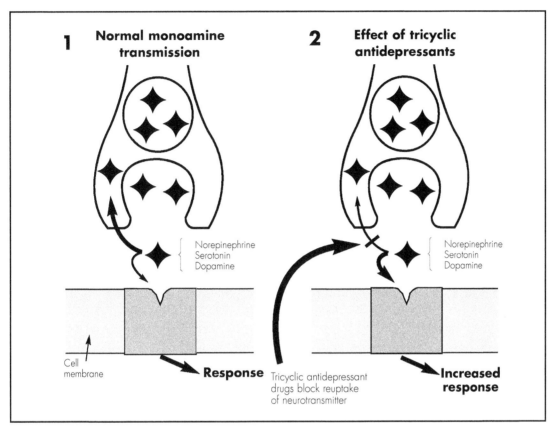

1 Normal monoamine transmission

2 Effect of tricyclic antidepressants

Norepinephrine
Serotonin
Dopamine

Norepinephrine
Serotonin
Dopamine

Cell membrane

Response

Tricyclic antidepressant drugs block reuptake of neurotransmitter

Increased response

Figure 5.10: Actions of tricyclic antidepressants. 1: In normal monoamine transmission, a monoamine (epinephrine, norepinephrine, and/or dopamine) is released by the presynaptic neuron and activates a receptor on the postsynaptic membrane. **2:** In the presence of a tricyclic antidepressant, reuptake of the monoamine is inhibited and therefore remains longer in the synaptic cleft ultimately increasing stimulation of the receptor.

Noradrenergic receptors may also be involved. Many other complex observations and theories of effects have also been theorized, but the bottom line is there are complex interactions between TCAs and the brain, and we are still exploring how they result in antidepressant activity.

DOSAGES

AMITRIPTYLINE, for *children*, for depressive disorders, initiate at 1 mg/kg/d given in 3 divided doses with increases to 1.5 mg/kg/d; doses up to 3 mg/kg/d have been proposed; for *adolescents*, for depressive disorders, initiate at 25-50 mg/d; may administer in divided doses; increase gradually to 100 mg/d. For *adults*, for depression, 50-150 mg/d single dose nocte or in divided doses; dose may be gradually increased up to 300 mg/d. For the *elderly*, for depression, initiate at 10-25 mg nocte; dose should be increased

in 10-25 mg increments weekly if tolerated to a usual dose range of 25-150 mg/d.

AMOXAPINE, for *children*, not established in children less than 16 years of age. For *adolescents*, initiate at 25-50 mg/d; increase gradually to 100 mg/d; may administer as divided doses or as a single dose at bedtime. For *adults*, initiate at 25 mg 2-3 times/d; if tolerated, dosage may be increased to 100 mg 2-3 times/d; may be given in a single bedtime dose when dosage <300 mg/d. For the *elderly*, initiate at 25 mg nocte increased by 25 mg weekly for outpatients and every 3 days for inpatients if tolerated; usual dose is 50-150 mg/d, but doses up to 300 mg may be necessary.

CLOMIPRAMINE, for *children* 10 years or older, for OCD, 25 mg/d; gradually increase, as tolerated, to a maximum of 3 mg/kg/d or 200 mg/d, whichever is smaller. For *adults*, initiate at 25 mg/d; gradually increase dose to 100 mg/d in the first 2 weeks; dosage may then be increased to a maximum of 250 mg/d.

DESIPRAMINE, for *children* 6-12 years, for depression (unlabeled use), 10-30 mg/d or 1-3 mg/kg/d in divided doses; do not exceed 5 mg/kg/d. For *adolescents*, for depression, initiate at 25-50 mg/d; gradually increase to 100 mg/d in single or divided doses; maximum dose is 150 mg/d. For *adults*, for depression, initiate at 75 mg/d in divided doses; increase gradually to 150-200 mg/d in divided or single dose; maximum dose is 300 mg/d. For the *elderly*, for depression, initiate at 10-25 mg/d; increase by 10-25 mg every 3 days for inpatients and every week for outpatients if tolerated; usual maintenance dose is 75-100 mg/d, but doses up to 150 mg/d may be necessary.

DOXEPIN, for *adults*, for depression or anxiety, initiate at 25-150 mg/d nocte or in 2-3 divided dose; may gradually increase up to 300 mg/d; single dose should not exceed 150 mg; for insomnia, 3-6 mg nocte. For the *elderly*, for depression and/or anxiety, initiate at 10-25 mg nocte; increase by 10-25 mg every 3 days for inpatients and weekly for outpatients if tolerated; rarely the maximum dose is more than 75 mg/d; for insomnia, 3 mg once nocte; increase to 6 mg prn.

IMIPRAMINE, for *children*, for enuresis, 6 years and older, initiate at 25 mg nocte; if inadequate after 1 week of therapy, increase by 25 mg per day; dose should not exceed 2.5 mg/kg/d or 50 mg nocte if 6-12 years of age or 75 mg nocte if 12 years of age or older; for *adolescents*, for depression, initiate at 30-40 mg/d; increase gradually to a maximum of 100 mg/d in single or divided doses. For *adults*, for depression, for outpatients, initiate at 75 mg/d; may increase gradually to 150 mg/d. May be given in divided doses or as a single bedtime dose; maximum dose is 200 mg/d; for inpatients, initiate at 100-150 mg/d; may increase gradually to 200 mg/d; if no response after 2 weeks, may increase to 250-300 mg/d; may be given in divided doses or as a single bedtime dose. For the *elderly*, for

depression, initiate at 25-50 mg nocte; may increase every 3 days for inpatients and weekly for outpatients if tolerated to a maximum of 100 mg/d.

MAPROTILINE, for *adults*, for depression/anxiety, initiate at 75 mg/d; increase by 25 mg every 2 weeks up to 150-225 mg/d, given in 3 divided doses or in a single daily dose. For the *elderly*, for depression/anxiety, initiate at 25 mg nocte; increase by 25 mg every 3 days for inpatients and weekly for outpatients if tolerated; usual maintenance dose is 50-75 mg/d; higher doses may be necessary in nonresponders.

NORTRIPTYLINE, for *children*, for nocturnal enuresis (unlabeled use), 10-20 mg/d; may increase to a maximum of 40 mg/d; for depression (unlabeled use), 1-3 mg/kg/d. For *adults*, for depression, 25 mg 3-4 times/d up to 150 mg/d; for myofascial pain, neuralgia, burning mouth syndrome (dental use), initiate at 10-25 mg nocte; dosage may be increased by 25 mg/d weekly if tolerated; usual maintenance dose is 75 mg as a single bedtime dose or 2 divided doses. For the *elderly*, for depression, initiate at 10-25 mg nocte, dosage can be increased by 25 mg every 3 days for inpatients and weekly for outpatients if tolerated; usual maintenance dose is 75 mg as a single bedtime dose or 2 divided doses.

PROTRIPTYLINE, for *adolescents*, 15-20 mg/d. For *adults*, 15-60 mg/d in 3-4 divided doses. For *elderly*, initiate at 5-10 mg/d; increase every 3-7 days by 5-10 mg; usual dose is 15-20 mg/d.

TRIMIPRAMINE, for *adolescents*, for depression, initiate at 50 mg nocte; gradually increase to 100 mg per day. For *adults*, for depression, for outpatients, initiate at 75 mg/d in divided doses; may increase to 150 mg/d, maximum dose is 200 mg/d; for inpatients, initiate at 100 mg per day in divided doses; may increase to 200 mg/d; if no improvement after 2-3 weeks, may increase to 250-300 mg/d. For the *elderly*, 50 mg/d; gradually increase to 100 mg/d.

ADVERSE EFFECTS

Many adverse effects can result from use of these agents. These include:

Antimuscarinic activity can cause blurred vision, **xerostomia**, urinary retention, constipation, and aggravation of glaucoma and epilepsy.

Orthostatic hypotension can result from blockage of α-adrenergic receptors. Reflex **tachycardia** may result. This is the most serious problem in elderly patients using TCAs.

Sedation may be common in the first several weeks of treatment.

Other common side effects include: epigastric distress, dizziness, tachycardia, palpitations, weight gain, weakness, and fatigue.

RED FLAGS

Cardiovascular effects due to increased **catecholamine** activity include cardiac overstimulation, which can be fatal in overdoses. Slowed atrioventricular conduction is a concern in the elderly. Reflex tachycardia may result in the elderly from blockage of α-adrenergic receptors. This is the most serious problem in elderly patients using TCAs.

TCAs have a narrow therapeutic index. For example, imipramine can be lethal at 5-6 times the maximum daily dose. Because of this, suicidal patients should only be given small amounts of these drugs and monitored closely.

The use of antidepressant drugs in patients with major depressive disorder and/or suicidal ideation can precipitate a suicide attempt. While patients may have suicidal thoughts in the middle of major depressive episodes, they often do not have enough energy to carry through on the thoughts. As an antidepressant starts to work, the patients will gain energy, but the antidepressant effects may not have fully engaged. In other words, they now have the energy to attempt suicide, but the medication hasn't worked well enough yet to change the thoughts of suicide. Careful oversight needs to be employed when using any antidepressant in patients with major depression to prevent suicide.

INTERACTIONS

TCAs should be used with caution in manic-depressive patients because they can unmask manic behaviors.

DRUG

Albumin binding by phenytoin, phenylbutazone, aspirin, aminopyrine, scopalamine, and phenothiazines may potentiate TCAs. They can also be potentiated from interference of liver metabolism by barbiturates; many anticonvulsant medications, especially carbamazepine; and cigarette smoking. Some serotonin reuptake inhibitors may also compete for metabolism and cause TCA levels to become toxic.

Combined use of ethanol or other sedatives with TCAs may cause toxic sedation.

TCAs potentiate the effects of direct-acting adrenergic agents because they prevent their removal from the synaptic cleft. Conversely, TCAs block the effects of indirect-acting adrenergic agents by preventing them from reaching their intracellular sites of action.

MAOIs and TCAs mutually enhance their effects and can cause hypertension, hyperpyrexia, convulsions, and coma.

HERB

Because of their narrow therapeutic index, caution should be used whenever tricyclic antidepressants are combined with herbs.

AMITRIPTYLINE
- *Guan Ye Lian Qiao* (St. John's wort) (C)–decreases blood concentrations (Zhou, Chan, Pan, Huang & Lee, 2004) Level 3b evidence; (Izzo & Ernst, 2009) Level 4 evidence.
- *Ma Huang* (Ephedra) (C)–hypertensive effects of ephedrine were blocked when used with amitriptyline in one human case report despite the possibility of hypertension and arrhythmias speculatively thought to occur when sympathomimetics and tricyclic antidepressants are combined (Stockley, 1996) Level 4 evidence.

TRICYCLIC ANTIDEPRESSANTS
- *Ma Huang* (Ephedra) (C)–hypertensive effects of ephedrine were blocked when used with amitriptyline in one human case report despite the possibility of hypertension and arrhythmias

Xerostomia: A dry mouth

Orthostatic hypotension: A period of reduced blood pressure due to standing rapidly from a seated or lying position, usually causes lightheadedness

Tachycardia: A rapid heart rate defined as over 100 bpm

Catecholamines: Sympathomimetic neurotransmitter family that includes epinephrine, norepinephrine, and dopamine

speculatively thought to occur when sympathomimetics and tricyclic antidepressants are combined (Stockley, 1996) Level 4 evidence.

- *Rou Cong Rong* (Cistanche) (Indeterminate) –may interact with sympathomimetics, MAOIs, SSRIs, and TCAs by increasing activities of neurotransmitters such as norepinephrine, dopamine, and serotonin (Chinese language article cited in Chen & Chen, 2004) Indeterminate level of evidence.
- *Ying Su Ke* (Opium husks) (D)–phenothiazines, monoamine oxidase inhibitors, and tricyclic antidepressants may exacerbate the depressant and CNS suppressive effects of *Ying Su Ke*, expert opinion (Chen & Chen, 2004) Level 5 evidence.

INTERACTION ISSUES

A:

D: Clomipramine is 97% protein bound; trimipramine is 95% bound.

M: Amitriptyline is a major substrate of CYP2D6; clomipramine is a major substrate of CYP1A2, 2C19, and 2D6 and is a moderate inhibitor of CYP2D6; doxepin is a major substrate of CYP2D6; imipramine is a major substrate of CYP2C19 and 2D6 and a moderate inhibitor of CYP2D6; trimipramine is a major substrate of CYP2C19, 2D6, and 3A4.

E:

TI: Some experts consider the entire category of tricyclic antidepressants to have a narrow therapeutic index.

Pgp:

CLASS 2:
SELECTIVE SEROTONIN REUPTAKE INHIBITORS:

CITALOPRAM (sye TAL oh pram) PR=C *(Celexa®)*

ESCITALOPRAM (es sye TAL oh pram) PR=C *(Lexapro®)*

FLUOXETINE (floo OKS e tene) PR=C *(Prozac®, Prozac® Weekly™, Sarafem®, Symbyax®7)*

FLUVOXAMINE (floo VOKS a mene) PR=C *(Luvox® CR)*

NEFAZODONE (nef AY zoe done) PR=C *(Serzone®)*

PAROXETINE (pa ROKS e tene) PR=D *(Paxil®, Paxil CR®, Pexeva®)*

SERTRALINE (SER tra lene) PR=C *(Zoloft®)*

TRAZODONE (TRAZ oh done) PR=C *(Oleptro™)*

VILAZODONE (vil AZ oh done) PR=C *(Viibryd™)*

SEROTONIN/NOREPINEPHRINE REUPTAKE INHIBITORS:

DESVENLAFAXINE (des VEN la FAX ene) PR=C *(Pristiq®)*

DULOXETINE (doo LOX e teen) *(Cymbalta®)*

MILNACIPRAN (mil NAY ci pran) PR=C *(Savella®)*

VENLAFAXINE (VEN la faks ene) PR=C *(Effexor®, Effexor XR®)*

SELECTIVE NOREPINEPHRINE REUPTAKE INHIBITORS:

ATOMOXETINE (AT oh mox e tene) PR=C *(Strattera®)*

FUNCTION

This class of drugs is used to treat depression. In addition, these drugs are used in many other disorders including GAD, panic disorder, PMDD, PTSD, social anxiety disorder, obsessive-compulsive disorder, pain, and fibromyalgia. Fluvoxamine is primarily used for the treatment of obsessive-compulsive disorder (OCD) but is used off-label for a variety of psychiatric disorders including major depression, panic disorder, a variety of anxiety disorders such as post-traumatic stress disorder (PTSD) and social anxiety disorder, dementia-associated agitation in non-psychotic patients, and paraphilias.

As the first and only agent of a relatively new class of drugs, selective norepinephrine reuptake inhibitors, atomoxetine is used to treat attention deficit/hyperactivity disorder (ADHD). It is included in this section because it uses a similar mechanism of action to other drugs here.

MECHANISMS OF ACTION

This class of agents specifically prevents the reuptake of serotonin from the synaptic cleft into the presynaptic neuron, allowing more serotonin to remain longer in the synaptic cleft. This is in contrast to TCAs that inhibit uptake of norepinephrine and serotonin and block muscarininc, H1-histaminic, and α1-adrenergic receptors. Because of this specificity, SSRIs tend to have a better adverse effect profile than TCAs. A subclass of this class of agents is the serotonin/norepinephrine reuptake inhibitors (SNRIs). These agents prevent the reuptake of norepinephrine in addition to serotonin. Their effects are similar to SSRIs, while their adverse effect profiles differ slightly.

These drug classes are very similar to TCAs in that the reuptake inhibition does not completely explain their effectiveness as antidepressants. They also can take 3-8 weeks of use before being fully effective indicating there are secondary effects to reuptake inhibition. These secondary effects are poorly understood, but several of the same theories of TCA effectiveness are being applied to these agents.

DOSAGES

Most SNRIs and SSRIs need to be tapered off when stopping their use.

ATOMOXETINE, for *children* 6 years and older and 70 kg or under, for treatment of ADHD, initiate at 0.5 mg/kg/d; increase after a minimum of 3 days to approximately 1.2 mg/kg/d; may administer as a single daily dose or bid; maximum daily dose is 1.4 mg/kg or 100 mg, whichever is less. For *adults*, for ADHD, initiate at 40 mg/d; increase after a minimum of 3 days to approximately 80 mg/d in a single dose 40 mg bid morning and late afternoon or early evening; may increase to a maximum dose of 100 mg/d in 2-4 additional weeks.

CITALOPRAM, for *adults*, initiate at 20 mg once daily; increase to a maximum of 40 mg after an interval of one week. For the *elderly*, initiate at 20 mg once daily, maximum dose is 20 mg/d.

DESVENLAFAXINE, for *adults*, 50 mg once daily.

DULOXETINE, for *adults*, for major depression, initiate at 40-60 mg/d in 1 or 2 doses; maximum dose is 120 mg/d though doses over 60 mg/d have not been shown to have increased effectiveness; for diabetic neuropathy, 60 mg once daily; for fibromyalgia, 30 mg once daily for 1 week, then increase to 60 mg once daily; for generalized anxiety disorder (GAD), initiate at 30-60 mg/d; when started at 30 mg/d should be increased to 60 mg/d after 1 week;maximum dose is 120 mg/d but doses over 60 mg/d have not been shown to have increased effectiveness; for chronic musculoskeletal pain, 30 mg once daily for 1 week, then increase to 60 mg once daily.

ESCITALOPRAM, for *children* with major depressive disorder, initiate at 10 mg/d; may increase to a maximum 20 mg/d after 3 weeks. For *adults* with major depressive disorder or generalized anxiety disorder (GAD), initiate at 10 mg/d; may increase to a maximum of 20 mg/d after 1 week. For the *elderly* with major depressive disorder or GAD, 10 mg/d.

FLUOXETINE, for *children*, for depression, 8-18 years, 10-20 mg/d; lower-weight children can be started at 10 mg/d; may increase to 20 mg/d after 1 week; for OCD, 7-17 years, initiate at 10 mg/d; may be increased to 20 mg/d after 2 weeks; usual range is 20-30 mg/d for lower-weight children and 20-60 mg/d in adolescents and heavier children. For *adults*, initiate at 20 mg/d mane; can be increased every several weeks by 20 mg/d up to a maximum of 80 mg/d. Doses over 20 mg can be given once or twice daily. Usual dose for bulimia nervosa is 60 mg/d; for OCD is 20-60 mg/d; for premenstrual dysphoric disorder 20 mg/d continuously or 20 mg/d starting 14 days before menses and through first full day; for panic disorder, start at 10 mg/d; and after one week, increase to 20 mg/d; may be increased every several weeks thereafter. For the *elderly*, some may require initiation at 10 mg/d; may increase 10-20 mg every several weeks.

FLUVOXAMINE, for *children* 8-17 years, initiate at 25 mg nocte; may adjust in 25 mg increments at 4-7 day intervals; usual dose range is 50-200 mg/d; maximum doses are: for *children* 8-11 years, 200 mg/d; for *adolescents*, 300 mg/d; lower dosing may be effective in female patients. Immediate release: initiate at 50 mg nocte; may be increased in 50 mg increments at 4-7 day intervals to a usual dose range of 100-300 mg/d and up to maximum 300 mg/d. When total daily dose is over 100 mg, it should be given in 2 doses with the largest at bedtime. Extended release: initiate at 100 mg nocte; may be increased in 50 mg increments at weekly or more intervals, usual dose range 100-300 mg/d with a maximum of 300 mg/d.

MILNACIPRAN, for *adults*, for fibromyalgia, should be initiated by a 12.5 mg dose on day 1, 2 12.5 mg bid on days 2 and 3, 25 mg/bid on days 4-7, and then 50 mg bid up to a maximum of 200 mg/d.

NEFAZODONE, for *adults*, initiate at 100 mg/bid; should be increased to 150-300 mg/bid. In the *elderly*, initiate at 50 mg bid and in 2 weeks increase to 100 mg bid; usual maintenance dose is 200-400 mg/d.

PAROXETINE, for *adults*, for depression, for Paxil® and Pexeva®, initiate at 20 mg mane;may increase by 10 mg/d increments in at least weekly intervals up to a maximum dose of 50 mg/d. Paxil CR® should be initiated at 25 mg once daily and may be increased by 12.5 mg/d in at least weekly intervals up to a maximum dose of 62.5 mg/d; for generalized anxiety disorder (Paxil®, Pexeva®), initiate at 20 mg mane; for obsessive-compulsive disorder (Paxil®, Pexeva®), initiate at 20 mg mane; may increase by 10 mg/d increments in at least weekly intervals; recommended dose is 40 mg/d; maximum dose is 60 mg/d; for panic disorder, Paxil®, Pexeva®: initiate at 10 mg mane; may increase in 10 mg/d increments in at least weekly intervals; recommended dose is 40 mg/d and maximum dose is 60 mg/d, Paxil CR®: initiate at 12.5 mg once daily; may increase 12.5 mg/d in at least weekly intervals up to a maximum dose of 75 mg/d; for premenstrual dysphoric disorder (Paxil CR®), initiate at 12.5 mg mane; may be increased to 25 mg/d after at least a week; may be given daily throughout the menstrual cycle or limited to the luteal phase; for post-traumatic stress disorder (Paxil®), initiate at 20 mg mane; may increase by 10 mg/d increments weekly to a usual range of 20-50 mg; for social anxiety disorder, Paxil®: initiate at 20 mg mane; doses over 20 mg may not have additional benefit, Paxil CR®: initiate at 12.5 mg mane; may increase by 12.5 mg/d in at least weekly intervals up to a maximum dose of 37.5 mg/d. In the *elderly*, Paxil®, Pexeva®: initiate at 10 mg/d; may increase by 10 mg/d increments in at least weekly intervals up to a maximum of 40 mg/d; Paxil CR®: initiate at 12.5 mg/d; may increase by 12.5 mg/d increments in at least weekly intervals up to maximum 50 mg/d.

SERTRALINE, for *children* and *adolescents*, for OCD, for 6-12 years, initiate at 25 mg once daily; for 13-17 years, initiate at 50 mg once daily; may increase at intervals of more than one week, to a maximum of 200 mg/d; if sleepiness is noted, give at bedtime. For *adults*, initiate at 50 mg/d; may be increased at intervals of at least one week to a maximum of 200 mg/d. Should be given at bedtime if sleepiness is noted; for panic disorder, PTSD, and social anxiety disorder, should be initiated at 25 mg once daily and increased to 50 mg after one week up to a maximum of 200 mg/d; for premenstrual dysphoric disorder (PMDD), 50 mg/d or limited to the luteal phase of the menstrual cycle; if non-responsive to this dose may increase in 50 mg/d increments to 150 mg/d or 100 mg/d , if used during luteal phase only. In the *elderly*, initiate at 25 mg/d and increase by 25 mg/d every 2-3 days to a usual dose of 50-100 mg/d; maximum dose 200 mg/ d.

TRAZODONE, for *adults*, initiate at 50 mg tid; may be increased by 50 mg/d every 3-7 days with a maximum of 600 mg/d. In the *elderly*, initiate at 25-50 mg nocte with 25-50 mg/d increases every 3 days until a usual dose of 75-150 mg/d is achieved.

VENLAFAXINE, for *children* and *adolescents*, for

ADHD, initiate at 12.5 mg/d; for *children* <40 kg, increase by 12.5 mg/week to maximum of 25 mg/bid, for *children* ≥40 kg, increase by 25 mg/week to maximum of 25 mg/tid. For *adults*, for depression, immediate release: initiate at 75 mg/d, administered in 2 or 3 divided doses; may increase in 75 mg/d or less increments every 4 or more days up to a maximum dose of 225-375 mg/d; extended release: initiate at 37.5-75 mg once daily; in patients who start at 37.5 mg once daily; may increase to 75 mg/d after 4 days; dose may be increased 75 mg/d or less at intervals of 4 or more days up to a maximum dose of 225 mg/d; for generalized anxiety disorder (GAD), extended release: initiate at 37.5-75 mg once daily; in patients who start at 37.5 mg once daily, may increase to 75 mg/d after 4 days; dose may be increased 75 mg/d or less at intervals of 4 or more days up to maximum of 225 mg/d; for panic disorder, extended release: initiate at 37.5 mg once daily for 1 week; may increase to 75 mg/d after 7 days; may be increased by 75 or less mg/d increments at intervals of 7 or more days up to a maximum dose of 225 mg/d; for social anxiety disorder, extended release: 75 mg/d.

VILAZODONE, for *adults*, initiate at 10 mg/d for 7 days, increase to 20 mg/d for 7 days, then to the recommended dose of 40 mg/d.

ADVERSE EFFECTS

Nausea and vomiting, sleep disturbances, and headaches are common side effects of SSRIs. Loss of libido, delayed ejaculation, and **anorgasmia** are common side effects that are generally underreported. Overdosage does not result in arrhythmias as in TCAs, but can cause seizures. In general, SSRIs are well tolerated and have better side effect profiles than other antidepressants.

Duloxetine has been shown to increase the risk of additional liver damage in patients with preexisting liver disease and should not be used in this patient population.

RED FLAGS

The use of antidepressant drugs in patients with major depressive disorder and/or suicidal ideation can precipitate a suicide attempt. While patients may have suicidal thoughts in the middle of a major depressive episode, they often do not have enough energy to carry through on the thoughts. As an antidepressant starts to work, the patient will gain energy but the antidepressant effects may not have fully engaged. In other words, they now have the energy to attempt suicide, but the medication hasn't worked well enough yet to change the thoughts of suicide. Careful oversight needs to be employed when using any antidepressant in patients with major depression to prevent suicide.

Recent studies have caused the FDA to issue a warning not to use paroxetine during pregnancy as it may increase the chance of congenital malformations.

INTERACTIONS

DRUG

SSRIs can interact with the metabolism of β-adrenergic receptor antagonists, caffeine, several antipsychotic agents, most TCAs, barbiturates, phenytoin, imipramine, benzodiazepines, and carbamazepine. Some serotonin reuptake inhibitors may compete for metabolism and cause TCA levels to become toxic when coadministered.

Combined use of ethanol or other sedatives with SSRIs may cause toxic sedation.

Coadministration of MAOIs and SSRIs can cause "serotonin syndrome." Symptoms of this include: **akathisia**-like restlessness, muscle **fasciculations**, **myoclonus**, hyperreflexia, sweating, penile erection, shivering, tremors, and ultimately seizures and coma. Other medications besides MAOIs may cause this syndrome, including: meperidine, pentazocine, dextromethorphan, fenfluramine, and rarely, TCAs.

HERB

FLUOXETINE

- *Guan Ye Lian Qiao* (St. John's wort) (C) and *Yin Guo Ye* (Ginkgo leaf)–were concurrently used with buspirone and fluoxetine. One case report reported that a hypomanic episode occurred in

Anorgasmia: Inability to have an orgasm

Akathisia: The inability to remain seated; includes motor restlessness and a feeling of muscle twitching; may be a side effect of antipsychotic medication

Fasciculations: Involuntary twitchings of muscle fibers

Myoclonus: A single or series of shock-like contractions of muscle groups

a patient, which ended with cessation of herbs (Spinella & Eaton, 2002) Level 4 evidence.

SELECTIVE SEROTONIN REUPTAKE INHIBITORS (SSRIS)

- *Guan Ye Lian Qiao* (St. John's wort) (D)– inhibits serotonin reuptake and may cause "serotonin syndrome" when used concurrently with an SSRI, expert opinion (Chen & Chen, 2004) Level 5 evidence.
- *Guan Ye Lian Qiao* (St. John's wort) (C-) and *Yin Guo Ye* (Ginkgo leaf)–were concurrently used with buspirone and fluoxetine. One case reported a hypomanic episode occurred in a patient, which ended with cessation of herbs (Spinella & Eaton, 2002) Level 4 evidence.
- *Guan Ye Lian Qiao* (St. John's Wort) (C)– decreases blood concentrations (Zhou, Chan, Pan, Huang & Lee, 2004) Level 2b evidence, (Izzo & Ernst, 2009) Level 4 evidence.
- *Rou Cong Rong* (Cistanche) (Indeterminate)– may interact with sympathomimetics, monoamine oxidase inhibitors, selective serotonin inhibitors, and tricyclic antidepressants by increasing the activities of neurotransmitters such as norepinephrine, dopamine, and serotonin (Chinese language article cited in Chen & Chen, 2004) Indeterminate level of evidence.
- *Yin Guo Ye* (Ginkgo leaf) (C-)and *Guan Ye Lian Qiao* (St. John's wort)–were concurrently used with buspirone and fluoxetine. One case report reported a hypomanic episode in a patient, which ended with cessation of herbs (Spinella & Eaton, 2002) Level 4 evidence.

TRAZODONE

- *Yin Guo Ye* (Gingko) (D)–clinical cases indicate interactions of ginkgo with antiepileptics, aspirin (acetylsalicylic acid), diuretics, ibuprofen, risperidone, rofecoxib, trazodone and warfarin (Izzo & Ernst, 2009) Level 4 evidence.

VENLAFAXINE

- *Guan Ye Lian Qiao* (St. John's wort) (C)– decreases blood concentrations (Izzo & Ernst, 2009) Level 3b evidence.

INTERACTION ISSUES

A:

D: Atomoxetine is 98% protein bound; fluoxetine is 95% protein bound; nefazodone is over 99% bound; paroxetine is 93-95% bound; sertraline is 98% bound; trazodone is 85-95% bound; vilazodone is 96-99% bound.

M: Atomoxetine is a major substrate of CYP2D6; citalopram and escitalopram are major substrates of CYP2C19 and 3A4; desvenlafaxine is a weak/moderate inducer of CYP3A4; duloxetine is a major substrate of CYP1A2 and both a major substrate of and a moderate inhibitor of 2D6; fluoxetine is a major substrate of CYP2C9 and 2D6, a moderate inhibitor of CYP1A2 and 2C19, and a strong inhibitor of CYP2D6; fluvoxamine is a major substrate of CYP1A2 and 2D6 and a strong inhibitor of CYP1A2 and 2C19; nefazodone is a major substrate of CYP2D6 and both a major substrate of and a strong inhibitor of CYP3A4; paroxetine is a major substrate of and a strong inhibitor of CYP2D6 and a moderate inhibitor of CYP2B6; sertraline is a major substrate of CYP2D6 and a moderate inhibitor of 2B6, 2C19, 2D6, and 3A4; trazodone is a major substrate of CYP3A4; venlafaxine is a major substrate of CYP2D6 and 3A4; vilazodone is a major substrate of CYP3A4 and is a weak/moderate inducer of 2C19.

E:

TI:

Pgp: Nefazodone and trazodone induce Pgp.

CLASS 3:
MONOAMINE OXIDASE INHIBITORS

ISOCARBOXAZID (eye soe kar BOKS a zid)
 PR=C *(Marplan®)*

PHENELZINE (FEN el zene) PR=C *(Nardil®)*

RASAGILINE AND SELEGILINE (See Section 1 above)

TRANYLCYPROMINE (tran il SIP roe mene)
 PR=not assigned *(Parnate®)*

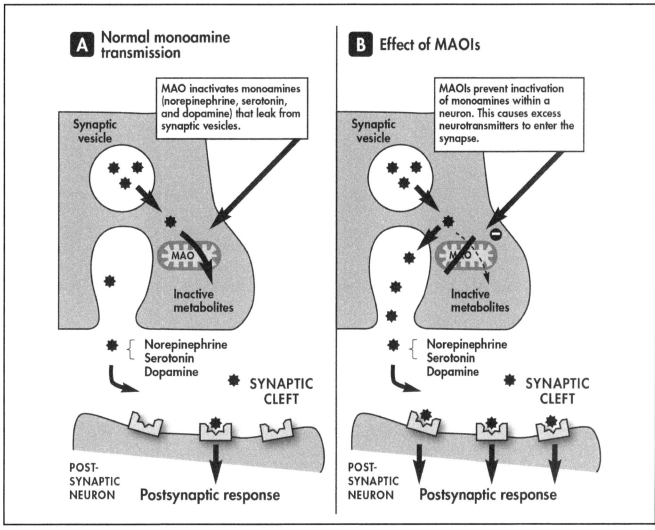

Figure 5.11 How monoamine oxidase inhibitors work.

FUNCTION

This class of drugs is used to treat depression. Selegiline targets more specific types of monoamine oxidases (MAOs) and is used more in the treatment of Parkinson's disease than as an antidepressant. Please refer to Section 1 of this chapter for more information about selegiline. While not as commonly used as other antidepressants due to its dietary restrictions and potential toxicities, these agents are used commonly in subsets of patients. These include patients unresponsive or allergic to TCAs and patients with strong anxiety, low psychomotor activity, phobias, and an interesting subcategory of depression known as atypical depression.

MECHANISMS OF ACTION

Monoamine oxidase (MAO) is an enzyme found in neurons as well as other tissues such as the intestines and liver. In the neuron, MAO deactivates excess monoamine neurotransmitters that leak out of the synaptic vesicles, which store the chemicals until they are needed. Monoamine transmitters include norepinephrine, dopamine, and serotonin. Inhibition of MAO causes more of these neurochemicals to be available both in the presynaptic neuron, allowing more of them to be released when an action potential occurs, and in the synaptic cleft as they leak out of the vesicles and presynaptic neuron. MAOIs may reversibly or irreversibly inactivate MAO.

Because the effects of MAO are not specific, inhibition can cause many adverse reactions to food substances that contain tyramine. Relatively severe diet restrictions are necessary when taking this agent. Foods to avoid are listed under interactions below.

MAOIs are similar to TCAs and SSRIs in that inhibition of MAO does not completely explain their effectiveness as antidepressants. They also need several weeks of use before being fully effective antidepressants. This indicates there are secondary effects. These secondary effects are poorly understood but several of the same theories of TCA effectiveness are being applied to these agents.

DOSAGES

ISOCARBOXAZID, for *adults*, initiate at 10 mg 2-4 times/d; may increase by 10 mg/d increments every 2-4 days up to 40 mg/d by the end of the first week in 2-4 doses; after first week, may increase by up to 20 mg/wk to a maximum dose of 60 mg/d.

PHENELZINE, for *adults*, 15 mg tid; may increase to 60-90 mg/d for maximum response, then reduce slowly for maintenance.

TRANYLCYPROMINE, for *adults*, 30 mg/d in divided doses; may increase by 10 mg increments at 1-3 week intervals up to a maximum dose of 60 mg/d.

ADVERSE EFFECTS

Foods that contain tyramine must be avoided to prevent toxic reactions. Tyramine-containing foods include aged cheeses, chicken, liver, beer, and red wines. Ingesting these while taking an MAOI can cause release of stored catecholamines and can result in headache, tachycardia, nausea, hypertension, cardiac arrhythmias, and stroke.

Other side effects of MAOIs include: drowsiness, orthostatic hypotension, blurred vision, dry mouth, constipation, and **dysuria**.

Given the toxic potential of MAOIs, their use in suicidal patients may be dangerous.

RED FLAGS

Eating tyramine-containing foods while taking MAOIs may result in arrhythmias, tachycardia,

Dysuria: Painful urination

Intracranial: Within the head

and stroke. Because of these toxic effects, MAOI use with suicidal patients may be dangerous. Orthostatic hypotension may induce life-threatening falls in the elderly.

Hypertensive episodes have rarely caused **intracranial** bleeding. However, any patient taking MAOIs who complains of a severe throbbing headache or a feeling of pressure in the head should be immediately evaluated for intracranial bleeding.

The use of antidepressant drugs in patients with major depressive disorder and/or suicidal ideation can precipitate a suicide attempt. While patienst may have suicidal thoughts in the middle of major depressive episodes, they often do not have enough energy to carry through on the thoughts. As an antidepressant starts to work, the patients will gain energy but the antidepressant effects may not have fully engaged. In other words, they now have the energy to attempt suicide, but the medication hasn't worked well enough yet to change the thoughts of suicide. Careful oversight needs to be employed when using any antidepressant in patients with major depression to prevent suicide.

INTERACTIONS

DRUG

Coadministration of MAOIs and SSRIs can cause "serotonin syndrome." Symptoms of this include: akathisia-like restlessness, muscle fasciculations, myoclonus, hyperreflexia, sweating, penile erection, shivering, tremors, and ultimately seizures and coma. Other medications besides SSRIs may cause this syndrome, including: meperidine, pentazocine, dextrometorphan, fenfluramine, and rarely TCAs.

The combined use of most antidepressants and ethanol or other sedatives may cause toxic sedation.

FOOD

Foods that contain tyramine must be avoided to prevent toxic reactions. Tyramine-containing foods include aged cheeses, chicken liver, beer, and red wines.

HERB

ISOCARBOXAZID

- *Ren Shen* (Ginseng) (D)–rare cases of manic-like symptoms have been documented with concurrent use of phenelzine. Use caution with concurrent use of *Ren Shen* with phenelzine or similar antidepressants, expert opinion (Fugh-Berman, 2000) Level 5 evidence.

MONOAMINE OXIDASE INHIBITORS (MAOI)

- *Gan Cao* (Licorice) (D)–may increase toxicity of MAOIs due to constituents that non-competitively inhibit MAO, bench research (Hatano, Fukuda, Miyase, Noro & Okuda, 1991) Level 5 evidence.
- *Ma Huang* (Ephedra) (B-)–based on ephedrine content, may cause hypertension with MAOI use, expert opinion (Blumenthal, 1998) Level 5 evidence. One case report described a patient who stopped a MAOI, phenelzine, and who ingested a combination pill of ephedrine, caffeine, and theophylline 24 hours later. She developed encephalopathy, neuromuscular irritability, sinus tachycardia, hypotension, rhabdomyolysis, and hyperthermia (Dawson, Earnshaw & Graham, 1995) Level 4 evidence. Other possible effects include arrhythmias, chest pain, hyperpyrexia, and death (Gruenwald, Brendler & Jaenicke, 2004). One human study showed an increase in cardiovascular symptoms (Dingemanse, 1993) Level 2c evidence. *Ma Huang* should be avoided for at least 2 weeks after stopping MAOIs (Brinker, 2001).
- *Ren Shen* (Ginseng) (D)–rare cases of manic-like symptoms have been documented with concurrent use of phenelzine. Use caution with concurrent *Ren Shen* and phenelzine or similar antidepressants, expert opinion (Fugh-Berman, 2000) Level 5 evidence.

- *Rou Cong Rong* (Cistanche) (Indeterminate)–may interact with sympathomimetics, MAOIs, SSRIs, and TCAs by increasing the activities of neurotransmitters such as norepinephrine, dopamine, and serotonin (Chinese language article cited in Chen & Chen, 2004) Indeterminate level of evidence.
- *Yin Guo Ye* (Gingko leaf) (B/C against potentiation)–theoretically may potentiate effects of MAOIs. Animal studies have substantiated this effect (Sloley, Urichuk, Morley *et al.*, 2000) Level 5 evidence; (White, Scates, & Cooper, 1996) Level 5 evidence, however, a human study did not (Fowler, Wang, Volkow, Logan, Franceschi, Franceschi *et al.*, 2000) Level 2c evidence.
- *Ying Su Ke* (Opium husks) (D)–phenothiazines, monoamine oxidase inhibitors, and tricyclic antidepressants may exacerbate the depressant and CNS suppressive effects of *Ying Su Ke*, expert opinion (Chen & Chen, 2004) Level 5 evidence.

PHENELZINE

- *Ren Shen* (Ginseng) (D)–rare cases of manic-like symptoms have been documented with concurrent use of phenelzine. Use caution with concurrent *Ren Shen* and phenelzine or similar antidepressants, expert opinion (Fugh-Berman, 2000) Level 5 evidence.

INTERACTION ISSUES

A:

D:

M: Tranylcypromine is a moderate inhibitor of CYP1A2, 2C19, and 2D6 and a strong inhibitor of 2A6.

E:

TI:

Pgp:

CLASS 4: ALPHA-2 ANTAGONISTS

MIRTAZAPINE (mir TAZ a pene) PR=C

(Remeron®, Remeron Soltab®)

▒ **FUNCTION**

This class of drugs is used to treat depression.

▒ **MECHANISMS OF ACTION**

These drugs work by antagonizing α-2-adrenergic receptors on the presynaptic neuron. Since these

Feedback inhibition: Where an intermediate or final product of a biological pathway stops or slows down an initiating step, eventually reducing the end results of that pathway

Hypomanic: similar to mania but less severe in its symptoms

Neutropenia: Reduction in the number of neutrophils, one type of immune cell, in the blood

Agranulocytosis: Extreme reduction in the number of leukocytes, or white blood cells, in the blood

receptors are used for **feedback inhibition**, antagonizing them causes more NE and 5-HT to be released from the presynaptic neuron into the synaptic cleft. More NE and 5-HT in the synaptic cleft means less depression.

▣ DOSAGES

MIRTAZAPINE, for *adults*, initiate at 15 mg nocte; increase up to 15-45 mg; incremental increases no more frequently than every 1-2 weeks.

▣ ADVERSE EFFECTS

May cause sedation and impaired performance of tasks requiring alertness. Appetite may be stimulated, and weight gain may occur. Other common side effects include constipation, xerostomia, weakness, and dizziness. May worsen psychosis in some patients. Can precipitate a manic or **hypomanic** shift in bipolar patients.

▣ RED FLAGS

May cause **neutropenia/agranulocytosis** and should be stopped immediately if signs or symptoms of these conditions occur.

The use of antidepressant drugs in patients with major depressive disorder and/or suicidal ideation can precipitate a suicide attempt. While patients may have suicidal thoughts in the middle of major depressive episodes, they often do not have enough energy to carry through on the thoughts. As an antidepressant starts to work, the patients will gain energ, but the antidepressant effects may not have fully engaged. In other words, they now have the energy to attempt suicide, but the medication has yet to work well enough to change the thoughts of suicide. Careful oversight needs to be employed when using any antidepressant

in patients with major depression to prevent suicide.

▣ INTERACTIONS

DRUG

The use of MAOIs and α-2 antagonists should not be initiated within 14 days of each other.

Metabolism may conflict with and cause increased activity of mirtazapine when combined with: amiodarone, ciprofloxacin, fluvoxamine, ketoconazole, norfloxacin, ofloxacin, rofecoxib, chlorpromazine, delaviridine, fluoxetine, miconazole, paroxetine, pergolide, quinidine, quinine, ritonavir, ropinirole, clarithromycin, dicolfenac, doxycycline, erythromycin, imatinib, isonazid, nefazodone, nicardipine, propofol, protease inhibitors, and verapamil.

Decreased effect of mirtazapine may occur when combined with: carbamazepine, phenobarbital, rifampin, clonidine, nafcillin, nevirapine, phenytoin, and rifamycin.

Combined use of most antidepressants and ethanol or other sedatives may cause toxic sedation.

HERB

α-2 RECEPTOR ANTAGONISTS

- *Gan Cao* (Licorice) (D)–theoretically may reduce effects of antihypertensive agents (α-1 adrenergic blockers, ACEI, α-2 receptor antagonists, β-adrenergic blockers, calcium channel blockers, clonidine, guanabenz, guanfacine, hydralazine, methyldopa, minoxidil, and reserpine). Undertake concurrent use with caution, expert opinion (Kowalak & Mills, 2001) Level 5 evidence.

INTERACTION ISSUES

A:
D:
M: Mirtazapine is a major substrate of CYP1A2, 2D6, and 3A4.
E:
TI:
Pgp:

CLASS 5:
DOPAMINE REUPTAKE INHIBITORS
BUPROPION (byoo PROE pee on) *(Aplenzin™,*

Budeprion SR®, Buproban®, Forfivo™ XL, Wellbutrin®, Wellbutrin SR®, Wellbutrin XL®, Zyban®)

FUNCTION

This class of drugs is used to treat depression. In addition, Zyban is specifically marketed for use in smoking cessation. Also, the FDA recently approved the use of bupropion for prevention of major depressive episodes in patients with a history of seasonal affective disorder (SAD). This is the first agent approved for use as a treatment for SAD.

MECHANISM OF ACTION

The mechanism of action of bupropion is not completely understood. It is a novel drug in that it has a dissimilar structure and is believed to have a different action than other antidepressants. It is thought that most of its antidepressant effects are due to reuptake inhibition of serotonin, norepinephrine, and dopamine. Unlike most antidepressants, current thinking is that most of its action is due to its effects on norepinephrine and/or dopamine rather than serotonin. It does inhibit MAO. Some metabolites of bupropion have amphetamine-like effects.

DOSAGES

BUPROPION, for *adults*, for depression, for immediate release: initiate at 100 mg bid; may increase to 100 mg tid after 3 days; if no clinical improvement for several weeks, may increase to 150 mg tid; for sustained release: initiate at 150 mg mane; may increase to 150 mg bid after 3 days; may increase, if no clinical improvement after several weeks, to a maximum of 200 mg bid; for extended release: initiate at 150 mg mane; may increase to 300 mg mane after 3 days; may increase, if no clinical improvement after several weeks, to a maximum of 450 mg once daily; Aplenzin™ should be initiated at 174 mg mane; may increase after 3 days to 348 mg once daily, maximum dose 522 mg/d; for seasonal affective disorder (SAD), initiate at 150 mg (Wellbutrin XL®) or 174 mg (Aplenzin™) mane; may increase after a week to 300 mg once daily (Wellbutrin XL®) or 348 mg once daily (Aplenzin™) mane; for smoking cessation, initiate at 150 mg once a day for 3 days

and then increase to 150 mg bid; treatment should continue for 7-12 weeks. For the *elderly*, for depression, initiate at 37.5 mg bid of immediate release or 100 mg daily of sustained release tablets; increase by 37.5-100 mg every 3-4 days to a maximum dose of 300 mg/d in divided doses.

ADVERSE EFFECTS

May cause dizziness, headache, insomnia, nausea, xerostomia, and agitation. Cardiovascular side effects occurred in a small population and include arrhythmias, hypertension, hypotension, palpations, syncope, and tachycardia. Because of these potential cardiac effects, cardiovascular patients should use bupropion with caution.

Seizures may occur when taking bupropion. The likelihood of this occurring is increased by higher doses, previous history, or other CNS events that may make a patient more susceptible to seizures such as head trauma, tumor, and so on.

As with most antidepressants, may precipitate a manic or hypomanic shift in bipolar patients. May worsen psychosis in some patients.

RED FLAGS

The use of antidepressant drugs in patients with major depressive disorder and/or suicidal ideation can precipitate a suicide attempt. While patients may have suicidal thoughts in the middle of major depressive episodes, they often do not have enough energy to carry through on the thoughts. As an antidepressant starts to work, the patients will gain energy, but the antidepressant effects may not have fully engaged. In other words, they now have the energy to attempt suicide, but the medication hasn't worked well enough yet to change the thoughts of suicide. Careful oversight needs to be employed when using any antidepressant in patients with major depression to prevent suicide.

INTERACTIONS

DRUG

The use of MAOIs and bupropion should not be initiated within 14 days of each other. Should not be used when patient is abruptly stopping ethanol or sedative use.

Metabolism may conflict with and cause increased activity of bupropion when combined with cimetidine. Risk of seizures may be increased when taken with antipsychotics, antidepressants, theophylline, and abrupt discontinuation of benzodiazepines and systemic steroids. The effects of warfarin may be altered by coadministration. Concurrent use of amantadine has been associated with increased side effects. Concurrent use of the following may increase the levels and effects of bupropion: desipramine, paroxetine, sertraline, orphenadrine, and cyclophosphamide.

Bupropion toxicity may be enhanced by levodopa and MAOIs.

Decreased effect of bupropion may occur when combined with: carbamazepine, nevirapine, phenytoin, phenobarbital, and rifampin.

The combined use of most antidepressants and ethanol or other sedatives may cause toxic sedation.

HERB

BUPROPION

- *Guan Ye Lian Qiao* (St. John's wort) (C)– decreases blood concentrations (Izzo & Ernst, 2009) Level 4 evidence.

INTERACTION ISSUES

A:

D:

M: Bupropion is a major substrate of CYP2B6 and a strong inhibitor of 2D6.

E:

TI:

Pgp:

SECTION 7: DRUGS FOR MANIA

LITHIUM (LITH ee um) PR=D *(Lithobid®)*

ATYPICAL ANTIPSYCHOTICS *(See Section 2, 3, or 7 of this Chapter)*

DRUGS USED TO TREAT EPILEPSY *(See Section 8 of this Chapter)*

According to the DSM-5-TM® (American Psychiatric Association, 2001), a manic episode is defined by a period of at least one week during which there is an abnormally and persistently elevated, expansive, or irritable mood. At least three of the following symptoms need to be present in order to meet this definition of a manic episode: inflated self-esteem or grandiosity, decreased need for sleep, pressured speech, flight of ideas, distractibility, psychomotor agitation, and excessive involvement in pleasurable activities with high potential for painful consequences. This last symptom often includes inappropriate sexual behavior, gambling, shopping, or other activities. A similar diagnosis is hypomania, which is similarly defined except that it lasts for a minimum of 4 days and is not severe enough to cause marked impairment in social or occupational functioning.

Manic episodes are commonly combined with depression in bipolar disorders. Bipolar I disorder is present when a patient has had manic episodes often with a past that includes major depressive episodes. Bipolar II disorder involves hypomania and major depressive episodes. Cyclothymic disorder involves numerous alternating episodes of hypomaniac and depressive symptoms.

FUNCTION

Lithium is used in the treatment of mania both acutely and prophylactically. In acute treatment, antipsychotic and antiseizure medication will often also be used because of the slow onset of action of lithium. Several atypical antipsychotics and antiseizure agents are useful in the management of mania as well as the treatment of acute episodes. Benzodiazepines can also be used for sedation during an acute episode.

MECHANISM OF ACTION

The mechanism of action of lithium is not well understood but is thought to involve an intracellular second messenger system. In animals, it has been shown that lithium decreases release of norepinephrine and dopamine into the synaptic cleft while not affecting the release of serotonin or possibly even increasing it.

DOSAGES

LITHIUM, for *adults*, 900-2400 mg/d in 3-4 divided doses. Extended release: 450-900 mg bid. In the *elderly*, initiate at 300 mg bid and increase weekly by 300 mg/d with monitoring. Rarely need to exceed 900-1200 mg/d.

ADVERSE EFFECTS

The therapeutic index of lithium is very low, and toxic effects are common. These include vomiting, acute diarrhea, ataxia, tremors, convulsions and coma, confusion, hyperreflexia, dysarthria, seizures, nerve damage, hypotension, albuminuria, cardiac arrhythmias, and death. More common side effects include nausea, diarrhea, drowsiness, polyuria, polydipsia, weight gain, fine tremor of the hand, and skin reactions including acne.

RED FLAGS

The therapeutic index of lithium is very low, and toxic effects are common. Toxic effects include vomiting, acute diarrhea, ataxia, tremors, convulsions and coma, confusion, hyperreflexia, dysarthria, seizures, nerve damage, hypotension, albuminuria, cardiac arrhythmias, and death.

INTERACTIONS

DRUG

Concurrent use of lithium and anticholinergic and other agents that affect gastrointestinal motility may alter Li^+ blood concentrations.

HERB

While there may not be a lot of specific drug-herb interactions documented, the narrow therapeutic index of this agent indicates that extreme caution be used when combined with herbs. It is the opinion of the authors that this drug should not be used with herbs without direct medical permission and supervision.

LITHIUM
- *Pu Gong Ying* (Dandelion) (D)–lithium toxicity may be worsened due to this herb's diuretic effect, enhancing sodium excretion as demonstrated in a rat study (two unobtainable studies cited in Brinker, 2001) Level 5 evidence.

INTERACTION ISSUES

A:
D:
M:
E:
TI: Lithium has a narrow therapeutic index.
Pgp:

SECTION 8: OPIOID ANALGESICS AND ANTAGONISTS

AGONISTS:

CARBETAPENTANE (kar bay ta PEN tane)
PR=C *(Carbaphen 12 Ped®,8 Carbaphen 12®8)*

CODEINE (KOE dene) PR=C *(Allfen CD,9 Allfen CDX,9 Ascomp® with Codeine,13 Capital® and Codeine,25 Cheratussin® DAC,14 Codar® D,15 Codar® GF,9 Dex-Tuss,9 Enda-Cof-DC,15 Fioricet® with Codeine,12 Fiorinal® with Codeine,13 Guaiatussin AC,9 Iophen C-NR,9 M-Clear,9 M-Clear WC,9 Mar-Cof® CG,9 Mytussin® DAC,14 Notuss®-DC,15 Phenylhistine DH [O],11 Robafen AC,9 Tricode® AR,11 Tricode® GF,14 Tylenol® with Codeine No. 3,10 Tylenol® with Codeine No. 410)*

DEXTROMETHORPHAN (deks troe meth OR fan) PR=C *(Alka-Seltzer Plus® Day Cold [O],33 All-Nite Multi-Symptom Cold/Flu Relief [O],58 Ambifed DM,39 Ambifed-G DM,39 Anaplex® DM,34 Bromaline® DM [O],34 Bromdex D,34 Bromfed® DM,34 Bromphenex™ DM [O],34 Brotapp-DM,34 Cardec™ DM [O],35 Cheracol® D [O],37 Cheracol® Plus [O],37 Comtrex®*

SECTION 8: OPIOID ANALGESICS AND ANTAGONISTS cont.

Maximum Strength, Non-Drowsy Cold & Cough [O],[33] Corfen-DM [O],[35] Coricidin HBP® Chest Congestion and Cough [O],[37] Coricidin® HBP Cough & Cold [O],[29] Creo-Terpin® [O], Creomulsion® Adult Formula [O], Creomulsion® for Children [O], Daytime Cold & Flu Relief Multi-Symptom [O],[33] De-Chlor DM [O],[35] Delsym® [O], Diabetic Siltussin-DM DAS-Na [O],[37] Diabetic Siltussin-DM DAS-Na Maximum Strength [O],[37] Diabetic Tussin® DM [O],[37] Diabetic Tussin® DM Maximum Strength [O],[37] Dicel® DM Chewables [O],[36] Dimetapp® Children's Long Acting Cough Plus Cold [O],[37] Double Tussin DM [O],[37] Ed A-Hist DM [O],[35] EndaCof [O],[35] ExeFen-DMX,[39] Father John's® [O], Father John's® Plus [O],[35] Fenesin DM IR [O],[37] Guaicon DMS [O],[37] Hold® DM [O], Iophen DM-NR [O],[37] Kidkare Children's Cough/Cold [O],[36] Kole-phrin® GG/DM [O],[37] LoHist PSB DM [O],[34] M-END DM [O],[36] Mapap® Multi-Symptom Cold [O],[33] Maxichlor PEH DM [O],[35] Maxichlor PSE DM [O],[36] Maxifed DM,[39] Maxifed DMX,[39] Maxiphen DM,[38] Maxiphen DMX,[38] Mucinex® Children's Multi-Symptom Cold [O],[38] Muci-nex® DM [O],[37] Mucinex® DM Maximum Strength [O],[37] Mucinex® Kid's Cough [O],[37] Mucinex® Kid's Cough Mini-Melts™ [O],[37] Nasohist™ DM Pediatric [O],[35] Neo DM,[34] Neo DM [O],[35] Neutrahist PDX [O],[36] Night Time Multi-Symptom Cold/Flu Relief [O],[58] NoHist DM [O],[35] Nuedexta™,[31] Nycoff [O], PE-Hist-DM [O],[35] Pedia Relief™ Cough-Cold [O],[36] Pedia Relief Cough and Cold [O],[40] PediaCare® Children's Long-Acting Cough [O], PediaCare® Children's Multi-Symptom Cold [O],[30] PediaHist DM,[34] Pediatric Cough & Cold [O],[36] Q-Tapp Cold & Cough [O],[34] Q-Tussin DM [O],[37] Refenesen™ DM [O],[37] Rescon DM [O],[36] Resperal-DM,[34] Robafen Cough [O], Robafen CF Cough & Cold [O],[38] Robafen DM [O],[37] Robafen DM Clear [O],[37] Robitussin® Children's Cough & Cold CF [O],[38] Robitussin® Children's Cough & Cold Long-Acting [O],[29] Robitussin® Children's Cough Long-Acting [O], Robitussin® Lingering Cold Long-Acting Cough [O], Robitussin® Linger-ing Cold Long-Acting CoughGels® [O], Robi-tussin® Peak Cold Cough + Chest Congestion DM [O],[37] Robitussin® Peak Cold Maximum Strength Cough + Chest Congestion DM [O],[37] Robitussin® Peak Cold Maximum Strength Multi-Symptom Cold [O],[38] Robitus-sin® Peak Cold Multi-Symptom Cold [O],[38] Robitussin® Peak Cold Sugar-Free Cough + Chest Congestion DM [O],[37] Safe Tussin® DM [O],[37] Safe-tussin® CD [O],[30] Scot-Tussin® Diabetes [O], Scot-Tussin® DM Maxi-Strength [O],[29] Scot-Tussin® Senior [O],[37] Silexin [O],[37] Silphen-DM [O], Siltussin DM [O],[37] Siltussin DM DAS [O],[37] Sudafed® Children's Cold & Cough [O],[40] Sudafed PE® Children's Cold & Cough [O],[30] Theraflu® Daytime Severe Cold & Cough [O],[33] Theraflu Warming Relief® Daytime Multi-Symptom Cold [O],[33] Theraflu Warming Relief® Daytime Severe Cold & Cough [O],[33] Triaminic® Children's Cough Long Acting [O], Triaminic® Children's Softchews® Cough & Runny Nose [O],[29] Triaminic® Daytime Cold & Cough [O],[30] Tylenol® Cold & Cough Night-time [O],[32] Tylenol® Cold Head Congestion Daytime [O],[33] Tylenol® Cold Multi-Symptom Daytime [O],[33] Tylenol® Cough & Sore Throat Nighttime [O],[32] Vicks® 44® Cough Relief [O], Vicks® 44E [O],[37] Vicks® DayQuil® Cold & Flu Multi-Symptom [O],[33] Vicks® DayQuil® Cough [O], Vicks® DayQuil® Mucus Control DM [O],[37] Vicks® Nature Fusion™ Cold & Flu Multi-Symptom Relief [O],[33] Vicks® Nature Fusion™ Cold & Flu Nighttime Relief [O],[32] Vicks® Nature Fusion™ Cough [O], Vicks® Nature Fusion™ Cough & Chest Congestion [O],[37] Vicks® NyQuil® Cold & Flu Nighttime Relief [O],[32] Vicks® Pediatric Formula 44E [O],[37] Virdec DM [O][35])

DIHYDROCODEINE (dye hye droe KOE dene) PR=C *(Coldcough PD,[16] Novahistine DH,[16] Synal-gos®-DC,[41] Trezix™,[17] Tusscough DHC™[16])*

FENTANYL (FEN ta nil) PR=C *(Abstral®, Actiq®, Duragesic®, Fentora®, Lazanda®, Onsolis®, Subsys®)*

HYDROCODONE (hye droe KOE done) PR=C *(Hycet®,[18] Hydromet®,[22] Ibudone®,[23] Lorcet® 10/650,[18] Lorcet® Plus,[18] Lortab®, Margesic®*

MIXED AGONIST-ANTAGONISTS AND PARTIAL AGONISTS:

BUTORPHANOL (byoo TOR fa nole) PR=C

NALBUPHINE (NAL byoo fene) PR=C

PENTAZOCINE (pen TAZ oh seen) PR=C
(Talacen®, Talwin®)

ANTAGONISTS:

ALVIMOPAN (al VI moe pan) PR=B *(Entereg®)*

METHYLNALTREXONE (meth il nal TREKS own) PR=B *(Relistor®)*

NALOXONE (nal OKS own) PR=C *(Suboxone®27)*

NALTREXONE (nal TREKS own) PR=C *(Depade®, ReVia®, Vivitrol™)*

Opioid analgesics are the drug of choice for moderate to severe, acute, or chronic pain management. These compounds are derived from or are similar to morphine. Opiates are drugs derived directly from the opium poppy such as morphine and codeine. Opioid is an all-encompassing term including these natural derivatives as well as synthetically derived morphine-like drugs. They are not used for **neurogenic** pain (tricyclic, SSRI, and SNRI antidepressants are most effective) or mild to moderate pain where NSAIDs are more appropriate.

For Oriental medical practitioners, opioid drugs are particularly interesting in that they activate natural opioid receptors. Acupuncture has been shown in numerous studies to release **endorphins**, **enkephalins**, and **dynorphins,** which activate the same opioid receptors and are thought to be the basis for the pain relief function of acupuncture.

FUNCTION

The main purpose of opioids is pain relief and the anxiety surrounding moderate to severe pain. They can also be used for reducing the cough reflex, intractable diarrhea, and illicitly for their euphoric effects. While they can be used to treat pain in opioid novice patients, the mixed agonist-antagonists and partial agonists are generally used for treating opioid addiction by reducing withdrawal symptoms.

Many opioids, such as codeine, dihydrocodeine, dextromethorphan, and hydrocodone are widely used as antitussives, usually in combination with an antihistamine or decongestant.

Opioid antagonists are used to reverse the effects of agonist overdose.

MECHANISMS OF ACTION

There are three major opioid receptors: μ (mu), κ (kappa), and Δ (delta). Opioid drugs have different affinities for each of these receptors.

Pain relief is mostly moderated by the μ receptors with some help from κ receptors in the dorsal horn of the spinal cord. In general, the receptors work by decreasing excitatory neurotransmitter release of the presynaptic neuron and dampening the response of the postsynaptic neuron (see Figure 5.12). In the spinal cord, opioids reduce the release of substance P, a major attenuator of pain.

A fourth opioid receptor has been recently discovered. The role of the N/OFQ receptor is still not completely understood but appears to enhance or decrease analgesia depending on where the receptor is located. How opioids affect this receptor is being studied.

Opioid receptors are located throughout the body, and their placement helps explain their beneficial as well as adverse effects:

- **BRAIN STEM:** Helps moderate respiration, blood pressure, cough, nausea and vomiting, miosis, and stomach secretions.
- **MEDIAL THALAMUS:** Helps moderate pain that has an emotional component and is poorly localized.
- **SPINAL CORD:** Initial integration of sensory information is performed here, and painful stimuli can be modified.
- **HYPOTHALAMUS:** Neuroendocrine effects are moderated here.

Neurogenic: Originating from the nervous system

Endorphins: Morphine-like pain-relieving chemicals produced naturally within the body

Enkephalins: A neurochemical that activates opiate receptors, increasing the threshold of pain

Dynorphins: A group of endogenous neurochemicals that includes endorphins and enkephalins that have morphine-like effects on the body

• **LIMBIC SYSTEM:** As part of the "emotional" system of the brain, opioid effects here are mainly modification of emotional behavior.

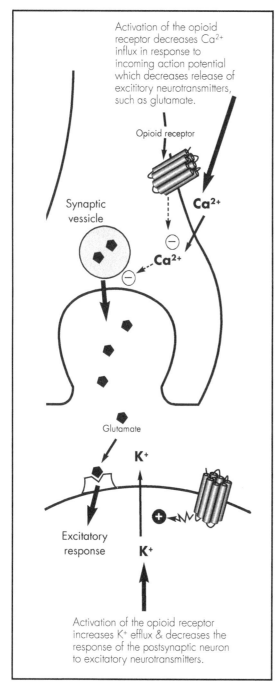

Activation of the opioid receptor decreases Ca²⁺ influx in response to incoming action potential which decreases release of excitatory neurotransmitters, such as glutamate.

Opioid receptor

Ca²⁺

Synaptic vessicle

⊖ Ca²⁺

⊖

Glutamate

K⁺

⊕

Excitatory response

K⁺

Activation of the opioid receptor increases K⁺ efflux & decreases the response of the postsynaptic neuron to excitatory neurotransmitters.

Figure 5.12: How an opioid acts on both the pre- and post-synaptic neuron. Opioid receptors on the presynaptic neuron slow calcium ion influx due to an action potential that in turn slows neurotransmitter release. On the postsynaptic opioid receptor, activation opens potassium ion channels, which makes it more difficult to initiate an action potential.

• **PERIPHERY:** May prevent inflammatory chemical release.

Methadone and buprenorphine have similar effects to morphine and heroin but with a longer duration of action and milder withdrawal symptoms.

Opioid antagonists work by competitively inhibiting binding at the opioid receptors and preventing activation of the receptors.

■ DOSAGES

ALVIMOPAN, for *adults*, for management of postoperative ileus, initiate at 12 mg administered 30 minutes to 5 hours prior to surgery;maintain at 12 mg bid beginning the day after surgery for a maximum of 7 days or until discharged; maximum treatment is 15 doses.

BUPRENORPHINE, for acute moderate to severe pain, for *children* 2-12, IM: 2-6 mcg/kg every 4-6 hours; for *children* 13 or older, refer to adult dosing. For *adults*, for acute moderate to severe pain, in the opiate naïve, 0.3 mg every 6-8 hours prn, initial dose may be repeated once in 30-60 minutes; usual dose range is 0.15-0.6 mg every 4-8 hours prn; for chronic moderate to severe pain, transdermal patch: initiate at 5 mcg/h every 7 days in opiate naïve patients; may increase after at least 72 hours; maximum dose is 20 mcg/h every 7 days, when discontinuing, taper off over 7 days to prevent withdrawal; for opioid dependence, sublingual tablet: on day 1, 8 mg, day 2 and subsequent induction days, 16 mg; usual induction dose range is 12-16 mg/d usually accomplished over 3-4 days; treatment should begin at least 4 hours after last use of heroin or other short-acting opioids, preferably when first signs of withdrawal appear; maintain at 16 mg/d; in some patients 12 mg/d may be effective; patients should be switched to the buprenorphine/naloxone combination product. For the *elderly*, for acute moderate to severe pain, IM: 0.15 mg every 6 hours; long-term use not recommended.

BUTORPHANOL, for *adults*, for acute moderate to severe pain, IM: initiate at 2 mg; may repeat every 3-4 hours prn; usual range is 1-4 mg every 3-4 hours prn; intranasal spray: also used for migraine headache pain, initiate at 1 spray in 1 nostril; an additional 1 spray in 1 nostril may be given in 60-90 minutes, if necessary; may repeat initial dose in 3-4 hours after the last as needed; as preoperative medication, IM: 2 mg 60-90 minutes before surgery; pain during labor when the fetus is over 37 weeks gestation and there are no signs of fetal distress, IM: 1-2 mg; may repeat in 4 hours. For the *elderly*, IM: initial dosage should generally be 1/2 of the adult recommended dose; repeated dosing must be based on patient's response; but generally should be at least 6 hours apart; nasal spray: initial dose should not exceed 1 mg; a second dose may be given after 90-120 minutes.

CARBETAPENTANE, only used in combination with other drugs and does not have individual dosing.

CODEINE, for *adults*, for pain management, immediate release: initiate at 15-60 mg every 4 hours prn; maximum daily dose 360 mg/d.

DEXTROMETHORPHAN, as a cough suppressant, for *children* 4-6 years, 2.5-7.5 mg every 4-8 hours, extended release: 15 mg bid up to a maximum of 30 mg per 24 hours, for *children* 6-12 years, 5-10 mg every 4 hours or 15 mg every 6-8 hours; extended release: 30 mg bid up to a maximum of 60 mg per 24 hours. For *children* over 12 years, and *adults*, as a cough suppressant, 10-20 mg every 4 hours or 30 mg every 6-8 hours, extended release: 60 mg bid up to a maximum of 120 mg per day.

DIHYDROCODEINE, HYDROCODONE, only used in combination with other drugs and does not have individual dosing.

FENTANYL, for *adults*, for surgical premedication, IM: 50-100 mcg 30-60 minutes prior to surgery; for breakthrough cancer pain, lozenge: initiate at 200 mcg; second dose may be started 15 minutes after first dose if necessary; only 1 additional dose can be given per pain episode, then the patient must wait at least 4 hours before treating another episode; no more than 4 units/d should be administered; buccal film (Onsolis®): initiate at 200 mcg; if an increase is necessary, do so in 200 mcg increments once per episode; separate single doses by at least 2 hours without exceeding 800 mcg simultaneously; if more is required, treat next episode with 1200 mcg film; usual single dose per episode is 200-1200 mcg; buccal tablet (Fentora®): initiate at 100 mcg; a second 100 mcg dose may be started 30 minutes after the start of the first, if needed; maximum of 2 doses per breakthrough episode every 4 hours; nasal spray (Lazanda®): initiate at one 100 mcg spray in one nostril; if pain is relieved within 30 minutes, maintain dosing in future episodes; if unrelieved, may increase in the following fashion: if no relief with 100 mcg, increase to one 100 mcg spray in each nostril; if no relief with 200 mcg, use one 400 mcg spray; if no relief with 400 mcg, use one 400 mcg spray in each nostril; must wait at least 2 hours before treating another episode with nasal spray; sublingual spray (Subsys®): initiate at 100 mcg; if unrelieved, 1 additional 100 mcg dose may be given 30 minutes after first dose; a maximum of 2 doses can be given per breakthrough pain episode and must wait at least 4 hours before treating with another; to maintain, follow these titration steps: if pain is relieved within 30 minutes, the same dose should be used to treat subsequent episodes; if unrelieved increase to 200 mcg per episode; if no relief with 200 mcg dose, increase to one 400 mcg unit; if no relief with 400 mcg dose, increase to one 600 mcg unit; if no relief with 600 mcg dose, increase to one 800 mcg unit, if no relief with 800 mcg dose, increase to two 600 mcg units; if no relief with 1200 mcg dose, increase to two 800 mcg units; sublingual tablet (Abstral®): initiate at 100 mcg for all patients, if unrelieved, a second dose may be given 30 minutes after first dose; a maximum of 2 doses can be given per episode, and one must wait at least 2 hours before treating another episode; may increase in 100 mcg increments up to 400 mcg over consecutive breakthrough episodes; if more is still needed over 400 mcg, increase in increments of 200 mcg, starting with 600 mcg dose; doses of over 800 mcg have not been evaluated. This agent can be used for chronic pain management in *children* 2 years or older and *adults*; however, dosing is complicated by transferring from a previous opioid to fentanyl and should be done using appropriate guidelines. It has been found that the *elderly* are about twice as sensitive to fentanyl as other patients, and a wide range of dosing may be used; but generally is lower than adult dosing.

HYDROMORPHONE, for *children* over 50 kg, please refer to adult dosing for moderate to severe acute pain. For *adults*, for moderate to severe acute pain, initiate at 2-4 mg every 4-6 hours prn; the American Pain Society recommends an initial dose of 4-8 mg in patients in severe pain; subcutaneous 0.8-1 mg every 3-4 hours prn; patients with prior opioid use may require larger initial doses; rectal: 3 mg every 6-8 hours prn; for chronic pain, extended release formulation (Exalgo®): for use in opioid tolerant patients only; dose range is 8-64 mg every 24 hours; pain relief and adverse events should be assessed frequently; do not increase more often than every 3-4 days. For the *elderly*, for acute pain, initiate at the lower end of the adult dosing.

LEVORPHANOL, for *adults*, for moderate to severe acute pain, initiate at 2 mg every 6-8 hours prn; patients with prior opiate exposure may require higher initial dose; usual dose range is 2-4 mg every 6-8 hours prn; for chronic pain, the appropriate dose is one that relieves pain without unmanageable side effects.

MEPERIDINE, not recommended as an analgesic and should only be used for 48 hours or less and a maximum of 600 mg/d. For *children*, for pain, oral, IM, or subcutaneous: 1.1-1.8 mg/kg every 3-4 hours prn; up to a maximum of 50-150 mg/dose, total maximum of 600 mg/d; as a preoperative analgesic IM or subcutaneous: 1.1-2.2 mg/kg given 30-90 minutes before the beginning of anesthesia up to a maximum of 50-150 mg/dose. For *adults*, for pain, oral, IM, or subcutaneous: 50-150 mg every 3-4 hours prn; as preoperative analgesia: IM or subcutaneous: 50-150 mg given 30-90 minutes before anesthesia; for obstetric analgesia: IM or subcutaneous: 50-100 mg when pain becomes regular; may repeat every 1-3 hours. Use should be avoided in the *elderly*.

METHADONE, the following are guidelines; state laws and regulations as well as individual responses should be taken into consideration when using this agent. For *adults*, for moderate to severe chronic pain, initiate at 2.5-10 mg every 8-12 hours; more frequent administration may be required when initiating to maintain adequate analgesia; for detoxification, initiate at 20-30 mg; lower doses should be considered in patients with lower tolerance; for example, those who have not taken opioids for 5 or more days, may be provided an additional 5-10 mg if withdrawal symptoms have not been suppressed or if symptoms reappear after 2-4 hours; total daily dose on the first day should not exceed 40 mg; maintain by establishing a dosage that prevents craving, attenuates the euphoric effect and tolerance to sedation; usual range is 80-120 mg/d; to withdraw, reduce dose by less than 10% of the maintenance dose; every 10-14 days. For the *elderly*, oral and IM: 2.5 mg every 8-12 hours.

METHYLNALTREXONE, for *adults*, for opioid-induced constipation, subcutaneous: dose according to body weight, administer 1 dose every other day prn, maximum of 1 dose/day; under 38 kg, 0.15 mg/kg (round dose up to nearest 0.1 mL of volume); 38 to less than 62 kg, 8 mg; 62-114 kg, 12 mg; over 114 kg, 0.15 mg/kg (round dose up to nearest 0.1 mL of volume).

MORPHINE, for *children* over 6 months and below 50 kg, for moderate to severe acute pain, 0.15-0.2 mg/kg every 3-4 hours prn; IM: 0.1-0.2 mg/kg every 3-4 hours prn. For *adults*, for moderate to severe acute pain, initiate at 10 mg every 4 hours prn; patients with prior opiate exposure may require higher initial doses; usual range is 10-30 mg every 4 hours prn; IM and subcutaneous: initiate at 5-10 mg every 4 hours prn; patients with prior opiate exposure may require higher initial doses;usual range is 5-20 mg every 4 hours prn; for chronic pain there is no optimal or maximal dose; the dose is whatever controls pain with manageable side effects.

NALBUPHINE, for adults, for pain management, IM or subcutaneous: 10 mg/70 kg every 3-6 hours; maximum single dose is 20 mg; maximum daily dose is 160 mg.

NALOXONE, for *adults*, for opioid overdose, IM or subcutaneous: initiate at 0.4-2 mg; may need to repeat every 2-3 minutes; after reversal, may need to dose again at a later time (20-60 minutes) depending on opioid used; if no response is observed after a total administration of 10 mg, consider other causes of respiratory depression; for reversal of respiratory depression with therapeutic opioid doses, IM or subcutaneous: initiate at 0.04-0.4 mg; may repeat until desired response achieved; if desired response is not achieved after 0.8 mg total, consider other causes of respiratory depression.

NALTREXONE, for *adults*, for alcohol or opioid dependence, do not initiate therapy until patient is opioid free for at least 7-10 days; initiate at 25 mg; if no withdrawal signs occur, administer 50 mg on the second day; maintenance dose is 50 mg/d; alternative maintenance regimens could be 50 mg on weekdays with a 100 mg dose on Saturday, 100 mg every other day, or 150 mg every 3 days; IM: 380 mg once every 4 weeks.

OPIUM TINCTURE, for *adults*, for diarrhea, usual dose is 6 mg of undiluted opium tincture (10 mg/mL) qid.

OXYCODONE, for *adults*, for pain management, initiate at 5-15 mg every 4-6 hours prn; dose range is 5-20 mg per dose; for severe chronic pain, should be taken on a regular schedule, every 4-6 hours, at the lowest dose that achieves adequate analgesia; controlled release: initiate at: 10 mg every 12 hours.

OXYMORPHONE, for *adults*, for analgesia, IM or subcutaneous, initiate at 1-1.5 mg, may repeat every 4-6 hours prn; for labor analgesia, IM: 0.5-1 mg; for acute pain, initiate at 5-10 mg every 4-6 hours prn; for chronic pain, extended release: initiate at 5 mg every 12 hours.

PAREGORIC, For *children*, 0.25-0.5 mL/kg 1-4 times/d. For *adults*, 5-10 mL 1-4 times/d.

PENTAZOCINE, for *children* 1-16 years, as a preoperative or preanesthetic, IM: .5 mg/kg. For *adults*, as an analgesic, IM or subcutaneous: 30-60 mg every 3-4 hours, maximum of 360 mg/d; for labor pain, IM 30 mg once.

TAPENTADOL, for *adults*, for moderate to severe acute pain, day 1: 50-100 mg every 4-6 hours prn; may administer a second dose no less than 1 hour after the first; maximum dose on first day is 700 mg daily; day 2 and after, 50-100 mg every 4-6 hours prn up to a maximum of 600 mg daily; for moderate to severe chronic pain and neuropathic pain associated with diabetic peripheral neuropathy, extended release: initiate at 50 mg bid.

TRAMADOL, for *adults*, for moderate to severe pain, 50-100 mg every 4-6 hours, maximum of 400 mg/d; for patients not requiring rapid onset, tolerability may be improved by starting at 25 mg/d and increasing by 25 mg every 3 days until reaching 25 mg qid; total daily dose may then be increased 50 mg every 3 days as tolerated to reach 50 mg qid; after that 50-100 mg may be given every 4-6 hours prn up to a maximum 400 mg/d; for orally disintegrating tablet (Rybix™ ODT): 50-100 mg every 4-6 hours with a maximum of 400 mg/d; for patients not requiring rapid onset, tolerability may be improved by starting dose at 50 mg/d and increasing dose by 50 mg every 3 days until reaching 50 mg qid; after that 50-100 mg may be given every 4-6 hours prn up to a maximum 400 mg/d; extended release: 100 mg once daily; maximum dose is 300 mg daily. For the *elderly* over 75 years, do not exceed 300 mg/d; extended release: use with great caution.

ADVERSE EFFECTS

Several major adverse effects may occur with opioid use. Respiratory depression is the main cause of death in opioid overdose. Addiction, in that opioids cause tolerance and physical dependence, is of major concern as well, though the probability of addiction with proper usage for pain relief is relatively small and should not be a major consideration when deciding on appropriate pain management. Withdrawal symptoms include tearing, runny nose, sweating, yawning, miosis, flushing, heart palpitations, twitching, shaking, fever, restlessness/irritability, spasms, N/V, hot/cold flashes, insomnia, HR changes.

Miosis is common with opioid usage. Constipation, sedation, menstrual changes, nausea and vomiting, and dysphoria are also common.

Opioids should not be used in patients with emphysema or cor pulmonale without respiration monitoring. Intracranial pressure can elevate rapidly in head injuries, and opioid use can enhance cerebral and spinal ischemia. Urinary retention may occur when used in patients with prostatic hypertrophy. Adrenal insufficiency and myxedema may reduce clearance. Use opioids with caution in patients with liver failure and asthma.

Opioid antagonists may initiate withdrawal in patients with opioid addictions (see Figure 5.13).

While tramadol is not an opioid, it works by binding the μ (mu) receptors and weakly prevents reuptake of serotonin and norepinephrine.

RED FLAGS

Respiratory depression can be life threatening. The potential for addiction can have profound effects on the patient's quality of life, and overdosage of any of these medications can result in death due to respiratory depression.

The FDA recently issued a warning for breast-feeding women taking codeine. In the small population of women who are rapid metabolizers of codeine (which is metabolized to morphine), enough morphine may be delivered in breast milk to cause serious and potentially fatal reactions in the breast-feeding infant. A clinical test can confirm the presence of rapid metabolism.

The FDA has issued a warning regarding methadone. If taken too often, if the dose is too high, or if taken with certain other medicines or

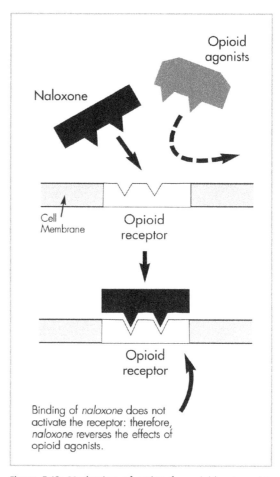

Figure 5.13: **Mechanism of action** for opioid antagonists such as naltrexone and naloxone.

supplements, slowed or stopped breathing, heart conduction pathologies (QT prolongation and Torsades de Pointes), and death have been reported. This is probably due to the difference between methadone's analgesic effect and half-life. It is analgesic for 4-8 hours, but its half-life is 8-59 hours. This means the dose of methadone potentially remains in the system for much longer than its effects. Health-care professionals should tell patients to take no more methadone than has been prescribed without first talking to their physician.

INTERACTIONS

DRUG

Depressant effects of opioids may be enhanced by antipsychotic agents, sedative hypnotics, MAOIs, and tricyclic antidepressants. Analgesia is enhanced by amphetamine and hydroxyzine through an unknown mechanism. Carbamazepine can increase metabolism of tramadol probably due to cytochrome P450 2D6 induction.

HERB

METHADONE

- *Guan Ye Lian Qiao* (St. John's wort) (C)–decreases blood concentrations (Zhou, Chan, Pan, Huang & Lee, 2004) Level 2b evidence; (Izzo & Ernst, 2009) Level 4 evidence.

NARCOTICS

- *Bai Jiang Cao* (Dahurian patrinia herb), *Lang Dan Cao* (Gentiana), *Zhi Zi* (Gardenia, cape jasmine fruit), and *Xi Jiao* (Rhinoceros horn) (Indeterminate)–all have a sedative effect and may increase sedative effects of drugs (Chinese language article cited in Chen & Chen, 2004) Indeterminate level of evidence.
- *Bai Shao* (White peony root) and *Tian Nan Xing* (Arisaema) (Indeterminate)–have a sedative and analgesic effect and may increase sedative effects of drugs (Chinese language article cited in Chen & Chen, 2004) Indeterminate level of evidence.
- *Chan Tui* (Cicada moulting), *Qin Jiao* (Gentiana macrophylla root) (Indeterminate)–both have an inhibitory effect on the CNS potentiating sedative drugs (Chinese language article cited in Chen & Chen, 2004) Indeterminate level of evidence.
- *Jiao Gu Lan* (Gynostemma) (Indeterminate)–has sedative, hypnotic, and analgesic effects and may increase sedative effects of drugs (Chinese language article cited in Chen & Chen, 2004) Indeterminate level of evidence.
- *Niu Huang* (Cow gallstone) (Indeterminate)– mild

sedative effect may increase sedative effects of drugs (Chinese language article cited in Chen & Chen, 2004) Indeterminate level of evidence.

- *Shen*-calming medicinals (D)–may have marked sedative and tranquilizing effects and may increase sedative effects of drugs, expert opinion (Chen & Chen, 2004) Level 5 evidence.
- *Wu Jia Pi* (Acanthopanax) (Indeterminate)–has a mild sedative effect and may increase sedative effects of drugs (Chinese language article cited in Chen & Chen, 2004) Indeterminate level of evidence.

OXYCODONE

- *Guan Ye Lian Qiao* (St. John's wort) (C)–decreases blood concentrations (Nieminen, Hagelberg, Saari, Neuvone *et al.,* 2010) Level 3b evidence.

INTERACTION ISSUES

A:

D: Buprenorphine is approximately 96% protein bound.

M: Buprenorphine is a major substrate of CYP3A4; codeine is a major substrate of CYP2D6; dextromethorphan is a major substrate of CYP2D6; fentanyl is a major substrate of CYP3A4; hydrocodone is a substrate CYP2D6 and 3A4; methadone is a major substrate of CYP2B6 and 3A4 and a moderate inhibitor of 2D6; oxycodone is a major substrate of CYP3A4; tramadol is a major substrate of CYP2D6 and 3A4.

E:

TI: Methadone has a narrow therapeutic index.

Pgp:

SECTION 9: DRUGS USED TO TREAT EPILEPSY

PRIMARY DRUGS:

ACETAZOLAMIDE (a set a ZOLE a mide) PR=C
(Diamox®, Sequels®)

CARBAMAZEPINE (kar ba MAZ e pene) PR=D
(Carbatrol®, Epitol®, Equetro®, Tegretol®, Tegretol®-XR)

CLONAZEPAM, CLORAZEPATE, DIAZEPAM

(See Section 2)

DIVALPROEX (dye VAL proe ex) PR=D
(Depakote®, Depakote® ER, Depakote® Sprinkle)

ETHOSUXIMIDE (eth oh SUKS i mide) PR=C
(Zarontin®)

ETHOTOIN (ETH oh toe in) PR=D *(Peganone®)*

continues on next page

SECTION 9: DRUGS USED TO TREAT EPILEPSY, cont.

LORAZEPAM *(See Section 2)*

METHSUXIMIDE (meth SUKS i mide) PR=C
(Celontin®)

OXCARBAZEPINE (ox car BAZ e pene) PR=C
(Oxtellar XR™, Trileptal®)

PHENOBARBITAL *(See Section 2)*

PHENYTOIN (FEN i toe in) PR=D *(Dilantin®,*
Dilantin–125®, Phenytek®)

PRIMIDONE *(See Section 2)*

VALPROIC ACID (val PROE ik AS id) PR=D
(Depacon®, Stanzor™)

ADJUNCT DRUGS:

FELBAMATE (FEL ba mate) PR=C *(Felbatol®)*

FOSPHENYTOIN (fos FEN i toe in) PR=D

GABAPENTIN (ga ba PEN tin) PR=C *(Gralise™,*
Neurontin®)

GABAPENTIN ENACARBIL (gab a PEN tin
en a KAR bil) PR=C *(Horizant™)*

LACOSAMIDE (la KOE sa mide) PR=C
(Vimpat®)

LAMOTRIGINE (la MOE tri jene) PR=C
(Lamictal®, Lamictal® ODT™, Lamictal® XR™)

LEVETIRACETAM (lee va tye RA se tam) PR=C
(Keppra®, Keppra XR®)

PERAMPANEL (per AM pa nel) PR=C

PREGABALIN *(See Chapter 11, Section 2)*

RUFINAMIDE (roo FIN a mide) PR=C *(Banzel™)*

TIAGABINE (tye AG a bene) PR=C *(Gabitril®)*

TOPIRAMATE (toe PYRE a mate) PR=C
(Qsymia™,[42] Topamax®)

VIGABATRIN (vye GA ba trin) PR=C *(Sabril®)*

ZONISAMIDE (zoe NIS a mide) PR=C
(Zonegran®)

Epilepsy is the second most common neurological disorder (behind stroke), affecting over 2.5 million individuals in the United States. By definition, epilepsy is a condition of recurrent seizures involving the sudden, excessive, and synchronous discharge of cerebral neurons. But there the similarities between different types of epilepsy end. Seizures are differentiated by where in the brain they occur, which determines the type of seizure, how often, and how severe they are. Drugs are the most effective means of controlling seizures with approximately half of epileptics gaining complete relief from drugs. Of the remaining patients about half receive meaningful improvement in their symptoms. Since most antiepileptic medications have substantial side effects, patient compliance becomes a substantial issue as do drug-drug interactions.

There are several schema for breaking down epilepsy into different types. The first breaks it down into primary and secondary epilepsy. Primary epilepsy is where an anatomical cause,

such as a tumor or trauma, is not apparent. It is inherited. Secondary epilepsy involves seizures due to reversible CNS injury from neoplasms, trauma, hypoglycemia, rapid alcohol withdrawal, and meningitis or from irreversible CNS injury such as trauma and CVAs.

Approximately 70% of epileptics have only one type of seizure, with the remaining 30% having 2 or more types of seizures. Seizures can be classified by whether they are partial or generalized. And each of these can be further broken down, as follows:

• **PARTIAL SEIZURES** are those where consciousness is maintained and generally involve smaller areas of the CNS. They may, however, continue to progress and become generalized tonic-clonic seizures.

• *Simple partial seizures* are where the focus of the seizure and the abnormal electrical activity is confined to single locus in the brain and does not spread. This results in specific limbs or muscle groups and sensory modes being affected. These can include flashes of light, chewing movements or smacking of gums, olfactory hallucinations, and so on. In Jacksonian seizures motor symptoms start in the hand and "march up" the arm.

• *Complex partial seizures* are similar to simple partial seizures but also alter consciousness with sensory hallucinations and mental distortion and may cause loss of consciousness.

• **GENERALIZED SEIZURES** begin at a small focus but rapidly spread throughout both hemispheres of the brain. They usually cause an immediate loss of consciousness.

• *Infantile seizures* occur in the first 3 years of life and then are replaced by other forms of seizures. They are characterized by sudden flexion of the arms and trunk and extension of the legs. Developmental abnormalities are often present.

• *Absence seizures* (previously called petit mal) are brief seizures causing a 10-30-second loss of consciousness and eyelid fluctuations with or without loss of **axial** muscle tone. These seizures are genetic, occur mostly in children, and may occur several times a day. They may be precipitated by hyperventilation and sitting quietly and rarely occur during exercise.

• *Tonic-clonic seizures* (also known as grand mal) begin with an outcry and involve loss of consciousness, falling, and **tonic then clonic contractions** of the limbs, trunk, and head. Urinary and fecal incontinence may occur. They typically last from 1 to 2 minutes. Confusion and exhaustion often occur **postictally**.

• *Atonic seizures* are brief seizures, primarily in children, where there is complete loss of muscle tone and consciousness. The greatest danger in this type of seizure is that the child falls and may suffer head or other trauma.

• *Myoclonic seizures* are brief, rapid jerking of a limb, multiple limbs, or the trunk that may be repetitive and lead to a tonic-clonic seizure. There is no loss of consciousness in this type of seizure. They are rare and often result from permanent neurological damage.

• *Febrile seizures* occur in children from 3 months to 5 years old when ill with a high fever. They consist of tonic-clonic seizures of short duration. They are benign, and while frightening to observe, do not indicate any serious or permanent damage and rarely require medication.

• *Lennox-Gastaut Syndrome* is a severe form of epilepsy that usually begins before the age of 4 and may involve tonic, atonic, absence, or myoclonic seizures. Most children with this syndrome have some form of intellectual impairment. It can be caused by brain malformations, perinatal **asphyxia**, severe head injury, central nervous system infection, and inherited conditions, although in 30-35% of cases a cause cannot be determined.

• *Status epilepticus* is the state where seizures follow one another without any refractory period between. It can be fatal and may result from overly rapid removal of anticonvulsant medications.

In general, patients are started on one drug in this class, usually a primary drug, and effectiveness is assessed. If the patient becomes seizure free, which occurs 47% of the time, then no further drugs are used. If not, the first drug is stopped and a second drug is tried. This eliminates seizures in another 13% of patients. If that fails, another drug is added, and two drug combinations are attempted. In general, monotherapy is preferred to polytherapy as there are fewer adverse effects and toxicity. The adjunct drugs have been developed in the last decade or two and, with a few exceptions, are used in polytherapy.

Axial: Pertaining to the central part of the body; not the limbs

Tonic convulsion: A prolonged generalized contraction of the voluntary muscles

Clonic convulsion: A convulsion characterized by rhythmic alternating contractions and relaxations of muscle groups

Postictal: Pertaining to the period after a convulsion

Asphyxia: Severe hypoxia leading to loss of consciousness and death

FUNCTION

The antiepileptic/anticonvulsant drugs are used for the prevention of seizures. Each drug tends to work best with a few of the different types of seizures as shown in Figure 5.14 on the next page.

In the benzodiazepine class of drugs, clon-

	Partial	Generalized					
	SIMPLE or COMPLEX	TONIC-CLONIC (grand mal)	ABSENCE (petit mal)	MYOCLONIC	INFANTILE SPASMS	STATUS EPILEPTICUS	LENNOX-GASTAUT SYNDROME
Barbiturates						Second	
Benzodiazepines				Alternative	Second	First	Alternative
Carbamazepine	Second						
Divalproex	Alternative	Second	First	First	Second		First
Ethosuximide			Alternative				
Felbamate							Alternative
Fosphenytoin						First	
Gabapentin	Alternative						
Lamotrigine	First	First	First	Second	Alternative		First
Levetiracetam	First	First		First			Second
Locosamide	Second						
Oxycarbazine	Alternative						
Phenytoin	Alternative						
Pregabalin	Second						
Rufinamide							First
Tiagabine	Alternative						
Topiramate	First	First	Second	Second	Second		First
Vigabatrin					First		Second
Zonisamide	Second	Second		Alternative	Alternative		Second

Figure 5.14: **Which drugs are useful for which type of epilepsy?** Drugs are classified as first choice, second choice, or alternative drugs. First choice drugs are used initially. If they fail or are not tolerated, second, choice drugs are attempted. If those are not useful, alternative drugs may be employed.

azepam and clorazepate are used in the treatment of chronic epilepsy. In contrast, diazepam and lorazepam are used in the acute treatment of status epilepticus.

Gabapentin is also used in treating postherpetic pain and diabetic neuropathic pain. Lamotrigine is used in treating bipolar disorder.

▪ MECHANISMS OF ACTION

All anticonvulsant drugs reduce the reactivity of neural cells so as to make them not as prone to creating an action potential. They do this in a variety of ways. Phenytoin does this by binding to voltage-gated sodium channels when they are in an inactive state and slowing their rates of recovery. Other drugs affect the sodium channel in similar ways as shown in Figure 5.15. Drugs that affect the sodium channel include carbamazepine, lamotrigine, levetiracetam, oxcarbazepine, topiramate, valproic acid, and zonisamide.

Some drugs affect GABA, a neurotransmitter that binds to chlorine channels causing influx that slows the onset of an action potential. Gabapentin increases the presynaptic release of GABA. Others drugs, such as valproate or valproic acid and tigabine, prevent the metabolism of GABA in the synaptic cleft. Others directly bind to the postsynaptic receptor allowing chlorine influx. This last category includes the benzodiazepines, such as clonazepam, clorazepate, diazepam, and lorazepam, and the barbiturates such as phenobarbital.

Felbamate potentiates the GABA response so that it enhances inhibition of action potential propagation. In addition, it also inhibits NMDA-triggered neural responses. NMDA is an excitatory neurotransmitter; therefore inhibition reduces the propagation of action potentials.

Some antiseizure medications reduce the influx of the calcium channels, which reduce the possibil-

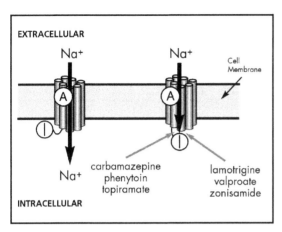

Figure 5.15: Shows sodium channel inhibition and therefore reduced opportunity for an action potential with specific antiseizure medications.

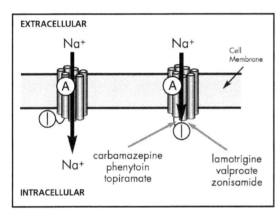

Figure 5.16: Valproate and ethosuxamide inhibition of calcium channels reduces the possibility of an action potential.

ity of an action potential in pacemaker cells that are particularly vulnerable in patients with absence seizures. These include valproic acid and ethosuximide. Figure 5.16 shows this mechanism.

▨ DOSAGES

ACETAZOLAMIDE, for *children*, for epilepsy, refer to *adult* dosing; for altitude illness, for prevention, 2.5 mg/kg/dose every 12 hours initiated preferably the day before or on the day of ascent; may be discontinued after staying at the same elevation for 2-3 days or upon starting the descent; maximum dose is 125 mg. It is not recommended that children use altitude sickness prevention drugs unless they have a history of acute mountain sickness and must

ascend rapidly; for treating altitude sickness, 2.5 mg/kg/dose every 8-12 hours; maximum dose is 250 mg. For *adults*, for altitude illness, 500-1000 mg/d in divided doses every 8-12 hours or divided every 12-24 hours if using extended release capsules); for edema, 250-375 mg once daily; for epilepsy, 8-30 mg/kg/d in divided doses; maximum dose is 30 mg/kg/d or 1 g/d, extended release capsules are not recommended for treating epilepsy; for chronic simple (open-angle) glaucoma, 250 mg 1-4 times/day or 500 mg extended release capsule bid; for secondary or acute (closed-angle) glaucoma, initiate at 250-500 mg, maintain at 125-250 mg every 4 hours. In the *elderly*, dosing should start on the lower end of *adult* dosing range.

CARBAMAZEPINE, for *children*, for epilepsy, <6 years: initiate at 10-20 mg/kg/d divided 2 or 3 times daily as tablets; increase dose every week until optimal response and therapeutic levels are achieved; maintenance dose is divided into 3-4 doses daily up to a maximum recommended dose of 35 mg/kg/d; for 6-12 years, initiate at 100 mg bid (tablets or extended release tablets); increase up to 100 mg/d at weekly intervals using a twice-daily regimen of other formulations until optimal response and therapeutic levels are achieved; usual maintenance is 400-800 mg/d up to a maximum recommended dose of 1000 mg/d. For *children* over 12 years and *adults*, for epilepsy, initiate at 200 mg bid (tablets, extended release tablets, or extended release capsules) or 100 mg of suspension qid; increase by up to 200 mg/d at weekly intervals using a twice-daily regimen of extended release capsules or tablets, or a 3-4 times/d regimen of other formulations until optimal response and therapeutic levels are achieved; usual dose is 800-1200 mg/d. For *adults*, for trigeminal or glossopharyngeal neuralgia, initiate at 100 mg bid with food, gradually increasing in increments of 100 mg bid prn; usual maintenance dose is 200-400 mg daily bid; maximum dose is 1200 mg/d;

for bipolar disorder, initiate at 200 mg/d bid; may adjust by 200 mg daily increments up to a maximum dose of 1600 mg/d.

DIVALPROEX, for *children*, for seizures, refer to *adult* dosing; younger children may require larger maintenance doses; for prevention of migraines in children 12 or older, refer to *adult* dosing. For *adults*, any doses of over 150 mg/d should be administered in divided doses; for simple and complex absence seizures, initiate at 15 mg/kg/d; increase by 5-10 mg/kg/d at weekly intervals until therapeutic levels are achieved; maximum dose is 60 mg/kg/d; for complex partial seizures, initiate at 10-15 mg/kg/d; increase by 5-10 mg/kg/d at weekly intervals until therapeutic levels are achieved up to a maximum of 60 mg/kg/d; for mania, Depakote® tablet: initiate at 750 mg/d in divided doses; should be adjusted as rapidly as possible to desired effect; maximum dose is 60 mg/kg/d; Depakote® ER: initiate at 25 mg/kg/d once daily; should be adjusted as rapidly as possible to desired effect; maximum dose is 60 mg/kg/d; for prevention of migraines, Depakote® tablet: 250 mg bid; may increase to 1000 mg/d; Depakote® ER: 500 mg once daily for 7 days, then increase to 1000 mg once daily; usual dose range is 500-1000 mg/d.

ETHOSUXIMIDE, for absence or petit mal seizures, for *children* 3-6, initiate at 250 mg/d; increase every 4-7 days to an usual maintenance dose of 20 mg/kg/d; maximum dose is 1.5 g/d in divided doses; for *children* 6 or older and *adults*, initiate at 500 mg/d; increase by 250 mg prn every 4-7 days up to 1.5 g/d in divided doses.

ETHOTOIN, for *children* 1 or older, as an anticonvulsant, maximum initial dose is 750 mg/d; usual maintenance dose is 0.5-1 g/d up to a maximum dose of 3 g/d. For *adults*, for generalized tonic-clonic or complex-partial seizures, initiate at 1 g/d or less; usual dose is 2-3 g/d.

FELBAMATE, as adjunctive therapy, for *children* 2-14, for Lennox-Gastaut syndrome, initiate

at 15 mg/kg/d in 3-4 divided doses; increase once per week by 15 mg/kg/d increments up to 45 mg/kg/d in 3-4 divided doses. For *children* over 14 years and *adults*, as an anticonvulsant, initiate at 1200 mg/d in 3-4 divided doses; increase the dosage under close supervision in 600 mg increments every 2 weeks to 2400 mg/d based on clinical response and thereafter to 3600 mg/d as clinically indicated; as an anticonvulsant used adjunctively, initiate at 1200 mg/d in 3-4 divided doses; increase once per week by 1200 mg/d increments up to 3600 mg/d in 3-4 divided doses.

FOSPHENYTOIN, for *adults*, dosing is IM or IV and is dispensed, uniquely, in what are known as phenytoin sodium equivalents (PE). This makes sense as fosphenytoin is a prodrug of phenytoin.

GABAPENTIN, for *children* 3-12 years, as an anticonvulsant, initiate at 10-15 mg/kg/d in 3 divided doses; increase to effective dose over ~3 days, dosages of up to 50 mg/kg/d have been tolerated in clinical studies; 3-4 years, effective dose is 40 mg/kg/d in 3 divided doses; 5-12 years, effective dose is 25-35 mg/kg/d in 3 divided doses. For *children* over 12 years and *adults*, as an anticonvulsant, initiate at 300 mg tid; may be increased up to 1800 mg/d; dosage range is 300-600 mg tid; up to a maximum of 800-1200 tid, for post herpetic neuralgia, day 1: 300 mg; day 2: 300 mg bid; day 3: 300 mg tid; dose may be increased prn for pain relie; usual range is 1800-3600 mg/d; daily doses >1800 mg do not generally show greater benefit.

GABAPENTIN ENACARBIL, for *adults*, for postherpetic neuralgia (PHN), initiate at 600 mg mane for 3 days, then increase to 600 mg bid, increasing to over 1200 mg/d provided no additional benefit; for restless legs syndrome (RLS), 600 mg once daily at approximately 5:00 pm.

LACOSAMIDE, for *adults*, for partial-onset seizures, initiate at 50 mg bid; may be increased at weekly intervals by 100 mg/d; maintain at 200-400 mg/d.

LAMOTRIGINE, for *children*, for adjunctive use in Lennox-Gastaut, primary generalized tonic-clonic seizures, or partial seizures, *children* under 30 kg will likely require maintenance doses to be increased as much as 50% regardless of regimen below; *children* 2-12 years, for regimens not containing carbamazepine, phenytoin, phenobarbital, primidone, or valproic acid, initiate in weeks 1 and 2 with 0.3 mg/kg/d in 1-2 divided doses; weeks 3 and 4 with 0.3 mg/kg bid; week 5 and after, increase by 0.6 mg/kg/d every 1-2 weeks; maintain at 4.5-7.5 mg/kg/d in 2 divided doses; maximum dose is 300 mg/d; regimens containing valproic acid, initiate in weeks 1 and 2 with 0.15 mg/kg/d in 1-2 divided doses; weeks 3 and 4 with 0.3 mg/kg/d in 1-2 divided doses; week 5 and after, increase by 0.3 mg/kg/d every 1-2 weeks; maintain at 1-5 mg/kg/d in 1 or 2 divided doses up to a maximum of 200 mg/d; for regimens containing carbamazepine, phenytoin, phenobarbital, or primidone and without valproic acid, initiate during weeks 1 and 2 at 0.3 mg/kg bid; in weeks 3 and 4 with 0.6 mg/kg bid; for week 5 and after, increase by 1.2 mg/kg/d every 1-2 weeks; maintain at 5-15 mg/kg/d in 2 divided doses up to a maximum of 400 mg/d; for *children* 13 years or older, refer to *adult* dosing. For *adults*, for adjunctive use in Lennox-Gastaut, primary generalized tonic-clonic seizures or partial seizures, regimens not containing carbamazepine, phenytoin, phenobarbital, primidone, or valproic acid, initiate during weeks 1 and 2 with 25 mg once daily; in weeks 3 and 4, 50 mg once daily; in week 5 and after, increase by 50 mg/d every 1-2 weeks; maintain at 225-375 mg/d in 2 divided doses; for regimens containing valproic acid, initiate during weeks 1 and 2 with 25 mg every other day; weeks 3 and 4, 25 mg once daily; week 5 and after, increase by 25-50 mg/d every 1-2 weeks; maintain at 100-200 mg/d; for regimens containing carbamazepine, phenytoin, phenobarbital, or primidone and without valproic acid, initiate during weeks 1 and 2, 50 mg once daily; weeks 3 and 4, 50 mg bid; week 5 and after, increase by 100 mg/d every 1-2 weeks; maintain at 150-250 mg bid; maximum dose is 700 mg/d; for adjunctive use with partial seizures and primary generalized tonic-clonic seizures, extended release: for regimens not containing carbamazepine, phenytoin, phenobarbital, primidone, or valproic acid, initiate during weeks 1 and 2, 25 mg once daily; weeks 3 and 4, 50 mg once daily; week 5, 100 mg once daily; week 6, 150 mg once daily; week 7, 200 mg once daily; maintain at 300-400 mg once daily; for regimens containing valproic acid, initiate during weeks 1 and 2, 25 mg every other day; weeks 3 and 4, 25 mg once daily; week 5, 50 mg once daily; week 6, 100 mg once daily; Week 7, 150 mg once daily, maintain at 200-250 mg once daily; regimens containing carbamazepine, phenytoin, phenobarbital, or primidone and without valproic acid, initiate during weeks 1 and 2, 50 mg once daily; weeks 3 and 4, 100 mg once daily; week 5, 200 mg once daily; week 6, 300 mg once daily; week 7, 400 mg once daily; maintain at 400-600 mg once daily; for bipolar disorder, for regimens not containing carbamazepine, phenytoin, phenobarbital, primidone, or valproic acid, initiate during weeks 1 and 2, 25 mg once daily; weeks 3 and 4, 50 mg once daily; week 5, 100 mg once daily; week 6 and maintain at 200 mg once daily; for regimens containing valproic acid, initiate during weeks 1 and 2, 25 mg every other day; weeks 3 and 4, 25 mg once daily; week 5, 50 mg once daily, week 6 and maintain at 100 mg once daily; for regimens containing carbamazepine, phenytoin, phenobarbital, or primidone and without valproic acid, initiate during weeks 1 and 2, 50 mg once daily; weeks 3 and 4, 100 mg/d in divided doses; week 5, 200 mg/d in divided doses; week 6, 300 mg/d in divided doses; maintain at up to 400 mg/d in divided doses.

LEVETIRACETAM, for *children* 4-16 years old, for partial-onset seizures (unlabeled use), 10-20 mg/kg/d in 2 divided doses; may increase weekly by 10-20 mg/kg up to a maximum of

60 mg/kg. For *children* >16 years and *adults*, for partial-onset seizure, initiate at 500 mg bid;additional dosing requirements may be given (1000 mg/d additional every 2 weeks) to a maximum recommended daily dose of 3000 mg; for bipolar disorder (unlabeled use), initiate at 500 mg bid; if tolerated, increase by 500 mg bid; dose may be increased every 3 days until target dose of 3000 mg/d is reached; maximum is 4000 mg/d.

METHSUXIMIDE, for *adults*, as an anticonvulsant, 300 mg/d for the first week; may increase by 300 mg/d at weekly intervals up to 1.2 g/d in 2-4 divided doses/d.

OXCARBAZEPINE, as adjunctive therapy for partial seizures, for *children* 2-3 years, initiate at 8-10 mg/kg/d; maximum dose is 300 mg bid; the maintenance dose should be achieved over 2-4 weeks and is dependent on patient weight, a maximum of 30 mg/kg bid; for *children* under 20 kg, initiate at 16-20 mg/kg/d;maximum maintenance dose is 60 mg/kg/d and should be achieved over 2-4 weeks; for *children* 4-16 years, 8-10 mg/kg/d up to maximum 300 mg bid; maintenance dose should be achieved over 2 weeks and is dependent on patient weight, according to the following: 20-29 kg: 450 mg bid; 29.1-39 kg: 600 mg bid; >39 kg: 900 mg bid; for children 6-17 years, extended release: initiate at 8-10 mg/kg once daily, maximum of 600 mg daily in the first week; maintenance dose should be achieved over 2-3 weeks with dose increases of 8-10 mg/kg/d increments at weekly intervals; maintenance dose depends on weight: 20-29 kg: 900 mg once daily; 29.1-39 kg: 1200 mg once daily; over 39 kg: 1800 mg once daily; for *children* 4-16, for induction of monotherapy, initiate at 4-5 mg/kg bid; maintenance doses by weight: 20 kg: 600-900 mg daily, 25-30 kg: 900-1200 mg daily; 35-40 kg: 900-1500 mg daily; 45 kg: 1200-1500 mg daily; 50-55 kg: 1200-1800 mg daily; 60-65 kg: 1200-2100 mg daily; 70 kg: 1500-2100 mg daily. For *adults*, as adjunctive therapy for partial seizures, initiate at 300 mg bid; dose may be increased by as much as 600 mg/d at weekly intervals; recommended daily dose is 600 mg bid; extended release: initiate at 600 mg once daily; dosage may be increased by 600 mg/d increments at weekly intervals; recommended dose is 1200-2400 mg once daily; for initiation of monotherapy for partial seizures, initiate at a dose of 300 mg bid; may increase dose by 300 mg/d every third day to a final dose of 600 mg bid. For the *elderly,* immediate release: see *adult* dosing; extended release: initiate at 300 mg or 450 mg once daily; may be increased by 300-450 mg daily increments at weekly intervals; maximum dose is 2400 mg daily.

PERAMPANEL, for *children* 12 or older and *adults*, as adjunctive treatment of partial seizures, when combined with most anticonvulsants, initiate at 2 mg nocte; may increase daily dose by 2 mg weekly; recommended dose is 8-12 mg nocte; when combined with phenytoin, carbamazepine, or oxcarbazepine, initiate at 4 mg nocte; may increase daily dose by 2 mg weekly; recommended dose is 8-12 mg nocte.

PHENYTOIN, for use as a non-emergency anticonvulsant, for *children*, as a loading dose use 10-15 mg/kg in 3 divided doses given every 2-4 hours; maintenance dose in *infants* and children, 5 mg/kg/d in 2-3 divided doses; usual range is 4-8 mg/kg/d; maximum dose is 300 mg/d. For *adolescents* and *adults*, as an anticonvulsant, as a loading dose use 10-15 mg/kg in 3 divided doses given every 2-4 hours; initiate maintenance dose at 100 mg tid; range is 300-600 mg/d.

RUFINAMIDE, for *children* 4 years or older, for adjunctive treatment of Lennox-Gastaut, initiate at 5 mg/kg bid; increase dose by approximately 10 mg/kg/d every other day to a target dose of 22.5 mg/kg or 1600 mg (whichever is lower) bid. For *adults,* for adjunctive treatment of Lennox-Gastaut, initiate at 200-400 mg bid; increase by 200-400 mg every other day up to a maximum dose of 1600 mg bid.

TIAGABINE, administer with food. For *children* 12-18 years, 4 mg once daily for 1 week; may increase to 4 mg bid for 1 week, then may increase by 4-8 mg weekly to response or up to 32 mg daily in 2-4 divided doses. For *adults*, 4 mg once daily for 1 week; may increase by 4-8 mg weekly to response or up to 56 mg daily in 2-4 divided doses.

TOPIRAMATE, for *children* 2-16 years, for partial seizures (adjunctive therapy), primary generalized tonic-clonic seizures (adjunctive therapy), or seizures associated with Lennox-Gastaut syndrome, initiate at 25 mg (or less, based on a range of 1-3 mg/kg/d) nightly for the first week; dosage may be increased in increments of 1-3 mg/kg/d (administered in 2 divided doses) at 1 or 2 week intervals to a total daily dose of 5-9 mg/kg/d. For *adults*, for partial-onset seizures (adjunctive therapy) and primary generalized tonic-clonic seizures (adjunctive therapy), initiate at 25-50 mg/d; increase in increments of 25-50 mg per week until an effective daily dose is reached; the daily dose may be increased by 25 mg at weekly intervals for the 4 first weeks;thereafter, the daily dose may be increased by 25-50 mg weekly to an effective daily dose (usually at least 400 mg); usual maximum dose is 1600 mg/d; for migraine prophylaxis, initiate at 25 mg/d, titrated weekly intervals in 25 mg increments up to the recommended total daily dose of 100 mg given in 2 divided doses.

VALPROIC ACID, for *adolescents* and *adults*, for preventing migraines, 250 mg bid; adjust based upon patient response up to 1000 mg/d. For *adults*, doses over 250 mg/d should be administered in divided doses; for simple and complex absence seizures, initiate at 15 mg/kg/d; increase by 5-10 mg/kg/d at weekly intervals; maximum dose is 60 mg/kg/d; for complex partial seizures, initiate at 10-15 mg/kg/d; increase by 5-10 mg/kg/d at weekly intervals; maximum dose is 60 mg/kg/d; for mania, initiate at 750 mg/d in divided doses; should be increased as rapidly as possible to desired effect; maximum dose is 60 mg/kg/d.

VIGABATRIN, for *children* 1 month to 2 years, for infantile spasms, initiate at 25 mg/kg bid; may increase by 25-50 mg/kg/day every 3 days to a maximum of 150 mg/kg/d. For *adolescents* 16 or older and *adults*, for refractory complex partial seizures, initiate at 500 mg bid; increase by 500 mg/d weekly, recommended dose is 3 g/d.

ZONISAMIDE, for *children* >16 years and *adults*, as adjunctive treatment of partial seizures, initiate at 100 mg/d; dose may be increased to 200 mg/d after 2 weeks, further dosage increases to 300 mg/d, and 400 mg/d can then be made with a minimum of 2 weeks between adjustments.

ADVERSE EFFECTS

This class of drugs has serious adverse effects. Common ones include nausea and vomiting, headache, behavioral changes such as confusion, hallucinations, sedation, ataxia, and nystagmus.

Phenytoin has some unique, serious adverse effects. These include megaloblastic anemia, inhibition of antidiuretic hormone, and hyperglycemia and glycosuria due to inhibition of insulin secretion. In children, phenytoin can cause gingival hyperplasia and coarsening of facial features. In gingival hyperplasia the gums overgrow the teeth, slowly receding with termination of the drug.

Carbamazepine may cause stupor, coma, respiratory depression, blurred vision, a characteristic rash, blood dyscrasias, liver toxicity, and hyponatremia (especially in the elderly). Frequent blood and liver function tests are highly recommended when taking this drug.

Phenobarbital and primidone may cause vertigo, acute psychotic reactions, morbilliform rash, agitation, and confusion. Rebound seizures may occur with cessation.

Valproic acid may induce tremors, rash, alopecia, thrombocytopenia, inhibition of platelet aggregation, and, rarely, liver failure. Ethosuximide may cause lethargy, dizziness, restlessness, agitation, anxiety, inability to concentrate, urticaria, leucopenia, aplastic anemia, and thrombocytopenia.

Lamotrigine can cause a rash that can progress to become life threatening. This reaction is more likely in those under 16 years of age, and therefore this drug is only used in this age group for Lennox-Gestaut syndrome. Levetiracetam may cause sleep disturbances and asthenia in addition to the common effects above.

Topiramate may cause impaired concentration, diplopia, somnolence, nervousness, weight loss, renal stones (in 1.5% of patients) and, rarely, glaucoma. Zonisamide may cause kidney stones, and cases of oligohidrosis have been reported in children who should be monitored for increased body temperature and decreased sweating, especially during the summer months.

RED FLAGS

Phenytoin is teratogenic. Fetal hydantoin syndrome includes cleft lip and palate, congenital heart disease, mental deficiency, and slowed growth. Topiramate has been shown to be teratogenic in animals and should be avoided in pregnant women.

A new FDA alert suggests that babies exposed to lamotrigine during the first three months of pregnancy may have a higher chance of being born with a cleft lip or cleft palate.

INTERACTIONS

DRUG

The following drugs inhibit phenytoin metabolism and increase plasma concentration: chloramphenicol, dicumarol, cimetidine, sulfonamides, and isonazid. Carbamazepine increases metabolism of phenytoin and lowers its plasma concentration. Phenytoin induces the cytochrome P450 system, which will increase metabolism of other antiepileptics, anticoagulants, oral contraceptive pills, cyclosporine, doxycycline, levodopa, methadone, mexiletine, and quinidine.

The following drugs reduce carbamazepine metabolism: cimetidine, diltiazem, erythromycin, isoniazid, and propoxyphene. Plasma levels may increase when carbamazepine is combined with these drugs, and toxic levels may occur.

Felbamate plasma levels may be reduced by

enzyme inducers such as phenytoin and carbamazepine. The half-life of lamotrigine, zonisamide, and tiagabine are similarly reduced by phenytoin and carbamazepine but increased by valproic acid.

Serum concentrations of topiramate are reduced by approximately 50% when used with metabolism inducers such as phenytoin and carbamazepine. It also decreases the concentration of ethinyl estradiol in oral contraceptive pills.

HERB

Due to its small therapeutic index, high protein binding, and interactions with numerous isozymes of cytochrome P450 (especially CYP3A4), it is the authors' recommendation that herbs should not be combined with phenytoin without supervision and written approval from a medical doctor.

ANTICONVULSANTS
- *Yin Guo Ye* (Gingko leaf) (D)–may precipitate epileptic seizures (Gruenwald, Brendler & Jaenicke, 2004) Level 5 evidence.

ANTISEIZURE DRUGS
- *Chen Pi* (Tangerine peel), *Qing Pi* (Citrus Viride), *Zhi Shi* (Aurantium Immaturus), and *Zhi Ke* (Aurantium fruit) (Indeterminate)– all these contain constituents that stimulate the sympathetic nervous system and should be used with caution in those taking antihypertensives, antidiabetic, antihyperthyroid, and/or antiseizure medications (Chinese language article cited in Chen & Chen, 2004) Indeterminate level of evidence.
- *Yin Guo Ye* (Gingko) (D)–clinical cases indicate interactions of ginkgo with antiepileptics, aspirin (acetylsalicylic acid), diuretics, ibuprofen, risperidone, rofecoxib, trazodone, and warfarin (Izzo & Ernst, 2009) Level 4 evidence.

CARBAMAZEPINE
- *Hu Zhang* (Bushy Knotweed) (D)–HLPC showed inhibition of CYP3A and increased concentration of carbamazepine when combined with Hu Zhang (Chi, Lin & Hou, 2012) Level 5 evidence.
- *Yin Guo Ye* (Gingko) (D)–An animal study showed significant decrease in pharmacologi-

cal measures of activity and plasma levels of carbamazepine when combined with two different doses of gingko leaf (Chandra, Rajkumar, Veeresham 2009) Level 5 evidence.

PHENYTOIN

- *Ding Xiang* (Clove) (D)–may cause a false increase on phenytoin assays, expert opinion (Gruenwald, Brendler & Jaenicke, 2004) Level 5 evidence.
- *Hei Hu Jiao* (Black pepper) (B-)–caused an increase in absorption kinetics and slowed elimination of phenytoin in a small cross-over study (Bano, Amla, Raina, Zutshi & Chopra, 1987) Level 3b evidence.

VALPROIC ACID

- *Bai Shao* (White peony root) (D)–*Huang Qin Tang* (with *Huang Qin, Bai Shao, Gan Cao,* and *Da Zao*) showed a marked decrease in plasma concentrations of valproic acid when coadministered in rats (Yu, Tsai, Kao, Chao & Hou, 2013) Level 5 evidence.
- *Da Zao* (Jujube) (D)–*Huang Qin Tang* (with *Huang Qin, Bai Shao, Gan Cao,* and *Da Zao*) showed a marked decrease in plasma concentrations of valproic acid when coadministered in rats (Yu, Tsai, Kao, Chao & Hou, 2013) Level 5 evidence.
- *Gan Cao* (Licorice) (D)–*Huang Qin Tang* (with *Huang Qin, Bai Shao, Gan Cao,* and *Da Zao*) showed a marked decrease in plasma concentrations of valproic acid when coadministered in rats (Yu, Tsai, Kao, Chao & Hou, 2013) Level 5 evidence.
- *Huang Qin* (Scutellaria) (D)–*Huang Qin Tang* (with *Huang Qin, Bai Shao, Gan Cao,* and *Da Zao*) showed a marked decrease in plasma concentrations of valproic acid when coadministered in rats (Yu, Tsai, Kao, Chao & Hou, 2013) Level 5 evidence.

INTERACTION ISSUES

A:

D: Fosphenytoin is 95-99% protein bound; perampanel is 95-99% bound; phenytoin is 90-95% bound; tiagabine is 96% bound.

M: Carbamazepine is a major substrate of CYP3A4 and a strong inducer of 1A2, 2B6, 2C8, 2C9, 2C19, and 3A4; divalproex is a weak/moderate inducer of CYP2A6; ethosuximide is a major substrate of CYP3A4; felbamate is a major substrate and a weak/moderate inducer of CYP3A4; methsuximide is a major substrate of CYP2C19; oxcarbazepine is a strong inducer of CYP3A4; perampanel is a major substrate and a weak/moderate inducer of CYP3A4; fosphenytoin and phenytoin are major substrates of CYP2C19 and 2C9 and strong inducers of CYP2B6, 2C19, 2C8, 2C9, and 3A4; rufinamide is a weak to moderate inducer of CYP3A4; tiagabine is a major substrate of CYP3A4; topiramate is a weak/moderate inducer of CYP3A4; valproic acid is a weak/ moderate inducer of CYP2A6; vigabatrin is a weak/moderate inducer of CYP2C9; zonisamide is a major substrate of CYP3A4.

E:

TI: Phenytoin has a narrow therapeutic index. Fosphenytoin is not listed on most lists of narrow therapeutic index drugs. However, it is a prodrug of phenytoin and thus should be considered as potentially having a narrow index.

Pgp: Carbamazepine is a substrate of Pgp.

ENDNOTES

[1] Combination of Levodopa and Carbidopa.
[2] Stalevo is a combination of Levodopa, Carbidopa, and Entacapone.
[3] Combination of Acetaminophen, Butalbital, Codeine, and Caffeine.
[4] Combination of Butalbital and Acetaminophen.
[5] Combination of Chlordiazepoxide and Clidinium.
[6] Combination of Ergotamine and Caffeine.
[7] Symbyax® is a combination of Olanzapine and Fluoxetine.
[8] Combination of Carbetapentane, Phenylephrine, and Chlorpheniramine.
[9] Combination of Guaifenesin and Codeine.
[10] Combination of Acetaminophen and Codeine.
[11] Combination of Chlorpheniramine, Pseudo-

ephedrine, and Codeine.

[12] Combination of Acetaminophen, Butalbital, Caffeine, and Codeine.

[13] Combination of Aspirin, Butalbital, Caffeine, and Codeine.

[14] Combination of Guaifenesin, Pseudoephedrine, and Codeine.

[15] Combination of Codeine and Pseudoephedrine.

[16] Combination of Phenylephrine, Chlorpheniramine, and Dihydrocodeine.

[17] Combination of Acetaminophen, Caffeine, and Dihydrocodeine.

[18] Combination of Acetaminophen and Hydrocodone.

[19] Combination of Chlorpheniramine, Pseudoephedrine, and Hydrocodone.

[20] Combination of Hydrocodone and Chlorpheniramine.

[21] Combination of Hydrocodone and Pseudoephedrine.

[22] Combination of Hydrocodone and Homatropine.

[23] Combination of Ibuprofen and Hydrocodone.

[24] Combination of Acetaminophen and Oxycodone.

[25] Combination of Oxycodone and Aspirin.

[26] Combination of Acetaminophen and Tramadol.

[27] Combination of Buprenorphine and Naloxone.

[28] Combination of Acetaminophen and Pentazocine.

[29] Combination of Dextromethorphan and Chlorpheniramine.

[30] Combination of Dextromethorphan and Phenylephrine.

[31] Combination of Dextromethorphan and Quinidine.

[32] Combination of Dextromethorphan, Acetaminophen, and Doxylamine.

[33] Combination of Dextromethorphan, Acetaminophen, and Phenylephrine.

[34] Combination of Dextromethorphan, Brompheniramine, and Pseudoephedrine.

[35] Combination of Dextromethorphan, Chlorpheniramine, and Phenylephrine.

[36] Combination of Dextromethorphan, Chlorpheniramine, and Pseudoephedrine.

[37] Combination of Dextromethorphan and Guaifenesin.

[38] Combination of Dextromethorphan, Guaifenesin, and Phenylephrine.

[39] Combination of Dextromethorphan, Guaifenesin, and Pseudoephedrine.

[40] Combination of Dextromethorphan and Pseudoephedrine.

[41] Combination of Dihydrocodeine, Aspirin, and Caffeine.

[42] Combination of Topiramate and Phentermine.

[43] Combination of Caffeine, Acetaminophen, and Aspirin.

■ CHINESE MEDICAL DESCRIPTIONS

The Chinese medical explanation of the drug categories in this chapter may be found in Chapter 15 on pages 385–418.

Drugs Affecting the Cardiovascular System

Antihypertensive agents are used to lower blood pressure. Blood pressure (BP) is determined by multiplying **cardiac output** (CO) and **total peripheral vascular resistance** (TPR). TPR is mostly based on blood vessel "tone," the state of the muscles in arteries and capillary beds. To a lesser degree, TPR is also determined by intravascular blood volume; more blood in the vessels means higher TPR. CO is itself a product of stroke volume (SV) and heart rate (HR). SV is how much blood is being pushed through contraction of the heart and is determined by heart muscle contractility (how hard the muscle squeezes) and the amount of venous blood that returns to the heart (called preload). The HR is simply how fast the heart is contracting. These equations look like the following:

$$BP = CO \times TPR$$
$$CO = SV \times HR$$

From these equations, there are three main controllers of blood pressure in the body: the heart, blood vessel tone, and the kidneys. The heart can control blood pressure by regulating the speed and force of contraction. Blood vessel tone changes TPR. The kidneys control blood volume and therefore can affect SV, CO, and TPR. (see figure 6.1)

All classes of drugs that affect blood pressure

> Cardiac output: The volume of blood ejected by the ventricles of the heart

> Total peripheral vascular resistance: Degree of resistance to blood flow from systemic blood vessels

CLASSIFICATION OF BLOOD PRESSURE (BP)*			
CATEGORY	SBP MMHG		DPB MMHG
NORMAL	<120	AND	<80
PREHYPERTENSION	120-139	OR	80-89
HYPERTENSION, STAGE 1	140-159	OR	90-99
HYPERTENSION, STAGE 2	≥160	OR	≥100

Figure 6.1: This table shows the different stages of hypertension.

act on the areas above. The most common antihypertensive agents are the diuretics, which work on the kidneys to reduce intravascular blood volume and therefore SV and TPR.

β-blockers decrease contractility of the heart muscle to reduce CO and affect the renin-angiotensin system to reduce blood volume and therefore SV, CO, and TPR. Angiotensin converting enzyme (ACE) inhibitors cause vasodilation and affect the renin-angiotensin system causing changes in TPR, SV, and CO. Angiotensin II antagonists act similarly to ACE inhibitors. Due to some recent studies, calcium channel blockers are not used as much as in the past for hypertension. They work by reducing the contractility of the myocardium and thus SV and CO. Other pharmaceuticals that are used in treating hypertension work in similar ways. These include adrenergic blockers, central acting adrenergic drugs, and vasodilators. (see Figure. 6.2 on the next page.)

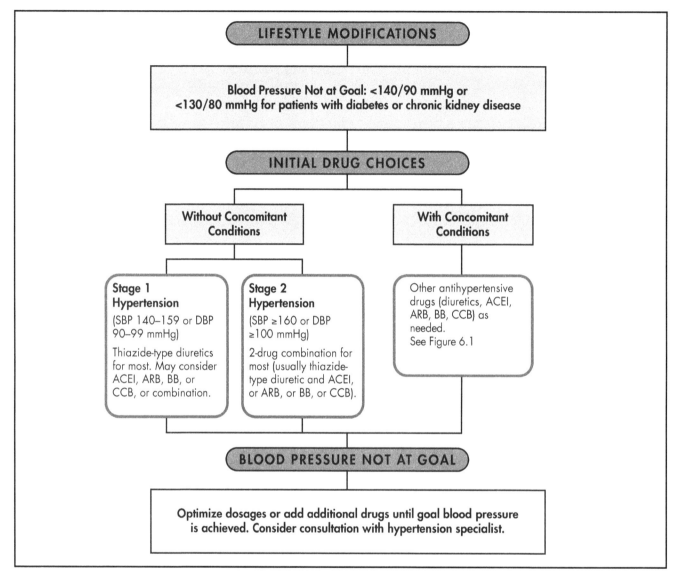

Figure 6.2 This figure shows how to treat hypertension depending on complications and staging. ACEI: ACE inhibitor, ARB: angiotensin receptor blocker, BB: beta blocker, CCB: calcium channel blocker, SBP: systolic blood bressure, DBP: diastolic blood pressure.

SECTION 1: RENIN-ANGIOTENSIN SYSTEM INHIBITORS

ANGIOTENSIN CONVERTING ENZYME INHIBITORS (ACEI):

BENAZEPRIL (ben AY ze pril) PR=D *(Lotensin®, Lotensin® HCT,[1] Lotrel®[2])*

CAPTOPRIL (cap TOE pril) PR=D

ENALAPRII (e NAL a pril) PR=D *(Vaseretic®,[17] Vasotec®)*

FOSINOPRIL (foe SIN oh pril) PR=C in the 1st trimester and D in the 2nd–3rd *(Monpril®)*

LISINOPRIL (lye SIN o pril) PR=D *(Prinivil®, Prinzide®,[22] Zestoretic®,[22] Zestril®)*

MOEXIPRIL (mo EKS i pril) PR=D *(Uniretic®,[25] Univasc®)*

PERINDOPRIL (per IN doe pril) PR=D *(Aceon®)*

QUINAPRIL (KWIN a pril) PR=D *(Accupril®, Accuretic®[3])*

RAMIPRIL (ram I pril) PR=D *(Altace®)*

TRANDOLAPRIL (tran DOE la pril) PR=D *(Mavik®, Tarka®4)*

ANGIOTENSIN RECEPTOR BLOCKERS:

AZILSARTAN (ay zil SAR tan) PR=D *(Darbi™, Edarbyclor™48)*

CANDESARTAN (can di SAR tan) PR=D *(Atacand®, Atacand HCT®)*

EPROSARTAN (ep roe SAR tan) PR=D *(Teveten®, Teveten® HCT6)*

IRBESARTAN (ir be SAR tan) PR=D *(Avalide®,7 Avapro®)*

LOSARTAN (loe SAR tan) PR=C in the 1st

trimester and D in the 2nd–3rd *(Cozaar®, Hyzaar®8)*

OLMESARTAN (ole me SAR tan) PR=D *(Azor™,26 Benicar®, Benicar HCT®,9 Tribenzor™30)*

TELMISARTAN (tel mi SAR tan) PR=D *(Micardis®, Micardis® HCT,10 Twynsta®31)*

VALSARTAN (val SAR tan) PR=D *(Diovan®, Diovan HCT®,11 Exforge®,35 Exforge HCT®36)*

RENIN INHIBITORS:

ALISKIREN (a-LIS-KYE-ren) PR=D *(Amturnide™,37 Tekamlo™,38 Tekturna®, Tekturna HCT®39)*

These drugs affect the renin-angiotensin system. As seen in Figure 6.3, renin helps convert angiotensinogen (an inactive precursor) to Angiotensin I, which in turn is converted to Angiotensin II by angiotensin converting enzyme. Angiotensin II stimulates aldosterone secretion. Aldosterone causes sodium retention and potassium secretion in the kidney tubules. And where sodium goes so goes water; therefore aldosterone increases intravascular blood volume, SV, CO, and, ultimately, BP. Several pharmaceutical drugs block this cascade so that blood volume decreases. This decrease in volume is very useful in several conditions including hypertension, heart failure, **arrhythmia**, and **myocardial infarction** (MI).

ACE inhibitors have been shown in clinical studies to lower the incidence of heart disease and lower **morbidity** and **mortality** of cardiac events. As the drugs in this class of antihypertensives are the only ones to show this reduction in heart disease (other antihypertensives show lower incidences of stroke but not necessarily heart events), they have become mainline drugs for controlling hypertension and are considered drugs of first choice by many doctors in treating it. They have been shown to be especially useful in controlling hypertension in patients with diabetes as they seem to have a **nephroprotective** effect.

Please note that all of the ACE inhibitors have a suffix of -pril, and the angiotensin receptor blockers all end with -sartan.

FUNCTION

Angiotensin converting enzyme inhibitors (ACE inhibitors, or ACEI) cause a decrease in blood volume and therefore decreased stroke volume and blood pressure. They reduce the effects of the sympathetic nervous system. In addition, they cause changes in the systemic vascular system that reduce total peripheral vascular resistance. All together this decreases cardiac output.

Arrhythmia: An irregular heartbeat

Myocardial infarction: Necrosis of part of the heart muscle; heart attack

Morbidity: Rate of illness or abnormality

Mortality: Rate of death

Nephroprotective: Protects the kidneys

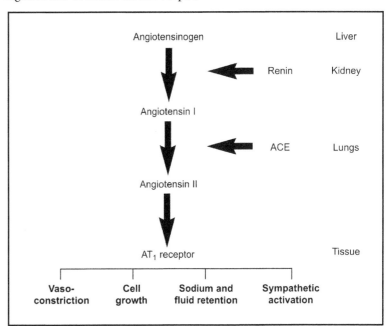

Figure 6.3: The renin-angiotensin system and the end results of the physiological cascade.

Angiotensin-receptor blockers (ARBs) have similar functions and are used primarily for hypertension and in heart failure when ACE inhibitors are not tolerated due to side effects. ARBs do not have much effect on the peripheral vasculature.

Aliskaren is a brand new agent and the first that inhibits renin. Because of this, it inhibits the renin-angiotensin system just like ACEIs and ARBs and is used to treat hypertension.

Both ACE inhibitors and ARBs are nephroprotective and can be used to prevent damage to the kidneys in diabetic patients. ACE inhibitors have been shown to be effective in protecting the kidneys of type 1 diabetic patients, but the results have been mixed with type 2 diabetes. ARBs, on the other hand, have been shown to be effective in protecting the kidneys in diabetes type 2 patients and are therefore the current drugs of choice in diabetic patients.

▓ MECHANISM OF ACTION

ACEIs lower blood volume by blocking conversion of angiotensin I to angiotensin II and thus blocking aldosterone secretion. This causes decreased sodium retention in the kidney tubules resulting in a decrease of intravascular blood volume, SV, and BP. In addition, ACE plays a role in the breakdown of bradykinin, a powerful vasodilator. By blocking the activity of ACE, more bradykinin remains in circulation and causes vasodilation especially in the arterioles. This adds to the reduction in TPR.

Angiotensin-receptor blockers act by blocking receptors of angiotensin type 1. Theoretically, ARBs create a more complete blockade of the renin-angiotensin system than ACE inhibitors and should be more effective in lowering blood pressure. However, they do not affect bradykinin, and many of the secondary beneficial effects of ACE inhibitors may not occur. For this reason and the fact that they have been researched more thoroughly, ACE inhibitors are usually employed before ARBs. It is currently unclear whether there is a significant difference between ACEIs and ARBs.

Renin inhibitors directly inhibit renin, therefore preventing conversion of angiotensinogen to angiotensin I, thus shutting down the renin-angiotensin cascade and decreasing blood pressure.

▓ DOSAGES

ALISKIREN, for *adults*, initiate at 150 mg once daily; this dose may be increased to 300 mg when necessary.

AZILSARTAN, for *adults*, for hypertension, 80 mg once daily; in patients with volume depletion such as patients receiving high doses of diuretics, consider starting at 40 mg once daily.

BENAZEPRIL, for *children* 6 years or older, initiate at 0.2 mg/kg/d as monotherapy; dose range is 0.1-0.6 mg/kg/d up to a maximum of 40 mg/d. For *adults*, initiate at 10 mg/d in patients not receiving a diuretic; 20-40 mg/d as a single dose or 2 divided doses. For the *elderly*, initiate at 5-10 mg/d in single or divided doses; usual range is 20-40 mg/d.

CANDESARTAN, for *adults*, for hypertension, usual dose is 4-32 mg once daily; dosage must be individualized; usual recommended starting dose of 16 mg once daily when it is used as monotherapy in patients who are not volume depleted; it can be administered once or twice daily; for congestive heart failure, initiate at 4 mg once daily; double the dose at 2-week intervals, as tolerated; target dose 32 mg.

CAPTOPRIL, for *infants*, initiate at 0.15-0.3 mg/kg/dose, increase to a maximum of 6 mg/kg/d in 1-4 divided doses; usual required dose 2.5-6 mg/kg/d. For *children*, initiate at 0.5 mg/kg/dose; increase to maximum of 6 mg/kg/d in 2-4 divided doses. For *older children*, initiate at 6.25-12.5 mg/ dose every 12-24 hours; increase to a maximum of 6 mg/kg/d. For *adolescents*, initiate at 12.5-25 mg/dose given every 8-12 hours; increase by 25 mg/dose to a maximum of 450 mg/d. For *adults*, for acute hypertension (urgency/emergency), 12.5-25 mg; may repeat as needed (may be given sublingually, but no therapeutic advantage demonstrated); for hypertension, initiate at 12.5-25 mg 2-3 times/d; may increase by 12.5-25 mg/dose at 1-2 week intervals up to 50 mg 3 tid; maximum dose is 150 mg tid; add diuretic before further dosage increases; usual dose range is 25-100 mg/d in 2 divided doses; for congestive heart failure, initiate at 6.25-12.5 mg tid in conjunction with cardiac glycoside and diuretic therapy; initial dose depends upon patient's fluid/electrolyte status; target dose is 50 mg tid; for LVD after myocardial infarction (MI), initiate at 6.25 mg followed by 12.5 mg, tid then increase to 25 mg tid during next several days and then over next several weeks to target dose of 50 mg tid; for diabetic nephropathy, 25 mg tid; other antihypertensives often given concurrently.

ENALAPRIL, for *children* 1 month to 16 years, for hypertension, initiate at 0.08 mg/kg (up to 5 mg) once daily; adjust dosage based on patient response; doses >0.58 mg/kg (40 mg) have not been evaluated in pediatric patients. For *adults*, for hypertension, 2.5-5 mg/d, then increase as required, usually at 1- to 2-week intervals; usual dose range is 2.5-40 mg/d in 1-2 divided doses; initiate with 2.5 mg if patient is taking a diuretic that cannot be discontinued; may add a diuretic if blood pressure cannot be controlled with enalapril alone; for heart failure, initiate at 2.5 mg once or twice daily; usual range is 2.5-20 mg/d bid; increase slowly at 1- to 2-week intervals; for asymptomatic left ventricular dysfunction, 2.5 mg bid; increase, as tolerated to 20 mg/d.

EPROSARTAN, for *adults*, for hypertension, dosage must be individualized; can administer once or twice daily with total daily doses of 400-800 mg; usual starting dose is 600 mg once daily as monotherapy.

FOSINOPRIL, for *children* >50 kg, for hypertension, initiate at 5-10 mg once daily. For *adults*, for hypertension, initiate at 10 mg/d; most patients are maintained on 20-40 mg/d; for heart failure, initiate at 10 mg/d; increase, as needed, to a maximum of 40 mg once daily over several weeks; usual dose is 20-40 mg/d.

IRBESARTAN, for *children*, 6-12 years, initiate at 75 mg once daily; may be increased to a maximum of 150 mg once daily. For *children* 13 years and older and *adults*, 150 mg once daily; may be increased to 300 mg once daily.

LISINOPRIL, for *children* ≥6 years, initiate at 0.07 mg/kg once daily (up to 5 mg); increase dose at 1- to 2-week intervals; doses >0.61 mg/kg or >40 mg have not been evaluated. For *adults*, for hypertension, usual dosage range is 10-40 mg/d; initiate at 10 mg/d; for congestive heart failure, initiate at 2.5-5 mg once daily, then increase by no more than 10 mg increments at intervals no less than 2 weeks to a maximum daily dose of 40 mg; usual maintenance is 5-40 mg/d as a single dose; for acute myocardial infarction (within 24 hours in hemodynamically stable patients), 5 mg immediately, then 5 mg at 24 hours, 10 mg at 48 hours, and 10 mg every day thereafter for 6 weeks. For the *elderly*, initiate at 2.5-5 mg/d; increase doses 2.5-5 mg/d at 1-2-week intervals up to a maximum daily dose of 40 mg.

LOSARTAN, for *children* 6-16 years, for hypertension, 0.7 mg/kg once daily, up to a maximum of 50 mg/d; adjust dose based on response, doses >1.4 mg/kg (maximum 100 mg) have not been studied. For *adults*, for hypertension, usual starting dose is 50 mg once daily; can be administered once or twice daily with total daily doses ranging from 25-100 mg.

MOEXIPRIL, for *adults*, for hypertension, initiate at 7.5 mg once daily (in patients not receiving diuretics), 1 hour prior to a meal; maintenance dose is 7.5-30 mg/d in 1 or 2 divided doses 1 hour before meals.

OLMESARTAN, for *adults*, initiate at 20 mg once daily; if initial response is inadequate, may be increased to 40 mg once daily after 2 weeks.

PERINDOPRIL, for *adults*, for hypertension, initiate at 4 mg/d but may increase to a usual range of 4-8 mg/d (may be given in 2 divided doses); increase at 1-to-2 week intervals to a maximum of 16 mg/d; for stable coronary artery disease, initiate at 4 mg once daily for 2 weeks; increase as tolerated to 8 mg once daily; for the *elderly*, for hypertension, over 65 years, initiate at 4 mg/d; maintenance dose is 8 mg/d; for stable coronary artery disease, over 70 years of age, initiate at 2 mg/d for 1 week; increase as tolerated to 4 mg/d for 1 week, then increase as tolerated to 8 mg/d.

QUINAPRIL, for *adults*, for hypertension, initiate

at 10-20 mg once daily, adjust according to blood pressure response at peak and trough blood levels; for congestive heart failure or post-MI, initiate at 5 mg once or twice daily, increased at weekly intervals to 10-20 mg bid, target dose is 20 mg bid. For the *elderly*, initiate at 2.5-5 mg/d, increase dosage at increments of 2.5-5 mg at 1- to 2-week intervals.

RAMIPRIL, for *adults*, for hypertension, 2.5-5 mg once daily up to a maximum of 20 mg/d for reduction in risk of MI, stroke, and death from cardiovascular causes; initiate at 2.5 mg once daily for 1 week, 5 mg once daily for the next 3 weeks, then increase as tolerated to 10 mg once daily (may be given as divided dose); for heart failure postmyocardial infarction, initiate at 2.5 mg bid; increase upward, if possible, to 5 mg bid.

TELMISARTAN, for *adults*, for hypertension, initiate at 40 mg once daily; usual maintenance dose range is 20-80 mg/d.

TRANDOLAPRIL, for *adults*, for hypertension, initiate at 1 mg/d (2 mg/d in black patients); adjust dosage according to the blood pressure response; make dosage adjustments at intervals of 1 week or greater; most patients have required dosages of 2-4 mg/d; for heart failure postmyocardial infarction or left ventricular dysfunction postmyocardial infarction, initiate at 1 mg/d; increase as tolerated towards the target dose of 4 mg/d.

VALSARTAN, for *adults*, for hypertension, initiate at 80 mg or 160 mg once daily (in patients who are not volume depleted); dose may be increased to achieve desired effect, maximum recommended dose is 320 mg/d; for heart failure, initiate at 40 mg bid; increase dose to 80-160 mg bid, as tolerated; maximum daily dose is 320 mg; for left ventricular dysfunction after MI, initiate at 20 mg bid; increase dose to target of 160 mg bid as tolerated; may initiate ≥12 hours following MI.

Hypotension: Lower than normal blood pressure. Can cause light-headedness, dizziness, and fainting

Macule: A flat area of skin that has changed color and is less than 1 cm in diameter

Papule: An elevated, firm area on the skin less than 1 cm diameter

Neutropenia: An abnormal decrease in blood neutrophils

Glycosuria: An abnormal increase of glucose in the urine

Hepatotoxicity: Toxic to the liver

BUN: Blood urea nitrogen

Hyperkalemia: Too much potassium in the blood

NSAID: Non-steroidal anti-inflammatory drug used in pain relief; examples include aspirin and ibuprofen

Asystole: Non-contraction of the heart

Fibrillation: Recurrent, abnormal muscle contraction that is not physiologically useful

Stenosis: Narrowing

ADVERSE EFFECTS

Hypotension can be precipitated upon first dose, especially in those that are sodium depleted, patients on multiple antihypertensive drugs, and patients who have congestive heart failure.

A cough can occur in approximately 5-20% of patients. This cough is dry, bothersome, and not dose related. This occurs more often in women and develops between 1 week and 6 months from initial dose. Stopping ACEI therapy will stop the cough usually within 4 days. While ARBs have similar side effects as ACE inhibitors, they do not cause this cough.

ACE inhibitors and ARBs of the renin-angiotensin system should not be used in pregnancy, especially in the second and third trimesters.

A **maculopapular** skin rash occasionally occurs. It may resolve on its own or respond to reduction of dose or use of antihistamines. Can occur with most ACEIs but especially captopril.

Dysgeusia, an alteration or loss of taste, may occur. This is reversible.

Neutropenia can rarely occur especially in patients with collagen-vascular or renal parenchymal disease. Initial symptoms of this serious reaction may include a sore throat or fever.

Glycosuria, or glucose in the urine, is exceedingly rare and reversible. This occurs in the absence of hyperglycemia.

Hepatotoxicity is also extremely rare and reversible.

Renin inhibitors may increase **BUN** or serum creatinine on lab tests and cause diarrhea, cough, or rash.

RED FLAGS

Hyperkalemia rarely occurs in patients with normal kidney function but can occur in patients with renal insufficiency, taking potassium-sparing diuretics, potassium supplements, β-adrenergic receptor blockers, or **NSAIDs.** Hyperkalemia can be life-threatening, as it interferes with normal cardiac muscle function causing ventricular **asystole** or **fibrillation.**

Acute renal failure can be caused in individuals with bilateral renal artery **stenosis** (or to the one remaining kidney), heart failure, dehydration due to diarrhea or use of diuretics, or congestive heart failure in *elderly* patients. With appropriate treatment renal function is usually recovered.

In 0.1% to 0.2% of patients, ACEIs can induce an edematous condition in the mouth and throat called angioneurotic edema. This reaction does not appear to be dose related and usually occurs within the first few hours after drug initiation but can occur within the first week of usage. This can be considered life-threatening, and immediate medical care is necessary. ARBs and renin inhibitors have a much lower incidence of this reaction than ACE inhibitors.

▨ INTERACTIONS

DRUG

Allopurinol hypersensitivity reactions may also increase with ACEI use.

Antacids may reduce bioavailability. ACEI-induced cough may be worsened by capsaicin. NSAIDs may reduce hypertensive effect.

Digoxin and lithium plasma levels may increase with ACEI use.

Potassium-sparing diuretics, renin inhibitors, and potassium supplements may exacerbate ACEI-induced hyperkalemia.

HERB

ACE INHIBITORS

• *Gan Cao* (Licorice) (D)–theoretically may reduce the effects of antihypertensive agents such as alpha-1-adrenergic blockers, ACEI, A$_2$ receptor antagonists, beta-adrenergic blockers, calcium channel blockers, clonidine, guanabenz, guanadrel, guanethidine, guanfacine, hydralazine, methyldopa, minoxidil, and reserpine, and concurrent use should be undertaken with caution, expert opinion (Kowalak & Mills, 2001) Level 5 evidence.

• *Ma Huang* (Ephedra) (D)–antihypertensives including ACE inhibitors and beta-blockers may be antagonized by *Ma Huang,* and severe hypertension may result. This is speculative (Mills & Bone, 2000) Level 5 evidence.

LOSARTAN

• *Bing Pian* (Borneol), *Dan Shen* (Salvia), and *San Qi* (Psuedoginseng) (D)–a rat study showed a compound danshen tablet containing *dan shen, san qi*, and *bing pian* affected metabolism and excretion of losartan (Yuan, Zhang, Ma, Sun *et al.,* 2013). Level 5 evidence.

ANTIHYPERTENSIVES

• *Chen Pi* (Tangerine peel), *Qing Pi* (Citrus Viride), *Zhi Ke* (Aurantium fruit), *Zhi Shi* (Aurantium immaturus) (Indeterminate)– contains constituents that stimulate the sympathetic nervous system and should be used with caution in those taking antihypertensives, antidiabetic, antihyperthyroid, and/or antiseizure medications (Chinese language article cited in Chen & Chen, 2004) Indeterminate level of evidence.

• *Gan Cao* (Licorice) (D)–theoretically may reduce effects of antihypertensive agents such as alpha-1-adrenergic blockers, ACEI, A$_2$-receptor antagonists, beta-adrenergic blockers, calcium channel blockers, clonidine, guanabenz, guanfacine, hydralazine, methyldopa, minoxidil, and reserpine, and concurrent use should be undertaken with caution (Kowalak & Mills, 2001) Level 5 evidence.

• *Ma Huang* (Ephedra) (C)–based on ephedrine content, antagonizes effects of antihypertensives (White, Gardner, Gurley, Marx, Wang & Estes) Level 3b evidence. Antihypertensives including ACE inhibitors and beta-blockers may be antagonized by *Ma Huang,* and severe hypertension may result. This is speculative (Mills & Bone, 2000) Level 5 evidence.

• *Sheng Ma* (Cimicifuga) (D)–may potentiate the effect of antihypertensive agents. Undertake concurrent use with caution, expert opinion (Gruenwald, Brendler & Jaenicke, 2004) Level 5 evidence.

INTERACTION ISSUES

A:

D: Azilsartan is greater than 99% protein bound; benazepril is approximately 97% protein bound,; candesartan is greater than 99% bound; eprosartan is 98% bound; fosinopril is

95% bound; losartan is 99.7% bound; olme-sartan is 99% bound; quinapril is 97% bound; telmisartan is >99.5% bound; valsartan is 95% bound.

M: Captopril is a major substrate of CYP2D6; irbesartan moderately inhibits CYP2C8 and

2C9; losartan is a major substrate of CYP2C9 and 3A4 and moderately inhibits 2C8 and 2C9.

E:

TI:

Pgp: Aliskiren is a substrate of Pgp.

SECTION 2: BETA ADRENERGIC BLOCKING AGENTS

This class, covered in Chapter 4, Section 8, has many affects on the cardiovascular system and is used in many diseases of that system including hypertension, heart failure, arrhythmias, and angina. It is useful for the cardiovascular system because of its **negative**

Negative inotrope: A drug that reduces the force of the heart's contraction

---

Negative chronotrope: A drug that reduces the rate of heartbeats

---

inotropic and **chronotropic** effects, which help reduce the amount of work the heart needs to do. Cardiac output is reduced consequently lowering blood pressure. Because of these varied effects, beta-blockers can play a role in most cardiovascular diseases.

SECTION 3: DIURETICS

THIAZIDE DIURETICS:

BENDROFLUMETHIAZIDE (ben droe floo meth EYE a zide) PR=C *(Corzide®[12])*

CHLOROTHIAZIDE (klor oh THYE a zide) PR=C *(Diuril®)*

CHLORTHALIDONE (klor THAL i done) PR=B *(Clorpres®,[13] Edarbyclor™,[48] Tenoretic®[14])*

HYDROCHLOROTHIAZIDE (hye droe klor oh THYE a zide) PR=B *(Accuretic®,[3] Aldacta-zide®,[41] Amturnide™,[37] Atacand HCT®,[5] Avalide®,[7] Benicar HCT®,[9] Diovan HCT®,[11] Dutoprol™,[16] Dyazide®,[15] Exforge HCT®,[36] Hyzaar®,[8] Lopressor HCT®,[16] Lotensin HCT,®[1] Maxzide®,[15] Maxzide®-25,[15] Micardis® HCT,[10] Microzide®, Prinzide®,[22] Tekturna HCT®,[39] Teveten® HCT[6] Tribenzor™,[30] Uniretic®,[25] Vaseretic®,[17] Zestoretic®,[22] Ziac®[40])*

METHYCLOTHIAZIDE (meth i kloe THYE a zide) PR=B

THIAZIDE-RELATED DIURETICS:

INDAPAMIDE (in DAP a mide) PR=B

METOLAZONE (me TOLE a zone) PR=B *(Zaroxolyn®)*

LOOP DIURETICS:

BUMETANIDE (byoo MET a nide) PR=C

ETHACRYNIC ACID (eth a KRIN ik AS id) PR=B *(Edecrin®, Sodium Edecrin®)*

FUROSEMIDE (fyoor OH se mide) PR=C *(Lasix®)*

TORSEMIDE (TORE se mide) PR=B *(Demadex®)*

POTASSIUM-SPARING DIURETICS:

AMILORIDE (a MIL oh ride) PR=B

EPLERENONE (e PLER en one) PR=B *(Inspra™)*

SPIRONOLACTONE (speer on oh LAK tone) PR=C *(Aldactazide®,[47] Aldactone®)*

TRIAMTERENE (trye AM ter een) PR=C *(Dya-zide®,[15] Dyrenium®, Maxzide,[15] Maxzide®-25[15])*

CARBONIC ANHYDRASE INHIBITORS:

ACETAZOLAMIDE (a set a ZOLE a mide) PR=C *(Diamox® Sequels®)*

METHAZOLAMIDE (meth a ZOE la mide) PR=C *(Neptazane™)*

Diuretics, by definition, are drugs that induce urination. All types of diuretics act on the kidneys. The kidneys are made up of nephrons, which are individual filtration units. Nephrons allow fluid, ions, and other chemicals to enter their lumen through both passive and active means. While this fluid passes within the lumen, blood vessels travel alongside it, and ultimately, in a properly functioning kidney, waste products and some fluid remains in the lumen and forms urine while nutrients, proteins, cells, and other beneficial constituents of the blood remain in the blood.

The nephron is broken down into several areas; each has a different function in the formation of urine. The first part of the nephron is the Bowman's capsule. This is where 16-20% of the blood plasma enters the nephron. Many constituents of the blood are also filtered and may or may not be reabsorbed later in the nephron. These constituents include glucose, sodium bicarbonate, amino acids, and sodium, potassium, and chlorine ions among others.

As the nephron continues, it narrows into small pipes called tubules. The proximal convoluted tubule reabsorbs into the blood almost all glucose, amino acids, and other metabolites. About two-thirds of sodium ions are also reabsorbed. Water follows the osmolarity changes: where salts are, water is found. Carbonic anhydrase is an enzyme produced by the luminal walls and proximal tubule cells. It modulates the reabsorption of bicarbonate. The proximal tubule is also where organic acids and bases are secreted from the blood. The acid secretory system secretes uric acid, antibiotics, and most diuretics. This system can be saturated, causing competition between certain drugs and waste products.

Distal to the proximal tubule are the descending and ascending loops of Henle. The main function of the descending loop of Henle is to reabsorb water from the tubule. This causes a much greater concentration of salts in the tubule. The ascending loop is impermeable to water. Sodium, potassium, and chlorine ions are reabsorbed by the Na+/K+/2Cl- cotransporter. Magnesium and calcium both enter the interstitium from the tubule in the ascending loop of Henle. About 25-30% of tubular sodium chloride enters the interstitium. Because of the large amount of salt reabsorption that occurs here, drugs affecting this area are among the strongest of the diuretic drugs.

Next in the nephron is the distal convoluted tubule. It is also impermeable to water. About 10% of the tubular sodium chloride is reabsorbed here through the Na+/Cl- transporter. Calcium is also transported from the tubule lumen. The Na+/Cl- transporter is sensitive to thiazide diuretics, and calcium reabsorption is affected by the parathyroid hormone.

Finally, the nephron exits into the collecting tubule and, ultimately, the collecting duct before continuing into the renal pelvis and ureters. The collecting tubule allows for transport of sodium, potassium, and water. Aldosterone affects the cells of the collecting tubules to promote sodium reabsorption and secretion of potassium. Antidiuretic hormone (also known as vasopressin) promotes water reabsorption in the collecting tubules and ducts.

For a summary of the action of the nephron on various ions and water, see Figure 6.4 on the next page.

The thiazide diuretics are the most commonly prescribed of all diuretics and are among the most prescribed of all medications.

▦ FUNCTION

Diuretics can be used to treat many different diseases. These can be broken down into two major types: edematous and nonedematous. Edematous states can be caused by retention of sodium chloride and therefore water. In heart failure, inadequate cardiac output causes the kidney to act as if there was **hypovolemia**. The kidney, in turn, causes compensation by retaining more sodium chloride and water. When the vascular space cannot hold the increased blood volume it leaks into the tissues and causes edema. Hepatic ascites is caused by cirrhosis of the liver, which raises portal blood pressure. Combined with the liver's impaired

Hypovolemia: Abnormally low blood volume

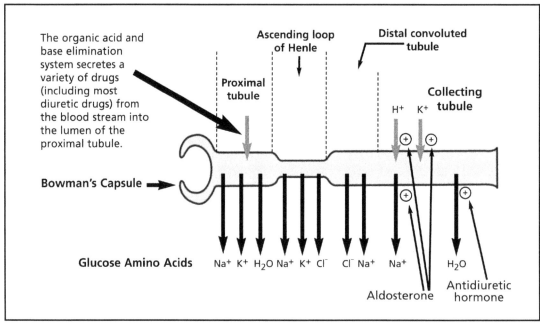

The organic acid and base elimination system secretes a variety of drugs (including most diuretic drugs) from the blood stream into the lumen of the proximal tubule.

Ascending loop of Henle

Distal convoluted tubule

Proximal tubule

Collecting tubule

H^+ K^+

Bowman's Capsule →

Glucose Amino Acids Na^+ K^+ H_2O Na^+ K^+ Cl^- Cl^- Na^+ Na^+ H_2O

Aldosterone

Antidiuretic hormone

Figure 6.4: A summary of the effects on water and various ions at different parts of a nephron.

ability to make proteins, especially albumin, which maintains osmotic pressure, fluid leaks into the abdominal cavity. Ascites may also be caused by secondary hyperaldosteronism. Aldosterone secretion is caused by decreased blood volume and causes sodium and water retention. In secondary hyperaldosteronism, the liver is not able to perform its normal function and inactivate aldosterone. This increases the amount of the active hormone and causes fluid accumulation. Loop diuretics are not generally useful in this condition, but spironolactone is. Another form of edema is caused by nephrotic syndrome, which is a disease of the kidneys that allows plasma proteins to be excreted with the urine. This in turn causes decreased osmotic pressure and allows edema. It is exacerbated by aldosterone secretion leading to sodium and water retention and aggravating the edema. Another condition that can cause edema is premenstrual edema. This is caused by imbalances of the hormones and can be treated with diuretics, if severe.

Diuretics are used in a variety of nonedematous states as well. Chief among these is hypertension. Thiazides are among the drugs of first choice in hypertension as they not only reduce blood volume but dilate arterioles. **Hypercalcemia** is a rapidly life-threatening condition that is treated with high doses of loop diuretics as they promote calcium excretion. Paradoxically, thiazide diuretics are used in treating **polydipsia** and **polyuria** associated with diabetes insipidus. They work by reducing plasma volume, which in turn causes a drop in glomerular filtration rate and increases reabsorption of sodium and water.

Thiazide diuretics may also be used in **hypercalciuria** and specifically in patients with urinary tract stones formed of calcium oxalate.

Loop diuretics are the drugs of choice in reducing pulmonary edema of heart failure and other emergency conditions. They are used in **hyperkalemia**, in addition to the common uses stated above.

Carbonic anhydrase inhibitors are used in glaucoma to reduce the intraocular pressure of open-angle glaucoma. Generally, they should not be used in an acute attack of glaucoma. Occasionally, they are used to prevent mountain sickness in healthy individuals who rapidly ascend above 10,000 feet.

In addition to treating hypertension, eplerenone is used to treat congestive heart failure after an acute myocardial infarct.

Hypercalcemia: Too much calcium in the blood

Polydipsia: Excessive thirst

Polyuria: Excessive urination

Hypercalciuria: Too much calcium in the urine

Hyperkalemia: Too much potassium in the blood

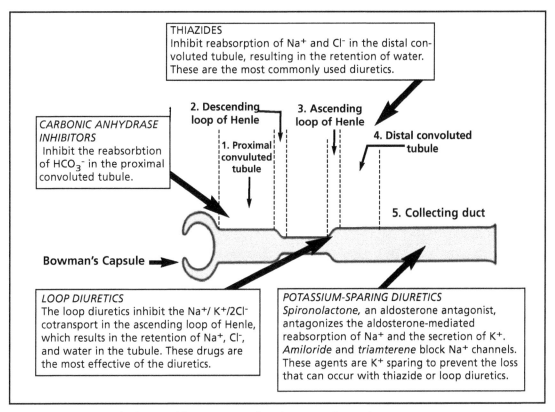

Figure 6.5: **Summary of where and how** common diuretics act on the nephron.

Osmotic diuretics are used to maintain urine flow in acute renal failure due to ingestion of toxic substances, shock, drug toxicities, and trauma. They are also commonly used to lower raised intracranial pressure.

▓ MECHANISM OF ACTION

In general, all diuretics work by affecting specific parts of the nephron. These effects are summarized in Figure 6.5.

Thiazide diuretics are excreted into the tubule lumen and are thought to inhibit the Na+/Cl- cotransporter in the distal convoluted tubule. They also appear to have a lesser but similar effect in the proximal tubule. These cause more sodium chloride to remain in the tubule, and hence more water remains in the tubule. Since they need to be excreted into the lumen before they are effective, thiazide diuretics lose efficacy with decreased kidney function. Other effects of thiazides include loss of potassium and magnesium, decreased urinary calcium excretion, and reduced peripheral vascular resistance due to

relaxation of the smooth muscles of the arterioles. Reduced calcium excretion is caused by increased calcium reabsorption. Studies have shown this to have a beneficial effect on bone density of the hip and spine.

Indapamide is metabolized and excreted by the gastrointestinal tract as well as the kidneys. It is therefore less likely to accumulate and have adverse effects due to kidney failure. Metolazone, unlike other thiazides, allows sodium excretion in renal-failure patients.

Loop diuretics are the most efficacious of the diuretics because they work at the ascending loop of Henle, which accounts for 25-30% of sodium chloride reabsorption. They act by inhibiting the Na+/K+/2Cl- cotransporter, thus increasing these ions and water in the tubule lumen. Loop diuretics, like the thiazides, also cause increased excretion of potassium and magnesium. However, they allow excretion of calcium, unlike the thiazides. In patients with normal serum calcium, however, most of this is reabsorbed in the distal tubule.

Potassium-sparing diuretics work in the collecting tubule and inhibit sodium reabsorption and potassium excretion. Generally, these drugs are used in combination with other diuretics, especially thiazides. However, they are used alone when aldosterone is in excess. Spironolactone and eplerenone work by antagonizing aldosterone and preventing the normal protein synthesis that stimulates Na+/K+ exchange. Other diuretics in this category affect this Na+/K+ exchange, but do not need to be in the presence of aldosterone to be effective. None of these are particularly strong diuretics and are often used with other diuretics, especially to counteract loss of potassium.

Carbonic anhydrase inhibitors work in the proximal tubule epithelial cells to prevent the formation of hydrogen and bicarbonate from carbon dioxide and water. Fewer hydrogen ions mean less exchange with sodium in the tubule. The increased luminal sodium causes more bicarbonate, potassium, and water to remain in the tubule lumen. pH increases due to the bicarbonate. Generally the diuretic actions of carbonic anhydrase inhibitors are quite weak, and they are used for other reasons.

DOSAGES

Generally dosing of diuretics should not take place too late in the evening as they can cause excessive **nocturia**.

ACETAZOLAMIDE, for *children*, for epilepsy, refer to *adult* dosing; for altitude sickness, prevention isn't recommended however, dosing would be 2.5 mg/kg every 12 hours starting the day before (preferred) or on the day of ascent; can be stopped after remaining at the same elevation for 2-3 days or if descent is started; maximum dose is 125 mg; to treat altitude sickness, 2.5 mg/kg every 8-12 hours up to a maximum dose of 250 mg. For *adults*, for altitude illness, 500-1000 mg/d in divided doses every 8-12 hours or divided every 12-24 hours for extended release capsules; for edema, 250-375 mg once daily; for epilepsy, 8-30 mg/kg/d in divided doses; max-

Nocturia: Excessive urination at night

imum dose is 30 mg/kg/d or 1 g/d; for chronic simple (open-angle) glaucoma, 250 mg 1-4 times/d or 500 mg extended release capsule bid; for secondary or acute (closed-angle) glaucoma, initiate at 250-500 mg; maintain at 125-250 mg every 4 hours.

AMILORIDE, for *elderly*, initially, 5 mg once daily or every other day.

BENDROFLUMETHIAZIDE, 5 mg once daily.

BUMETANIDE, for *infants* and *children*, for edema, oral and IM: 0.015-0.1 mg/kg every 6-24 hours up to a maximum of 10 mg/d. For *adults*, in edema, 0.5-2 mg 1-2 times/d up to a maximum of 10 mg/d; IM: 0.5-1 mg; if initial dose is inadequate, may repeat in 2-3 hours for up to 2 doses up to a maximum of 10 mg/d.

CHLOROTHIAZIDE, for *infants* <6 months, 10-20 mg/kg/bid (maximum dose: 375 mg/d). Infants >6 months and *children*, 5-10 mg/kg bid; maximum dose is 375 mg/d in children under 2 years or 1 g/d in children 2-12 years. For *adults*, for hypertension, 500-2000 mg/d divided in 1-2 doses; doses of 125-500 mg/d have also been recommended. For edema, 250-1000 mg once or twice daily; intermittent treatment (e.g., therapy on alternative days) may be appropriate for some patients. Maximum daily dose: 1000 mg. For *elderly*, 500 mg once daily or 1 g 3 times/wk.

CHLORTHALIDONE, for *adults*, for hypertension, 25-100 mg/d or 100 mg 3 times/week; usual dosage range: 12.5-25 mg/d. For edema, initiate at 50-100 mg/d or 100 mg on alternate days; maximum dose: 200 mg/d. For heart-failure-associated edema, 12.5-25 mg once daily; maximum daily dose: 100 mg. For the *elderly*, initiate at 12.5-25 mg/d or every other day; there is little advantage to using doses >25 mg/d.

EPLERENONE, for *adults*, for hypertension, initiate at 50 mg once daily; may increase to 50 mg bid if response is not adequate; may take up to 4 weeks for full therapeutic response; for congestive heart failure (post-MI), initiate at 25 mg once daily; increase dosage to 50 mg once daily within 4 weeks, as tolerated.

ETHACRYNIC ACID, for *children*, 1 mg/kg once

daily; increase at intervals of 2-3 days prn to a maximum of 3 mg/kg/d. For *adults*, 50-200 mg/d in 1-2 divided doses; may increase in increments of 25-50 mg at intervals of several days; doses up to 200 mg bid may be required with severe, refractory edema.

FUROSEMIDE, for *infants* and *children*, for edema or heart failure, 1-2 mg/kg increased in increments of 1 mg/kg with each succeeding dose until satisfactory effect is achieved up to a maximum of 6 mg/kg no more frequently than 6 hours; IM: initiate at 1 mg/kg; if response is inadequate, may increase dose in increments of 1 mg/kg and administer more than 2 hours after previous dose; may administer maintenance dose at intervals of every 6-12 hours; maximum dose is 6 mg/kg. For *adults*, for edema or heart failure, 20-80 mg initially increased in increments of 20-40 mg at intervals of 6-8 hours; usual maintenance dose interval is twice daily or every day; may be increased to 600 mg/d with severe edematous states; IM: initiate at 20-40 mg; if response is inadequate, may repeat the same dose or increase dose in increments of 20 mg and administer 1-2 hours after previous dose up to a maximum of 200 mg; this dose should then be given once or twice daily, although some patients may initially require dosing as frequent as every 6 hours; for resistant hypertension, 10-40 mg bid. For the *elderly*, oral or IM: initiate at 20 mg/d and increase slowly.

HYDROCHLOROTHIAZIDE, for *children* <6 months, 2-3 mg/kg/d in 2 divided doses; over 6 months, 1 mg/kg/d bid. For *adults*, for edema, 25-100 mg/d in 1-2 doses; maximum 200 mg/d. For hypertension, 12.5-50 mg/d. For the *elderly*, 12.5-25 mg once daily.

INDAPAMIDE, for *adults*, for edema: 2.5-5 mg/d; for hypertension, 1.25 mg mane; may increase to 5 mg/d by increments of 1.25-2.5 mg.

METHAZOLAMIDE, for *adults*, 50-100 mg 2-3 times/d.

METHYCLOTHIAZIDE, for edema, 2.5-10 mg/d; for hypertension: 2.5-5 mg/d.

METOLAZONE, for edema, 2.5-20 mg/dose every 24 hours; for hypertension, 2.5-5 mg/dose every 24 hours, Mykrox®, 0.5 mg/d; if response is not adequate, increase dose to maximum of 1 mg/d.

SPIRONOLACTONE, to reduce delay in onset of effect, a loading dose of 2 or 3 times the daily dose may be administered on the first day of therapy. For *adults*, for edema and hypokalemia, 25-200 mg/d in 1-2 divided doses; for hypertension, 25-50 mg/d in 1-2 divided doses; for diagnosis of primary aldosteronism, 100-400 mg/d in 1-2 divided doses; for CHF, severe (with ACE inhibitor and a loop diuretic ± digoxin), 12.5-25 mg/d; maximum daily dose is 50 mg (higher doses may occasionally be used). For the *elderly*, initially 25-50 mg/d in 1-2 divided doses, increasing by 25-50 mg every 5 days as needed.

TORSEMIDE, for *adults*, for congestive heart failure, 10-20 mg once daily; may increase gradually for chronic treatment by doubling dose until diuretic response is apparent to a maximum daily oral dose of 200 mg; for chronic renal failure: 20 mg once daily; increase as described above; for hepatic cirrhosis, 5-10 mg once daily with an aldosterone antagonist or a potassium-sparing diuretic; increase as described above; for hypertension, 2.5-5 mg once daily; increase to 10 mg after 4-6 weeks if an adequate hypotensive response is not apparent; if still not effective, an additional antihypertensive agent may be added.

TRIAMTERENE, for *adults*, 100-300 mg/d in 1-2 divided doses; maximum dose is 300 mg/d; usual dosage range is 50-100 mg/d.

ADVERSE EFFECTS

Potassium depletion is a concern for both thiazide and loop diuretics. Increased sodium in the tubule allows more potassium and sodium exchange to occur and with it, the possibility of hypokalemia. Diet alone may be able to slow down or reverse potassium loss. Dietary suggestions include increasing potassium-containing foods, such as bananas, citrus fruits, and prunes, as well as restricting sodium. Spironolactone and triamterene can also be coadministered to reduce the chances of hypokalemia.

Thiazide diuretics can also cause the following effects: hyperuricemia, which can lead to gout; volume depletion causing orthostatic hypotension; hypercalcemia; and hyperlipidemia. In diabetics, thiazides can cause hyperglycemia and reduced control of sugar levels. And they very rarely cause hypersensitivity reactions such as bone marrow suppression, necrotizing vasculitis, interstitial nephritis, and dermatitis. Patients allergic to sulfa drugs may also be allergic to thiazides. Central nervous system effects are rare but include vertigo, headaches, paresthesias, and weakness. May cause erectile dysfunction.

Loop diuretics can be **ototoxic**, permanently affecting hearing and possibly balance. This risk is minimized by oral administration. They can also cause **hypomagnesemia** and hypocalcemia especially in the elderly. They can also cause hyperuricemia leading to gout, hyperglycemia, hyperlipidemia, skin rashes, photosensitivity, paresthesias, bone marrow depression, and gastrointestinal disturbances. If used in excessive quantities they could cause reduced glomerular filtration rate (GFR); circulatory collapse; **thromboembolic** episodes; and in patients with liver disease, hepatic **encephalopathy**.

Spirolonolactone may cause peptic ulcers and gastric upset. Due to its similarity chemically with some sex hormones, it may induce **gynecomastia** in men and menstrual disturbances in women among other sexual trait disruptions. Because of this it should not be administered in high doses chronically. Other possible adverse effects include hyperkalemia, nausea, lethargy, and mental confusion. Triamterene may cause leg cramps and increased blood urea nitrogen (BUN), uric acid, and hyperkalemia. Eplerenone can cause **hypertriglyceridemia**.

Carbonic anhydrase inhibitors may cause mild

Ototoxic: Having a harmful effect on the ear or Cranial Nerve VIII

Hypomagnesemia: Abnormally low magnesium in the blood

Thromboembolism: Blockage of a blood vessel due to a piece of a clot breaking off from another location and preventing blood flow

Encephalopathy: Pathology of the structure or tissues of the brain

Gynecomastia: Abnormal enlargement of one or two breasts in men

Hypertriglyceridemia: Abnormally high amounts of triglycerides in the blood

Acidosis: Abnormal increase in hydrogen ions in the body

metabolic **acidosis**, hypokalemia, renal stones, drowsiness, and paresthesias. Patients allergic to sulfonamides may also be allergic to these drugs. They should not be used with liver cirrhosis because it can decrease ammonia excretion.

Osmotic diuretics can cause dehydration and hypernatremia. Mannitol can cause hyponatremia before diuresis occurs.

RED FLAGS

Hypokalemia is a life-threatening possibility for both thiazide and loop diuretics. Hyponatremia, excessive loss of sodium, is another life-threatening effect of thiazide diuretics.

Loop diuretics may precipitate a rapid and severe loss of blood volume and can result in such serious conditions as hypotension, shock, and cardiac arrhythmias.

Hyperkalemia is also a life-threatening risk with potassium-sparing drugs, especially in patients who have renal failure, are taking ACE inhibitors, or are taking potassium supplements.

INTERACTIONS

DRUG

Probenacid can interfere with excretion of thiazide diuretics and may increase the uric acid levels in the blood. Thiazides may also decrease the effects of anticoagulants, agents used to treat gout, sulfonylureas, and insulin. They may increase the effects of anesthetics, diazoxide, digitalis glycosides, lithium, and vitamin D. NSAIDs reduce the effect of thiazides. A lethal drug reaction occurs between thiazide diuretics and quinidine.

Loop diuretics have many potential drug interactions. Aminoglycoside antibiotics, cisplatin, and ethacrynic acid may potentiate their ototoxicity. Use with furosemide and ethacrynic acid may cause hyperuricemia and gout. They can potentiate anticoagulants; there may be increased digitalis-induced arrhythmias when used with digitalis glycosides. Lithium levels may increase when coadministered. Propranolol may have increased blood levels. Sulfonylureas are not as effective. Use with high doses of NSAIDs may blunt diuretic response and cause salicylate toxicity. When given with amphotericin B may increase potential for nephrotoxicity and electrolyte imbalances.

HERB

ACETAZOLAMIDE

- *Ma Huang* (Ephedra) (C)–based on ephedrine content, acetazolamide may increase the serum concentrations of ephedrine from *Ma Huang* (Wilkinson & Beckett, 1968) Level 4 evidence.

ANTIHYPERTENSIVES

- *Chen Pi* (Tangerine peel), *Qing Pi* (Citrus Viride), *Zhi Ke* (Aurantium fruit), *Zhi Shi* (Aurantium immaturus), (Indeterminate)– all contain constituents that stimulate the sympathetic nervous system and should be used with caution in those taking antihypertensives, antidiabetic, antihyperthyroid, and/ or antiseizure medications (Chinese language article cited in Chen & Chen, 2004) Indeterminate level of evidence.
- *Gan Cao* (Licorice) (D)–theoretically may reduce effects of antihypertensive agents such as alpha-1-adrenergic blockers, ACEI, A_2 receptor antagonists, beta-adrenergic blockers, calcium channel blockers, clonidine, guanabenz, guanfacine, hydralazine, methyldopa, minoxidil, and reserpine. Undertake concurrent use with caution (Kowalak & Mills, 2001) Level 5 evidence.
- *Ma Huang* (Ephedra) (C)–based on ephedrine content, antagonizes the effects of antihypertensives (White, Gardner, Gurley, Marx, Wang, & Estes) Level 3b evidence. Antihypertensives including ACE inhibitors and beta-blockers may be antagonized by *Ma Huang,* and severe hypertension may be result. This is speculative (Mills & Bone, 2000) Level 5 evidence.
- *Sheng Ma* (Cimicifuga) (D)–may potentiate the effect of antihypertensive agents. Undertake concurrent use with caution. Expert opinion (Gruenwald, Brendler & Jaenicke, 2004) Level 5 evidence.

DICHLORPHENAMIDE

- *Ma Huang* (Ephedra) (D)–based on ephedrine content, dichlorphenamide may cause ephedrine and pseudoephedrine toxicity from *Ma Huang* due to alkalinization of the urine and decreased urinary excretion, expert opinion (Gruenwald, Brendler & Jaenicke, 2004) Level 5 evidence.

DIURETICS

- *Bai Ji Li* (Tibulus) (D)–has a mild diuretic effect in rats and may lead to increased elimination of water and/or electrolytes (Chen, 1998/1999) Level 5 evidence.
- *Bai Mao Gen* (Imperata), *Bai Zhu* (White Atractylodes), *Ban Bian Lian* (Lobelia), *Bian Xu* (Common knotgrass), *Cang Zhu* (Red Actractylodes), *Che Qian Zi* (Plantago seed), *Dan Zhu Ye* (Lophatherum), *Fen Fang Ji* (Stephania), *Fu Ling* (Poria), *Gui Zhi* (Cinnamon twigs), *Jin Qian Cao* (Lysimachia), *Jue Ming Zi* (Cassia seed), *Long Dan Cao* (Gentiana), *Ma Huang* (Ephedra), *Mi Meng Hua* (Buddleja), *Qu Mai* (Dianthus), *Sang Ji Sheng* (Taxillus), *Tong Cao* (Tetrapanax), *Yu Mi Xu* (Corn silk), *Yuan Zhi* (Polygala), *Ze Lan* (Lycopus), *Ze Xie* (Alsima), *Zhi Shi* (Aurantium immaturus), *Zhu Ling* (Polyporus), and other water-regulating and damp-resolving herbs (D)–all have a diuretic effect that may lead to increased elimination of water and/or electrolytes (Chen, 1998/1999) Level 5 evidence.
- *Fan Xie Ye* (Senna) (Indeterminate)–can cause increased loss of potassium from diuretics if overused. Examples include chlorothiazide, hydrochlorothiazide, furosemide, bumetanide, and torsemide (unobtainable article as cited in Chen & Chen, 2004) Indeterminate level of evidence.
- *Gan Cao* (Licorice) (C)–may increase potassium loss and cause hypertension when used with diuretics (Harada *et al.,* 2002) Level 4 evidence; (de Klerk, Nieuwenhuis, Beutler, 1997) Level 4 evidence; (Folkersen, Knudsen, Teglbjaerg, 1996) Level 4 evidence; (Hussain, 2003), Level 5 evidence; (Lin *et al.,* 2003), and

(Shintani *et al.*, 1992) Level 4 evidence.

- *Lu Hui* (Aloe) (D)–can increase potassium loss due to thiazide diuretics and corticosteroids (Blumenthal, 1998); (Gruenwald, Brendler & Jaenicke, 2004) Level 5 evidence.
- *Shan Zhu Yu* (Cornus) (D)–has been shown to have a diuretic effect in dogs that may lead to increased elimination of water and/or electrolytes in humans (Chen, 1998/1999) Level 5 evidence.
- *Ting Li Zi* (Descurainia), *Xuan Fu Hua* (Inula flowers) (D)–both have a mild diuretic effect that may lead to increased elimination of water and/or electrolytes (Chen, 1998/1999) Level 5 evidence.
- *Yin Guo Ye* (Gingko) (D)–clinical cases indicate interactions of ginkgo with antiepileptics, aspirin (acetylsalicylic acid), diuretics, ibuprofen, risperidone, rofecoxib, trazodone, and warfarin (Izzo & Ernst, 2009) Level 4 evidence.

FUROSEMIDE

- *Gan Cao* (Licorice) (C)–a case was reported of congestive heart failure and hypokalemia in a patient taking *Gan Cao*, furosemide, and digoxin (Harada, Ohtaki, Misu, Sumiyoshi & Hosada, 2002) Level 4 evidence.

LOOP DIURETICS, THIAZIDE DIURETICS

- *Lu Hui* (Aloe) (D)–can increase potassium loss due to thiazide and loop diuretics and corticosteroids, expert opinions (Blumenthal, 1998) (Gruenwald, Brendler, & Jaenicke, 2004) Level 5 evidence.

THIAZIDE DIURETICS

- *Yin Guo Ye* (Ginkgo leaf) (C-)–may have increased blood pressure as reported by a single case report (Saw, Leon, Kolev, & Murray, 1997) Level 4 evidence.

INTERACTION ISSUES

A:

D: Bumetanide is 94-96% protein bound, furosemide is 91-99% bound; metolazone is 95% bound; spironolactone is 91-98% bound; torsemide is over 99% bound.

M: Eplerenone is a major substrate of CYP3A4; torsemide is a major substrate of CYP2C9.

E: All diuretics could theoretically increase elimination because of increased urination. However, this may or may not be true given that there may be other rate-limiting steps, such as needing to be metabolized by the liver, before elimination can occur.

TI:

Pgp:

SECTION 4: VASODILATORS

AMBRISENTAN (am bri SEN tan) PR=X *(Letairis®)*

AMYL NITRITE (AM il NYE trite) PR=C

BOSENTAN (boe SEN tan) PR=X *(Tracleer®)*

DIAZOXIDE (dye az OKS ide) PR=C *(Proglycem®)*

DIPYRIDAMOLE (dye peer ID a mole) PR=B *(Aggrenox®,[19] Persantine®)*

HYDRALAZINE (hye DRAL a zeen) PR=C *(BiDil®[20])*

ILOPROST (EYE loe prost) PR=C *(Ventavis®)*

ISOSORBIDE DINITRATE (eye soe SOR bide dye NYE trate) PR=C *(BiDil®,[20] Dilatrate® SR, IsoDitrate® ER, Isordil®, Titradose™)*

ISOSORBIDE MONONITRATE (eye soe SOR bide mon oh NYE trate) PR=B/C *(Imdur®)*

ISOXSUPRINE (eye SOKS syoo prene) PR=C

MINOXIDIL (mi NOKS i dil) PR=C

NITROGLYCERIN (nye troe GLI ser in) PR=C *(Minitran™, Nitro-Bid®, Nitro-Dur®, Nitro-Time®, Nitrolingual®, NitroMist®, Nitrostat®, Rectiv®)*

PAPAVERINE (pa PAV er ene) PR=C

RANOLAZINE (RAY-no-lah-zene) PR=C *(Ranexa)*

FUNCTION

While these compounds all fall under the category of vasodilators, they have different functions. Organic nitrates such as isosorbide mono- and dinitrates and nitroglycerin are used in treating angina pectoralis. They can also be used for congestive heart failure and myocardial infarction. The others in this category are primarily used for treatment of moderately severe to malignant hypertension.

However, in the category of vasodilators, diazoxide is only used as an antihypertensive in intravenous injections. As an oral drug, it is used to treat hypoglycemia due to neoplastic disease affecting pancreatic islet cells.

Isoxsuprine is used to treat peripheral vascular diseases including Raynaud's disease and arteriosclerosis obliterans. Minoxidil is also used topically to grow hair. Dipyridamole is primarily used with warfarin to prevent thromboemboli in patients with cardiac valve replacement. Isosorbide dinitrate is used in treating congestive heart failure. Nitroglycerin, besides treating angina, is also used in treating congestive heart failure, pulmonary hypertension, and hypertensive emergencies.

Papaverine is used to treat ischemia due to arterial spasms in addition to myocardial **ischemia** complicated by arrhythmias.

Ranolazine is a relatively new agent for treating chronic angina. As it affects the heart's electrical conduction, it should only be used when other anti-anginal agents are not effective.

MECHANISM OF ACTION

Vasodilators work by causing smooth muscle relaxation in blood vessels. Where they work depends on each individual drug.

Diazoxide treats hypertension by peripheral arteriole smooth muscle relaxation causing blood pressure decreases and an increase in the heart rate and cardiac output.

Dipyridamole works by inhibiting certain enzymes that break down vasodilating mediators. These mediators cause vasodilation especially in the heart. In addition, they inhibit platelet aggregation and thus provide this drug's clinical usefulness.

Hydralazine and minoxidil work by relaxing systemic arterioles and thus reducing total peripheral resistance, which in turn reduces blood pressure.

Isosorbide dinitrate, isosorbide mononitrate, and nitroglycerin work by causing both venous and arterial relaxation. This results in some pooling of blood in the veins and thus decreases preload on the heart and lessens the amount of work the heart needs to do. The arterial vasodilation drops total peripheral resistance and blood pressure. The coronary arteries are also dilated, and this increases oxygenated blood flow to the heart and counteracts any ischemia. Esophageal smooth muscle is also relaxed.

While the mechanism of action for isoxsuprine is not entirely certain, it is believed that it has an effect on beta-receptor stimulation as well as a direct effect on dilating vascular smooth muscle.

Papaverine's mechanism of action is not completely understood. It causes systemic and widespread smooth muscle relaxation: vasodilation, bronchiolar muscle relaxation, and gastrointestinal sphincter relaxation. It also increases blood flow to the brain.

How ranolazine works is not understood.

DOSAGES

AMBRISENTAN, for *adults*, for pulmonary arterial hypertension, initiate at 5 mg once daily; if tolerated, may increase to a maximum of 10 mg once daily.

AMYL NITRITE, for *adults*, for angina, inhalation: 2-6 nasal inhalations from 1 crushed ampule, may repeat in 3-5 minutes.

BOSENTAN, for *adolescents* over 12 and *adults*, for pulmonary artery hypertension, for patients under 40 kg, 62.5 mg bid; in patients 40 kg or heavier, initiate at 62.5 mg bid for 4 weeks; increase to maintenance dose of 125 mg bid.

DIAZOXIDE, for hyperinsulinemic hypoglycemia, use lowest dose listed as initial dose; for *newborns* and *infants*, 8-15 mg/kg/d in divided doses every 8-12 hours. For *children* and *adults*, use 3-8 mg/kg/d in divided doses every 8-12 hours.

DIPYRIDAMOLE, for *children*, for proteinuria (unlabeled use), 4-10 mg/kg/d; for mechanical

Ischemia: Decreased blood flow to an organ/body part, often accompanied by pain and dysfunction

prosthetic heart valves (unlabeled use), 2-5 mg/kg/d. For *adults*, 75-100 mg qid.

HYDRALAZINE, for *children*, initiate at 0.75-1 mg/kg/d in 2-4 divided doses; increase over 3-4 weeks to a maximum of 7.5 mg/kg/day in 2-4 divided doses; maximum daily dose is 200 mg/d. For *adults*, for hypertension, initiate at 10 mg qid for first 2-4 days; increase to 25 mg qid for the balance of the first week; increase by 10-25 mg/dose gradually to 50 mg qid; maximum dose is 300 mg/d; usual dose range is 12.5-50 mg/d bid; for congestive heart failure, initiate at 10-25 mg 3-4 times/d; dosage must be adjusted based on individual response, target dose is 225-300 mg/d in divided doses; use in combination with isosorbide dinitrate. For the *elderly*, initiate at 10 mg 2-3 times/d; increase by 10-25 mg/d every 2-5 days.

ILOPROST, for *adults*, for pulmonary arterial hypertension (PAH), inhalation: initiate at 2.5 mcg; if tolerated, increase to 5 mcg; administer 6-9 times daily in intervals of 2 hours or more; maintain at 2.5-5 mcg/dose up to a maximum daily dose of 45 mcg.

ISOSORBIDE DINITRATE, for *adults*, for angina, 5-40 mg qid or 40 mg every 8-12 hours in sustained-release dosage form; in sublingual form, 2.5-5 mg every 5-10 minutes for maximum of 3 doses in 15-30 minutes; may also use prophylactically 15 minutes prior to activities that may provoke an attack; for congestive heart failure, initiate at 20 mg 3-4 times per day; target dose, 120-160 mg/d in divided doses; use in combination with hydralazine.

ISOSORBIDE MONONITRATE, for *adults* and the *elderly*, regular tablet, 5-10 mg bid with the two doses given 7 hours apart to decrease tolerance development; then increase to 10 mg bid in first 2-3 days; extended release tablet, initiate at 30-60 mg given in morning as a single dose; titrate upward as needed, giving at least 3 days between increases; maximum daily single dose of 240 mg.

ISOXSUPRINE, for *adults*, 10-20 mg 3-4 times/d. Start with lower dose in the *elderly* due to potential hypotension.

MINOXIDIL, for *children* less than 12 years old, for hypertension, initiate at 0.1-0.2 mg/kg once daily up to a maximum of 5 mg/d; increase gradually every 3 days; usual dosage is 0.25-1 mg/kg/d in 1-2 divided doses up to a maximum of 50 mg/d. For *children* older than 12 and *adults*, for hypertension, initiate at 5 mg once daily; increase gradually every 3 days up to a maximum of 100 mg/d; usual dose range is 2.5-80 mg/d in 1-2 divided doses. For the *elderly*, initiate at 2.5 mg once daily and increase gradually.

NITROGLYCERIN, for *adults*, 2.5-9 mg 2-4 times/d (up to 26 mg qid); as an ointment, 1/2 upon rising and 1/2 six hours later; the dose may be doubled and even doubled again as needed; for the patch/transdermal application, initiate at 0.2-0.4 mg/hr, increase to doses of 0.4-0.8 mg/hr; tolerance is minimized by using a patch-on period of 12-14 hours and patch-off period of 10-12 hours; for sublingual use, 0.2-0.6 mg every 5 minutes for maximum of 3 doses in 15 minutes; may also use prophylactically 5-10 minutes prior to activities that may provoke an attack; translingually, 1-2 sprays into mouth under tongue every 3-5 minutes for maximum of 3 doses in 15 minutes, may also be used prophylactically 5-10 minutes prior to activities which may provoke an attack.

PAPAVERINE, for *adults*, 30-120 mg; may repeat every 3 hrs.

RANOLAZINE, for *adults*, 500 mg bid; may increase to 1000 mg and up to a maximum of 2000 mg/d.

ADVERSE EFFECTS

Organic nitrates, such as isosorbide mono- and dinitrate and nitroglycerin, commonly cause headaches, with high doses causing postural hypotension, facial flushing, and tachycardia. Tolerance is a major issue for these drugs; therefore a drug-free period must occur every day, usually overnight.

Diazoxide can cause hypotension, dizziness, nausea and vomiting, and muscular weakness.

Hydralazine can cause headaches, nausea, sweating, arrhythmia, and precipitation of angina. With high doses, a lupus-like syndrome may occur, reversible upon discontinuation of the drug.

Minoxidil causes serious water and sodium retention, which can lead to hypervolemia, edema, and congestive heart failure. This drug should always be used with a diuretic and beta-blocker in order to avoid these effects.

Isoxsuprine and papaverine may cause hypotension, tachycardia, dizziness, nausea and vomiting, and a skin rash.

Ranolazine may cause dizziness, headache, GI issues, tinnitus, vertigo, peripheral edema, and dyspnea. Can lengthen QT interval and therefore a baseline with regular ECG monitoring is necessary.

RED FLAGS

Hydralazine and minoxidil may cause a reflex stimulation of the heart, which in turn causes increased contractility, heart rate, and oxygen consumption that may precipitate angina pectoralis and myocardial infarction in predisposed individuals.

INTERACTIONS

Ranolazine should not be used in patients with pre-existing QT prolongation.

DRUG

Sildenafil potentiates the organic nitrates and can cause dangerous hypotension.

Ranolazine requires CYP3A4 for metabolism, so strong inhibitors of this enzyme should be avoided. These include diltiazem, ketoconazole, and grapefruit juice.

HERB

DIPYRIDAMOLE

- *Bai Hua She* (Bungarus snake) (D)–has an antiplatelet effect; use with caution in those taking anticoagulants or antiplatelets (Chen, 1998/1999) Level 5 evidence.
- *Bai Shao* (White peony root) (D)–has a mild antiplatelet effect; use with caution in those taking anticoagulants or antiplatelets (Chen, 1998/1999) Level 5 evidence.
- *Bai Zhu* (White Atractylodes) (D)–has an antiplatelet effect and should be used with caution in those taking anticoagulants or antiplatelets

(Chen, 1998/1999) Level 5 evidence.
- *Ban Lan Gen* (Isatis root) (D)–has an antiplatelet effect; use with caution in those taking anticoagulants or antiplatelets (Chen, 1998/1999) Level 5 evidence.
- *Chi Shao* (Red peony root) (D)–has an antiplatelet effect; use with caution in those taking anticoagulants or antiplatelets (Chen, 1998/1999) Level 5 evidence.
- *Chuan Xiong* (Cnidium, Sichuan Lovage rhizome) (D)–may potentiate anticoagulant and antiplatelet effects and should be used with caution in patients taking these medications (Chen, 1998/1999) Level 5 evidence.
- *Ci Wu Jia* (Siberian ginseng) (D)–may potentiate the effects of anticoagulant, antiplatelet, and thrombolytic agents (Yun-Choi, Kim & Lee, 1987) Level 5 evidence.
- *Da Suan* (Garlic) (D)–may potentiate anticoagulant and antiplatelet effects; use with caution in patients taking anticoagulant and antiplatelet agents, thrombolytic agents, and low molecular weight heparins, expert opinion (Gruenwald, Brendler & Jaenicke, 2004) Level 5 evidence.
- *Da Suan* (Garlic) (D)–potentiates anticoagulant and antiplatelet effects of indomethacin and dypiridamole in bench research (Apitz-Castro, Escalante, Vargas & Jain, 1986) Level 5 evidence.
- *Dang Gui* (Angelica Sinensis) (D)–may potentiate anticoagulant and antiplatelet effects and should be used with caution in patients taking anticoagulant and antiplatelet agents, thrombolytic agents, and low molecular weight heparins, expert opinion (Gruenwald, Brendler & Jaenicke, 2004) Level 5 evidence.
- *Di Bie Chong* (Eupolyphaga) (D)–may potentiate anticoagulant and antiplatelet effects; use with caution in patients taking these medications (Chen, 1998/1999) Level 5 evidence.
- *Ding Xiang* (Clove) (D)–may potentiate anticoagulant and antiplatelet effects and should be used with caution in patients taking anticoagulant and antiplatelet agents, thrombolytic agents, and low molecular weight heparins, expert opinion (Gruenwald, Brendler & Jaenicke, 2004) Level 5 evidence.

- *Ding Xiang* (Clove) (D)–may potentiate anti-coagulants due to platelet aggregation inhibition (Mills & Bone, 2000) Level 5 evidence.
- *Du Huo* (Pubescent angelica root) (D)–has an antiplatelet effect and should be used with caution in those taking anticoagulants or anti-platelets (Chen, 1998/1999) Level 5 evidence.
- *E Zhu* (Cucuma zedoaria), *Hong Hua* (Safflower, Carthamus), *Ge Gen* (Pueraria root) (D)–these may potentiate anticoagulant and antiplatelet effects; use with caution in patients taking these medications (Chen, 1998/1999) Level 5 evidence.
- *Gan Cao* (Licorice) (D)–may potentiate anti-coagulant and antiplatelet effects (Norred & Brinker, 2001). In addition, *Gan Cao* has coumarin-like constituents (Heck, Dewitt & Lukes, 2000), and glycyrhizzin, a major constituent of *Gan Cao*, has been shown to have some in vitro thrombin inhibition (Francis-chetti, Monteiro & Guimaraes, 1997) and should be used with caution in patients taking anticoagulant and antiplatelet agents, throm-bolytic agents, and low molecular weight heparins, expert opinion (Gruenwald, Brendler & Jaenicke, 2004) Each of these studies is Level 5 evidence.
- *Gan Jiang/Sheng Jiang* (Ginger) (D)–extract of ginger may speculatively enhance anticoag-ulation of warfarin and other anticoagulants (Mills & Bone, 2000; Gianni & Dreitlein, 1988) Level 5 evidence. A single dose of 2 grams *Gan Jiang* in 8 men did not affect bleeding time, platelet count, or aggregation (Lumb, 1994) Level 2b evidence. Ten grams of extract did affect platelet aggregation, while taking 4 grams daily for 3 months did not show significant anticoagulation activity (Bordia, Verma & Srivastava, 1997) Level 3b evidence.
- *Gou Teng* (Cat's claw) (D)–may potentiate anticoagulant and antiplatelet effects; use with caution in patients taking anticoagulant and antiplatelet agents, thrombolytic agents, and low molecular weight heparins, expert opin-

ion (Gruenwald, Brendler & Jaenicke, 2004) Level 5 evidence.
- *Hou Po* (Magnolia bark), *Mao Dong Qing* (Ilex pubescentis) (D)–both have a mild anti-platelet effect; use with caution in those taking anticoagulants or antiplatelets (Chen, 1998/1999) Level 5 evidence.
- *Hu Tai Ren* (Walnut) (D)–has antiplatelet and thrombolytic effects; use with caution in those taking anticoagulants or antiplatelets (Chen, 1998/1999) Level 5 evidence.
- *Huang Qi* (Astragulus) (D)–may potentiate anticoagulant and antiplatelet effects and should be used with caution in patients taking anticoagulant and antiplatelet agents, throm-bolytic agents, and low molecular weight heparins, expert opinion (Gruenwald, Brendler & Jaenicke, 2004) Level 5 evidence.
- *Jiang Huang* (Tumeric) (D)–may potentiate anticoagulant and antiplatelet effects; use with caution in patients taking these medications (Chen, 1998/1999) Level 5 evidence.
- *Jiang Huang* (Turmeric) (D)–may potentiate anticoagulant and antiplatelet effects; use with caution in patients taking anticoagulant and antiplatelet agents, thrombolytic agents, and low molecular weight heparins (Srivastava, Puri, Srimal & Dhawan, 1986) Level 5 evi-dence.
- *Pu Huang* (Bulrush, cattail pollen) (D)–uniquely both increases blood circulation and stops bleeding and may interfere with antico-agulant and antiplatelet medications (Chen, 1998/1999) Level 5 evidence.
- *Qian Hu* (Peucedanum, white-flowered hog-fen-nel root) (D)–has an antiplatelet effect; use with caution in those taking anticoagulants or antiplatelets (Chen, 1998/1999) Level 5 evidence.
- *San Leng* (Sparganium, Common burreed rhizome) (D)–may potentiate anticoagulant and antiplatelet effects and should be used with caution in patients taking these medica-tions (Chen, 1998/1999) Level 5 evidence.
- *San Qi* (Indeterminate)–uniquely both in-creases blood circulation and stops bleeding;

may interfere with anticoagulant and anti-platelet medications (Chinese language study cited in Chen & Chen, 2004) Indeterminate level of evidence.

- *Sang Ji Sheng* (Taxillus), *Sha Ren* (Amomum), *Shui Zhi* (Medicinal leech) (D)–all have an antiplatelet effect, and caution should be used in those taking anticoagulants or antiplatelets (Chen, 1998/1999) Level 5 evidence.
- Stop-bleeding herbs (D)–may counteract anti-platelet and anticoagulant effects; use with caution in patients taking these medications, expert opinion (Chen & Chen, 2004) Level 5 evidence.
- *Su He Xiang* (Styrax), *Tao Ren* (Peach seed), *Xie Bai* (Bakeri, long-stamen onion bulb), *Yu Jin* (Turmeric tuber), *Xia Tian Wu* (Decumbent corydalis rhizome), *Ye Ju Hua* (Wild chrysanthemum flower), *Yi Mu Cao* (Motherwort herb) (D)–all may potentiate anticoagulant and antiplatelet effects; use with caution in patients taking these medications (Chen, 1998/1999) Level 5 evidence.
- *Yin Guo Ye* (Ginkgo leaf) (D)–may potentiate anticoagulant and antiplatelet effects and should be used with caution in patients taking anticoagulant and antiplatelet agents, thrombolytic agents, and low molecular weight heparins, expert opinion (Gruenwald, Brendler, & Jaenicke, 2004) Level 5 evidence. In fact, a Level 2b study (Engelsen, Nielsen & Hansen, 2003) showed no change in coagulation (INR levels) when using warfarin and gingko.
- *Zhi Ke* (Aurantium fruit, bitter orange) (D)–

has an antiplatelet effect; use with caution in those taking anticoagulants or antiplatelets (Chen, 1998/1999) Level 5 evidence.

HYDRALAZINE, MINOXIDIL

- *Gan Cao* (Licorice) (D)–theoretically may reduce the effects of antihypertensive agents such as alpha-1 adrenergic blockers, ACEI, A_2 receptor antagonists, beta-adrenergic blockers, calcium channel blockers, clonidine, guanabenz, guanfacine, hydralazine, methyldopa, minoxidil, and reserpine, and concurrent use should be undertaken with caution (Kowalak & Mills, 2001) Level 5 evidence.

PAPAVERINE

- *Yin Guo Ye* (Ginkgo leaf) (D)–may increase adverse effects associated with papaverine, expert opinion (Gruenwald, Brendler & Jaenicke, 2004) Level 5 evidence.

INTERACTION ISSUES

A:

D: Ambrisentan is 99% protein bound; bosentan is over 98% bound; dipyridamole is 91-99% bound.

M: Bosentan is a major substrate and strong inducer of CYP2C9 and 3A4; isosorbide dinitrate and mononitrate are major substrates of CYP3A4; ranolazine is a major substrate of CYP3A4.

E:

TI:

Pgp: Ambrisentan is a substrate of P-glycoprotein; dipyridamole inhibits Pgp; ranolazine is a substrate of and inhibits Pgp.

SECTION 5: ANTIARRHYTHMIC AGENTS

CARDIAC GLYCOSIDES:

DIGOXIN (di JOKS in) PR=C *(Lanoxin®)*

CLASS I, SODIUM CHANNEL BLOCKERS:

CLASS IA:

DISOPYRAMIDE (dye soe PEER a mide) PR=C
  (Norpace®, Norpace® CR)

PROCAINAMIDE (proe kane A mide) PR=C

QUINIDINE (KWIN i deen) PR=C

CLASS IB:

MEXILETINE (meks IL e tene) PR=C

CLASS 1C:

Continues on next page

SECTION 5: ANTIARRHYTHMIC AGENTS cont.

FLECAINIDE (fle KAY nide) PR=C *(Tambocor™)*

PROPAFENONE (proe pa FEEN one) PR=C *(Rythmol®, Rythmol® SR)*

CLASS II, BETA-ADRENORECEPTOR BLOCKERS: *(See Chapter 4, Section 8)* **ACEBUTOLOL, ATENOLOL, BETAXOLOL, BISOPROLOL, CARVEDILOL, METOPROLOL, NADOLOL, PROPRANOLOL, SOTALOL**

CLASS III, POTASSIUM CHANNEL BLOCKERS:

AMIODARONE (a MEE oh da rone) PR=D *(Cordarone®, Nexterone®, Pacerone®)*

DOFETILIDE (doe FET il ide) *(Tikosyn™)* **PR=C**

DRONEDARONE (droe NE da rone) PR=X *(Multaq®)*

SOTALOL *(See Chapter 4, Section 8)*

CLASS IV, CALCIUM CHANNEL BLOCKERS: *(See Section 7 below).* **DILTIAZEM, VERAPAMIL**

An arrhythmia is an abnormality to impulse formation and conduction in the heart muscle. These can fall into several possibilities. Sinus bradycardia is when the heart rate is too slow. The rate can be too fast, which can be caused by sinus or ventricular tachycardia, atrial or ventricular premature depolarization, or atrial flutter. The cardiac muscle may respond to impulses originating from sites other than the sinoatrial (SA) node or it may be caused by responding to impulses traveling down extra pathways that lead to inappropriate depolarizations such as in AV

reentry or Wolff-Parkinson-White syndrome.

Arrhythmias may have several causes. Abnormal automaticity can cause arrhythmias when normal cardiac cells are changed so that they set the pace of impulses supplanting the normal function of the SA node. These abnormal cardiac cells are often caused by damage from hypoxia, potassium imbalance, or other reasons. They cause abnormal automatic discharges because they depolarize more slowly than other cells and are therefore faster to hit the firing threshold.

The most common cause of arrhythmias is

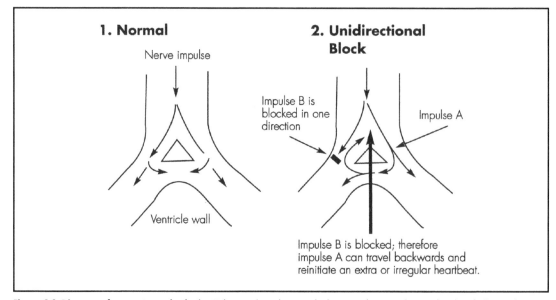

Figure 6.6: Diagram of a re-entry arrhythmia. When an impulse travels down pathway A, it can also depolarize pathway B, which then reenters pathway A and starts another impulse.

reentry. This is where a unidirectional block occurs in damaged myocardial cell(s) resulting in an abnormal conduction pathway. If a normal pathway has two directions and one has a unidirectional block, it may allow the other to act in a retrograde fashion and reenter the pathway and cause a re-excitation of the myocardia. This is shown in Figure 6.6 on the previous page.

TYPES OF ARRHYTHMIAS

Arrhythmias may be broken down into a number of types including where they take place, how fast they are, or how they are caused. Arrhythmias are generally diagnosed with electrocardiograms (ECGs). A list of common or important arrhythmias follows.

ATRIAL FIBRILLATION: A rapid, irregularly irregular atrial rhythm. It causes considerable symptoms including palpitations and occasional weakness and presyncope. Thrombi can form and embolize to the brain causing a CVA.

ATRIAL FLUTTER: A rapid regular atrial rhythm due to an atrial reentrant circuit. The main symptom is palpitations. Thrombi may form and embolize.

AV BLOCK: Where there is a partial or incomplete transmission of the impulse from the atria to the ventricles. These are broken down into different degrees. A first degree AV block is where the PR interval on the ECG is longer than normal. This can be physiological in young patients and in well-trained athletes and is always asymptomatic and requires no treatment. Second-degree AV block is where some but not all P waves (atrial impulses) are not necessarily followed by ventricular conduction and contraction. There are several subtypes of second-degree AV blocks. A third-degree AV block is a complete block where there is no connection between P waves (atrial impulses) and QRS complexes (ventricular conduction and contractions).

BRADYARRHYTHMIA: An arrhythmia that has an overall rate slower than 60 beats per minute (bpm).

ECTOPIC SUPRAVENTRICULAR RHYTHM: Where cells in the atria become pacemaker-like cells causing a discharge similar to the SA node that triggers an extra heartbeat. Many are asymptomatic and require no intervention.

JUNCTIONAL ARRHYTHMIA: An arrhythmia originating from the junction of the atria and ventricles.

PREMATURE VENTRICULAR CONTRACTION (PVC): An abnormal heart rhythm caused by the ventricle initiating depolarization before it is expected.

SINUS ARRHYTHMIA: An arrhythmia with its origin in a dysfunction of the sinoatrial (SA) node.

SUPRAVENTRICULAR TACHYCARDIA (SVT): An arrhythmia that originates above the ventricle, either in the SA node, atria, or atrioventricular (AV) junction.

TACHYARRHYTHMIA: Arrhythmias with an overall rate of over 100 bpm.

TORSADE DE POINTES: A specific type of ventricular tachycardia characterized by rapid irregular QRS complexes. It may end spontaneously or degenerate into ventricular fibrillation. It causes significant blood flow compromise and often causes death.

VENTRICULAR FIBRILLATION: Causes uncoordinated quivering of the ventricle without any useful contractions. Immediate syncope occurs and death happens within minutes.

VENTRICULAR PREMATURE BEAT (VPB): A single impulse in the ventricle caused by reentry or abnormal automaticity of ventricular cells. VPBs are asymptomatic or can cause palpitations and usually require no intervention.

WOLFF-PARKINSON-WHITE (WPW) SYNDROME: The most common reentrant supraventricular tachycardia. When combined with atrial fibrillation, WPW is a medical emergency.

Arrhythmias can be treated by various drugs and are broken down into four classes of agents with one class (Class I) having three subtypes. In general, drugs are being used less to control arrhythmias, especially Class I and some II agents, due to adverse effects and toxicities. Further hastening this decreased use is the advent of implantable pacemakers which are more reliable and have fewer side effects (see figure 6.7).

FUNCTION

In general, antiarrhythmics modify action potential generation and conduction thus diminishing, eliminating, or reducing the potential for arrhythmias. Many types of arrhythmias exist and can be treated by these agents. These can be broken down into atrial arrhythmias, including flutters and fibrillations; supraventricular tachycardias, including AV nodal reentry; acute supraventricular tachycardia, and ventricular tachycardias; including acute ventricular tachycardia and ventricular fibrillation.

The cardiac glycosides are used in treating congestive heart failure, atrial fibrillation, atrial flutter, paroxysmal atrial **tachycardia**, and cardiogenic shock.

Class I drugs are being used less and less due to their potential to cause rather than assist arrhythmias. In contrast, Class II and III agents are being used more as this proarrhythmia tendency is much less and these drugs are better tolerated. However, none of these drugs have been investigated in large trials, and their overall potential to prolong life has not been well established. Class I drugs should not be used in patients with ischemic heart disease or reduced left ventricular function as the potential

Tachycardia: A rapid heart rate defined as over 100 bpm

Defibrillation: Reversal of ventricular fibrillation by applying an electric shock to the heart

Sinus rhythm: A heart rhythm initiated by the SA node; a normal rhythm

for causing arrhythmias is greatly increased in this patient population.

Class Ia drugs are useful in a wide variety of arrhythmias including atrial, AV-junctional, and ventricular arrhythmias. They can be used after **defibrillation** of atrial flutter or fibrillation to maintain **sinus rhythm**. These agents are also used to prevent ventricular tachycardia.

Since Class Ib agents do not slow conduction, they are not effective on artial or AV-junction arrhythmias. They are, however, useful for prevention of ventricular arrhythmias after a myocardial infarction.

Class Ic agents are only approved for treating refractory ventricular arrhythmias, especially premature ventricular contractions (PVCs); however, recent studies have seriously questioned the safety of these agents.

Class II drugs are useful in treating tachyarrhythmias caused by increased sympathetic activation. They are also useful in treating atrial flutter and fibrillation and AV nodal reentry tachycardia.

Class III drugs can be used in a wide variety of arrhythmias. Amiodarone is used to treat severe refractory supraventricular and ventricular tachyarrhythmias. Unfortunately, this drug can be quite toxic, which limits its clinical usefulness. In addition, studies have shown that it does not reduce the incidence of sudden death or increase long-term survival in congestive heart failure patients. Sotalol has been compared with several other agents

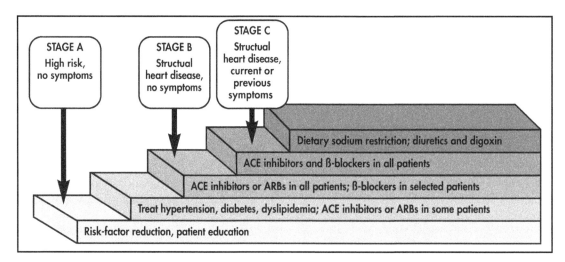

Figure 6.7: This figure shows the various stages of heart failure and the recommended treatment protocols for each stage.

(imipramine, mexiletine, procainamide, propafenone, and quinidine) and was more effective in preventing the recurrence of arrhythmias and extending life in patients with sustained ventricular tachycardia. It has strong antifibrillary effects that work especially well in ischemic heart muscle.

Class IV antiarrhythmics are more effective in treating atrial arrhythmias than ventricular arrhythmias and are used in reentrant supraventricular tachycardias and in reducing the ventricular rate in atrial flutter and fibrillation. In addition to their antiarrhythmic effects, these agents are used to treat hypertension and angina.

Digoxin is used to reduce ventricular response to atrial flutter and fibrillation.

Quinidine is used in treating malaria when other agents have failed.

MECHANISMS OF ACTION

Different classes of antiarrhythmia drugs act in different ways to modify the contraction and conduction process. They act on the action potential as conducted through Purkinje fibers. The normal action potential has five phases. Phase 0 is the fast upstroke where sodium "fast channels" open and cause a rapid depolarization. Phase 1 is the phase of partial repolarization where sodium channels close and potassium channels open. Phase 2 is where the voltage-sensitive calcium channels open and antagonize the already open potassium channels with little net change in voltage. Phase 3 is repolarization where the calcium channels are closed and potassium channels remain open. And finally there is Phase 4, forward current, where there is a slow depolarization due to sodium permeability. These phases of the action potential are graphically shown in Figure 6.8.

No matter the mechanism, all antiarrhythmic drugs have in common that they act on the action potential albeit in different phases. These are summarized in the table above.

In treating arrhythmias, cardiac gly-

Drug Class	Mechanism of Action	Action
IA	Sodium channel blocker	Slows Phase 0 depolarization
IB	Sodium channel blocker	Shortens Phase 3 repolarization
IC	Sodium channel blocker	Markedly slows Phase 0 depolarization
II	Beta-adrenoreceptor blocker	Suppresses Phase 4 depolarization
III	Potassium channel blocker	Prolongs Phase 3 repolarization
IV	Calcium channel blocker	Shortens action potential

cosides work by suppressing the atrioventricular node conduction, which increases the refractory period, allowing more cardiac muscle recovery between beats, a positive inotropic effect, enhanced parasympathetic activation, and a decreased heart rate.

Class I drugs act by blocking the sodium channels. They act on open or inactivated sodium channels; thus they have a propensity for frequently depolarizing cells and therefore work most effectively on the cells that need it the most.

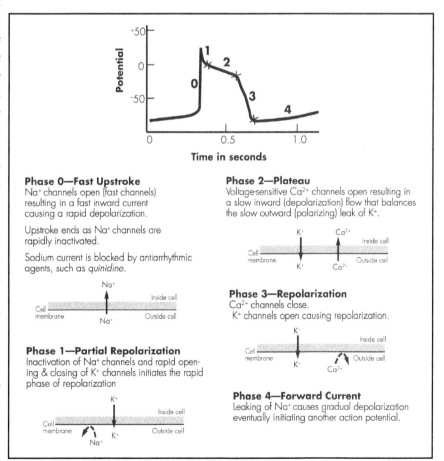

Phase 0—Fast Upstroke
Na⁺ channels open (fast channels) resulting in a fast inward current causing a rapid depolarization.

Upstroke ends as Na⁺ channels are rapidly inactivated.

Sodium current is blocked by antiarrhythmic agents, such as *quinidine*.

Phase 1—Partial Repolarization
Inactivation of Na⁺ channels and rapid opening & closing of K⁺ channels initiates the rapid phase of repolarization

Phase 2—Plateau
Voltage-sensitive Ca²⁺ channels open resulting in a slow inward (depolarization) flow that balances the slow outward (polarizing) leak of K⁺.

Phase 3—Repolarization
Ca²⁺ channels close.
K⁺ channels open causing repolarization.

Phase 4—Forward Current
Leaking of Na⁺ causes gradual depolarization eventually initiating another action potential.

Figure 6.8: A normal depolarization of a cardiac cell involves five phases.

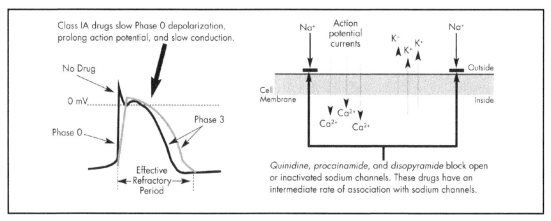

Figure 6.9: Class IA antiarrhythmic drugs act on Phase 0 and ultimately increase the refractory period for cardiac depolarization.

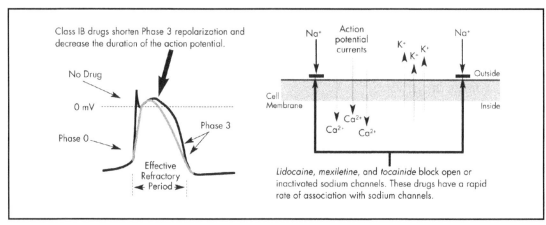

Figure 6.10: Class IB antiarrhythmic drugs act by shortening Phase 3 and shorten the whole action potential.

Class I drugs are further broken down into three subclasses.

CLASS IA agents slow the rate of Phase 0 depolarization and prolong the entire action potential, making the **refractory period** longer. They have an intermediate speed of binding and unbinding with sodium channels. Figure 6.9 shows these effects. In general, the use of class I agents have been declining due to their potential to cause arrhythmias especially in patients with ischemic heart disease and reduced left ventricular function.

CLASS IB drugs have little effect on depolarization and exert their primary effects by shortening the Phase 3 repolarization and hence shortening the overall action potential. They rapidly bind with sodium channels. These actions are shown in Figure 6.10.

CLASS IC agents act solely in Phase 0 depolar-

> **Refractory period:** Referring to the period after an event has occurred and before another can be initiated again

ization and markedly slow the rate of depolarization causing considerable conduction slowing without affecting the overall length of the action potential or refractory period. They slowly bind to sodium channels. Figure 6.11 illustrates this.

CLASS II drugs act on Phase 4 depolarization, reducing it and depressing automaticity, prolonging AV conduction, and decreasing contractility (negative inotrope) and heart rate. They are especially useful in treating rapid arrhythmias due to increased sympathetic activation, atrial flutter and fibrillation, and tachycardia due to AV node reentry. These agents are increasing in use. Sotalol is an interesting agent in that it is a beta-adrenergic blocker and thus belongs in Class II antiarrhythmics, but it also has Class III effects and thus is also included in that section.

CLASS III agents act by prolonging Phase 3 repolarization by blocking potassium channels. The

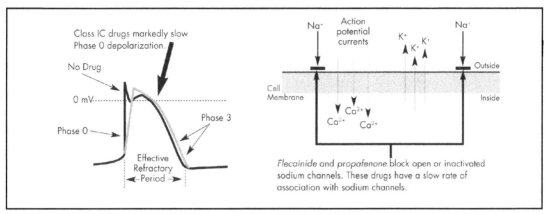

Figure 6.11: Class IC antiarrhythmic drugs act by slowing Phase 0 deplolarization, which slows conduction without changing the length of the action potential or refractory period.

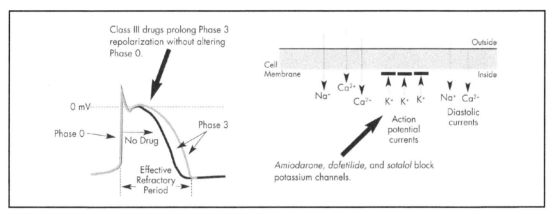

Figure 6.12: Class III antiarrhythmic drugs act by prolonging Phase 3 repolarization, which prolongs the action potential and beneficially increases the refractory period.

benefit of these drugs is that they prolong the duration of the action potential without affecting Phase 0 depolarization or the resting membrane potential. This is shown in Figure 6.12. Ultimately, their strength is in prolonging the effective refractory period. Unfortunately, these drugs do have the potential to induce an arrhythmia.

CLASS IV agents, calcium channel blockers, work by decreasing the rate of Phase 4 spontaneous depolarization. In addition, they slow conduction in other tissues dependent on calcium for their effects. An example of this is the AV node. Figure 6.13 on the next page shows the mechanism of action of Class IV agents.

While there are many tissues that are calcium channel dependent, calcium channel blockers primarily affect vascular smooth muscle and the heart.

DOSAGES

AMIODARONE, for *adults*, for ventricular arrhythmias, 800-1600 mg/d in 1-2 doses for 1-3 weeks; then when adequate arrhythmia control is achieved, decrease to 600-800 mg/d in 1-2 doses for 1 month; maintain at 400 mg/d; lower doses are recommended for supraventricular arrhythmias.

DIGOXIN, dose per table on the next page. Initial doses should be given one-half upon initiation; and one-quarter each in 2 doses at 8-12 hour intervals. An ECG should be obtained 6 hours after each dose to assess toxicity. Mainten-ance doses in *children* under 10 should be given in divided doses over 12 hours and once daily to those over 10 and to *adults*.

DISOPYRAMIDE, for *children*, under 1 year, 10-30 mg/kg/d in 4 divided doses;;1-4 years, 10-20

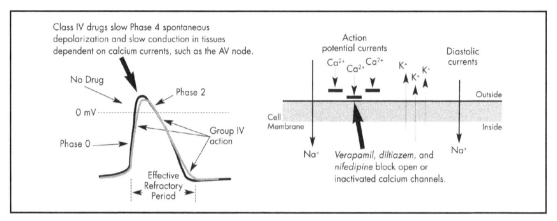

Figure 6.13: **Class IV** antiarrhythmic drugs act on Phase 4 and decrease the rate of spontaneous depolarization.

Age	Initial Doses	Maintenance Doses
Preterm infant	20-30 mcg/kg	5-7.5 mcg/kg
Full-term infant	25-35 mcg/kg	6-10 mcg/kg
1 month-2 years	35-60 mcg/kg	10-15 mcg/kg
2-5 years	30-40 mcg/kg	7.5-10 mcg/kg
5-10 years	20-35 mcg/kg	5-10 mcg/kg
>10 years	10-15 mcg/kg	2.5-5 mcg/kg
Adults	0.75-1.5 mg	0.125-.5 mg

mg/kg/d in 4 divided doses; 4-12 years, 10-15 mg/kg/d in 4 divided doses; 12-18 years, 6-15 mg/kg/d in 4 divided doses. For *adults*, <50 kg: 100 mg every 6 hours or 200 mg every 12 hours (controlled release); >50 kg: 150 mg every 6 hours or 300 mg every 12 hours (controlled release); may increase to 200 mg every 6 hours; maximum dose required for patients with severe refractory ventricular tachycardia is 400 mg every 6 hours.

DOFETILIDE, for *adults*, initiate at 500 mcg bid. Further dosing is dependent on ECG values.

DRONEDARONE, for *adults*, for atrial fibrillation/atrial flutter, 400 mg bid.

FLECAINIDE, for *children*, initiate at 3 mg/kg/d or 50-100 mg/m²/d in 3 divided doses; usual dose of 3-6 mg/kg/d or 100-150 mg/m²/d in 3 divided doses up to 11 mg/kg/d or 200 mg/m²/d. For *adults*, for life-threatening ventricular arrhythmias, initiate at 100 mg every 12 hours; increase by 50-100 mg/d (given in 2 doses/d) every 4 days up to a maximum of 400 mg/d; for prevention of paroxysmal supraventricular arrhythmias in patients with disabling symptoms but no structural heart disease, initiate at 50 mg every 12 hours; increase by 50 mg bid at

4-day intervals up to a maximum of 300 mg/d.

MEXILETINE, for *adults*, for arrhythmias, initiate at 200 mg every 8 hours; may load with 400 mg; can adjust every 2-3 days; usual dose is 200-300 mg every 8 hours up to a maximum of 1.2 g/d.

PROCAINAMIDE, for *children*, 15-50 mg/kg/d divided every 3-6 hours. For *adults*, 50 mg/kg/d; maximum dose of 5 g/d; immediate release formulation: 250-500 mg/dose every 3-6 hours; extended release formulation: 500 mg to 1 g every 6 hours.

PROPAFENONE, for *adults*, immediate release tablet, initiate at 150 mg every 8 hours; increase at 3- to 4-day intervals up to 300 mg every 8 hours; for extended release capsule, initiate at 225 mg every 12 hours; dosage increase may be made at a minimum of 5-day intervals; may increase to 325 mg every 12 hours; if further increase is necessary, may increase to 425 mg every 12 hours.

QUINIDINE, for *children*, test dose for idiosyncratic reaction: 2 mg/kg or 60 mg/m², quinidine sulfate: 15-60 mg/kg/d in 4-5 divided doses or 6 mg/kg every 4-6 hours; usual 30 mg/kg/d or 900 mg/m²/d given in 5 daily doses. For *adults*, test dose: 200 mg administered several hours before full dosage; sulfate: 100-600 mg/dose every 4-6 hours; initiate at 200 mg and increase to desired effect up to a daily maximum of 3-4 g; gluconate: 324-972 mg every 8-12 hours.

ADVERSE EFFECTS

Any antiarrhythmic agent can potentially exacerbate the arrhythmia.

Cardiac glycosides often cause anorexia, nausea, and vomiting. Other adverse effects include headache, fatigue, confusion, blurred vision, skin rashes, and visual disturbances.

Class IC drugs can cause dizziness, blurred vision, headache, and nausea. They can potentially cause life-threatening, treatment-resistant ventricular tachycardia.

Class II agents can cause arrhythmias if suddenly stopped, along with sexual impairment and metabolic disturbances such as reduced glycogenolysis and glucagon secretion, which can cause fasting hypoglycemia. Cold extremities, fatigue, insomnia, nightmares, and depression may also occur. Beta-blockers may increase the symptoms of peripheral vascular disease or cause Raynaud's phenomenon.

Class IV agents, calcium channel blockers, are contraindicated in patients with reduced cardiac function due to their negative inotropic effects. They may also reduce blood pressure due to peripheral vasodilation. While this is a beneficial effect in hypertensive patients, it can cause light-headedness, dizziness, and postural hypotension in some patients.

Amiodarone has a variety of toxic effects. Over half of patients taking it long term have adverse effects severe enough to discontinue use. These effects include interstitial pulmonary fibrosis, gastrointestinal intolerance, tremor, ataxia, dizziness, thyroid and liver problems, photosensitivity, muscle weakness, neuropathy, and iodine accumulation in the skin causing a blue discoloration.

Disopyramide and, to a lesser degree, quinidine have anticholinergic effects such as dry mouth, urinary retention, blurred vision, and constipation. Disopyramide should not be used in heart-failure patients. This agent and procainimide are usually used when other agents cannot be tolerated due to toxicity.

Procainimide, with chronic use, has a high potential for adverse effects, including the development of a reversible lupus **erythematous**-like syndrome in 25-30% of patients. Toxic concentrations can induce **asystole** or ventricular arrhythmias. CNS effects include depression, hallucination, and psychosis. There is greater GI tol-

erance for this drug than others in its class.

Quinidine may cause SA or AV node block or asystole, and at toxic levels it may induce ventricular tachycardia. These effects can be exacerbated by hyperkalemia. Other common side effects include nausea, vomiting, and diarrhea. Large doses may induce symptoms of **cinchonism**, blurred vision, **tinnitus**, head-ache, disorientation, and **psychosis**.

Sotalol has been shown to have the fewest acute or long-term adverse effects of any agents in this section. However, 3-4 % of patients, develop the syndrome of Torsade de Pointes.

▨ RED FLAGS

Digitalis toxicity is common with the cardiac glycosides and can be life threatening in the extreme. Initial symptoms include nausea and vomiting and progress to anorexia, diarrhea, abdominal discomfort, headache, weakness, drowsiness, visual disturbances, mental depression, confusion, restlessness, disorientation, seizures, and hallucinations. Cardiac abnormalities include ventricular tachycardia, **premature ventricular complexes**, excessive slowing of the pulse rate, atrioventricular blocks of varying degrees, ECG abnormalities, and occasional atrial fibrillation. Ventricular fibrillation is a common cause of death. Hypokalemia, hypercalcemia, and hypomagnesemia can all predispose one to digitalis toxicity. Hypothyroidism, hypoxia, renal failure, and myocarditis may also increase the possibility for toxicity.

Beta-blockers should not be discontinued abruptly as they can exacerbate angina pectoralis and increase the risk of sudden death. Since these agents can cause bronchoconstriction, they can be life threatening if given to patients with chronic obstructive pulmonary disease or asthma. They can also induce congestive heart failure in susceptible patients with impaired myocardial function such as compensated heart

Erythema: Redness or inflammation of the skin

Asystole: Non-contraction of the heart

Cinchonism: A condition characterized by deafness, headache, tinnitus, and cerebral congestion

Tinnitus: Ringing in the ears

Psychosis: A severe emotional and behavioral disorder that includes symptoms of gross distortion of mental capacity, inability to recognize reality, inability to relate to others, or perform ADLs

Premature ventricular complexes: An abnormal heart rhythm caused by the ventricle initiating depolarization before it is expected

Cardiomegaly: An enlarged heart

Glycogenolysis: Splitting of glycogen to release glucose

failure, acute myocardial infarction, and **cardiomegaly**. However, several studies have indicated that beta- blocker treatment is beneficial in mild to moderate cases of congestive heart failure. Beta-blockers can decrease **glycogenolysis** and glucagon secretion. This can cause insulin-dependent diabetics to have severe hypoglycemia after insulin injection. In addition, beta-blockers may increase the normal response to hypoglycemia. Because of these effects, while beta-blockers may still be used in insulin-dependent diabetics, caution and close monitoring is necessary. While bradycardia is a normal effect of these drugs, they can cause life-threatening bradyarrhythmias in patients with atrioventricular conduction defects and drugs that may reduce AV node conduction such as verapamil.

Dofetilide has a large potential for causing arrhythmias. Therefore it is only initiated in an inpatient setting, and only doctors who have received special manufacturer training may prescribe it.

INTERACTIONS

DRUG

Quinidine can displace digoxin from tissue-binding sites and decrease renal clearance, both of which increase the concentration of digoxin potentially to toxic levels. Patients taking phenytoin may need higher doses of quinidine.

Beta-blockers can induce life-threatening bradyarrhythmias in patients taking drugs that may reduce AV node conduction such as verapamil.

Amiodarone, erythromycin, quinidine, tetracycline, and verapamil may contribute to digitalis toxicity not only by displacing the glycosides from the protein binding sites but also by competing for renal excretion. Corticosteroids, thiazide, and loop diuretics can decrease blood levels of potassium and also increase the potential for toxicity.

HERB

AMIODARONE

- *Cao Wu* (Aconite, Kusnezoff monks' hood root), *Chuan Wu* (Sichuan aconite, mother root of common monks' hood), *Fu Zi* (Aconite, prepared daughter root of common monks' hood) (D)–may have positive inotropic and chronotropic effects; use with extreme caution in patients on antiarrhythmics (Chen, 1998/1999) Level 5 evidence.
- *Zhi Shi* (Aurantium) (D)–a rat study showed a significant increase in amiodarone peak plasma concentration when co-administered with *Zhi Shi.* (Rodrigues, Alves & Falcão, 2013). Level 5 evidence.

ANTIARRHYTHMICS

- *Cao Wu* (Aconite, Kusnezoff monks' hood root) (D)–may have positive inotropic and chronotropic effects and should be used with extreme caution in patients on antiarrhythmics (Chen, 1998/1999) Level 5 evidence.
- *Chuan Wu* (Sichuan aconite, mother root of common monks' hood) and *Fu Zi* (Aconite, prepared daughter root of common monks' hood) (D)–may have positive inotropic and chronotropic effects and should be used with extreme caution in patients on antiarrhythmics (Chen, 1998/1999) Level 5 evidence.
- *Fan Xie Ye* (Senna) (D)–may, with prolonged use, cause loss of potassium and potentiate arrhythmias when used with antiarrhythmic drugs, expert opinion, (Gruenwald, Brendler & Jaenicke, 2004) Level 5 evidence.
- *Gan Cao* (Licorice) (D)–may increase potassium loss and interfere with effects of antiarrhythmics (Kowalak & Mills, 2001) Level 5 evidence.
- *Lu Hui* (Aloe) (D)–misuse can lead to potassium loss and increased toxicity of antiarrhythmic drugs (Blumenthal, 1998) and cardiac glycosides (Blumenthal, 1998; Wichtl, 1995) Level 5 evidence.
- *Lu Hui* (Aloe) (D)–can cause potassium loss and increase effects of cardiac glycosides and antiarrhythmic drugs, expert opinion (Gruenwald, Brendler & Jaenicke, 2004) Level 5 evidence.
- *Shan Zha* (Hawthorn) (D)–has a similar effect to class III antiarrhythmics, expert opinion (Gruenwald, Brendler & Jaenicke, 2004) Level 5 evidence.

CARDIAC GLYCOSIDES

- *Da Huang* (Rhubarb root) (D)–prolonged use

may cause loss of potassium and increased cardiac glycoside toxicity, expert opinions (Chen & Chen, 2004) (Gruenwald, Brendler & Jaenicke, 2004) Level 5 evidence.

- *Fan Xie Ye* (Senna leaves) (D)–can cause excessive loss of potassium and increase cardiac glycoside toxicity, expert opinions (Chen & Chen, 2004) (Gruenwald, Brendler & Jaenicke, 2004) Level 5 evidence.
- *Gan Cao* (Licorice) (D)–may cause potassium loss and increase the toxicity of cardiac glycosides, expert opinions (Chen & Chen, 2004) Level 5 evidence.
- *Lu Hui* (Aloe) (D)–misuse can lead to potassium loss and increased toxicity of antiarrhythmic drugs and cardiac glycosides, expert opinions (Blumenthal, 1998); (Wichtl, 1995); (Chen & Chen, 2004) (Gruenwald, Brendler & Jaenicke, 2004) Level 5 evidence.
- *Ma Huang* (Ephedra) (D)–based on ephedrine content, may cause arrhythmias when used with cardiac glycosides, expert opinions (Brinker, 2001) (Chen & Chen, 2004) (Gruenwald, Brendler & Jaenicke, 2004) Level 5 evidence.
- *Shan Zha* (Hawthorn berry) (B-)–may potentiate the action of cardiac glycosides though the cited small human study (Tankanow, Tamer, Streetman, Smith, Welton, Annesley *et al.*, 2003) showed no significant interactions. Level 3b evidence.

DIGOXIN
- *Ci Wu Jia* (Acanthopanax root) (C)–caused increased serum levels of digoxin in a single patient. Unclear whether it was caused by interference, a false test result, or conversion of a component of ginseng into digoxin; however, the link was well established with multiple starts and stops of ginseng use and concomitant rise in digoxin levels (McRae, 1996) Level 4 evidence.
- *Ci Wu Jia* (Acanthopanax root) (D)–there have been reports of falsely raised digoxin levels on assay without actual elevation. However, further investigation showed that *Ci Wu Jia* may not actually be in the capsules but a common

substitute (Periploca sepium). This throws into doubt other studies that show a link between *Ci Wu Jia* and digoxin such as McRae, 1996. Expert opinion (Awang, 1996) Level 5 evidence.
- *Da Huang* (Rhubarb root) (D)–prolonged use may cause loss of potassium and increased cardiac glycoside toxicity, expert opinions (Chen & Chen, 2004) (Gruenwald, Brendler & Jaenicke, 2004) Level 5 evidence.
- *Dan Shen* (Salvia root) (D)–has been shown to have digoxin-like immunoreactivity and may interfere with serum assays of digoxin. Digoxin should be monitored with free digoxin concentration assays when taking *Dan Shen* (Wahed & Dasgupta, 2001) Level 5 evidence.
- *Fan Xie Ye* (Senna leaves) (D)–can cause excessive loss of potassium and increase cardiac glycoside toxicity, expert opinion (Chen & Chen, 2004); (Gruenwald, Brendler & Jaenicke, 2004) Level 5 evidence.
- *Gan Cao* (Licorice) (D)–may cause potassium loss and increase the toxicity of cardiac glycosides, expert opinion (Chen & Chen, 2004) Level 5 evidence.
- *Gan Cao* (Licorice) (D)–*Gan Cao, Ren Shen,* and *Shan Zha,* may interfere with digoxin either pharmacodynamically or with digoxin monitoring, expert opinions, (Miller, 1998) Level 5 evidence.
- *Gan Cao* (Licorice) (C)–a case was reported of congestive heart failure and hypokalemia in a patient taking *Gan Cao,* furosemide, and digoxin (Harada, Ohtaki, Misu, Sumiyoshi & Hosoda, 2002) Level 4 evidence.
- *Guan Ye Lian Qiao* (St. John's wort) (B/C)–was found to distort distribution of digoxin showing a significant ineterference with time in a small single-blind, placebo-controlled parallel study. Concommitant use should be avoided (Johne, Brockmöller, Bauer, Maurer, Lang-heinrich & Roots, 1999) Level 2b evidence.
- *Guan Ye Lian Qiao* (St. John's wort, hypericum) (D)–may induce the cytochrome P450 system and increase metabolism and reduce

plasma concentration of several drugs including digoxin, cyclosporine, theophylline, and phenprocoumon, expert opinion (Fugh-Berman, 2000) Level 5 evidence.

- *Guan Ye Lian Qiao* (St. John's Wort) (C)–decreases blood concentrations of digoxin (Zhou, Chan, Pan *et al.,* 2004) Level 3b evidence; (Izzo & Ernst 2009) Level 3a evidence.
- *Lu Hui* (Aloe) (D)–misuse can lead to potassium loss and increased toxicity of antiarrhythmic drugs (Blumenthal, 1998) and cardiac glycosides, expert opinions (Blumenthal, 1998); (Wichtl, 1995); (Chen & Chen, 2004); (Gruenwald, Brendler & Jaenicke, 2004) Level 5 evidence.
- *Ma Huang* (Ephedra) (D)–based on ephedrine content, may cause arrhythmias when used with cardiac glycosides, expert opinions (Brinker, 2001); (Chen & Chen, 2004); (Gruenwald, Brendler & Jaenicke, 2004) Level 5 evidence.
- *Ren Shen* (Ginseng) (D)–*Gan Cao, Ren Shen,* and *Shan Zha* may interfere with digoxin either pharmacodynamically or with digoxin monitoring, expert opinion (Miller, 1998) Level 5 evidence.
- *Ren Shen* (Siberian ginseng) (C)–*Ren shen* increased the serum concentration of digoxin in a single case study (Hu, Yang, Ho, Chan *et al.,* 2005) Level 2b evidence.
- *Shan Zha* (Hawthorn berry) An in vitro study demonstrated that *Shan Zha* interfered with one assay of digoxin levels (Digoxin III) but not another (Tina-Quant); (Dasgupta, Kidd, Poindexter & Bick 2010) Level 5 evidence.
- *Shan Zha* (Hawthorn berry) (B-)–may potentiate the action of cardiac glycosides though the cited small human study (Tankanow, Tamer, Streetman, Smith, Welton, Annesley *et al.,* 2003) showed no significant interactions (Gruenwald, Brendler & Jaenicke, 2004) Level 3b evidence.
- *Shan Zha* (Hawthorn berry) (D)–has a strong cardiotonic effect; use with caution with digoxin to avoid possible side effects, expert opinion (Miller, 1998) level 5 evidence.

DISOPYRAMIDE

- *Cao Wu* (Aconite, Kusnezoff monks' hood root), *Chuan Wu* (Sichuan aconite, mother root of common monks' hood), *Fu Zi* (Aconite, prepared daughter root of common monks' hood) (D)–may have positive inotropic and chronotropic effects and should be used with extreme caution in patients on antiarrhythmics (Chen, 1998/1999) Level 5 evidence.

FLECAINIDE

- *Cao Wu* (Aconite, Kusnezoff monks' hood root), *Chuan Wu* (Sichuan Aconite, mother root of common monks' hood), *Fu Zi* (Aconite, prepared daughter root of common monks' hood) (D)–may have positive inotropic and chronotropic effects and should be used with extreme caution in patients on antiarrhythmics (Chen, 1998/1999) Level 5 evidence.

PROCAINAMIDE

- *Cao Wu* (Aconite, Kusnezoff monks' hood root), *Chuan Wu* (Sichuan aconite, mother root of common monks' hood), *Fu Zi* (Aconite, prepared daughter root of common monks' hood) (D)–may have positive inotropic and chronotropic effects and should be used with extreme caution in patients on antiarrhythmics (Chen, 1998/1999) Level 5 evidence.
- *Gan Cao* (Licorice) (D)–may increase potassium loss and interfere with effects of antiarrhythmics (Kowalak & Mills, 2001) Level 5 evidence.

PROPAFENONE

- *Cao Wu* (Aconite, Kusnezoff monks' hood root), *Chuan Wu* (Sichuan aconite, mother root of common monks' hood), *Fu Zi* (Aconite, prepared daughter root of common monks' hood) (D)–may have positive inotropic and chronotropic effects and should be used with extreme caution in patients on antiarrhythmics (Chen, 1998/1999) Level 5 evidence.

QUINIDINE

- *Cao Wu* (Aconite, Kusnezoff monks' hood root), *Chuan Wu* (Sichuan aconite, mother root of common monks' hood), *Fu Zi* (Aconite, prepared daughter root of common monks' hood) (D)–may have positive inotropic and chronotropic effects and should be used with extreme caution in patients on antiarrhythmics (Chen, 1998/1999) Level 5 evidence.

- *Gan Cao* (Licorice) (D)–may increase potassium loss and interfere with the effects of antiarrhythmics (Kowalak & Mills, 2001) Level 5 evidence.

INTERACTION ISSUES

A:

D: Amiodarone is 96% protein bound; dronedarone is over 98% bound; propafenone is 95% bound.

M: Amiodarone is a major substrate of CYP2C8 and 3A4 and a moderate inhibitor of 2A6, 2C9, 2D6, and 3A4; disopyramide is a major substrate of CYP3A4; dronedarone is a major substrate of CYP3A4 and a moderate inhibitor of 2D6 and 3A4; flecainide is a major substrate of CYP2D6; procainamide and propafenone are major substrates of CYP2D6; quinidine is a major substrate of CYP3A4 and a strong inhibitor of 2D6.

E:

Pgp: Amiodarone and quinidine are substrates and inhibitors of Pgp; dronedarone is an inhibitor of Pgp.

SECTION 6: CALCIUM CHANNEL BLOCKERS

BENZOTHIAPENES:

DILTIAZEM (dil TYE a zem) PR=C *(Cardizem®, Cardizem® CD, Cardizem® LA, Cartia XT®, Dilacor® XR, Dilt-CD, Dilt-XR®, Diltia XT®, Diltzac, Matzim® LA, Taztia XT®, Tiazac®)*

DIHYDROPYRIDINES:

AMLODIPINE (am LOE di pene) PR=C *(Amturnide™, Azor™,[26] Caduet®,[21] Exforge®,[35] Exforge HCT®,[36] Lotrel®,[2] Norvasc®, Tarka®,[4] Tekamlo™,[38] Tribenzor™,[30] Twynsta®[31])*

FELODIPINE (fe LOE di pene) PR=C

ISRADIPINE (iz RA di pene) PR=C

NICARDIPINE (nye KAR de pene) PR=C *(Cardene® I.V., Cardene® SR)*

NIFEDIPINE (nye FED i peen) PR=C *(Adalat® CC, Afeditab® CR, Nifediac® CC, Nifedical® XL, Procardia®, Procardia® XL)*

NIMODIPINE (nye MOE di pene) PR=C

NISOLDIPINE (NYE sole di pene) PR=C *(Sular®)*

DIPHENYLALKYLAMINES:

VERAPAMIL (ver AP a mil) *(Calan®, Calan® SR, Isoptin® SR, Tarka®,[4] Verelan®, Verelan® PM)*

▨ FUNCTION

Calcium channel blockers are used primarily as second line antihypertensives when preferred agents are ineffective or contraindicated. They are especially useful in patients with asthma, diabetes, angina, or peripheral vascular disease. Some calcium channel blockers are very useful in treating arrhythmias and others in treating Raynaud's disease.

The diphenylalkylamines are also used to treat angina, supraventricular tachyarrhythmias, and migraines.

Benzothiazepines have a favorable adverse effect profile and are less negatively inotropic than verapamil.

Amlodipine and nicardipine have minimal interactions with other cardiovascular drugs such as digoxin and warfarin, and are therefore advantageous in patients on multiple drugs.

▨ MECHANISMS OF ACTION

Calcium channel blockers, independent of their chemical class, work by blocking voltage-gated calcium channels that allow the influx of calcium ions and trigger contractions in the smooth muscles of the heart and peripheral vasculature. This causes relaxation of the muscles, negative inotropic effects, and reduced peripheral resistance. The different chemical classes differ in how they block the channels, their antiarrhythmic effects, and their affinity for the myocardium and peripheral vasculature. Figure 6.14 shows these actions.

▣ DOSAGES

AMLODIPINE, for *children* 6-17 years, for hypertension, 2.5-5 mg once daily. For *adults*, for hypertension, initiate at 5 mg once daily; increase in 2.5 mg increments over 7-14 days up to a usual dosage range of 2.5-10 mg once daily; for angina, usual dose is 5-10 mg. In the *elderly*, dosing should start at the lower end of dosing range due to possible increased incidence of hepatic, renal, or cardiac impairment; for hypertension, 2.5 mg once daily; for angina, 5 mg once daily.

DILTIAZEM, for *adults*, for angina, capsule, extended release (Cardizem® CD, Cartia XT™, Dilacor® XR, Diltia XT®, Tiazac®): initiate at 120-180 mg once daily (maximum dose: 480 mg/d); tablet, extended release (Cardizem® LA): 180 mg once daily; may increase at 7-14 day intervals (maximum recommended dose: 360 mg/d); tablet, immediate release (Cardizem®): usual starting dose is 30 mg qid; usual range is between 180-360 mg/d; for hypertension, capsule, extended release (Cardizem® CD, Cartia XT™, Dilacor® XR, Diltia XT®, Tiazac®): initiate at 180-240 mg once daily; dose adjustment may be made after 14 days; usual dose range is 180-420 mg/d; Tiazac®: usual dose range is 120-540 mg/d; capsule, sustained release (Cardizem® SR): initiate at 60-120 mg bid; dose adjustment may be made after 14 days to a usual range of 240-360 mg/d; tablet, extended release (Cardizem® LA): initiate at 180-240 mg once daily; dose adjustment may be made after 14 days to a usual dose range of 120-540 mg/d.

FELODIPINE, for *adults*, initiate at 5 mg, increase by 5 mg at 2-week intervals as needed up to a usual dose of 2.5-10 mg once daily; usual dose range for hypertension is 2.5-20 mg once daily. For the *elderly*, begin with 2.5 mg/d.

ISRADIPINE, for *adults*, 2.5 mg bid; increase dose at 2- to 4-week intervals in 2.5-5 mg increments; usual dose range is 1.25-5 mg bid.

NICARDIPINE, for *adults*, immediate release, initiate at 20 mg tid up to a usual dose of 20-40 mg tid (allow 3 days between dose increases); sustained release, initiate at 30 mg bid; increase to 60 mg bid.

NIFEDIPINE, for *children*, for hypertrophic cardiomyopathy, 0.6-0.9 mg/kg/d in 3-4 divided doses. For *adolescents* and *adults*, initiate at 30 mg once daily as sustained release formulation, or if indicated, 10 mg tid as capsules; usual dose is 10-30 mg tid as capsules or 30-60 mg once daily as sustained release; maximum dose ranges from 120-180 mg/d; increase sustained release at 7-14 day intervals.

NIMODIPINE, for *adults*, for subarachnoid hemorrhage 60 mg every 4 hours for 21 days; start therapy within 96 hours after hemorrhage.

NISOLDIPINE, for *adults*, initiate at 20 mg once daily, then increase by 10 mg/wk (or longer intervals); usual dose range is 10-40 mg once daily; doses over 60 mg once daily are not rec-

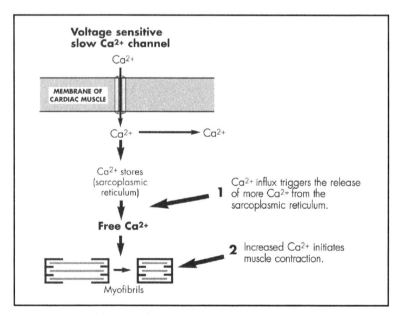

Figure 6.14: Normal function of calcium on myocardial and peripheral vasculature muscle cells. 1: An influx of calcium causes calcium release from the sarcoplasmic reticulum. 2: Muscle contraction is initiated by this extra calcium. All calcium channel blockers act by reducing the amount of intracellular calcium, which in turn makes for a weaker muscular contraction.

ommended. For the *elderly*, a starting dose not exceeding 10 mg/d is recommended.

VERAPAMIL, for *children*, 1-5 years, 4-8 mg/kg/d in 3 divided doses or 40-80 mg every 8 hours; >5 years: 80 mg every 6-8 hours. For *adults*, for angina, initiate at 80-120 mg tid up to a usual range of 240-480 mg/d in 3-4 divided doses; for hypertension, immediate release: 80 mg tid; usual dose range is 40-160 mg bid; sustained release: 240 mg/d; usual dose range is 120-360 mg/d in 1-2 divided doses; extended release: Verelan® PM: usual dose range of 200-400 mg nocte. For the *elderly*, for angina, 40 mg tid; for hypertension, 120 mg/d.

ADVERSE EFFECTS

Common adverse effects of calcium channel blockers include hypotension, fatigue, vertigo, constipation, and headache. Less common adverse effects include peripheral edema, coughing, wheezing, and pulmonary edema.

Nimodipine in large doses may produce muscle cramps.

RED FLAGS

These drugs, especially verapamil, should not be used in congestive heart failure patients due to their negative inotropic effects.

High doses of short-acting calcium channel blockers should be avoided as they may cause an increased risk of myocardial infarction.

INTERACTIONS

HERB

CALCIUM CHANNEL BLOCKERS

• *Gan Cao* (Licorice) (D)–theoretically may reduce the effects of antihypertensive agents such as alpha-1-adrenergic blockers, ACEI, A$_2$ receptor antagonists, beta-adrenergic blockers, calcium channel blockers, clonidine, guanabenz, guanfacine, hydralazine, methyldopa, minoxidil, and reserpine. Undertake concurrent use with caution, expert opinion (Kowalak & Mills, 2001). Level 5 evidence.

• *Qing Hao* (Artemesia, sweet wormwood herb)

(D)–a metabolite of *Qing Hao* may interfere with effectiveness of verapamil specifically, calcium channel blockers in general, and bufuralol and azole antifungals due to activation of CYP2D6 and competitive inhibition at CYP3A4 and possibly CYP3A5 (Grace, Skanchy & Aguilar, 1999) Level 5 evidence.

ISRADIPINE

• *Hong Qu* (Red yeast rice) (D)–due to increased hepatic blood flow, isradipine may increase clearance of *Hong Qu* constituents such as lovastatin and its metabolites, expert opinion (Chen & Chen, 2004) Level 5 evidence.

NICARDIPINE

• *Yin Guo Ye* (Ginkgo leaf) (D)–reduced the hypotensive effect of nicardipine in rats, possibly due to cytochrome P450 3A2 induction (Shinozuka, Umegaki, Kubota, Tanaka, Mizuno, Yamauchi *et al.*, 2002) Level 5 evidence.

NIFEDIPINE

• *Bai Zhi* (D)–has an inhibitory effect on cytochrome P450 in rats, which can lead to increased plasma concentration of testosterone, diazepam, tolbutamide, nifedipine, bufuralol, and potentially other drugs (Ishihara, Kushida, Yuzurihara, Wakui, Yanagisawa *et al.*, 2000) Level 5 evidence.

• *Guan Ye Lian Qiao* (St. John's wort) (C)–decreases blood concentrations (Izzo & Ernst, 2009) Level 2b evidence.

• *Yin Guo Ye* (Gingko leaf) (D)–may increase nifedipine's mean plasma concentration, expert opinion (Gruenwald, Brendler & Jaenicke, 2004) Level 5 evidence.

VERAPAMIL

• *Gan Cao* (Licorice) (D)– licorice decreased verapamil blood concentrations in rabbits when coadministered (Al-Deeb, Arafat & Irshaid, 2010) Level 5 evidence.

• *Guan Ye Lian Qiao* (St. John's wort) (C)–decreases blood concentrations (Izzo & Ernst, 2009) Level 2b evidence.

• *Qing Hao* (Artemesia, sweet wormwood herb) (D)–a metabolite of *Qing Hao* may interfere with the effectiveness of verapamil specifically, calcium channel blockers in general, as well as bufuralol, and azole antifungals due to activation of CYP2D6 and competitive inhibition at CYP3A4 and possibly CYP3A5 (Grace, Skanchy & Aguilar, 1999) Level 5 evidence.

INTERACTION ISSUES

A:

D: Amlodipine is 93-98% protein bound; felodipine is over 99% bound; isradipine is 95% bound; nicardipine is greater than 95% bound; nifedipine is 92-98% bound; nimodipine is greater than 95% bound; nisoldipine is greater than 99% bound.

M: Amlodipine is a major substrate of CYP3A4 and a moderate inhibitor of 1A2; diltiazem is a major substrate and a moderate inhibitor of CYP3A4; felodipine is a major substrate of CYP3A4 and a moderate inhibitor of 2C8; isradipine is a major substrate of CYP3A4; nicardipine is a major substrate of CYP3A4, moderate inhibitor of 2C19 and 2D6, and a strong inhibitor of 2C9 and 3A4; nifedipine is a major substrate of CYP3A4 and a moderate inhibitor of 1A2; nimodipine and nisoldipine are major substrates of CYP3A4; verapamil is a major substrate and a moderate inhibitor of CYP3A4.

E:

Pgp: Diltiazem and nicardipine are substrates of Pgp; verapamil is a substrate and an inhibitor of Pgp.

SECTION 7: OTHER ANTIHYPERTENSIVES

RESERPINE (re-SER-pene) PR=C

ENDOTHELIN RECEPTOR ANTAGONISTS (ETRAs):

AMBRISENTAN (am-bri-SEN-tan) PR=X (Letairis®)

BOSENTAN (boe-SEN-tan) PR=X (Tracleer®)

FUNCTION

Reserpine is used to treat schizophrenia in addition to hypertension.

Ambrisentan is an approved "orphan" drug to treat pulmonary arterial hypertension. The orphan drug act was designed to speed approval of drugs for rare diseases. Bosentan is also used for pulmonary arterial hypertension.

MECHANISMS OF ACTION

Reserpine acts by depleting stores of catecholamines and 5-HT in the presynaptic neuron. This causes less of these neurotransmitters to be released. Less catecholamine release is thought to reduce sympathetic action and decrease the heart rate and arterial blood pressure. This, with reduction of 5-HT in the brain, is thought to be the cause of this agent's sedative and tranquilizing effects and usefulness in treating schizophrenia.

Endothelin receptor antagonists (ETRAs) act by blocking endothelin receptors. Normally, endothelin is a potent vasoconstrictor. Physiologically, there are two main types of endothelin receptors: ETA and ETB, located in the endothelium and vascular smooth muscle. ETA causes vasoconstriction, while ETB is counter-regulatory and causes vasodilation. Blocking endothelin receptors ultimately causes vasodilation and reduction of hypertension. Bosentan, a first-generation ETRA, binds both types of receptors. In contrast, ambrisentan, the first second-generation ETRA, preferably binds ETA.

DOSAGES

AMBRISENTAN is available in 5.0 mg and 10 mg once-daily tablets.

BOSENTAN initiate at 62.5 mg bid for 4 weeks and then increase to maintenance dose of 125 mg bid.

RESERPINE, for *children*, not recommended, but if used, initiate at 20 mcg/kg up to a maximum of .25 mg daily. For *adults*, for hypertension, initiate at .5 mg daily for 1-2 weeks; maintenaince dose is .1-.25 mg daily; for psychiatric disorders, initiate at .5 mg daily; usual dose range is .1-1.0 mg daily.

ADVERSE EFFECTS

Ambrisentan's most common side effects include swelling of legs and ankles, nasal congestion, sinusitis, and facial flushing.

Bosentan can cause the same adverse effects as ambrisentan as well as headache, hypotension, palpitations, dyspepsia, fatigue, and pruritis. Dose-related decreases can occur to hemoglobin and hematocrit, and these lab tests should be monitored.

Reserpine can cause GI disturbances, arrhythmias, syncope, weight gain, decreased libido, gynecomastia, and rarely, parkinsonian syndrome and other extrapyramidal signs and symptoms.

RED FLAGS

Bosentan has an FDA box warning noting two serious concerns. The first is that it can cause serious liver injury, and liver enzymes should be closely monitored. In addition, it has been determined that it is very likely to produce major birth defects if used by pregnant women, and hence its use is prohibited in pregnant women.

INTERACTIONS

Reserpine is teratogenic in mice and therefore not recommended for use in pregnant women. In addition, it is present in breast milk, and lactating mothers should not use it.

DRUG

Bosentan is metabolized by CYP2C9 and CYP3A4. Therefore CYP2C9 inhibitors such as fluconazole or amiodarone and CYP3A4 inhibitors such as ketoconazole, itraconazole, or ritonavir should be avoided. Warfarin and HMG-CoA reductase inhibitors (simvastatin, lovastatin, and atorvastatin) show increased blood levels due to CYP interference. Increased blood levels of cyclosporin A, OCPs, and tacrolimus can be caused by co-administration.

MAOIs, tricyclic antidepressants, and sympathomimetics should be used with caution with reserpine. Cardiac arrhythmias have occurred when combined with digitalis and quinidine.

HERB

RESERPINE
• *Gan Cao* (Licorice) (D)–theoretically may reduce the effects of antihypertensive agents such as alpha-1-adrenergic blockers, ACEI, A_2 receptor antagonists, beta-adrenergic blockers, calcium channel blockers, clonidine, guanabenz, guanfacine, hydralazine, methyldopa, minoxidil, and reserpine. Undertake concurrent use with caution, expert opinion (Kowalak & Mills, 2001). Level 5 evidence.

INTERACTION ISSUES

A:

D: Amrisentan is 99% protein bound; bosentan is over 98% bound; reserpine is 96% protein bound.

M: Bosentan is a major substrate and a strong inducer of CYP2C9 and 3A4.

E:

Pgp: Ambrisentan is a substrate of Pgp; reserpine inhibits Pgp

SECTION 8: PLATELET INHIBITORS

ASPIRIN, ALSO KNOWN AS ACETYLSALICYLIC ACID (ASA) PR=C/D in 3rd trimester of pregnancy
(Aggrenox®,[19] Anacin® Advanced Headache Formula[44] [O], Ascomp® with Codeine,[28]

Ascriptin® Maximum Strength [O], Ascriptin® Regular Strength [O], Aspercin [O], Aspergum® [O], Aspir-low [O], Aspirtab [O], Bayer® Aspirin Extra Strength [O], Bayer® Aspirin Regimen Adult Low Strength [O],

Continues on next page

SECTION 8: PLATELET INHIBITORS cont.

Bayer® Aspirin Regimen Children's [O], Bayer® Aspirin Regimen Regular Strength [O], Bayer® Genuine Aspirin [O], Bayer® Plus Extra Strength [O], Bayer® PM[43] [O], Bayer® Women's Low Dose Aspirin [O], Buffasal [O], Bufferin® [O], Bufferin® Extra Strength [O], Buffinol [O], Ecotrin® Arthritis Strength [O], Ecotrin® Low Strength [O], Ecotrin® [O], Endodan®,[29] Excedrin® Extra Strength[44] [O], Excedrin® Migraine[44] [O], Fem-Prin®[44] [O], Fiorinal®,[27] Fiorinal® with Codeine,[28] Goody's® Extra Strength Headache Powder[44] [O], Goody's® Extra Strength Pain Relief[44] [O], Halfprin® [O], Pain-Off[44] [O], Percodan®,[29] St Joseph® Adult Aspirin [O], Synalgos®-DC,[45] Tri-Buffered Aspirin [O],

Vanquish® Extra Strength Pain Reliever[44] [O])

CLOPIDOGREL (kloh PID oh grel) PR=B *(Plavix®)*

DIPYRIDAMOLE *(See Section 4 in this chapter)*

PRASUGREL (PRA sue grel) PR=B *(Effient®)*

SALSALATE (SAL sa late) PR=C *(Amigesic®, Salflex®)*

TICAGRELOR (tie KA grel or) PR=C *(Brilinta™)*

TICLOPIDINE (tye KLOE pi dene) PR=B

PHOSPHODIESTERASE ENZYME INHIBITORS:

CILOSTAZOl (sil OH sta zol) PR=C *(Pletal®)*

FUNCTION

These drugs are useful in treating and preventing cardiovascular occlusive diseases, maintaining vascular grafts, keeping arteries patent, and as adjunctive treatment to thrombin inhibitors and thrombolytic therapy in myocardial infarction. Many of these agents are also used to treat pain.

Aspirin is also used in preventing transient cerebral ischemia, recurrent myocardial infarcts, and to decrease mortality in pre- and post-myocardial infarction patients.

MECHANISMS OF ACTION

When healthy, intact endothelial cells are damaged, a cascade of chemicals result that activate platelets to release more chemicals and adhere to one another forming a platelet plug to help seal the break in the endothelial cells. Agents in this category act by preventing this platelet aggregation.

Aspirin and salsalate work by inactivating the platelet enzyme cyclooxygenase 1 (COX-1), which prevents the transformation of arachidonic acid to prostaglandin H_2, ultimately inhibiting the aggregation of platelets. These effects are shown in Figure 6.15. Even though this drug irreversibly inactivates COX-1, platelets have a life

span of approximately 7-10 days. Aspirin also appears to act on the hypothalamus heat-regulating center in order to reduce fever.

Ticlopidine and clopidogrel work by preventing adenosine diphosphate (ADP) from binding to platelets and activating glycoprotein (GP) IIb/IIIa receptors necessary for allowing platelets to bind to fibrinogen, which is needed for platelet aggregation. Figure 6.16 shows normal platelet aggregation, while Figure 6.17 shows how it is affected by these agents.

The particular phosphodiesterase inhibited (type III) directly inhibits platelet aggregation. In

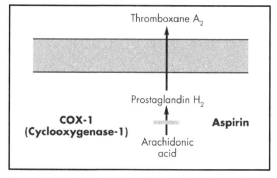

Figure 6.15: Aspirin inhibits COX-1-mediated transformation of arachidonic acid to prostaglandin H_2, which causes platelet aggregation inhibition.

addition, this agent also causes vasodilation due to increased cAMP.

Cilostazol works by inhibiting phosphodiesterase, which normally breaks down cAMP. Increased intracellular cAMP ultimately allows for increased calcium flow from the exterior to the interior of the cell by activating a calcium channel. Beta-adrenergic agonists (see Chapter 4, Section 4), also have positive inotropic effects and work in the same cascade as the phosphodiesterase inhibitors except that they increase cAMP by activating beta-adrenergic receptors. See Figure 6.18 for a summary of these actions.

DOSAGES

ASPIRIN, for *children*, for analgesia and as an antipyretic, 10-15 mg/kg/dose every 4-6 hours up to a total of 4 g/d; as an anti-inflammatory, initiate at 60-90 mg/kg/d in divided doses; usual dose of 80-100 mg/kg/d divided every 6-8 hours; it is necessary to monitor serum levels; for antiplatelet effects, suggested doses have ranged from 3-5 mg/kg/d to 5-10 mg/kg/d given as a single daily dose; for mechanical prosthetic heart valves, 6-20 mg/kg/d given as a single daily dose; as an antirheumatic, 60-100 mg/kg/d in divided doses every 4 hours. For *adults*, for analgesia and as an antipyretic, 325-650 mg every 4-6 hours up to 4 g/d; as an anti-inflammatory, initiate at 2.4-3.6 g/d in divided doses and maintain at 3.6-5.4 g/d; it is necessary to monitor serum concentrations; for myocardial infarction prophylaxis, 75-325 mg/d, may be reduced in patients receiving ACE inhibitors; for acute myocardial infarction, 160-325 mg/d; for coronary artery bypass graft (CABG), 75-325 mg/d starting 6 hours following procedure; if bleeding prevents administration at 6 hours after CABG, initiate as soon as possible; for percutaneous transluminal coronary angioplasty (PTCA), initiate at 80-325 mg/d starting 2 hours before procedure; for stent implantation, 325 mg 2 hours

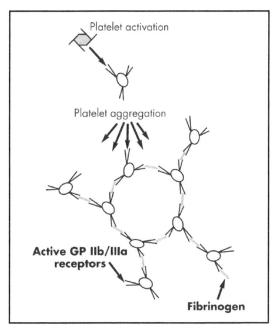

Figure 6.16: Normal platelet aggregation is facilitated by fibrinogen and active GP IIb/IIIa receptors.

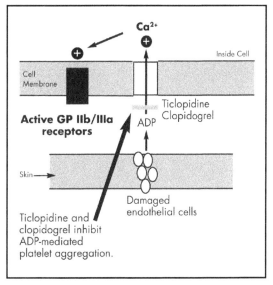

Figure 6.17: Inhibition of GP IIb/IIIa receptors by ticlopidine or clopidogrel induced inhibition of ADP binding. This ultimately results in reduced platelet aggregation.

prior to implantation and 160-325 mg daily thereafter; for carotid endarterectomy, 81-325 mg/d preoperatively and daily thereafter; for acute stroke, 160-325 mg/d, initiated within 48 hours (in patients who are not candidates for thrombolytics and are not receiving systemic

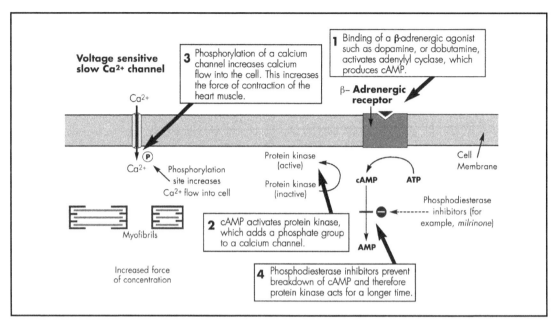

Figure 6.18 Function of cAMP on myocardial function. 1: Adenylyl cyclase is activated by a β-adrenergic agonist and converts intercellular ATP to cAMP. 2: cAMP activates a protein kinase, which activates a calcium channel. 3: Calcium channel activation causes more influx of calcium and increased myocardial contraction. 4: cAMP is normally broken down by phosphodiesterase; inhibiting this enzyme causes more cAMP to remain active and more activation of this whole cascade.

anticoagulation); for stroke prevention/transient ischemic attacks (TIA), 30-325 mg/d.

CILOSTAZOL, for *adults*, 100 mg bid taken at least one-half hour before or 2 hours after breakfast and dinner.

CLOPIDOGREL, for recent MI, stroke, or established arterial disease, 75 mg once daily; for acute coronary syndrome, initiate at 300 mg followed by 75 mg once daily (in combination with aspirin 75-325 mg once daily).

PRASUGREL, for *adults*, for acute coronary syndrome (ACS), for percutaneous coronary intervention (PCI) for ACS, load at 60 mg administered promptly and no later than 1 hour after PCI; maintain at 10 mg once daily with aspirin. Use not recommended in patients 75 or older, who may be considered in high-risk situations.

SALSALATE, 3 g/d in 2-3 divided doses.

TICAGRELOR, for *adults*, for acute coronary syndrome (ACS), for unstable angina, non-ST-segment elevation myocardial infarction (NSTEMI), ST-segment elevation myocardial infarction (STEMI), initiate with a 180 mg loading dose; maintain at 90

mg bid starting 12 hours after loading dose.

TICLOPIDINE, for stroke prevention, 250 mg bid with food; for coronary artery stenting, 250 mg bid with food (in combination with antiplatelet doses of aspirin) for up to 30 days.

ADVERSE EFFECTS

Many of aspirin's adverse effects are based on the fact that it prolongs bleeding time and include hemorrhagic stroke and gastrointestinal bleeding. These effects are more pronounced at higher dosages.

Both clopidogrel and ticlopidine can cause thrombocytopenic purpura.

Cilostazol can cause headaches, abnormal stools, diarrhea, rhinitis, infection, peripheral edema, palpitations, tachycardia, dizziness, and GI disturbances.

RED FLAGS

Ticlopidine can cause neutropenia, and frequent blood monitoring is necessary. While clopidogrel can cause neutropenia, it is much rarer than with ticlopidine.

INTERACTIONS

DRUG

Both clopidogrel and ticlopidine can inhibit cytochrome P450 and may interfere with the metabolism of phenytoin, tolbutamide, warfarin, fluvastatin, and tamoxifen.

New evidence shows that combining aspirin and ibuprofen counteracts the heart benefits of aspirin.

HERB

ANTIPLATELETS, ASPIRIN, CLOPIDOGREL

- *Bai Hua She* (Bungarus snake) (D)–has an antiplatelet effect and should be used with caution in those taking anticoagulants or antiplatelets (Chen, 1998/1999) Level 5 evidence.
- *Bai Shao* (White peony root) (D)–has a mild antiplatelet effect and should be used with caution in those taking anticoagulants or antiplatelets (Chen, 1998/1999) Level 5 evidence.
- *Bai Zhu* (White Atractylodes) (D)–has an antiplatelet effect and should be used with caution in those taking anticoagulants or antiplatelets (Chen, 1998/1999) Level 5 evidence.
- *Ban Lan Gen* (Isatis root) (D)–has an antiplatelet effect and should be used with caution in those taking anticoagulants or antiplatelets (Chen, 1998/1999) Level 5 evidence.
- *Chi Shao* (Red peony root) (D)–has an antiplatelet effect and should be used with caution in those taking anticoagulants or antiplatelets (Chen, 1998/1999) Level 5 evidence.
- *Chuan Xiong* (Cnidium, Sichuan Lovage rhizome) (D)–may potentiate anticoagulant and antiplatelet effects and should be used with caution in patients taking these medications (Chen, 1998/1999) Level 5 evidence.
- *Ci Wu Jia* (Siberian ginseng) (D)–may potentiate the effects of anticoagulant, antiplatelet, and thrombolytic agents (Yun-Choi, Kim & Lee, 1987) Level 5 evidence.
- *Da Suan* (Garlic) (D)–may potentiate anticoagulant and antiplatelet effects and should be used with caution in patients taking anticoag-

ulant and antiplatelet agents, thrombolytic agents, and low molecular weight heparins (Gruenwald, Brendler & Jaenicke, 2004) Level 5 evidence.

- *Dan Shen* (Red-rooted Sage, Salvia root) (C for warfarin, D for other anticoagulants)–may potentiate anticoagulants due to platelet aggregation inhibition (Brinker, 2001). There was a case study that showed interaction with warfarin (Yu, Chan & Sanderson, 1997) Level 4 evidence. Another case report showed severe anticoagulation (Izzat, Yim & El-Zufari, 1998) Level 4 evidence. Finally, a third case report showed interactions between warfarin, *Dan Shen*, and methyl salicylate (Tam, Chan, Leung & Critchley, 1995) Level 4 evidence.
- *Dang Gui* (Angelica sinensis) (D)–may potentiate anticoagulant and antiplatelet effects and should be used with caution in patients taking anticoagulant and antiplatelet agents, thrombolytic agents, and low molecular weight heparins (Gruenwald, Brendler & Jaenicke, 2004) Level 5 evidence.
- *Di Bie Chong* (Eupolyphaga) (D)–may potentiate anticoagulant and antiplatelet effects and should be used with caution in patients taking these medications (Chen, 1998/1999) Level 5 evidence.
- *Ding Xiang* (Clove)–(D) may potentiate anticoagulant and antiplatelet effects and should be used with caution in patients taking anticoagulant and antiplatelet agents, thrombolytic agents, and low molecular weight heparins (Gruenwald, Brendler,& Jaenicke, 2004) Level 5 evidence.
- *Ding Xiang* (Clove) (D)–may potentiate anticoagulants due to platelet aggregation inhibition (Mills & Bone, 2000) Level 5 evidence.
- *Du Huo* (Pubescent Angelica root) (D)–has an antiplatelet effect and should be used with caution in those taking anticoagulants or antiplatelets (Chen, 1998/1999) Level 5 evidence.
- *E Zhu* (Curcuma zedoaria) (D)–may potentiate anticoagulant and antiplatelet effects and should be used with caution in patients taking

these medications (Chen, 1998/1999) Level 5 evidence.

- *Gan Cao* (Licorice) (D)–may potentiate anticoagulant and antiplatelet effects (Norred & Brinker, 2001). In addition, *Gan Cao* has coumarin-like constituents (Heck, Dewitt & Lukes, 2000), and glycyrhizzin, a major constituent of *Gan Cao*, has been shown to have some in vitro thrombin inhibition (Francischetti, Monteiro & Guimaraes, 1997) and should be used with caution in patients taking anticoagulant and antiplatelet agents, thrombolytic agents, and low molecular weight heparins (Gruenwald, Brendler & Jaenicke, 2004). Each of these studies is Level 5 evidence.
- *Gan Jiang/Sheng Jiang* (Ginger) (D)–extract of ginger may speculatively enhance anticoagulation of warfarin and other anticoagulants (Mills & Bone, 2000); (Gianni & Dreitlein, 1988) Level 5 evidence, though a single dose of 2 grams *Gan Jiang* in 8 men did not affect bleeding time, platelet count or aggregation. (Lumb, 1994) Level 2b evidence, 10 grams of extract did affect platelet aggregation, while taking 4 grams daily for 3 months did not show significant anticoagulation activity (Bordia, Verma & Srivastava, 1997) Level 3b evidence.
- *Ge Gen* (Pueraria root) (D)–has an antiplatelet effect and should be used with caution in those taking anticoagulants or antiplatelets (Chen, 1998/1999) Level 5 evidence.
- *Gou Teng* (Cat's claw) (D)–may potentiate anticoagulant and antiplatelet effects and should be used with caution in patients taking anticoagulant and antiplatelet agents, thrombolytic agents, and low molecular weight heparins (Gruenwald, Brendler & Jaenicke, 2004) Level 5 evidence.
- *Hong Hua* (Safflower, Carthamus) (D)–may potentiate anticoagulant and antiplatelet effects and should be used with caution in patients taking these medications (Chen, 1998/1999) Level 5 evidence.
- *Hou Po* (Magnolia bark) (D)–has a mild antiplatelet effect and should be used with caution

in those taking anticoagulants or antiplatelets (Chen, 1998/1999) Level 5 evidence.

- *Hu Tao Ren* (Walnut) (D)–has antiplatelet and thrombolytic effects and should be used with caution in those taking anticoagulants or antiplatelets (Chen, 1998/1999) Level 5 evidence.
- *Huang Qi* (Astragulus) (D)–may potentiate anticoagulant and antiplatelet effects and should be used with caution in patients taking anticoagulant and antiplatelet agents, thrombolytic agents, and low molecular weight heparins (Gruenwald, Brendler & Jaenicke, 2004) Level 5 evidence.
- *Jiang Huang* (Turmeric) (D)–may potentiate anticoagulant and antiplatelet effects and should be used with caution in patients taking these medications (Chen, 1998/1999) Level 5 evidence.
- *Jiang Huang* (Turmeric) (D)–may potentiate anticoagulant and antiplatelet effects and should be used with caution in patients taking anticoagulant and antiplatelet agents, thrombolytic agents, and low molecular weight heparins (Srivastava, Puri, Srimal & Dhawan, 1986) Level 5 evidence.
- *Mao Dong Qing* (Ilex pubescentis) (D)–has mild anticoagulant effect and may potentiate anticoagulant and antiplatelet effects and should be used with caution in patients taking these medications (Chen, 1998/1999) Level 5 evidence.
- *Pu Huang* (Bulrush, cattail pollen) (D)–uniquely both increases blood circulation and stops bleeding and may interfere with anticoagulant and antiplatelet medications (Chen, 1998/1999) Level 5 evidence.
- *Qian Hu* (Peucedanum, White-flowered hog-fennel root) (D)–has an antiplatelet effect and should be used with caution in those taking anticoagulants or antiplatelets (Chen, 1998/1999) Level 5 evidence.
- *San Leng* (Sparganium, common burr-reed rhizome) (D)–may potentiate anticoagulant and antiplatelet effects and should be used with caution in patients taking these medications (Chen, 1998/1999) Level 5 evidence.

- *San Qi* (Pseudoginseng) (Indeterminate)– uniquely both increases blood circulation and stops bleeding and may interfere with anticoagulant and antiplatelet medications (Chinese study cited in Chen & Chen, 2004) Indeterminate level of evidence.
- *Sang Ji Sheng* (Taxillus) (D)–has an antiplatelet effect and should be used with caution in those taking anticoagulants or antiplatelets (Chen, 1998/1999) Level 5 evidence.
- *Sha Ren* (Amomum) (D)–has an antiplatelet effect and should be used with caution in those taking anticoagulants or antiplatelets (Chen, 1998/1999) Level 5 evidence.
- *Shan Zha* (Hawthorn berry) (D)–theoretically may increase the risk of bleeding associated with anitplatelet usage (Gruenwald, Brendler & Jaenicke, 2004) Level 5 evidence.
- *Shui Zhi* (Medicinal leech) (D)–may potentiate anticoagulant and antiplatelet effects and should be used with caution in patients taking these medications (Chen, 1998/1999) Level 5 evidence.
- Stop-bleeding herbs (D)–may counteract antiplatelet and anticoagulant effects and should be used with caution in patients taking these medications, expert opinion (Chen & Chen, 2004) Level 5 evidence.
- *Su He Xiang* (Styrax) (D)–has an antiplatelet effect and should be used with caution in those taking anticoagulants or antiplatelets (Chen, 1998/1999) Level 5 evidence.
- *Tao Ren* (Peach seed), *Yu Jin* (Turmeric tuber) (D)–both may potentiate anticoagulant and antiplatelet effects and should be used with caution in patients taking these medications (Chen, 1998/1999) Level 5 evidence.
- *Xia Tian Wu* (Decumbent corydalis rhizome) (D)–has an antiplatelet effect and should be used with caution in those taking anticoagulants or antiplatelets (Chen, 1998/ 1999) Level 5 evidence.
- *Xie Bai* (Bakeri, long-stamen onion bulb) (D)–has an antiplatelet effect and should be used with caution in those taking anticoagulants or antiplatelets (Chen, 1998/1999) Level 5 evidence.
- *Ye Ju Hua* (Wild chrysanthemum flower) (D)– has an antiplatelet effect and should be used with caution in those taking anticoagulants or antiplatelets (Chen, 1998/1999) Level 5 evidence.
- *Yi Mu Cao* (Motherwort herb) (D)–may potentiate anticoagulant and antiplatelet effects and should be used with caution in patients taking these medications (Chen, 1998/1999) Level 5 evidence.
- *Yin Guo Ye* (Ginkgo leaf) (D)–may potentiate anticoagulant and antiplatelet effects and should be used with caution in patients taking anticoagulant and antiplatelet agents, thrombolytic agents, and low molecular weight heparins (Gruenwald, Brendler & Jaenicke, 2004) Level 5 evidence. In fact, in a Level 2b study (Engelsen, Nielsen & Hansen, 2003), showed no change in coagulation (INR levels) with using warfarin and gingko.
- *Zhi Ke* (Aurantium fruit, bitter orange) (D)– has an antiplatelet effect and should be used with caution in those taking anticoagulants or antiplatelets (Chen, 1998/1999) Level 5 evidence.

INTERACTION ISSUES

A:

D: Cilostazol is 95-98% protein bound; clopidogrel is 98% bound; prasugrel is approximately 98% bound; ticagrelor is over 99% bound, Ticlopidine is 98% bound.

M: Cilostazol is a major substrate of CYP2C19 and 3A4; clopidogrel is a major substrate of CYP2C19 and a moderate inhibitor of 2C9; ticagrelor is a major substrate of CYP3A4 and a moderate inhibitor of 2C9; ticlopidine is a major substrate of CYP3A4, a moderate inhibitor of 2B6 and 2D6, and a strong inhibitor of 2C19.

E:

Pgp:

SECTION 9: ANTICOAGULANTS

Many of the drugs in this category are only available in injection form and are therefore not covered in this book.

WARFARIN (WAR far in) PR=X[46] *(Coumadin®, Jantoven®)*

Note: There is a whole other category of drugs, **Thrombolytics,** *used to break up a clot once it has formed. All of the drugs in this class, however, are injections and are therefore not covered in this book.*

FUNCTION

These agents are used in the prevention and treatment of venous thrombosis, pulmonary embolism, and thromboembolic disorders. They are also used with atrial fibrillation when there is a risk of embolism and as an adjunct in the prevention of systemic embolism after a myocardial infarct.

MECHANISM OF ACTION

Vitamin K is a necessary cofactor in the liver's production of many of the factors (II, VII, IX, and X) involved in coagulation reactions. These agents inhibit vitamin K epoxide reductase which regenerates vitamin K after it is used in one of these reactions. Therefore this inhibition prevents the formation of the necessary factors, and the ability to coagulate is reduced. It usually takes about eight to twelve hours after administration for the effects to be seen. Vitamin K can be used to reverse the effects of these agents, but it can take up to 24 hours for this reversal.

DOSAGES

A communication from the FDA and change in the prescribing information for Warfarin states that dosing can be controlled better and adverse effects reduced if genetic testing is used to determine if a patient has one of two genes involved with the metabolism or regulation of Warfarin in the body. This is the first time that genetic testing is being recommended as a determinant for dosing of a pharmaceutical drug.

WARFARIN, for *infants* and *children*, 0.05-0.34 mg/kg/d, for *infants* <12 months of age may require doses at or near the high end of this range, consistent anticoagulation may be difficult to maintain in *children* <5 years of age. For *adults*, initial dosing must be individualized, consider the patient (hepatic function, cardiac function, age, nutritional status, concurrent therapy, risk of bleeding) in addition to prior dose response (if available) and the clinical situation, start at 5-10 mg daily for 2 days and adjust dose according to international normalized ratio (INR) results, usual dose ranges from 2-10 mg daily.

ADVERSE EFFECTS

The primary adverse effect is hemorrhage. Frequent monitoring, in the form of blood tests, is necessary. Bleeding can be stopped by administration of vitamin K and, if severe enough, this can be administered through intravenous injection. Blood transfusion may be necessary in extreme cases. Certain conditions may potentiate warfarin's effects including vitamin K deficiency, liver disease impairs clotting factor synthesis, and hypermetabolic states affecting these factors.

RED FLAGS

Warfarin is teratogenic and an abortifactant and therefore should never be used during pregnancy.

A new patient medication guide recommends seeing a doctor if any of the following occur while taking warfarin:

- pain, swelling or discomfort
- headaches, dizziness, or weakness
- unusual bruising
- nose bleeds
- bleeding gums

- bleeding from cuts takes a long time to stop
- menstrual bleeding or vaginal bleeding that is heavier than normal
- pink or brown urine
- red or black stools
- coughing up blood/vomiting blood or material that looks like coffee grounds

INTERACTIONS

DRUG

A number of drug interactions have been noted with warfarin. These are summarized in Figure 6.19.

HERB

Warfarin has a narrow therapeutic index in addition to being highly protein bound. Because of both of these, it is the authors' recommendation that herbs not be combined with warfarin without the supervision of and written consent from a medical doctor. INR and prothrombin time lab tests must be carefully monitored if herbs and warfarin are combined to assess proper anticoagulation without unduly raising the risk of hemorrhage.

WARFARIN & ANTICOAGULANTS

- *Bai Hua She* (Bungarus snake), *Bai Shao* (White peony root), *Bai Zhu* (White Atractylodes), *Ban Lan Gen* (Isatis root), *Chi Shao* (Red peony root), *Chuan Xiong* (Cni-dium, Sichuan Lovage rhizome) (D)–have an antiplatelet effect and should be used with caution in those taking anticoagulants or antiplatelets (Chen, 1998/1999) Level 5 evidence.
- *Ci Wu Jia* (Siberian Ginseng) (D)–may potentiate the effects of anticoagulant, antiplatelet, and thrombolytic agents (Yun-Choi, Kim & Lee, 1987) Level 5 evidence.
- *Da Suan* (Garlic) (D)–may potentiate anticoagulant and antiplatelet effects and should be used with caution in patients taking anticoagulant and antiplatelet agents, thrombolytic agents, and low molecular weight heparins (Gruenwald, Brendler & Jaenicke, 2004) Level 5 evidence.

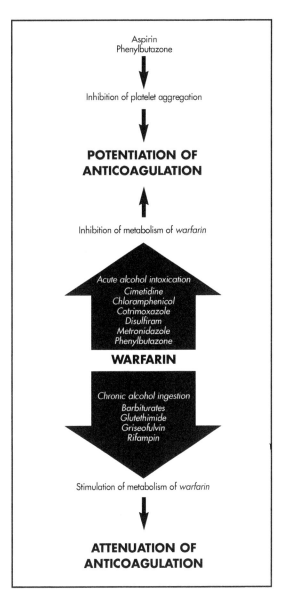

Figure 6.19: Diagram of drugs that interact with warfarin.

- *Dan Shen* (Red-rooted Sage, Salvia root) (C for warfarin, D for other anticoagulants)–may potentiate anticoagulants due to platelet aggregation inhibition (Brinker, 2001). There was a case study that showed interaction with warfarin (Yu, Chan & Sanderson, 1997) Level 4 evidence. Another case report showed severe anticoagulation (Izzat, Yim & El-Zufari, 1998) Level 4 evidence. Finally, a third case report showed interactions between warfarin, *Dan Shen*, and methyl salicylate (Tam, Chan, Leung & Critchley, 1995) Level 4 evidence.

- *Dang Gui* (Angelica sinensis) (D)–may potentiate anticoagulant and antiplatelet effects and should be used with caution in patients taking anticoagulant and anti-platelet agents, thrombolytic agents, and low molecular weight heparins (Gruenwald, Brendler & Jaenicke, 2004) Level 5 evidence.
- *Di Bie Chong* (Eupolyphaga) (D)–may potentiate anticoagulant and antiplatelet effects and should be used with caution in patients taking these medications (Chen, 1998/1999) Level 5 evidence.
- *Ding Xiang* (Clove)–(D) may potentiate anticoagulant and antiplatelet effects and should be used with caution in patients taking anticoagulant and antiplatelet agents, thrombolytic agents, and low molecular weight heparins (Gruenwald, Brendler & Jaenicke, 2004) Level 5 evidence.
- *Ding Xiang* (Clove) (D)–may potentiate anticoagulants due to platelet aggregation inhibition (Mills & Bone, 2000) Level 5 evidence.
- *Du Huo* (Pubescent Angelica root) (D)–has an antiplatelet effect and should be used with caution in those taking anticoagulants or antiplatelets (Chen, 1998/1999) Level 5 evidence.
- *E Zhu* (Curcuma zedoaria) (D)–may potentiate anticoagulant and antiplatelet effects and should be used with caution in patients taking these medications (Chen, 1998/1999) Level 5 evidence.
- *Gan Cao* (Licorice) (D)–may potentiate anticoagulant and antiplatelet effects (Norred & Brinker, 2001). In addition, *Gan Cao* has cou-marin-like constituents (Heck, Dewitt & Lukes, 2000), and glycyrhizzin, a major constituent of *Gan Cao*, has been shown to have some in vitro thrombin inhibition (Francischetti, Monteiro & Guimaraes, 1997) and should be used with caution in patients taking anticoagulant and antiplatelet agents, thrombolytic agents, and low molecular weight heparins (Gruenwald, Brendler & Jaenicke, 2004). Each of these studies is Level 5 evidence.
- *Gan Jiang/Sheng Jiang* (Ginger) (D)–extract of ginger may speculatively enhance anticoagulation of warfarin and other anticoagulants (Mills & Bone, 2000); (Gianni & Dreitlein, 1988) Level 5 evidence, though a single dose of 2 grams *Gan Jiang* in 8 men did not affect bleeding time, platelet count or aggregation (Lumb, 1994) Level 2b evidence; 10 grams of extract did affect platelet aggregation, while taking 4 grams daily for 3 months did not show significant anticoagulation activity (Bordia, Verma & Srivastava, 1997) Level 3b evidence.
- *Ge Gen* (Pueraria root) (D)–has an antiplatelet effect and should be used with caution in those taking anticoagulants or antiplatelets (Chen, 1998/1999) Level 5 evidence.
- *Gou Qi Zi* (Goji) (C)–One equivocal case study discusses a decrease in coagulation ability in a woman drinking goji berry juice (Rivera, Ferro, Bursua & Gerber, 2012). Level 4 evidence.
- *Gou Teng* (Cat's claw) (D)–may potentiate anticoagulant and antiplatelet effects and should be used with caution in patients taking anticoagulant and antiplatelet agents, thrombolytic agents, and low molecular weight heparins (Gruenwald, Brendler & Jaenicke, 2004) Level 5 evidence.
- *Guan Ye Lian Qiao* (St. John's wort) (C)–*Guan ye lian qiao* decreases blood concentrations of warfarin (Zhou, Chan, Pan, Huang *et al.,* 2004) Level 3b evidence (Izzo & Ernst, 2009) Level 4 evidence.
- *Hong Hua* (Safflower, Carthamus) (D)–may potentiate anticoagulant and antiplatelet effects and should be used with caution in patients taking these medications (Chen, 1998/1999) Level 5 evidence.
- *Hou Po* (Magnolia bark) (D)–has a mild antiplatelet effect and should be used with caution in those taking anticoagulants or antiplatelets (Chen, 1998/1999) Level 5 evidence.
- *Hu Tao Ren* (Walnut) (D)–has antiplatelet and thrombolytic effects and should be used with caution in those taking anticoagulants or antiplatelets (Chen, 1998/1999) Level 5 evidence.

- *Huang Qi* (Astragulus) (D)–may potentiate anticoagulant and antiplatelet effects and should be used with caution in patients taking anticoagulant and antiplatelet agents, thrombolytic agents, and low molecular weight heparins (Gruenwald, Brendler & Jaenicke, 2004) Level 5 evidence.
- *Jiang Huang* (Turmeric) (D)–may potentiate anticoagulant and antiplatelet effects and should be used with caution in patients taking these medications (Chen, 1998/1999) Level 5 evidence.
- *Jiang Huang* (Turmeric) (D)–may potentiate anticoagulant and antiplatelet effects and should be used with caution in patients taking anticoagulant and antiplatelet agents, thrombolytic agents, and low molecular weight heparins (Srivastava, Puri, Srimal & Dhawan, 1986) Level 5 evidence.
- *Mao Dong Qing* (Ilex pubescentis) (D)–has mild anticoagulant effect and may potentiate anticoagulant and antiplatelet effects and should be used with caution in patients taking these medications (Chen, 1998/1999) Level 5 evidence.
- *Pu Huang* (Bulrush, cattail pollen) (D)–both increase blood circulation and stop bleeding and may interfere with anticoagulant and antiplatelet medications (Chen, 1998/1999) Level 5 evidence.
- *Qian Hu* (Peucedanum, White-flowered hogfennel root) (D)–has an antiplatelet effect and should be used with caution in those taking anticoagulants or antiplatelets (Chen, 1998/1999) Level 5 evidence.
- *San Leng* (Sparganium, common burr-reed rhizome) (D)–may potentiate anticoagulant and antiplatelet effects and should be used with caution in patients taking these medications (Chen, 1998/1999) Level 5 evidence.
- *San Qi* (Pseudoginseng) (Indeterminate)– increases blood circulation and stops bleeding and may interfere with anticoagulant and antiplatelet medications (Chinese study cited in Chen & Chen, 2004) Indeterminate level of evidence.

- *Sang Ji Sheng* (Taxillus) (D)–has an antiplatelet effect and should be used with caution in those taking anticoagulants or antiplatelets (Chen, 1998/1999) Level 5 evidence.
- *Sha Ren* (Amomum) (D)–has an antiplatelet effect and should be used with caution in those taking anticoagulants or antiplatelets (Chen, 1998/1999) Level 5 evidence.
- *Shan Zha* (Hawthorn berry) (D)–theoretically may increase the risk of bleeding associated with anitplatelet usage (Gruenwald, Brendler & Jaenicke, 2004) Level 5 evidence.
- *Shui Zhi* (Medicinal leech) (D)–may potentiate anticoagulant and antiplatelet effects and should be used with caution in patients taking these medications (Chen, 1998/1999) Level 5 evidence.
- Stop-bleeding herbs (D)–may counteract antiplatelet and anticoagulant effects and should be used with caution in patients taking these medications, expert opinion (Chen & Chen, 2004) Level 5 evidence.
- *Su He Xiang* (Styrax) (D)–has an antiplatelet effect and should be used with caution in those taking anticoagulants or antiplatelets (Chen, 1998/1999) Level 5 evidence.
- *Tao Ren* (Peach seed) (D)–may potentiate anticoagulant and antiplatelet effects and should be used with caution in patients taking these medications (Chen, 1998/1999) Level 5 evidence.
- *Xi Yang Shen* (American ginseng) (C)–a small double-blinded, randomly controlled trial demonstrated a lower INR when American ginseng was combined with warfarin than when warfarin was administered alone. This indicates an interaction that counteracts the effects of warfarin (Qi, Wang, Du, Zhang et al., 2011, November 1). Level 2b evidence.
- *Xia Tian Wu* (Decumbent corydalis rhizome) (D)–has an antiplatelet effect and should be used with caution in those taking anticoagulants or antiplatelets (Chen, 1998/1999) Level 5 evidence.
- *Xie Bai* (Bakeri, long-stamen onion bulb) and *Ye Ju Hua* (Wild chrysanthemum flower) (D)–both have an antiplatelet effect and

should be used with caution in those taking anticoagulants or antiplatelets (Chen, 1998/1999) Level 5 evidence.

- *Yi Mu Cao* (Motherwort herb) (D)–may potentiate anticoagulant and antiplatelet effects and should be used with caution in patients taking these medications (Chen, 1998/1999) Level 5 evidence.
- *Yin Guo Ye* (Ginkgo leaf) (D)–may potentiate anticoagulant and antiplatelet effects and should be used with caution in patients taking anticoagulant and antiplatelet agents, thrombolytic agents, and low molecular weight heparins (Gruenwald, Brendler & Jaenicke, 2004) Level 5 evidence. In fact, a level 2b study (Engelsen, Nielsen & Hansen, 2003), showed no change in coagulation (INR levels) with using warfarin and Gingko.

- *Yu Jin* (Turmeric tuber) (D)–may potentiate anticoagulant and antiplatelet effects and should be used with caution in patients taking these medications (Chen, 1998/1999) Level 5 evidence.
- *Zhi Ke* (Aurantium fruit, bitter orange) (D)– has an antiplatelet effect and should be used with caution in those taking anticoagulants or antiplatelets (Chen, 1998/1999) Level 5 evidence.

INTERACTION ISSUES

A:

D: Warfarin is 99% protein bound.

M: Warfarin is a major substrate of CYP2C9.

E:

Pgp:

TI: Warfarin has a narrow therapeutic index.

SECTION 10: DRUGS USED TO TREAT BLEEDING

AMINOCAPROIC ACID (a mee noe ka PROE ik AS id) PR=C *(Amicar®)*

DESMOPRESSIN (des moe PRES in) PR=B *(DDAVP®, Stimate™)*

PHYTONADIONE, also known as Vitamin K, (fye toe na DYE one) PR=C *(Mephyton®)*

TRANEXAMIC ACID (tran eks AM ik AS id) PR=B *(Cyklokapron®, Lysteda™)*

▓ FUNCTION

These agents are used in stopping bleeding in patients. Many in this category, including the various factors used to treat forms of hemophilia, are injectables and are not covered.

Desmopressin's hemostatic effects occur primarily through injection. When used orally, it treats diabetes insipidus and primary nocturnal enuresis.

▓ MECHANISMS OF ACTION

Aminocaproic acid works by inhibiting plasminogen activation to plasmin, a necessary step in forming a blood clot.

Desmopressin is an analog of the endogenous hormone vasopressin and therefore has similar effects: water conservation, release of blood coagulation factors (VIII and von Willebrand), and possibly smooth muscle contraction in the gas-

trointestinal tract and vasculature. Water conservation occurs by increasing the permeability of collecting duct cells.

Vitamin K is a necessary cofactor in the liver's production of many of the factors (II, VII, IX, and X) involved in coagulation reactions. Therefore, phytonadione is replaced when there is a deficiency of vitamin K or to counteract warfarin's effects.

▓ DOSAGES

AMINOCAPROIC ACID, for *adults*, for acute bleeding syndrome, 4-5 g in the first hour, followed by 1 g/hr for 8 hours or until bleeding is controlled up to a maximum daily dose of 30 g.

DESMOPRESSIN, for *children*, for diabetes insipidus, 4 years or older, initiate at 0.05 mg bid; total daily dose should be increased or decreased as needed to obtain adequate antidiuresis, usual range is 0.1-1.2 mg divided 2-3 times/d; for nocturnal enuresis, 0.2 mg nocte; dose may be titrated up to 0.6 mg to achieve desired response. For *children* 12 years or older and *adults*, for diabetes insipidus, initiate at 0.05 mg bid; total daily dose should be increased or decreased as needed to obtain adequate antidiuresis; usual range is 0.1-1.2 mg divided 2-3 times/d.

PHYTONADIONE, for *children*, 1-3 years: 30 mcg/d; 4-8 years: 55 mcg/d; 9-13 years: 60 mcg/d; 14-18 years: 75 mcg/d. For *adults*, in males use 120 mcg/d, in females use 90 mcg/d; for hypo-pro-thrombinemia due to drugs (other than coumarin derivatives) or factors limiting absorption or synthesis, initiate at 2.5-25 mg (rarely up to 50 mg), for vitamin K deficiency secondary to coumarin derivative; dosage is quite complicated and variable based on symptoms and INR.

TRANEXAMIC ACID, for *adults*, for menorrhagia, 1300 mg tid for up to 5 days during menstruation.

ADVERSE EFFECTS

Aminocaproic acid may cause a wide variety of adverse effects including gastrointestinal and central nervous system complaints. Rare effects include agranulocytosis, renal failure, and **myoglobinuria**.

Desmopressin may cause various serious cardiovascular events including thrombosis and myocardial infarction. Minor complaints include various gastrointestinal and central nervous system effects.

Myoglobinuria: Abnormal presence of myoglobin in the urine

RED FLAGS

Aminocaproic acid may cause intravascular thrombosis with life-threatening sequelae.

INTERACTIONS

DRUG, HERB

No major interactions noted.

SECTION 11: DRUGS USED TO TREAT ANEMIA

CYANOCOBALAMIN (sye an oh koe BAL a min) PR=C *(Ener-B® [O], FaBB,[32] Folastin,[32] Folbee®,[32] Folbic™,[32] Folcaps™,[32] Folgard RX®,[32] Folplex 2.2,[32] Foltabs™ 800 [O],[32] Homocysteine Guard [O],[32] Lev-Tov [O],[32] Nascobal®, Tri-B® [O],[32] Tricardio B,[32] Twelve Resin-K [O]) Virt-Vite Forte,[32] Vita-Respa®,[32])*

FOLIC ACID (FOE lik AS id) PR=A *(FaBB,[32] Folastin,[32] Folbee®,[32] Folbic™,[32] Folcaps™,[32] Folgard RX®,[32] Folplex 2.2,[32] Foltabs™ 800 [O],[32] Homocysteine Guard [O],[32] Lev-Tov [O],[32] Tri-B® [O],[32] Tricardio B,[32] Virt-Vite Forte,[32] Vita-Respa®[32])*

PYRIDOXINE (peer i DOKS ene) PR=A in quantities lower than recommended daily intake and C in higher doses *(FaBB,[32] Folastin,[32] Folbee®,[32] Folbic™,[32] Folcaps™,[32] Folgard RX®,[32] Folplex 2.2,[32] Foltabs™ 800 [O],[32] Homocysteine Guard [O],[32] Lev-Tov [O],[32] Tri-B® [O],[32] Tricardio B,[32] Virt-Vite Forte,[32] Vita-Respa®[32])*

AGENTS USED TO TREAT IRON OVERLOAD: DEFERASIROX (de FER a sir ox) PR=C *(Exjade®)*

DEFEROXAMINE (de fer OKS a mene) PR=C *(Desferal®)*

Iron is a commonly used agent to treat microcytic, iron-deficiency anemia. Erythropoietin and its derivatives are used to treat anemia by stimulating red blood cell production. These agents, however, are injectables and therefore not covered here. In addition, various blood transfusion products can be used to acutely treat serious anemia.

FUNCTION

These agents are used to treat anemia.

Deferasirox is used in chronic iron overload due to blood transfusions.

MECHANISMS OF ACTION

These agents are used to treat anemia by replacing internal deficiencies of vitamins that are necessary for proper production of red blood cells.

Deferasirox acts by binding iron in the intestine. This bound complex is then excreted through the stool.

DOSAGES

CYANOCOBALAMIN, dosing of this vitamin is dependent on all dietary sources. Supplementation in *children* and *adults* should be administered at levels to complete recommended daily intake.

DEFERASIROX, for *children* 2 and over and *adults*, initiate at 20 mg/kg daily and adjust dose every 3-6 months based on serum levels of ferritin; maximum dose is 30 mg/kg/d.

DEFEROXAMINE, for *children* 3 or over, for acute iron toxicity, IM: 90 mg/kg/dose every 8 hours up to a maximum of 6000 mg/d; for chronic iron overload, SubQ: 20-40 mg/kg/d over 8-12 hours up to a maximum of 1000-2000 mg/d. For *adults*, for acute iron toxicity, IM: initiate at 1000 mg; may be followed by 500 mg every 4 hours for 2 doses; doses of 500 mg can be given every 4-12 hours prn; maximum recommended dose is 6000 mg/d; for chronic iron overload, IM: 500-1000 mg/d up to a maximum of 1000 mg/d; SubQ: 1000-2000 mg/d or 20-40 mg/kg/d over 8-24 hours.

FOLIC ACID and PYRIDOXINE. See instructions for CYANOCOBALAMIN above.

ADVERSE EFFECTS

Excess of these agents is generally harmlessly excreted in the urine and has no known adverse effects.

Common adverse effects of deferasirox include fever, headache, GI disturbances, cough, and flu. Hepatotoxicity, ocular disturbances, and a dose-related rash have also been reported.

RED FLAGS

The FDA has issued a warning regarding deferasirox. There have been several cases involving acute renal failure and cytopenias resulting in deaths among critically ill patients taking this agent. Serum creatinine should be monitored closely both before and after initiation of deferasirox.

INTERACTIONS

DRUG, HERB

None noted.

INTERACTION ISSUES

A:

D: Deferasirox is approximately 99% protein bound.

M: Deferasirox is a moderate inhibitor of CYP1A2 and 2C8 and a weak/moderate inducer of 3A4.

E:

Pgp:

TI:

SECTION 12: DRUGS USED TO TREAT SICKLE CELL DISEASE

HYDROXYUREA (hye droks ee yoor EE a)
PR=D *(Droxia®, Hydrea®)*

Sickle cell disease is a common genetic disease that causes abnormal hemoglobin (HbS), which is a necessary component of red blood cells and blood oxygen transport. The abnormal hemoglobin causes different HbS strands to aggregate and block capillaries causing extreme pain and tissue hypoxia. This is called sickle cell crisis.

FUNCTION

Besides treating recalcitrant sickle cell disease, hydroxyurea is used to treat various malignancies including melanoma, chronic myelocytic leukemia, ovarian cancer, and squamous cell cancer. Unlabeled uses include treating HIV, psoriasis, essential thrombocytopenia, polycythemia vera, hypereosinophilia, brain tumors, and other cancers such as uterine, cervical, and non-small-cell lung, renal, and prostate.

MECHANISMS OF ACTION

In sickle cell disease, hydroxyurea appears to work by increasing the production of fetal hemoglobin, which dilutes the amount of circulating HbS and reduces the incidence of sickle cell crisis. In treatment of cancers, it is thought to interfere with synthesis of DNA without interfering with RNA synthesis.

DOSAGES

HYDROXYUREA, for *adults*, dose should always be titrated to patient response and WBC counts; usual dose ranges from 10-30 mg/kg/d or 500-3000 mg/d; if WBC count falls to <2500 cells/mm^3, or the platelet count to <100,000/ mm^3, therapy should be stopped for at least 3 days and resumed when values rise towards normal; for solid tumors, for intermittent therapy, 80 mg/kg as a single dose every third day; for continuous therapy, 20-30 mg/kg/d given as a single dose per day; for resistant chronic myelocytic leukemia, for continuous therapy, 20-30 mg/kg as a single daily dose; for sickle cell disease, initiate at 15 mg/kg/d; increase by 5 mg/kg every 12 weeks if blood counts are in an acceptable range until the maximum tolerated dose of 35 mg/kg/d is achieved.

ADVERSE EFFECTS

There are many adverse effects of this drug including but not limited to: edema, dizziness, fever, hallucinations, headache, various dermatological effects, nausea and vomiting, constipation, diarrhea, **myelosuppression**, **thrombocytopenia**, and other hematologic disorders.

RED FLAGS

None noted.

INTERACTIONS

DRUG

Hydroxyurea should not be combined with didanosine as it may increase the latter's risk of inducing pancreatitis, hepatotoxicity, or neuropathy.

> Myelosuppression: A decrease in blood cell production from the bone marrow

> Thrombocytopenia: A decreased number of platelets in the blood

---

SECTION 13: HMG-COA REDUCTASE INHIBITORS

ATORVASTATIN (a TORE va sta tin) PR=X (Caduet®,[21] Lipitor®)

FLUVASTATIN (FLOO va sta tin) PR=X (Lescol®, Lescol® XL)

LOVASTATIN (LOE va sta tin) PR=X (Advicor®,[33] Altoprev®, Mevacor®)

PITAVASTATIN (pi TA va sta tin) PR=X (Livalo®)

PRAVASTATIN PR=X (PRA va stat in) (Pravachol®)

ROSUVASTATIN (roe SOO va sta tin) PR=X (Crestor®)

SIMVASTATIN (SIM va stat in) PR=X (Juvisync™,[47] Simcor®,[48] Vytorin®,[34] Zocor®)

The drugs in this class are commonly known as statins, as that is the last part in each agent's name. The herb *Hong Qu* (red yeast rice) has been found to include several of the statins as natural constituents. It is a potential whole food alternative to a statin drug. Be advised, however, that dosing is critical, with several studies showing beneficial effects at 2.4 g a day.

FUNCTION

These drugs are used in hyperlipidemia including hypertriglyceridemia and hypercholesterolemia.

▩ MECHANISMS OF ACTION

The agents in this class have two major mechanisms for reducing LDL and VLDL cholesterol. The first mechanism is by inhibiting 3-hydroxy-3-methylglutarate (HMG) coenzyme A (CoA) reductase, which is an enzyme necessary to produce cholesterol. Some of these agents do this directly, and others need to be metabolized to the active agent.

The second mechanism of action for these drugs is due to a reduction of LDL cholesterol in the cell due to the inhibition of HMG-CoA reductase. The cell starts to produce more LDL receptors on the cell surface that bind and reduce LDL that is in the blood. These effects are summarized in Figure 6.20.

Besides these effects, HMG-CoA reductase inhibitors also tend to raise HDL (the "good" cholesterol) cholesterol, stabilize plaques so that they don't break off and form an emboli, improve cardiac endothelial function, inhibit platelet thrombus synthesis, and have some anti-inflammatory effects. All of these are very beneficial in preventing or minimizing coronary heart disease, even though the exact mechanisms of these actions are not completely understood.

▩ DOSAGES

ATORVASTATIN, adjustments should be made at intervals of 2-4 weeks. For *children* 10-17 years: 10 mg once daily; may increase to 20 mg once daily; doses >20 mg have not been studied. For *adolescents* >17 years and *adults*, initiate at 10-20 mg once daily;;patients who require a reduction of >45% in LDL-C may be started at 40 mg once daily; recommended dosage range is 10-80 mg/d.

FLUVASTATIN, for *adolescents* 10-16 years, initiate at 20 mg once daily; may increase every 6 weeks based on tolerability and response to a maximum recommended dose of 80 mg/d, given in 2 divided doses (immediate release capsule) or as a single daily dose (extended release tablet). For *adults*, for patients requiring ≥25% decrease in LDL, 40 mg capsule nocte or 80 mg extended release tablet once

daily (anytime), or 40 mg capsule bid; for patients requiring <25% decrease in LDL, initiate at: 20 mg capsule nocte; may increase based on tolerability and response to a maximum recommended dose of 80 mg/d, given in 2 divided doses (immediate release capsule) or as a single daily dose (extended release tablet).

LOVASTATIN, for *children* and *adolescents* 10-17 years, initiate at, using immediate release formulation, 10 mg once daily,;increase to 20 mg once daily after 8 weeks and 40 mg once daily after 16 weeks as needed. Girls must be at least 1 year post menarche. For *adults*, using immediate release tablet, initiate at 20 mg once daily and adjust dosage at 4-week intervals to a usual range of 10-80 mg/d in a single or 2 divided doses; for extended release tablet, initiate at 20 mg once daily and adjust dosage at 4-week intervals up to a maximum dose of 60 mg/d.

PITAVASTATIN, for *adults*, for primary hyperlipidemia and mixed dyslipidemia, initiate at 2 mg once daily; may be increased to a maximum of 4 mg once daily.

PRAVASTATIN, for *children*, 8-13 years, 20 mg/d; 14-18 years, 40 mg/d. For *adults*, initiate at 40 mg once daily; usual dose range is 10-80 mg with a maximum dose of 80 mg once daily.

ROSUVASTATIN, for *adults*, initiate at 10 mg once daily (20 mg in patients with severe hypercholesterolemia or 5 mg in patients requiring less aggressive treatment or predisposed to myopathy); after 2 weeks, may be increased by 5-10 mg once daily; usual dosing range is 5-40 mg/d up to a maximum dose of 40 mg once daily

SIMVASTATIN, adjustments should be made at intervals of 4 weeks or more. For *children* 10-17 years (females >1 year post menarche), 10 mg once daily in the evening increasing to a usual dose range of 10-40 mg/d and a daily maximum of 40 mg. For *adults*, 20-40 mg once daily in the evening, changing to a usual range of 5-80 mg/d.

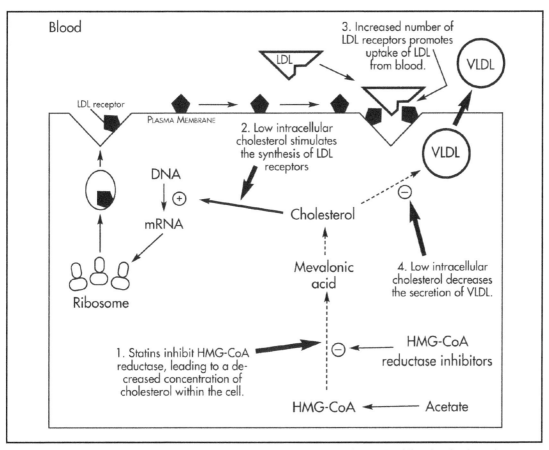

Figure 6.20: Effects of HMG CoA reductase inhibitors (statins). 1: HMG-CoA reductase is inhibited and reduces the amount of cholesterol produced in the cell. 2: Reduced cholesterol initiates LDL receptor synthesis. 3: An increased number of LDL receptors on the cell membrane increases the amount of cholesterol removed from the blood and hence lowers circulating LDL. 4: Low intracellular VLDL lowers secretion into the blood.

ADVERSE EFFECTS

In general, these drugs are considered relatively safe, and the incidence of adverse effects is minimal. With that said, there are some serious, if rare, adverse effects. These include liver failure, muscle abnormalities, and **rhabdomyolysis**. These last two effects are more prominent in patients who have renal issues or were taking other drugs with the statin. The drugs showing this increased risk include cyclosporine, itraconazole, erythromycin, gemfibrozil, and niacin. These drugs should not be used during pregnancy or breastfeeding, and only under specific conditions should they be used in children and teenagers.

Rosuvastatin has been implicated by several FDA scientists as having more adverse effects than other statins, and the agency has gone public with suggestions to take it off the market.

RED FLAGS

None noted.

INTERACTIONS

DRUG

Taking a statin with cyclosporine, itraconazole, erythromycin, gemfibrozil, or niacin may increase the risk of myopathies and rhabdomyolysis. These agents also increase warfarin levels, and increased observation of prothrombin times is warranted.

HERB

ANTICHOLESTEROL AGENTS

- *Da Suan* (Garlic) (D)–may potentiate cholesterol lowering agents as shown in meta-analysis of human clinical trials (Silagy & Neil, 1994) Level 5 evidence.
- *Hu Lu Ba* (Fenugreek) (D)–may potentiate

> **Rhabdomyolysis:** An acute, potentially fatal disease of destruction of skeletal muscle; signs include myoglobinemia and myoglobinuria

cholesterol lowering agents as shown in several small human studies and one dog study (Mills & Bone, 2000) Level 5 evidence.

ATORVASTATIN

- *Guan Ye Lian Qiao* (St. John's wort) (C)–decreases blood concentrations (Izzo & Ernst, 2009) Level 2b evidence.

LOVASTATIN

- *Hong Qu* (Red yeast rice) (D)–should not be used with gemfibrozil or lovastatin as severe rhabdomyolysis and myopathy have been reported, expert opinion (Chen & Chen, 2004) Level 5 evidence.

OTHER SUPPLEMENTS

- CoQ-10 is an excellent supplement to administer with statins. It has been found to reduce the amount of adverse effects.

SIMVASTATIN

- *Guan Ye Lian Qiao* (St. John's wort) (C)–decreases blood concentrations (Zhou, Chan,

Pan, Huang & Lee, 2004) Level 2b evidence, (Izzo & Ernst, 2009) Level 4 evidence.

INTERACTION ISSUES

A:

D: Atorvastatin is at least 98% protein bound; fluvastatin is greater than 98% bound; lovastatin is over 95% bound; pitavastatin is greater than 99% bound; simvastatin is approximately 95% bound.

M: Atorvastatin is a major substrate of CYP3A4; fluvastatin is a moderate inhibitor of CYP2C9; lovastatin and simvastatin are major substrates of CYP3A4.

E:

Pgp: Atorvastatin is a substrate and inhibitor of Pgp; lovastatin and pravastatin are substrates of Pgp.

TI:

SECTION 14: OTHER AGENTS FOR HYPERLIPIDEMIA

BILE ACID SEQUESTRANTS:

CHOLESTYRAMINE RESIN (koe LES teer a mene REZ in) PR=C *(Prevalite®, Questran®, Questran® Light)*

COLESEVELAM (koh le SEV a lam) PR=B *(Welchol®)*

COLESTIPOL (koe LES ti pole) PR=N *(Colestid®, Colestid® Flavored)*

FIBRATES:

FENOFIBRATE (fen oh FYE brate) PR=C *(Antara®, Fenoglide®, Lipofen®, Lofibra®, TriCor®, Triglide®)*

FENOFIBRIC ACID (fen oh FYE brik AS id) PR=C *(Fibricor®, TriLipix®)*

GEMFIBROZIL (jem FI broe zil) PR=C *(Lopid®)*

OTHERS:

EZETIMIBE (ez ET i mibe) PR=C *(Vytorin™,[34] Zetia™)*

ICOSAPENT ETHYL (eye KOE sa pent ETH il) PR=C *(Vascepa™)*

NIACIN (NYE a sin) PR=C *(Niacin-Time® [O], Niacor®, Niaspan®, Simcor®,[48] Slo-Niacin® [O])*

OMEGA-3-ACID ETHYL ESTERS (oh MEG a three AS id ETH il ES ters) PR=C *(Lovaza®)*

FUNCTION

These agents, through disparate means, all work to reduce the risks of hyperlipidemia in the development of coronary heart disease (CHD) or coronary artery disease (CAD). These agents are often used in addition to HMG-CoA reductase inhibitors. Figure 6.21 summarizes the effects of various hyperlipidemic drugs and their relative effectiveness at clearing LDL and triglycerides and increasing HDL.

Niacin is the best agent to shift VLDL and LDL cholesterol to HDL cholesterol, which in turns minimizes CHD risk.

MECHANISMS OF ACTION

Bile acid sequestrants work by binding in the small

intestine with bile acids and salts from the gall-bladder. These acids are formed by cholesterol in the liver, and binding causes them to be excreted in the feces. The liver reacts by increasing the production of LDL receptors on the cell surfaces. The uptake of cholesterol from the blood is increased; therefore, there is less circulating cholesterol. This increased uptake yields an increase in the amount of bile acid production. The normal functioning of the liver in this cascade is shown in Figure 6.22 with the changes that happen in the presence of a bile acid sequestrant.

Fibrates work by activating peroxisome proliferator-activated receptors that cause an increase in lipoprotein lipase. Lipase is an enzyme that breaks down circulating VLDL and other fatty acid structures and promotes storage of free fatty acids in adipose and other tissues. Ulti-mately, this causes increased breakdown of LDL and, through the increased expression of other genes, increases HDL. This is summarized in Figure 6.23.

Ezetimibe is the sole agent in a new class of drugs known as cholesterol absorption inhibitors. It works by inhibiting the absorption of cholesterol from the intestine. This in turn reduces the amount of cholesterol delivered to the liver, which responds by increasing the uptake of cholesterol from the blood. While this agent alone has a small effect on hyperlipidemia, when combined with other agents, especially HMG-CoA reductase inhibitors, it has been shown to have a synergistic effect.

Niacin acts in the adipose tissue. These tissues synthesize free fatty acids that circulate in the blood stream until the liver eventually processes them and creates VLDL and LDL. Niacin blocks the initial formation of fatty acids and prevents VLDL and LDL production later in this cascade. This is shown in Figure 6.24.

DOSAGES

CHOLESTYRAMINE RESIN, for *children*, 80 mg/kg/d tid. For *adults*, 4 g 1-2 times/d up to a maximum of 24 g/d and 6 doses/d.

COLESEVELAM, 3 tablets bid with meals or 6 tablets once daily with a meal.

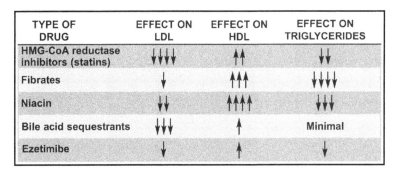

TYPE OF DRUG	EFFECT ON LDL	EFFECT ON HDL	EFFECT ON TRIGLYCERIDES
HMG-CoA reductase inhibitors (statins)	↓↓↓↓	↑↑	↓↓
Fibrates	↓	↑↑↑	↓↓↓↓
Niacin	↓↓	↑↑↑↑	↓↓↓
Bile acid sequestrants	↓↓↓	↑	Minimal
Ezetimibe	↓	↑	↓

Figure 6.21: Comparison of various hyperlipidemic agents on different types of lipids.

COLESTIPOL, granules: 5-30 g/d given once or in divided doses 2-4 times/d; initiate at 5 g 1-2 times/d; increase by 5 g at 1- to 2-month intervals; tablets: 2-16 g/d; initiate at 2 g 1-2 times/d; increase by 2 g at 1- to 2-month intervals.

EZETIMIBE, for *children* 10 or over and *adults*, for hyperlipidemia, 10 mg/d.

FENOFIBRATE, for *adults*, for hypertriglyceridemia, initiate at: Antara™: 43-130 mg/day; Lipofen™: 50-150 mg/d up to a max-

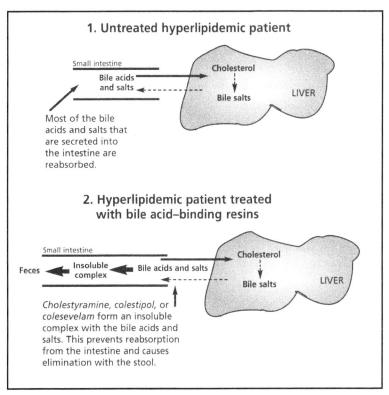

Figure 6.22: How bile acid sequestrants work to reduce cholesterol. 1: Normally the liver secretes bile acids and salts into the intestines, and then they are reabsorbed back into the liver. **2:** In the presence of a bile acid sequestrant, the bile acid is made into a complex that cannot be reabsorbed and is secreted in the stool. This reduces the overall cholesterol in the body.

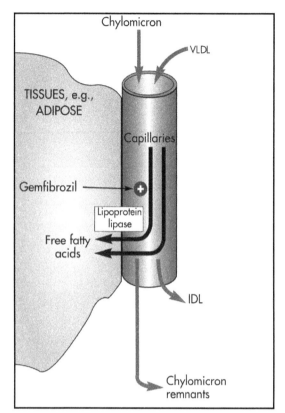

Figure 6.23: Action of gemfibrozil on cholesterol metabolism. Gemfibrozil increases activation of lipoprotein lipase, which increases breakdown of VLDLs and ultimately increases the amount of IDLs and HDLs.

imum dose of 150 mg/d; Lofibra™: 67 mg/day with meals up to 200 mg/d; TriCor®: 48 mg/d; up to 145 mg/d; Triglide™: 50-160 mg/d; for hypercholesterolemia or mixed hyperlipidemia, Antara™: 130 mg/day, Lipofen™: 150 mg/d; Lofibra™: 200 mg/d with meals; TriCor®: 145 mg/d; Triglide™: 160 mg/d. For the *elderly*, initiate at: Antara™: 43 mg/d; Lipofen™: 50 mg/d; Lofibra™: 67 mg/d; TriCor®: 48 mg/d, Triglide™: 50 mg/d.

FENOFIBRIC ACID, for *adults*, for mixed dyslipidemia when administered with a statin, TriLipix™: 135 mg once daily; for hypertriglyceridemia; Fibricor®: initiate at 35-105 mg once daily; TriLipix™: initiate at 45-135 mg once daily; for primary hypercholesterolemia or mixed dyslipidemia, Fibricor®: 105 mg once daily; TriLipix™: 135 mg once daily.

GEMFIBROZIL, for *adults*, 600 mg bid, 30 minutes before breakfast and dinner.

ICOSAPENT ETHYL, for *adults*, for hypertriglyceridemia, 1 g bid.

NIACIN, for *children*, recommended daily allowances: 0-0.5 years: 5 mg/d; 0.5-1 year: 6 mg/d; 1-3 years: 9 mg/d; 4-6 years: 12 mg/d; 7-10 years: 13 mg/d. For *children* and *adolescents*, recommended daily allowances: *Male:* 11-14 years: 17 mg/d; 15-18 years: 20 mg/d; 19-24 years: 19 mg/d; *Female:* 11-24 years: 15 mg/d. For *adults*, recommended daily allowances: *Male:* 25-50 years: 19 mg/d; >51 years: 15 mg/d; *Female:* 25-50 years: 15 mg/d; >51 years: 13 mg/d; for hyperlipidemia, usual target dose is .5-2 g/tid with or after meals; extended release: 375 mg to 2 g nocte; regular release formulation (Niacor®), initiate at 250 mg once daily (with evening meal); increase frequency and/or dose every 4-7 days to desired response or first-level therapeutic dose (1.5-2 g/d in 2-3 divided doses), after 2 months, may increase at 2-4 week intervals to 1 g tid; extended release formulation (Niaspan®), 500 mg nocte for 4 weeks, then 1 g nocte for 4 weeks; adjust dose to response

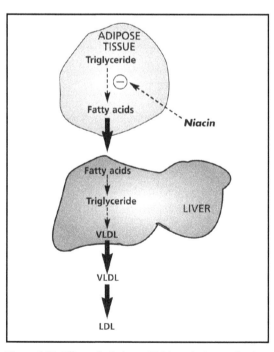

Figure 6.24: Effect of niacin on VLDL and LDL production. Niacin lowers conversion of triglycerides into fatty acids in adipose tissue. Ultimately, these fatty acids would be transformed into LDLs and VLDLs by the liver.

and tolerance; can increase to a maximum of 2 g/d but only at 500 mg/d at 4-week intervals; for niacin deficiency, 10-20 mg/d up to a maximum of 100 mg/d.

OMEGA-3-ACID ETHYL ESTERS, for *adults*, for hypertriglyceridemia, 4 g/d as a single daily dose or in 2 divided doses.

ADVERSE EFFECTS

Bile acid sequestrants commonly cause gastrointestinal disturbances including constipation, nausea, and flatulence. Colesevelam has fewer of these effects than others in this subclass. With the exception of colesevelam, these agents can, at high doses, interfere with the absorption of fat-soluble vitamins (A, D, E, and K).

Fibrates can cause abdominal distress, which lessens with use. They can increase the risk of cholelithiasis. Inflammation of muscles can occur, and any muscle weakness or pain should be investigated.

The most common complaint about niacin is that it produces an extremely uncomfortable flushing of the skin with a sensation of heat and intense itching. Patient compliance is a real concern due to this adverse effect. Taking aspirin before niacin may minimize this reaction. Other adverse effects include nausea, abdominal pain, and hyperuricemia, which can lead to gout.

RED FLAGS

Fibrates should not be used in pregnant or lactating women, or patients with hepatic or renal dysfunction or gallbladder disease.

Ezetimibe should not be used in patients with moderate to severe hepatic insufficiency.

INTERACTIONS

DRUG

With the exception of colesevelam, bile acid sequestrants can interfere with the intestinal absorption of many drugs including tetracycline, phenobarbital, digoxin, warfarin, pravastatin, fluvastatin, aspirin, and thiazide diuretics. These drugs should be taken 1 to 2 hours before, or 4 to 6 hours after bile acid sequestrants.

Fibrates may attenuate warfarin and sulfonylureas. An increased incidence of myopathy and rhabdomyolysis has been reported with concomitant use of gemfibrozil and lovastatin.

VITAMINS

Bile-acid sequestrants can interfere with absorption of fat-soluble vitamins (A, D, E, and K).

HERB

ANTICHOLESTEROL AGENTS

- *Da Suan* (Garlic) (D)–may potentiate cholesterol lowering agents as shown in meta-analysis of human clinical trials (Silagy & Neil, 1994) Level 5 evidence.
- *Hu Lu Ba* (Fenugreek) (D)–may potentiate cholesterol lowering agents as shown in several small human studies and one dog study (Mills & Bone, 2000) Level 5 evidence.

BILE-ACID SEQUESTRANTS

- *Hong Qu* (Red yeast rice) (D)–contains a precursor of lovastatin and should be taken 1 hour before or 4 hours after bile-acid sequestrants as they may decrease bioavailability of lovastatin, expert opinion (Chen & Chen, 2004) Level 5 evidence.

CHOLESTYRAMINE

- *Hong Qu* (Red yeast rice) (D)–contains a precursor of lovastatin and should be taken 1 hour before or 4 hours after bile-acid sequestrants as they may decrease bioavailability of lovastatin, expert opinion (Chen & Chen, 2004) Level 5 evidence.

GEMFIBROZIL

- *Hong Qu* (Red yeast rice) (D)–should not be used with gemfibrozil or lovastatin as severe rhabdomyolysis and myopathy have been reported, expert opinion (Chen & Chen, 2004) Level 5 evidence.

INTERACTION ISSUES

A: Theoretically, bile-acid sequestrants could interfere with absorption by binding with fat soluble drugs and herbs and excreting them.

D: Fenofibrate is over 99% protein bound; fenofibric acid is approximately 99% bound; gemfibrozil is 99% bound.

M: Fenofibric acid is a moderate inhibitor of

CYP2C9; gemfibrozil is a moderate inhibitor of CYP1A2 and a strong inhibitor of 2C8, 2C9, and 2C19.

E:

Pgp:

TI:

ENDNOTES

1. Combination of Benazepril and Hydrochlorothiazide.

2. Combination of Benazepril and Amlodipine.

3. Combination of Quinapril and Hydrochlorothiazide.

4. Combination of Trandolapril and Verapamil.

5. Combination of Candesartan and Hydrochlorothiazide.

6. Combination of Eprosartan and Hydrochlorothiazide.

7. Combination of Irbesartan and Hydrochlorothiazide.

8. Combination of Losartan and Hydrochlorothiazide.

9. Combination of Olmesartan and Hydrochlorothiazide.

10. Combination of Telmisartan and Hydrochlorothiazide.

11. Combination of Valsartan and Hydrochlorothiazide.

12. Combination of Bendroflumethiazide and Nadolol.

13. Combination of Chlorthalidone and Clonidine.

14. Combination of Atenolol and Chlorthalidone.

15. Combination of Hydrochlorothiazide and Triamterene.

16. Combination of Hydrochlorothiazide and Metoprolol.

17. Combination of Enalapril and Hydrochlorothiazide.

18. Combination of Dorzolamide and Timolol.

19. Combination of Dipyridamole and Aspirin.

20. Combination of Isosorbide and Hydralazine.

21. Combination of Amlodipine and Atorvastatin.

22. Combination of Lisinopril and Hydrochlorothiazide.

23. Combination of Trandolapril and Verapamil.

24. Combination of Aspirin and Dipyridmole.

25. Combination of Moexipril and Hydrochlorothiazide.

26. Combination of Olmesartan and Amlodipine.

27. Combination of Aspirin, Caffeine, and Butalbital, a barbiturate.

28. Combination of Butalbital, Aspirin, Caffeine, Codeine.

29. Combination of Oxycodone and Aspirin.

30. Combination of Olmesartan, Amlodipine, and Hydrochlorothiazide.

31. Combination of Telmisartan and Amlodipine.

32. Combination of Folic Acid, Cyanocobalamin, and Pyridoxine, all of which are vitamins.

33. Combination of Lovastatin and Niacin.

34. Combination of Ezetimibe and Simvastatin.

35. Combination of Valsartan and Amlodipine

36. Combination of Valsartan, Amlodipine, and Hydrochlorothiazide.

37. Combination of Aliskiren, Amlodipine, and Hydrochlorothiazide.

38. Combination of Aliskiren and Amlodipine.

39. Combination of Aliskiren and Hydrochlorothiazide.

40. Combination of Bisoprolol and Hydrochlorothiazide.

41. Combination of Hydrochlorothiazide and Spironolactone.

42. Combination of Azilsartan and Chlorthalidone.

43. Combination of Aspirin and Diphenhydramin.

44. Combination of Aspirin, Acetaminophen, and Caffeine.

45. Combination of Aspirin, Dihydrocodeine, and Caffeine.

46. The pregnancy risk of Coumadin is X except in women with mechanical heart valves where it is D.

47. Combination of Simvastatin and Sitagliptin.

48. Combination of Simvastatin and Niacin.

CHINESE MEDICAL DESCRIPTIONS

The Chinese medical explanation of the drug categories in this chapter may be found in Chapter 15 on pages 385–417.

Drugs Affecting the Endocrine System 7

At some level, almost everything involved with the endocrine system involves the hypothalamus and pituitary. A little review of this is therefore necessary before getting into the various drugs that affect the endocrine system.

The hypothalamus is part of the brain that, as its name implies, sits just below the thalamus. It generally secretes hormones (most often called releasing hormones) that directly affect the pituitary and drive release of pituitary hormones. Hypothalamic hormones include: growth hormone releasing hormone (GHRH), corticotropin releasing hormone (CRH), thyrotropin releasing hormone (TRH), gonadotropin releasing hormone (GnRH, also called LHRH, luteinizing hormone releasing hormone), prolactin inhibiting hormone (PIH, dopamine), and prolactin releasing hormone (PRH).

The hypothalamus is directly connected with the pituitary through the hypophyseal portal system. A portal system is a loop of the circulatory system that has two capillary beds rather than one. In this case, the first is in the hypothalamus and is where its hormones are released into the blood stream. The second is in the pituitary. This allows for a direct connection speeding up the action of the hypothalamic hormones' effects on the pituitary and maximizing the impact of the hormones. This happens since the hormones do not need to go through the entire circulatory system with only a very small fraction of the released hormone making it back to the pituitary.

The pituitary then releases an array of hormones affecting various areas of the body. These hormones are usually broken down into those released from the anterior pituitary and those released from the posterior. Anterior pituitary hormones include: growth hormone, adrenocorticotropic hormone (ACTH), thyrotropin stimulating hormone (TSH), follicle stimulating hormone (FSH), luteinizing hormone (LH), and prolactin. The hormones of the anterior pituitary cannot be administered orally, as they are peptide based and will be broken down in the digestive system before absorption. The posterior pituitary hormones are vasopressin and oxytocin.

This is summarized in Figure 7.1.

SECTION 1: HORMONES OF THE PITUITARY AND THYROID GLANDS

HORMONES OF THE POSTERIOR PITUITARY:

DESMOPRESSIN (des moe PRES in) PR=B *(DDAVP®, Stimate®)*

DRUGS AFFECTING THE THYROID:
LEVOTHYROXINE (lee voe thye ROKS ene) PR=A *(Levothroid®, Levoxyl®, Synthroid®, Tirosint®; Unithroid®)*

LIOTHYRONINE (lye oh THYE roe nene) PR=A *(Cytomel®, Triostat®)*

LIOTRIX (LYE oh triks) PR=A *(Thyrolar®)*

METHIMAZOLE (meth IM a zole) PR=D

(Tapazole®)

POTASSIUM IODIDE (poe TASS ee um EYE oh dide) PR=D *(iOSAT™ [O], SSKI® ThyroSafe® [O], Thyroshield® [O])*

PROPYLTHIOURACIL (proe pil thye oh YOOR a sil) PR=D

SODIUM IODIDE I¹³¹ (SOW dee um EYE oh dide) PR=X *(Hicon™, Iodotope®)*

THYROID (THYE roid) PR=A *(Armour® Thyroid, Nature-Throid™, Westhroid™)*

BETA-BLOCKERS: *(See Chapter 4, Section 8)*

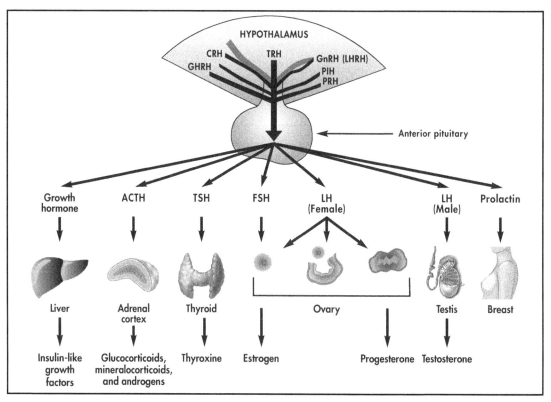

Figure 7.1 Hypothalamus hormones. This figure shows the hormones released from the hypothalamus and anterior pituitary as well as the target organs. GHRH: growth hormone releasing hormone, CRH: corticotropin releasing hormone, TRH: thyrotropin releasing hormone, GnRH: gonadotropin releasing hormone, PIH: prolactin inhibiting hormone, PRH: prolactin releasing hormone, ACTH: adrenocorticotropic hormone, TSH: thyrotropin stimulating hormone, FSH: follicle stimulating hormone, LH: luteinizing hormone.

FUNCTION

Desmopressin, when used orally, treats diabetes insipidus and primary nocturnal enuresis. Its hemostatic effects occur primarily through injection. It is an analogue of **endogenous** vasopressin.

The thyroid drugs break down into two major uses. Those in the first group, which includes levothyroxine, liothyronine, liotrix, and thyroid, are analogs to normal thyroid hormones and therefore promote the normal functioning of the thyroid and treat hypothyroidism. These drugs can also be used diagnostically to determine where in the hypothalamus-pituitary-thyroid axis there is pathology. Those in the second group, which includes methimazole, potassium iodide, propylthiouracil, and sodium iodide I^{131}, are antithyroid medications and work to blunt normal thyroid functioning or actually ablate it. They are used in treating hyperthyroidism.

Potassium iodide, in addition to aiding hyperthyroidism, is also used as an expectorant to thin mucus in the lungs and to prevent thyroid cancer after radiation exposure.

Sodium iodide I^{131} can also be used to test thyroid gland function and may treat specific cases of thyroid cancer. Generally, this causes permanent destruction of the thyroid gland, and patients often have to be on a pro-thyroid drug for the rest of their lives.

Beta-blockers that lack **sympathomimetic** activity, such as propranolol, can be used to blunt the effects of hyperthyroidism. In the case of thyroid storm, they are used intravenously. If beta-blockers are contraindicated, such as in patients with severe heart failure or asthma, the calcium channel blocker diltiazem is used.

Endogenous: Originating from within the body

Sympathomimetic: Either mimicking or stimulating the sympathetic nervous system

MECHANISM OF ACTION

Desmopressin is an analog of the endogenous hormone vasopressin and therefore has similar effects: water conservation, release of blood coagulation factors (VIII and von Willebrand), and possibly smooth muscle contraction in the gastrointestinal tract and vasculature. Water conservation occurs by increasing the permeability of collecting duct cells.

The pro-thyroid drugs primarily are animal or recombinant forms or analogues of the endogenous thyroid hormones, triiodothyronine (T3) and thyroxine (T4). Therefore these agents work similarly to their endogenous counterparts.

Propylthiouracil and methimazole are both thioamides and have similar actions. They become concentrated in the thyroid where they inhibit the addition of iodine to forming T3 and T4. Since thyroid hormone is stored in thyroglobulin, these agents may take a while to exert their effects as the release of thyroid hormone continues until these stores are dissipated.

Potassium iodide aids the treatment of hyperthyroidism by causing colloid accumulation in the thyroid follicles, which inhibits thyroid hormone formation. It reduces viscosity of mucus in the lungs and therefore aids expectoration. In radiation exposure, it competes for iodide uptake sites in the thyroid gland and reduces the uptake of radioisotopes, which can become concentrated in the thyroid gland and increase the risk of cancer. The free radioisotopes can be more easily excreted by the body.

Sodium iodide I^{131} works by being absorbed by the thyroid. In the case of diagnosis, small amounts are used with x-ray imaging to determine appropriate gland function. In large doses, the gland continues to absorb this agent, and the radiation destroys the gland and/or cancer.

DOSAGES

DESMOPRESSIN, for *children*, for diabetes insipidus, ≥4 years, initiate at 0.05 mg bid; total daily dose should be increased or decreased as needed to obtain adequate antidiuresis; usual range is 0.1-1.2 mg divided 2-3 times/d; for nocturnal enuresis, 0.2 mg nocte; dose may be titrated up to 0.6 mg to achieve desired response. For *children* ≥12 years and *adults*, for diabetes insipidus, initiate at 0.05 mg bid; increase or decrease total daily dose as needed to obtain adequate antidiuresis; usual range is 0.1-1.2 mg divided 2-3 times/d.

LEVOTHYROXINE, for *newborns*, for hypothyroidism, initiate at 10-15 mcg/kg/d; lower doses of 25 mcg/d should be considered in newborns at risk for cardiac failure; newborns with T4 levels <5 mcg/dL should be started at 50 mcg/d; adjust dose at 4- to 6-week intervals. For *infants* and *children*, for hypothyroidism, 0-3 months, 10-15 mcg/kg/d; 3-6 months, 8-10 mcg/kg/d; 6-12 months, 6-8 mcg/kg/d; 1-5 years, 5-6 mcg/kg/d; 6-12 years, 4-5 mcg/kg/d; over 12 years, 2-3 mcg/kg/d. For *adults*, for hypothyroidism, 1.7 mcg/kg/d in otherwise healthy adults <50 years old, *children* in whom growth and puberty are complete, and *older adults* who have been recently treated for hyperthyroidism or who have been hypothyroid for only a few months, increase dose every 6 weeks; average starting dose is approximately 100 mcg; usual doses are ≤200 mcg/d; doses ≥300 mcg/d are rare (consider poor compliance, malabsorption, and/or drug interactions); for severe hypothyroidism, initiate at 12.5-25 mcg/d, adjust dose by 25 mcg/d every 2-4 weeks as appropriate; for subclinical hypothyroidism (if treated), 1 mcg/kg/d; for TSH suppression, for well-differentiated thyroid cancer, highly individualized with doses >2 mcg/kg/d may be needed to suppress TSH to <0.1 mU/L; for benign nodules and nontoxic multinodular **goiter**, goal TSH suppression is 0.1-0.3 mU/L. For the *elderly*, for hypothyroidism, >50 years without cardiac disease or <50 years with cardiac disease, initiate at 25-50 mcg/d; adjust dose at 6- to 8-week intervals prn; for >50 years with cardiac disease, initiate at 12.5-25 mcg/d; adjust dose by 12.5-25 mcg increments at 4-6 week intervals.

Goiter: An enlarged thyroid gland. The gland may be hypo-, hyper- or euthyroid

LIOTHYRONINE, for *children*, for congenital hypothyroidism, 5 mcg/d; increase by 5 mcg every 3-4 days until the desired response is achieved; usual maintenance dose is 20 mcg/d for *infants*, 50 mcg/d for *children* 1-3 years of age, and adult dose for *children* >3 years. For *adults*, for hypothyroidism, 25 mcg/d; increase by increments of 12.5-25 mcg/d every 1-2 weeks up to a maximum of 100 mcg/d; usual maintenance dose is 25-75 mcg/d; for T3 suppression test, 75-100 mcg/d for 7 days; for **myxedema**, initiate at 5 mcg/d; increase in increments of 5-10 mcg/d every 1-2 weeks; when 25 mcg/d is reached, dosage may be increased at intervals of 5-25 mcg/d every 1-2 weeks; usual maintenance dose is 50-100 mcg/d; for simple (nontoxic) goiter, initiate at 5 mcg/d; increase by 5-10 mcg every 1-2 weeks, after 25 mcg/d is reached, may increase dose by 12.5-25 mcg; usual maintenance dose is 75 mcg/d. For the *elderly*, 5 mcg/d; increase by 5 mcg/d every 2 weeks.

Myxedema: The most severe form of hypothyroidism, may lead to coma or death

Euthyroid: A thyroid gland that is functioning within normal limits; not hypo- or hyperthyroid

LIOTRIX, for *children*, for congenital hypothyroidism, 0-6 months, 8-10 mcg/kg or 25-50 mcg/d; 6-12 months, 6-8 mcg/kg or 50-75 mcg/d; 1-5 years, 5-6 mcg/kg or 75-100 mcg/d; 6-12 years, 4-5 mcg/kg or 100-150 mcg/d; >12 years, 2-3 mcg/kg or >150 mcg/d. For *adults*, for hypothyroidism, 30 mg/d (15 mg/d if cardiovascular impairment), increasing by increments of 15 mg/d at 2-3-week intervals up to a maximum of 180 mg/d; usual maintenance dose is 60-120 mg/d. For the *elderly*, initiate at 15 mg; adjust dose at 2-4 week intervals by increments of 15 mg.

METHIMAZOLE, administer in 3 equally divided doses at approximately 8-hour intervals. For *children*, initiate at 0.4 mg/kg/d in 3 divided dose;, maintenance dose is 0.2 mg/kg/d in 3 divided doses up to 30 mg/d maximum; alternatively, initiate at 0.5-0.7 mg/kg/d or 15-20 mg/m^2/d in 3 divided doses; maintenance dose is one-third to two-thirds of the initial dose beginning when the patient is **euthyroid**, up to a maximum of 30 mg/d. For *adults*, initiate at 15 mg/d for mild hyperthyroidism; 30-40 mg/d in moderately severe hyperthyroidism; 60 mg/d in severe hyperthyroidism; maintenance range is 5-15 mg/d.

POTASSIUM IODIDE, for *children*, to reduce risk of thyroid cancer following nuclear accident (Iosat™, ThyroSafe™, ThyroShield™); dosing should continue until risk of exposure has passed or other measures are implemented, (see adult dose for *children* >68 kg); for *infants* <1 month, 16.25 mg once daily; for 1 month to 3 years, 32.5 mg once daily; for 3-18 years, 65 mg once daily; for thyrotoxic crisis, for *infants* <1 year, 150-250 mg (3-5 drops SSKI®) tid. For *children* and *adults*, for preoperative thyroidectomy, 50-250 mg (1-5 drops SSKI®) tid; administer for 10 days before surgery. For *adults*, as an expectorant, 325-650 mg tid; SSKI®, 300-600 mg 3-4 times/d; to reduce risk of thyroid cancer following nuclear accident (Iosat™, ThyroSafe™, ThyroShield™); dosing should continue until risk of exposure has passed or other measures are implemented; for *children* >68 kg and *adults* (including pregnant/lactating women), 130 mg once daily.

PROPYLTHIOURACIL, administer in 3 equally divided doses at approximately 8-hour intervals. For *children*, initiate at 5-7 mg/kg/d or 150-200 mg/m^2/d in divided doses every 8 hours; 6-10 years: 50-150 mg/d; over 10 years: 150-300 mg/d; maintenance is determined by patient response or one-third to two-thirds of the initial dose in divided doses every 8-12 hours. For *adults*, initiate at 300 mg/d tid; in patients with severe hyperthyroidism, very large goiters, or both, the initial dosage is usually 450 mg/d; an occasional patient will require 600-900 mg/d; maintenance range is 100-150 mg/d in divided doses every 8-12 hours. For the *elderly*, initiate at 150-300 mg/d. Therapy should be withdrawn gradually with evaluation of the patient every 4-6 weeks for the first 3 month, then every 3 months for the first year after discontinuation of therapy to detect any reoccurrence of a hyperthyroid state.

SODIUM IODIDE I¹³¹, for *adults*, for diagnostic procedures, thyroid uptake, 0.185-0.555 megabecquerels (5-15 microcuries); scintiscanning, 1.85-3.7 megabecquerels (50-100 microcuries); localization of extra-thyroid metastases, 37 megabecquerels (1000 microcuries); for treating hyperthyroidism, 148-370 megabecquerels (4-10 millicuries); for thyroid cancer, ablation of normal thyroid tissue, 1850 megabecquerels (50 millicuries); subsequent therapeutic doses, 3700-5500 megabecquerels (100-150 millicuries).

THYROID, for *children*, for congenital hypothyroidism, 0-6 mo, 15-30 mg, or 4.8-6 mg/kg,;6-12 mo, 30-45 mg, or 3.6-4.8mg/kg; 1-5 y, 45-60 mg, or 3-3.6 mg/kg; 6-12 y, 60-90 mg, or 2.4-3 mg/kg; >12 y, or >90 mg, 1.2-1.8 mg/kg. For *adults*, initiate at 15-30 mg; increase in 15 mg increments every 2-4 weeks; use 15 mg in patients with cardiovascular disease or myxedema; maintenance dose range is 60-120 mg/d.

ADVERSE EFFECTS

Desmopressin may cause various serious cardiovascular events including thrombosis and **myocardial infarction.** Minor complaints include various gastrointestinal and central nervous system effects.

The biggest adverse affect of the pro-thyroid drugs is that they can cause hyperthyroidism, or even **thyroid storm,** if there is a change in the dosing or just more in the blood circulation for any number of reasons. Dosing can be quite an issue and generally does not remain incredibly stable, so bouts of hypo- and hyperthyroidism occur with all the attendant symptoms including angina, arrhythmia, blood pressure changes, insomnia, anxiety, fatigue, fever, headache, irritability, nervousness, GI disturbances, **diaphoresis**, and heat intolerance, among others. Extreme adverse effects include myocardial infarction, heart failure, **angioedema**, and seizures.

Thyroid hormone blockers generally do not have a large amount of adverse effects but can, rarely, cause **agranulocytosis**, rash, and edema.

Potassium iodide side effects are relatively minor. These include rashes, a metallic taste in the mouth, a sore mouth and throat, and ulcers of the mucous membranes.

RED FLAGS

The pro-thyroid effects can become extreme and life threatening.

INTERACTIONS

DRUG

The pro-thyroid drugs use the P450 system for metabolism so any drugs that affect this system can affect these drugs. P450 inducers that can accelerate the thyroid hormones include phenytoin, rifampin, and phenobarbital.

HERB

ANTIHYPERTHYROIDS

- *Chen Pi* (Tangerine peel), *Qing Pi* (Citrus Viride), *Zhi Ke* (Aurantium fruit), *Zhi Shi* (Aurantium immaturus) (Indeterminate)–all these contain constituents that stimulate the sympathetic nervous system and should be used with caution in those taking antihypertensives, antidiabetic, antihyperthyroid, and/ or antiseizure medications (Chinese language article cited in Chen & Chen, 2004) Indeterminate level of evidence.

LEVOTHYROXINE

- *Dan Dou Chi* (Fermented soybean) (D)–may decrease the effects of levothyroxine, expert opinion (Gruenwald, Brendler & Jaenicke, 2004) Level 5 evidence.

INTERACTION ISSUES

A:
D: Levothyroxine is over 99% protein bound; T4 component of both liotrix and desiccated thyroid is over 99% bound.
M:
E:
Pgp:
TI:

Myocardial infarction: Necrosis of part of the heart muscle; heart attack

Thyroid storm: A crisis of uncontrolled hyperthyroidism characterized by high fever, rapid pulse, respiratory distress, apprehension, restlessness, and irritability; can lead to delirium, coma, or fatal heart failure

Diaphoresis: The act of perspiring or sweating

Angioedema: Large circumscribed area of subcutaneous edema of sudden onset frequently caused by an allergic reaction

Agranulocytosis: The extreme reduction in the number of leukocytes or white blood cells in the blood

SECTION 2: ANTIDIABETIC DRUGS

INSULINS

Rapid-acting

INSULIN ASPART (IN soo lin AS part) PR=B
(NovoLog®, NovoLog® Mix 70/30[28])

**INSULIN GLULISINE (IN soo lin gloo LIS ene)
PR=C** *(Apidra®)*

INSULIN LISPRO (IN soo lin LYE sproe) PR=C
*(Humalog®, Humalog® Mix 50/50™,[29]
Humalog® Mix 75/25™[30])*

Short-acting

**INSULIN REGULAR (IN soo lin REG yoo ler)
PR=B** *(Humulin® 50/50,[31] Humulin®70/30,[32]
Humulin® R (Concentrated) U-500, Humulin®
R, Novolin® 70/30,[32] Novolin® R)*

Intermediate-acting

INSULIN NPH PR=B *(Humulin® 50/50,[31]
Humulin® 70/30,[32] Humulin® N, Novolin®
70/30,[32] Novolin® N)*

Intermediate to long-acting

INSULIN DETEMIR (IN soo lin DE te mir) PR=B
(Levemir®)

Long-acting

INSULIN GLARGINE (IN soo lin GLAR jene) PR=C
(Lantus®)

ALPHA-GLUCOSIDASE INHIBITORS:

ACARBOSE (AY car bose) PR=B *(Precose®)*

MIGLITOL (MIG li tol) PR=B *(Glyset®)*

BIGUANIDES:

METFORMIN (met FOR min) PR=B
*(Actoplus Met®,[1] Actoplus Met® XR,[1]
Avandamet®,[2] Fortamet®, Glucophage®,
Glucophage® XR, Glucovance®,[5] Glumetza®,
Janumet®,[24] Janumet® XR,[24] Jentadueto™,[21]
Kazano™,[20] Kombiglyze™ XR, Metaglip™,[4]
PrandiMet®,[22] Riomet®)*

SGLT-2 INHIBITORS:

CANAGLIFLOZIN (KAN-a-gli-FLOW-zin) PR=C

(Invokana®)

DAPAGLIFLOZIN (DAP-a-gli-FLOw-zin) *PR=C*
(FarxigaTM)

EMPAGLIFLOZIN ((EM-pa-gli-FLOE-zin) *PR=C*
(Jardiance®)

DPP-IV INHIBITORS:

ALOGLIPTIN (al oh GLIP tin) PR=B
(Kazano™,[20] Nesina™, Oseni™[25])

LINAGLIPTIN (lin a GLIP tin) PR=B
(Jentadueto™,[21] Tradjenta™)

SAXAGLIPTIN (sax a GLIP tin) PR=B
(Kombiglyze™ XR,[23] Onglyza™)

SITAGLIPTIN (si TAG li pin) PR=B *(Janumet®,[24]
Janumet® XR,[24] Januvia®, Juvisync™[48])*

MEGLITINIDE DERIVATIVES:

NATEGLINIDE (na te GLYE nide) PR=C *(Starlix®)*

REPAGLINIDE (re pa GLI nide) PR=C
(PrandiMet®,[22] Prandin®)

SULFONYLUREAS:

CHLORPROPAMIDE (klor PROE pa mide) PR=C

GLIMEPIRIDE (GLYE me pye ride) PR=C
(Amaryl®, Avandaryl®,[27] Duetact™[26])

GLIPIZIDE (GLIP i zide) PR=C *(Glucotrol®,
Glucotrol® XL, Metaglip™)*

GLYBURIDE (GLYE byoor ide) PR=B/C
(DiaBeta®, Glucovance®,[5] Glynase®, PresTab®)

TOLAZAMIDE (tole AZ a mide) PR=C

TOLBUTAMIDE (tole BYOO ta mide) PR=C

THIAZOLIDINEDIONES *(aka peroxisome pro-
liferator-actived receptor [PPAR] gamma agonists)*

PIOGLITAZONE (pye oh GLI ta zone) PR=C
*(Actoplus Met®,[1] Actoplus Met® XR,[1] Actos®,
Duetact™,[26] Oseni,[25])*

ROSIGLITAZONE (roh si GLI ta zone) PR=C
(Avandamet™,[2] Avandaryl™,[3] Avandia®)

Diabetes mellitus (DM) is a disease of increased blood glucose. In type I, this is due to lack of insulin production in the pancreas and usually starts early in childhood. Type 2 usually affects older adults, though age of onset is becoming earlier and is caused by a combination of insulin resistance (lack of receptors on cells) and inadequate production of insulin by the pancreas. Type 2 is considered one of the fastest growing diseases of modern societies, affecting 20 million people in the United States, and is caused by genetic factors, aging, and obesity. Treatment of type 1 includes lifelong injections of insulin analogs. Type 2 may be treated by insulin injections in advanced cases but can be controlled by dietary changes, weight loss, exercise, and a variety of medications that are covered in this class of drugs. Table 7.1 summarizes the differences between Type I and II diabetes mellitus.

Insulin is a polypeptide hormone. Injected insulins in the past have been derived from beef or pork pancreas and had many side effects. Currently most injectable insulins are derived from human

	MECHANISM OF ACTION	EFFECT ON PLASMA INSULIN	RISK OF HYPO-GLYCEMIA	COMMENTS
First-generation sulfonylureas Tolazamide Tolbutamide Chlorpropramide	Stimulates insulin secretion	Increases	Yes	Weight gain can occur. Well-established history of effectiveness.
Second-generation Glimepiride Glipizide Glyburide	Stimulates insulin secretion	Increases	Yes	Weight gain can occur. Well-established history of effectiveness.
Meglitinide analogs Nateglinide Repaglinide	Stimulates insulin secretion	Increases	Yes (rarely)	Short action with less hypoglycemia either at a missed meal or at night.
SGLT-2 inhibitors Canagliflozin Dapagliflozin Empagliflozin	Inhibits reabsorption of glucose resulting in greater urinary excretion	No change	No	Often, has become the second drug after metformin fails to adequately control plasma levels.
Biguanides Metaformin	Decreased endogenous hepatic production of glucose	Decreases	No	Agent of first choice for Type 2 diabetes. Weight loss may occur. Established history of effectiveness.
Thiazolidinediones (glitazones) Pioglitazone Rosiglitazone	Binds to peroxisome proliferator-activated receptor-γ in muscle, fat, and liver to decrease insulin resistance	Greatly decreases	No	Effective in highly insulin-resistant patients. Once-daily dosing.
α–Glucosidase inhibitors Acarbose Miglitol	Decreased glucose absorption	Minimal or no change	No	Taken with meals. Adverse gastro-intestinal effects.
DPP-IV inhibitors Alogliptin Lindagliptin Sitagliptin	Decreases secretion of glucagon. Increases glucose-dependent insulin release	Increases	No	Well tolerated. Once-daily dosing. May be taken with or without food.

Figure 7.2: Summary of **antidiabetic agents** and their effects and risks of hypoglycemia.

	Type 1	Type 2
Age of onset	Usually childhood or puberty	Commonly over age 35
Nutritional status	Undernourished	Usually obese
Prevalence	5-10% of diabetics	90-95% of diabetics
Genetic predisposition	Moderate	Very strong
Pathology	No insulin production due to destroyed β (beta) cells	Insulin resistance, reduced β cell production of insulin, other defects

Table 7:1 This table shows major differences between type 1 and type 2 diabetes mellitus.

recombinant DNA. By making a few changes in the amino acid sequence, insulins used in the treatment of diabetes can have different pharmacokinetic properties and can be shorter or longer acting than regular insulin. Since polypeptides are rapidly broken down in the gastrointestinal tract, administration of insulin cannot be oral and is currently injected subcutaneously. Exubra, an inhaled insulin, was taken off the market in October 2007 after being introduced in January 2006. Pfizer, the pharmaceutical company, pulled the agent after poor consumer adoption and poor sales. In April 2008, it was announced that it could increase the risk of lung cancer.

FUNCTION

These drugs reduce blood glucose levels through various means. Insulins are used as the primary intervention in diabetes type 1 and as treatment of last choice when type 2 diabetes becomes severe enough. They are analogs of endogenous insulin normally secreted by the pancreas.

Metformin is considered the drug of choice for type 2 diabetics because it not only reduces glucose in the blood but has beneficial cardiac effects such as lowering hyperlipidemia. It may also cause weight loss by causing loss of appetite. It is the only oral hypoglycemic agent shown to decrease mortality from cardiovascular causes.

Sodium-glucose cotransporter 2 (SGLT2) inhibitors have become a common drug in the arsenal against type II DM. Since they have relatively few side effects, many of which are actually beneficial (such as lowering blood pressure), they have often become the next drug added after metformin does not show enough control. They are particularly useful in that

they do not work until blood glucose levels are relatively high. They therefore do not cause hypoglycemia.

Metformin and thiazolidinediones are used to lower the insulin resistance in women with polycystic ovary disease and supports ovulation and pregnancy.

DPP-IV inhibitors are a relatively recent class of antidiabetic for type II DM that can be monotherapy or combined with metformin or a thiazolidinedione.

MECHANISM OF ACTION

Insulins are analogs of endogenous insulin and act similarly to normally occurring insulin. While the mechanism of action may be similar, their pharmacokinetics, how fast they act, and how long they remain in the body may differ.

All oral hypoglycemic agents can be broken down into two major categories: those that increase the secretion of insulin and those that do not. This is an important distinction as those agents that do cause insulin release have the serious adverse effect of potentially causing hypoglycemia, while the others do not. A summary of which classes of drugs cause insulin release as well as a summary of their mechanisms of action and effects is in Figure 7.2 on the previous page.

Alpha-glucosidase inhibitors act by inhibiting α-glucosidase on the intestinal brush border. This enzyme breaks down **oligosaccharides** into glucose and other sugars for absorption. The overall effect of this inhibition is to blunt the **postprandial** increase of glucose in the blood. Acarbose also inhibits pancreatic α-amylase, which breaks down starches into oligosaccharides.

Biguanides, of which metformin is the only one currently available, act by inhibiting **gluconeogenesis** in the liver. This in turn decreases the overall output of glucose from the liver and ultimately the level of glucose in the blood.

Sodium-glucose cotransporter 2 (SGLT2) inhibitors act on SGLT2 in the proximal renal tubule of the nephron. Inhibition of this cotransporter prevents reabsorption of glucose from the lumen of the tubule causing greater urinary excretion of glucose and reduction of blood glucose levels.

DPP-IV inhibitors work by inhibiting the DPP-IV enzyme, which inactivates incretin. Therefore these agents increase the active levels of incretin, which ultimately causes an increase in insulin synthesis and release from pancreatic beta cells and decreases glucagon secretion from pancreatic alpha cells. Lowered **glucagon** secretion results in decreased hepatic glucose production. Under normal physiologic, circumstances, incretin hormones are released by the intestine throughout the day, and levels are increased in response to a meal.

Meglitinide derivatives and sulfonylureas act on the pancreas similarly. While they have slightly different binding sites, they both bind to and block ATP-sensitive potassium channels. This results in depolarization and calcium influx and release of insulin from the β-cells of the pancreas.

While this explains the mechanism of action for both of these agents, they do have significant differences. Meglitinide derivatives have a faster onset and shorter duration than sulfonylureas and are more effective in the rapid insulin increase that occurs just after eating. Therefore, these agents are considered postprandial glucose regulators.

Sulfonylureas also reduce glucagon levels and increase binding of insulin to target tissues and receptors.

While the exact mechanism of action of thiazolidinediones is not quite understood, it is known that they affect peroxisome proliferator-activated receptor-γ (PPARγ), which plays a role in fat cell production, secretion of fatty acids, and

glucose metabolism. These effects result in increased sensitivity of insulin receptors in the fat cells, liver, and skeletal muscles. These drugs also have beneficial effects on **hypertriglyceridemia** and HbA1C, a marker for long-term **hyperglycemia**. Both agents in this category raise HDL, but LDL is not affected by pioglitazone, and rosiglitazone raises it. Both agents increase subcutaneous fat.

DOSAGES

ACARBOSE, for *adults*, initiate at 25 mg tid with the first bite of each main meal; maintenance dose should be adjusted at 4-8 week intervals based on 1-hr postprandial glucose levels and tolerance; may be increased from 25 mg tid to 50 mg tid; some patients may benefit from increasing the dose to 100 mg tid; maintenance dose range is 50-100 mg tid; maximum dose: ≤60 kg, 50 mg tid, >60 kg, 100 mg tid.

ALOGLIPTIN. 25 mg once daily.

CANAGLIFLOZIN, for adults, initiate at 100 mg once daily prior to first meal of the day; may increase to 300 mg as needed.

CHLORPROPAMIDE, for *adults*, initiate at 250 mg/d in mild-to-moderate diabetes in middle-aged, stable diabetics. For the *elderly*, initiate at 100-125 mg/d. Subsequent dosages may be increased or decreased by 50-125 mg/d at 3-5 day intervals; usual maintenance dose is 100-250 mg/d; severe diabetics may require 500 mg/d; avoid doses over 750 mg/d.

DAPAGLIFLOZIN, for adults, initiate at 5 mg once daily prior to first meal of the day; may increase to 10 mg as needed.

GLIMEPIRIDE, for *adults*, initiate at 1-2 mg once daily, administered with breakfast or the first main meal; usual maintenance dose is 1-4 mg once daily; after a dose of 2 mg once daily, increase in increments of 2 mg at 1-2 week intervals based upon the patient's blood

Oligosaccharids: A compound made up of a small number of monosaccharides such as glucose

Postprandial: After a meal

Gluconeogenesis: The formation of glucose from fatty acids and proteins rather than carbohydrates

Glucagon: A pancreatic hormone that causes the breakdown of glycogen and elevates serum glucose levels

Hypertriglyceridemia: Abnormally high amounts of triglycerides in the blood

Hyperglycemia: Too much glucose in the blood

glucose response to a maximum of 8 mg once daily.

GLIPIZIDE, allow several days between dose titrations. For *adults*, initiate at 5 mg/d; adjust dosage at 2.5-5 mg daily increments as determined by blood glucose response at intervals of several days; immediate release tablet: maximum recommended once-daily dose is 15 mg; extended release tablet (Glucotrol® XL): maximum recommended dose is 20 mg. For the *elderly*, initiate at 2.5 mg/d, increase by 2.5-5 mg/d at 1-2 week intervals.

GLYBURIDE, for *adults*, initiate at 2.5-5 mg/d, administered with breakfast or the first main meal of the day; in patients who are more sensitive to hypoglycemic drugs, start at 1.25 mg/d; increase in increments of no more than 2.5 mg/d at weekly intervals based on the patient's blood glucose response; maintenance dose is 1.25-20 mg/d given as single or divided doses up to a maximum of 20 mg/d; For the *elderly*, initiate at 1.25-2.5 mg/d; increase by 1.25-2.5 mg/d every 1-3 weeks. Micronized tablets (Glynase®, PresTab®): for *adults*, initiate at 1.5-3 mg/d, administered with breakfast or the first main meal of the day; in patients who are more sensitive to hypoglycemic drugs, start at 0.75 mg/d; increase in increments of no more than 1.5 mg/d in weekly intervals based on patient's blood glucose response; maintenance range is 0.75-12 mg/d given as a single dose or in divided doses; some patients (especially those receiving over 6 mg/d) may have a more satisfactory response with twice-daily dosing.

INSULINS, doses for insulins vary greatly among individuals and their diets. While standard protocols exist, they are supposed to be modified according to frequent blood glucose readings. In general, doses include combinations of various insulins with different pharmacokinetics. These are often broken down into three broad categories.

Rapid-onset and ultrashort-acting preparations are used to give an insulin just before or after a meal to prevent hyperglycemia from a meal. Naturally occurring insulin would fall into this category. Intermediate-acting insulins and prolonged-acting insulin preparations are longer-acting insulins that prevent a large peak of insulin but provide a longer-term, lower level of insulin. Standard treatment involves a combination of rapid-onset and longer-acting insulins twice daily.

LINAGLIPTIN, for *adults*, for type 2 diabetes, 5 mg once daily.

METFORMIN, allow 1-2 weeks between dose titrations. Generally, clinically significant responses are not seen at doses under 1500 mg daily; however, a lower recommended starting dose and a gradually increased dosage are recommended to minimize gastrointestinal symptoms. For children 10-16 years, for management of type 2 diabetes mellitus, initiate at 500 mg bid (given with the morning and evening meals); increases in daily dosage should be made in increments of 500 mg at weekly intervals, given in divided doses, up to a maximum of 2000 mg/d. For adults ≥17 years, for management of type 2 diabetes mellitus, initiate at 500 mg bid (give with the morning and evening meals) or 850 mg once daily; increase dosage incrementally, increasing dosing recommendations based on dosage form: 500 mg tablet, one tablet/d at weekly intervals; 850 mg tablet: one tablet/d every other week; oral solution, 500 mg bid every other week. Doses of up to 2000 mg/d may be given twice daily; if a dose over 2000 mg/d is required, it may be better tolerated in 3 divided doses. Maximum recommended dose is 2550 mg/d. Extended release tablet: initiate at 500 mg once daily (with the evening meal); dosage may be increased by 500 mg weekly; up to a maximum dose of 2000 mg once daily; if glycemic control is not achieved at maximum dose, may divide dose to 1000 mg bid; if doses over 2000 mg/d are needed, switch to regular release tablets and increase to maximum dose of 2550 mg/d. For the *elderly*, initial and maintenance dosing should be conservative, due to the potential for decreased renal function; generally, *elderly* patients should not be increased to the maximum dose of metformin; do not use in patients over 80 years of age unless normal renal function has been established.

MIGLITOL, for *adults*, 25 mg tid with the first bite of food at each meal; the dose may be increased to 50 mg tid after 4-8 weeks; maximum recommended dose is 100 mg tid.

NATEGLINIDE, for *adults*, for management of type 2 diabetes mellitus, initial and maintenance dose is 120 mg tid 10-30 minutes before meals; patients close to HbA1c goal may be started at 60 mg tid.

PIOGLITAZONE, for *adults*, initiate at 15-30 mg once daily, if response is inadequate, the dosage may be increased in increments up to 45 mg once daily up to a maximum recommended dose of 45 mg once daily.

REPAGLINIDE, for *adults*, should be taken within 15 minutes of the meal, but time may vary from immediately preceding the meal to as long as 30 minutes before the meal; for patients not previously treated or whose HbA1c is <8%, the starting dose is 0.5 mg; for patients previously treated with blood glucose lowering agents whose HbA1c is ≥8%, the initial dose is 1-2 mg before each meal; determine dosing adjustments by blood glucose response, usually fasting blood glucose; may double the preprandial dose up to 4 mg until satisfactory blood glucose response is achieved; at least 1 week should elapse to assess response after each dose adjustment; usual dose range is 0.5-4 mg taken with meals; may be dosed preprandial 2, 3, or 4 times/d in response to changes in the patient's meal pattern; maximum recommended daily dose is 16 mg.

ROSIGLITAZONE, initiate at 4 mg daily as a single daily dose or in divided doses twice daily; if response is inadequate after 8-12 weeks of treatment, the dosage may be increased to 8 mg daily as a single daily dose or in divided doses twice daily.

SAXAGLIPTIN, for *adults*, for type 2 diabetes, 2.5-5 mg once daily.

SITAGLIPTIN, for *adults*, for Type 2 diabetes, 100 mg once daily.

TOLAZAMIDE, for *adults*, for type 2 diabetes, doses over 500 mg/d should be given in 2 doses; initiate at 100-250 mg/d with breakfast or the first main meal of the day; can increase in increments of 100-250 mg/d at weekly intervals, maximum dose is 1 g.

TOLBUTAMIDE, initiate at 1-2 g/d as a single dose in the morning or in divided doses throughout the day; total doses may be taken in the morning; however, divided doses may allow increased gastrointestinal tolerance, maintenance dose is 0.25-3 g/d; however, a maintenance dose >2 g/d is seldom required. For the *elderly*, initiate at 250 mg 1-3 times/d; usual range is 500-2000 mg up to a maximum of 3 g/d.

ADVERSE EFFECTS

As mentioned above, one of the more serious adverse effects of the drugs that increase insulin secretion is the possibility of developing hypoglycemia. This can happen with sulfonylureas and meglitinide derivatives and possibly DPP-IV inhibitors. Theoretically DPP-IV inhibitors increase plasma levels of insulin. However, pre-marketing studies show an approximately equal rate of hypoglycemia between those on an inhibitor and those on a placebo.

Adverse reactions to injected insulin include **lipodystrophy** and allergic reactions. Only regular insulin is considered safe to use during pregnancy.

> Lipodystrophy: A medical condition characterized by abnormal or degenerative conditions of the body's adipose tissue

Sulfonylureas can cause weight gain, hyperinsulinemia, and hypoglycemia. These agents are contraindicated in patients with liver or kidney impairment.

While meglitinide derivatives can cause hypoglycemia, they appear to do so less frequently than sulfonylureas. The incidence of weight gain is also less in these agents. They should be used with caution in patients with liver impairment.

Biguanides tend to cause GI disturbances. Rarely, lactic acidosis has occurred and been fatal. For this reason, diabetics being treated with medications for heart failure should not take metformin. Long-term use may lower vitamin B12 absorption. These drugs are contraindicated in diabetics with liver or kidney disease, cardiac or respiratory insufficiency, severe infection, pregnancy, or a history of alcohol abuse.

Sodium-glucose cotransporter 2 (SGLT2) inhibitors, because of the increased amount of glucose in the urine, can cause a greater chance of urinary tract infections and genitourinary fungal infections. Since they may increase urinary output, they also can cause thirst and hypotension.

DPP-IV inhibitors can cause headache, upper respiratory tract infections (URTIs), and nasopharyngitis. One of the original thiazolidinediones, troglitazone, now discontinued, caused deaths due to liver toxicity. Because of this, it is recommended that patients on other drugs in this class be regularly monitored for aberrations in their liver enzymes. Weight gain can occur due to increased subcutaneous fat and/or fluid retention. Because of this potential for fluid retention, caution should be exercised when these agents are used in heart-failure patients. Other adverse effects include anemia and headache.

Alpha-glucosidase inhibitors commonly cause GI disturbances such as flatulence, diarrhea, and cramping. They are contraindicated in patients with inflammatory bowel disease (IBD), colon ulcers, or intestinal obstruction.

▮ RED FLAGS

Insulin, sulfonylureas, and meglitinide derivatives can commonly cause hypoglycemia, which can be life threatening. Symptoms include tachycardia, confusion, vertigo, and **diaphoresis**. DPP-IV may also cause hypoglycemia.

Diaphoresis: The state of perspiring profusely

▮ INTERACTIONS

DRUG

Many drugs can interact with the insulins to either decrease or increase their hypoglycemic effects. The following may decrease hypoglycemic effects: oral contraceptives, corticosteroids, dextrothyroxine, diltiazem, dobutamine, niacin, smoking, thiazide diuretics, and thyroid hormone. Alcohol may increase hypoglycemic effects as can alph- and beta-blockers, clofibrate, guanethidine, MAO inhibitors, pentamidine, phenylbutazone, salicylates, sulfinpyrazone, and tetracyclines.

Many drugs can potentiate the hypoglycemic effects of sulfonylureas. This is caused by many mechanisms. Clofibrate, phenylbutazone, salicylates, and sulfonamides potentiate sulfonylureas by displacing them from plasma proteins. Allopurinol, probenacid, phenylbutazone, salicylates, and sulfonamides decrease the urinary excretion. And dicumerol, chloramphenicol, monoamine oxidase inhibitors, and phenylbutazone reduce metabolism of sulfonylureas in the liver.

Repaglinide utilizes the CYP3A4 enzyme for metabolism; drugs that inhibit this enzyme may potentiate the hypoglycemic effects of these agents. These include ketoconazole, itraconazole, erythromycin, fluconazole, and clarithromycin. Drugs such as barbiturates, carbamazepine, and rifampin that increase the levels of CYP3A4 may inhibit the hypoglycemic effects. In addition, combining repaglinide with gemfibrozil may cause severe hypoglycemia.

Metformin's effects may be potentiated by cimetidine, furosemide, nifedipine, and other drugs.

Combining thiazolidinediones and oral contraceptive pills (OCP) should be done with caution as these agents can reduce blood concentrations of the contraceptives.

Alpha-glucosidase inhibitors may decrease the bioavailablity of metformin, and these agents should not be used together.

HERB

ANTIDIABETIC MEDICATIONS

- *Bai Shao* (White peony root) (D)–may lower plasma glucose levels and may potentiate antidiabetic medications causing hypoglycemia (Chen, 1998/1999) Level 5 evidence.
- *Cang Er Zi* (Xanthium fruit, Siberian cocklebur fruit) (D)–lower plasma glucose levels and may potentize antidiabetic medications

causing hypoglycemia (Chen, 1998/1999) Level 5 evidence.

- *Cang Zhu* (Atractylodes) (D)–lowers plasma glucose levels and may potentize antidiabetic medications causing hypoglycemia (Chen, 1998/1999) Level 5 evidence.
- *Chen Pi* (Tangerine peel), *Qing Pi* (Citrus Viride), *Zhi Ke* (Aurantium fruit, bitter orange), *Zhi Shi* (Aurantium immaturus) (Indeterminate)–all these contain constituents that stimulate the sympathetic nervous system. Use with caution in those taking antihypertensive, antidiabetic, antihyperthyroid, and/or antiseizure medications (Chinese language article cited in Chen & Chen, 2004) Indeterminate level of evidence.
- *Ci Wu Jia* (Siberian ginseng) (D)–may po-tentiate effects of antidiabetic medications as shown in an animal study (Hikino, Takahashi, Otake & Konno, 1986) Level 5 evidence.
- *Da Suan* (Garlic) (D)–lowers plasma glucose levels in mice and may potentiate antidiabetic medications causing hypoglycemia (Chen, 1998/1999) Level 5 evidence.
- *Di Gu Pi* (Lycium root bark, Chinese wolfberry root bark) (D)–lowers plasma glucose levels in rabbits and may potentiate antidiabetic medications causing hypoglycemia (Chen, 1998/1999) Level 5 evidence.
- *Gan Cao* (Licorice) (D)–may reduce the effects of antidiabetic medications causing hyperglycemia, expert opinion (Gruenwald, Brendler & Jaenicke, 2004) Level 5 evidence.
- *Ge Gen* (Pueraria root) (D)–lowers plasma glucose levels and may potentize antidiabetic medications causing hypoglycemia (Chen, 1998/1999) Level 5 evidence.
- *Hu Lu Ba* (Fenugreek seed) (D)–may lower plasma glucose levels and potentiate antidiabetic medications causing hypoglycemia, expert opinion (Gruenwald, Brendler & Jaenicke, 2004) Level 5 evidence.
- *Hu Zhang* (Polygonum cuspidatum) (D)–lowers plasma glucose levels and may potentiate antidiabetic medications causing hypoglycemia (Chen, 1998/1999) Level 5 evidence.

- *Ku Gua* (Bitter melon) (D)–lowers plasma glucose levels and may potentiate antidiabetic medications causing hypoglycemia, expert opinion based on extrapolations of other studies (Brinker, 2001) Level 5 evidence.
- *Kun Bu* (Laminaria, kelp) (D)–lowers plasma glucose levels and may potentiate antidiabetic medications causing hypoglycemia (Chen, 1998/1999) Level 5 evidence.
- *Li Zhi He* (Lychee seed) (D)–lowers plasma glucose levels and may potentiate antidiabetic medications causing hypoglycemia (Chen, 1998/1999) Level 5 evidence.
- *Lu Hui* (Aloe) (D)–may lower plasma glucose levels and potentiate antidiabetic medications causing hypoglycemia, expert opinion (Gruenwald, Brendler & Jaenicke, 2004) Level 5 evidence.
- *Mai Ya* (Barley sprouts) (D)–lowers plasma glucose levels and may potentiate antidiabetic medications causing hypoglycemia (Chen, 1998/1999) Level 5 evidence.
- *Mo Yao* (Myrrh) (D)–may have hypoglycemic effects and interfere with antidiabetic medications, expert opinion (Gruenwald, Brendler & Jaenicke, 2004) Level 5 evidence.
- *Niu Bang Zi* (Arctium, burdock seed) (D)–lowers plasma glucose levels and may potentize antidiabetic medications causing hypoglycemia (Chen, 1998/1999) Level 5 evidence.
- *Nu Zhen Zi* (Ligustrum, glossy privet herb) (D)–lowers plasma glucose levels; may potentiate antidiabetic medications causing hypoglycemia (Chen, 1998/1999) Level 5 evidence.
- *Ren Shen* (Ginseng) (D)–may cause hypoglycemia when used with diabetes mellitus drugs due to association with reduction of fasting blood glucose levels, expert opinion (Chen & Chen, 2004) Level 5 evidence.
- *Shan Yao* (Dioscorea, common yam rhizome) (D)–lowers plasma glucose levels; may potentiate antidiabetic medications causing hypoglycemia (Chen, 1998/1999) Level 5 evidence.
- *Xuan Shen* (Scrophularia, figwort root) (D)–lowers plasma glucose levels in rabbits; may potentize antidiabetic medications causing

hypoglycemia (Chen, 1998/'99) Level 5 evidence.

- *Zhi Mu* (Anemarrhena) (D)–lowers plasma glucose levels and may potentize antidiabetic medications causing hypoglycemia (Chen, 1998/1999) Level 5 evidence.

GLIPIZIDE, GLYBURIDE

- *Bai Shao* (White peony root) (D)–may lower plasma glucose levels and may potentiate antidiabetic medications causing hypoglycemia (Chen, 1998/1999) Level 5 evidence.
- *Ban Lan Gen* (Isatis root, indigo woad root) (D)–those allergic to sulfonylureas and sulfonamides may also be allergic to *Ban Lan Gen*, expert opinion (Chen & Chen, 2004) Level 5 evidence.
- *Cang Er Zi* (Xanthium fruit, Siberian cocklebur fruit) (D)–lower plasma glucose levels and may potentize antidiabetic medications causing hypoglycemia (Chen, 1998/1999) Level 5 evidence.
- *Cang Zhu* (Atractylodes) (D)–lowers plasma glucose levels and may potentize antidiabetic medications causing hypoglycemia (Chen, 1998/1999) Level 5 evidence.
- *Chen Pi* (Tangerine peel), *Qing Pi* (Citrus Viride), *Zhi Ke* (Aurantium fruit, bitter orange), *Zhi Shi* (Aurantium immaturus) (Indeterminate)–all contain constituents that stimulate the sympathetic nervous system and should be used with caution in those taking antihypertensives, antidiabetic, antihyperthyroid, and/or antiseizure medications (Chinese language article cited in Chen & Chen, 2004) Indeterminate level of evidence.
- *Ci Wu Jia* (Siberian ginseng) (D)–may potentiate the effects of antidiabetic medications as shown in an animal study (Hikino, Takahashi, Otake & Konno, 1986) Level 5 evidence.
- *Da Qing Ye* (Isatis leaves, indigo woad leaves) (D)–those allergic to sulfonylureas and sulfonamides may also be allergic to *Da Qing Ye*, expert opinion (Chen & Chen, 2004) Level 5 evidence.
- *Da Suan* (Garlic) (D)–lowers plasma glucose levels in mice and may potentiate antidiabetic

medications causing hypoglycemia (Chen, 1998/1999) Level 5 evidence.

- *Di Gu Pi* (Lycium root bark, Chinese wolfberry root bark) (D)–lowers plasma glucose levels in rabbits and may potentiate antidiabetic medications causing hypoglycemia (Chen, 1998/1999) Level 5 evidence.
- *Gan Cao* (Licorice) (D)–may reduce the effects of antidiabetic medications causing hyperglycemia, expert opinion (Gruenwald, Brendler & Jaenicke, 2004) Level 5 evidence.
- *Ge Gen* (Pueraria root) (D)–lowers plasma glucose levels and may potentize antidiabetic medications causing hypoglycemia (Chen, 1998/1999) Level 5 evidence.
- *Hu Lu Ba* (Fenugreek seed) (D)–may lower plasma glucose levels and potentiate antidiabetic medications causing hypoglycemia, expert opinion (Gruenwald, Brendler & Jaenicke, 2004) Level 5 evidence.
- *Hu Zhang* (Polygonum cuspidatum) (D)–lowers plasma glucose levels and may potentiate antidiabetic medications causing hypoglycemia (Chen, 1998/1999) Level 5 evidence.
- *Ku Gua* (Bitter melon) (D)–lowers plasma glucose levels and may potentiate antidiabetic medications causing hypoglycemia, expert opinion based on extrapolations of other studies (Brinker, 2001) Level 5 evidence.
- *Kun Bu* (Laminaria, kelp) (D)–lowers plasma glucose levels and may potentiate antidiabetic medications causing hypoglycemia (Chen, 1998/1999) Level 5 evidence.
- *Li Zhi He* (Lychee seed) (D)–lowers plasma glucose levels and may potentiate antidiabetic medications causing hypoglycemia (Chen, 1998/1999) Level 5 evidence.
- *Lu Hui* (Aloe) (D)–may lower plasma glucose levels and potentiate antidiabetic medications causing hypoglycemia, expert opinion (Gruenwald, Brendler & Jaenicke, 2004) Level 5 evidence.
- *Mai Ya* (Barley sprouts) (D)–lowers plasma glucose levels and may potentiate antidiabetic medications causing hypoglycemia (Chen, 1998/1999) Level 5 evidence.

- *Mo Yao* (Myrrh) (D)–may have hypoglycemic effects and interfere with antidiabetic medications, expert opinion (Gruenwald, Brendler & Jaenicke, 2004) Level 5 evidence.
- *Niu Bang Zi* (Arctium, burdock seed) (D)–lowers plasma glucose levels and may potentize antidiabetic medications causing hypoglycemia (Chen, 1998/1999) Level 5 evidence.
- *Nu Zhen Zi* (Ligustrum, glossy privet herb) (D)–lowers plasma glucose levels; may potentiate antidiabetic medications causing hypoglycemia (Chen, 1998/1999) Level 5 evidence.
- *Qing Dai* (Indigo) (D)–those allergic to sulfonylureas and sulfonamides may also be allergic to *Qing Dai,* expert opinion (Chen & Chen, 2004) Level 5 evidence.
- *Ren Shen* (Ginseng) (D)–may cause hypoglycemia when used with diabetes mellitus drugs due to association with reduction of fasting blood glucose levels, expert opinion (Chen & Chen, 2004) Level 5 evidence.
- *Shan Yao* (Dioscorea, common yam rhizome) (D)–lowers plasma glucose levels; may potentiate antidiabetic medications causing hypoglycemia (Chen, 1998/1999) Level 5 evidence.
- *Xi Yang Shen* (American ginseng) (C)–reduced blood sugar levels in seven type 2 diabetics who were being treated with sulfonylureas or both sulfonylureas and metformin when the powdered root was given prior to a glucose challenge test (Vuksan *et al.,* 2000) Level 3b evidence.
- *Xuan Shen* (Scrophularia, figwort root) (D)–Lowers plasma glucose levels in rabbits; may potentize antidiabetic medications causing hypoglycemia (Chen, 1998/1999) Level 5 evidence.
- *Zhi Mu* (Anemarrhena) (D)–lowers plasma glucose levels and may potentize antidiabetic medications causing hypoglycemia (Chen, 1998/1999) Level 5 evidence.

INSULIN
- *Bai Guo (Ye)* (Gingko leaf) (C)–a small study showed potential interference with insulin metabolism in normal individuals. Theoretically, may alter blood glucose levels and affect insulin use (Kudolo, 2000) Level 2b evidence.

- *Bai Shao* (White peony Root) (D)–may lower plasma glucose levels and may potentiate antidiabetic medications causing hypoglycemia (Chen, 1998/1999) Level 5 evidence.
- *Cang Er Zi* (Xanthium fruit, Siberian cocklebur fruit) (D)–lower plasma glucose levels and may potentiate antidiabetic medications causing hypoglycemia (Chen, 1998/1999) Level 5 evidence.
- *Cang Zhu* (Atractylodes) (D)–lowers plasma glucose levels and may potentiate antidiabetic medications causing hypoglycemia (Chen & Chen, 2004) Level 5 evidence.
- *Che Qian Zi*–may inhibit carbohydrate absorption and necessitate changes in insulin dosage (Chen & Chen, 2004)
- *Ci Wu Jia* (Siberian ginseng) (D)–may potentiate the effects of antidiabetic medications as shown in an animal study (Hikino, Takahashi, Otake & Konno, 1986) Level 5 evidence.
- *Da Suan* (Garlic) (D)–lowers plasma glucose levels in mice and may potentiate antidiabetic medications causing hypoglycemia (Chen, 1998/1999) Level 5 evidence.
- *Di Gu Pi* (Lycium root bark, Chinese wolfberry root bark) (D)–lowers plasma glucose levels in rabbits and may potentiate antidiabetic medications causing hypoglycemia (Chen, 1998/1999) Level 5 evidence.
- *Gan Cao* (Licorice) (D)–may reduce effects of antidiabetic medications causing hyperglycemia (Gruenwald, Brendler & Jaenicke, 2004) Level 5 evidence.
- *Ge Gen* (Pueraria root) (D)–Lowers plasma glucose levels and may potentiate antidiabetic medications causing hypoglycemia (Chen, 1998/1999) Level 5 evidence.
- *Hu Lu Ba* (Fenugreek seed) (D)–may lower plasma glucose levels and potentiate antidiabetic medications causing hypoglycemia (Gruenwald, Brendler & Jaenicke, 2004) Level 5 evidence.
- *Hu Zhang* (Polygonum cuspidatum) (D)–lowers plasma glucose levels and may potentiate antidiabetic medications causing hypoglycemia (Chen, 1998/1999) Level 5 evidence.

- *Ku Gua* (Bitter melon) (B)–lowers plasma glucose levels and may potentiate antidiabetic medications causing hypoglycemia (Leatherdale, Panesar, Singh, Atkins, Bailey & Bignell, 1981) Level 2C evidence; (Welihinda, Karunanayake, Sheriff & Jayasinghe, 1986), Level 2C evidence; (Srivastava, Venkatakrishna-Bhatt, Verma, Venkaiah & Raval, 1993) Level 5 evidence.
- *Kun Bu* (Laminaria, kelp) (D)–lowers plasma glucose levels and may potentiate antidiabetic medications causing hypoglycemia (Chen, 1998/1999) Level 5 evidence.
- *Li Zhi He* (Lychee seed) (D)–lowers plasma glucose levels and may potentiate antidiabetic medications causing hypoglycemia (Chen, 1998/1999) Level 5 evidence.
- *Lu Hui* (Aloe) (D)–may lower plasma glucose levels and potentiate antidiabetic medications causing hypoglycemia (Gruenwald, Brendler & Jaenicke, 2004) Level 5 evidence.
- *Mai Ya* (Barley sprouts) (D)–lowers plasma glucose levels and may potentiate antidiabetic medications causing hypoglycemia (Chen, 1998/1999) Level 5 evidence.
- *Mo Yao* (Myrrh) (D)–may have hypoglycemic effects and interfere with antidiabetic medications (Gruenwald, Brendler & Jaenicke, 2004) Level 5 evidence.
- *Niu Bang Zi* (Arctium, burdock seed) (D)–lowers plasma glucose levels and may potentiate antidiabetic medications causing hypoglycemia (Chen, 1998/1999) Level 5 evidence.
- *Nu Zhen Zi* (Ligustrum, glossy privet herb) (D)–lowers plasma glucose levels; may potentiate antidiabetic medications causing hypoglycemia (Chen, 1998/1999) Level 5 evidence.
- *Qing Pi* (Citrus Viride) (Indeterminate)–contains constituents that stimulate the sympathetic nervous system. Use with caution in those taking antihypertensive, antidiabetic, antihyperthyroid, and antiseizure medications (Chen & Chen, 2004) Indeterminate level of evidence.
- *Ren Shen* (Ginseng) (D)–may cause hypoglycemia when used concomitantly with diabetes mellitus drugs due to association with reduction of fasting blood glucose levels (Chen & Chen, 2004) Level 5 evidence.
- *Shan Yao* (Dioscorea, common yam rhizome) (D)–lowers plasma glucose levels; may potentiate antidiabetic medications causing hypoglycemia (Chen, 1998/1999) Level 5 evidence.
- *Xi Yang Shen* (American ginseng) (D)–may alter the effects of insulin as inferred from a mice study (Oshima, Sato & Hikino, 1987) Level 5 evidence.
- *Xuan Shen* (Scrophularia, figwort root) (D)–lowers plasma glucose levels in rabbits; may potentiate antidiabetic drugs causing hypoglycemia (Chen, 1998/1999) Level 5 evidence.
- *Zhi Mu* (Anemarrhena) (D)–lowers plasma glucose levels and may potentiate antidiabetic medications causing hypoglycemia (Chen, 1998/1999) Level 5 evidence.

METFORMIN

- *Xi Yang Shen* (American ginseng) (C)–reduced blood sugar levels in seven type 2 diabetics who were being treated with sulfonylureas or both sulfonylureas and metformin when the powdered root was given prior to a glucose challenge test (Vuksan *et al.*, 2000) Level 3b evidence.

SULFONYLUREAS

The herb interactions for these drugs are the same as the list for **Glipizide** and **Glyburide** shown above.

TOLBUTAMIDE

The herb interactions for these drugs are the same as the list for **Glipizide** and **Glyburide** shown above, with the following additions:

- *Chai Hu* (in *Xiao Chai Hu Tang* formula, not as an individual herb) (Bupleurum, Chinese throwax root) (D)–shown to decrease overall bioavailability of tolbutamide in rats (Nishimura, Naora, Hirano & Iwamoto, 1999) Level 5 evidence.
- *Yin Guo Ye* (Gingko) (D)–decreases blood concentrations of this medication (Izzo & Ernst, 2009) Level 2b evidence.

INTERACTION ISSUES

A:

D: Canagliflozin is 99% protein bound;

glimepiride is over 99.5% protein bound; glipizide is 98 to 99% bound; glyburide is over 99% bound; nateglinide is 98% protein bound; pioglitazone is over 99% bound; repaglinide is over 98% bound; rosiglitazone is 98.8% bound; tolbutamide is approximately 95% bound.

M: Chlorpropamide, glimepiride, glipizide, and glyburide are major substrates of CYP2C9; linagliptin is a major substrate of CYP3A4; nateglinide is a major substrate of CYP 2C9 and 3A4; pioglitazone is major substrate and

a moderate inhibitor of CYP2C8 and a weak/moderate inducer of 3A4; Repaglinide is a major substrate of CYP2C8 and 3A4; rosiglitazone is a major substrate and a moderate inhibitor of CYP2C8; saxagliptin is a major substrate of CYP3A4; tolbutamide is a major substrate and a strong inhibitor of CYP2C9.

E:

Pgp: Linagliptin, saxagliptin, and sitagliptin are substrates of Pgp.

TI:

SECTION 3: SEX HORMONES

ANDROGENS:

DANAZOL (DA na zole) PR=X

FLUOXYMESTERONE (floo oks i MES te rone) PR=X *(Androxy™)*

METHYLTESTOSTERONE (meth il tes TOS te rone) PR=X *(Android®, Covaryx®,[11] Covaryx® H.S.,[11] EEMT™,[11] EEMT™ HS,[11] Estratest®,[11] Methitest™, Testred®, Syntest D.S.,[11] Virilon®)*

OXANDROLONE (oks AN droe lone) PR=X *(Oxandrin®)*

OXYMETHOLONE (oks i METH oh lone) PR=X *(Anadrol®[50])*

TESTOSTERONE (tes TOS ter own) PR=X *(Androderm®, AndroGel®, Axiron®, Delatestryl®, Depo®-Testosterone, First®-Testosterone, First®-Testosterone MC, Fortesta™, Striant®, Testim®, Testopel®)*

ANTIANDROGENS:

ABIRATERONE ACETATE (a bir A ter own AS e tate) PR=X *(Zytiga®)*

BICALUTAMIDE (bye ka LOO ta mide) PR=X *(Casodex®)*

DUTASTERIDE (doo TAS teer ide) PR=X *(Avodart®, Jalyn™[33])*

ENZALUTAMIDE (en za LOO ta mide) PR=X *(Xtandi®)*

FINASTERIDE (fi NAS teer ide) PR=X *(Propecia®, Proscar®)*

FLUTAMIDE (FLOO ta mide) PR=D

NILUTAMIDE (ni LOO ta mide) PR=C *(Nilandron®)*

ANTIPROGESTIN:

MIFEPRISTONE (mi FE pris tone) PR=X *(Korlym™, Mifeprex®)*

ESTROGENS:

ESTRADIOL (es tra DYE ole) PR=X *(Activella®,[6] Alora®, Angeliq®,[7] Climara®, ClimaraPro®,[8] CombiPatch®,[6] Delestrogen®, Depo®-Estradiol, Divigel®, Elestrin®, Estrace®, Estrasorb®, Estring®, EstroGel®, Evamist®, Femring®, Femtrace®, Menostar®, Mimvey™,[6] Minivelle™, Natazia®,[34] Prefest™,[9] Vagifem®, Vivelle-Dot®)*

ESTROGENS (Conjugated A/Synthetic) (ES troe jenz) PR=X *(Cenestin®)*

ESTROGENS (Conjugated B/Synthetic) (ES troe jenz) PR=X *(Enjuvia™)*

ESTROGENS (Conjugated/Equine) (ES troe jenz) PR=X *(Premarin®, Premphase®,[10] Prempro™[10])*

ESTROGENS (Esterified) (ES troe jenz) PR=X *(Covaryx®,[11] Covaryx® H.S.,[11] EEMT™,[11] EEMT™ HS,[11] Menest®)*

ESTROPIPATE (ES troe pih pate) PR=X *(Ogen®)*

ETHINYL ESTRADIOL (ETH in il es tra DYE ole) PR=X *(Altavera™,[12] Alyacen 1/35,[19] Alyacen 7/7/7,[19] Amethia™,[12] Amethia™ Lo,[12] Amethyst™,[12] Apri®,[13] Aranelle®,[19] Aviane™,[12] Azurette™,[13] Balziva™,[19]*

...continued on the following page

SECTION 3: SEX HORMONES cont.

Beyaz™,[37] Brevi-con®,[19] Briellyn,[19] Camrese™,[12] Caziant®; Chateal™,[12] Cryselle® 28,[15] Cyclafem™ 1/35,[19] Cyclafem™ 7/7/7,[19] Cyclessa®,[13] Dasetta™ 1/35,[19] Dasetta™ 7/7/7,[19] Daysee™,[12] Deso-gen®,[13] Emoquette™,[13] Enpresse®,[12] Esta-rylla™,[17] Estrostep® Fe,[19] Falmina™,[12] Fem-con® Fe,[19] femhrt®,[19] femhrt® Lo,[19] Gen- eress™ Fe,[19] Gianvi™,[18] Gildess® FE 1.5/30,[19] Gildess® FE 1/20,[19] Introvale™,[12] Jinteli™,[19] Jolessa™,[12] Junel® 1.5/30,[19] Junel® 1/20,[19] Junel® Fe 1.5/30,[19] Junel® Fe 1/20,[19] Kari-va®,[13] Kelnor™,[16] Kurvelo™,[12] Leena®,[19] Levonest™,[12] Levora®,[12] Lo Lessina®,[12] Lo/Ov-ral®-28,[15] Loestrin®,[21] Loestrin™ Fe,[19] Loes-trin®21 1/20,[19] Loestrin® 24 Fe,[19] Loestrin® Fe 1.5/30,[19] Loestrin® Fe 1/20,[19] Loryna™,[18] LoSeason-ique®,[12] Lutera®,[12] Low-Oges-trel®,[15] Lybrel®,[12] Marlissa,[12] Microges-tin®1.5/30,[19] Microgestin® 1/20,[19] Micro-gestin® Fe 1.5/30,[19] Microgestin® Fe 1/20,[19] Mircette®,[13] Modicon®,[19] MonoNessa®,[17] Myzilra™,[12] Natazia®, Necon® 0.5/35,[19] Necon® 1/35,[19] Necon® 10/11,[19] Necon® 7/7/7,[19] Norinyl® 1+35,[19] Nortrel® 0.5/35,[19] Nortrel®1/35,[19] Nortrel® 7/7/7,[19] NuvaRing®,[35] Ocella™,[18] Ogestrel®,[15] Orsythia™,[12] Ortho-Cept®,[13] Ortho-Cyclen®,[17] Ortho Evra®,[36] Ortho-Novum® 1/35,[19] Ortho-Novum® 7/7/7,[19] Ortho Tri-Cyclen®,[17] Ortho Tri-Cyclen® Lo,[17] Ovcon® 35,[19] Portia®,[12] Previfem®,[17] Quasense®,[12] Safyral™,[37] Seasonique®,[12] Sprintec®,[17] Sronyx®,[12] Trivora® Reclipsen®,[13] Syeda™,[18] Tilia™ Fe,[19] Tri-Estarylla™,[17] Tri-Legest™ Fe,[19] Tri-Norinyl®,[19] Tri-Previfem®,[17] Tri-Sprintec®,[17] TriNessa®,[17] Velivet™,[13] Vestura™,[18] Viorele,[13] Wera™,[19] Wymzya™ Fe,[19] Yasmin®,[18] Yaz®,[18] Zarah®,[18] Zenchent®,[19] Zenchent Fe™,[19] Zeosa™,[19] Zovia®[16])

LEVOMEFOLATE (lee voe me FOE late) PR=X

PROGESTINS:

DESOGESTREL (des oh JES trel) PR=X
(Apri®,[13] Azurette™,[13] Caziant®,[13] Cyclessa®,[13] Desogen®,[13] Emoquette™,[13] Kariva™,[13] Mircette®,[13] Ortho-Cept®,[13] Reclipsen™,[13] Velivet™,[13] Viorele[13])

DROSPIRENONE (droh SPYE re none) PR=X
(Angeliq®,[7] Beyaz™,[37] Gianvi™,[18] Loryna™,[18] Ocella™,[18] Safyral™,[37] Syeda™,[18] Vestura™,[18] Yasmin®,[18] Yaz,[18] Zarah®[18])

ETHYNODIOL DIACETATE (e thye noe DYE ole dye AS e tate) PR=X *(Kelnor™,[16] Zovia™[16])*

ETONOGESTREL (e toe noe JES trel) PR=N
(Implanon, Nexplanon)

HYDROXYPROGESTERONE CAPROATE (hye droks ee proe JES te rone CAP ro ate) PR=B
(Makena)

LEVONORGESTREL (LEE voe nor jes trel) PR=X
(Altavera™,[12] Amethia™,[12] Amethia™ Lo,[12] Amethyst™,[12] Aviane™,[12] Camrese™,[12] Cha-teal™,[12] ClimaraPro®,[8] Daysee™,[12] Enpresse®,[12] Falmina™,[12] Introvale™,[12] Jolessa™,[12] Kurvelo™,[12] Lessina®,[12] Levo-nest™,[12] Levora®,[12] LoSeasonique®,[12] Lutera®,[12] Lybrel®,[12] Marlissa,[12] Mirena, My Way, Myzilra™,[12] Next Choice 1-Dose, Orsy-thia™,[12] Plan B, Plan B 1-Step, Portia®,[12] Quasense®,[12] Seasonique®,[12] Skyla, Sronyx®,[12] Trivora®[12])

MEDROXYPROGESTERONE (me DROKS ee proe JES te rone) PR=X *(Depo-Provera®, Depo-SubQ Provera 104, Premphase®,[10] Prempro™,[10] Provera®)*

MEGESTROL (me JES trole) PR=D (tablet)/X (suspension) *(Megace® ES, Megace® Oral)*

MESTRANOL (MES tra nole) PR=X *(Necon® 1/50,[19] Norinyl®1+50[19])*

NORETHINDRONE (nor eth IN drone) PR=X
(Activella®,[6] Alyacen 1/35,[14] Alyacen 7/7/7,[14] Aranelle®,[14] Aygestin, Balziva™,[14] Brevi-con®,[14] Briellyn,[14] Camila, CombiPatch®,[6] Cyclafem™ 1/35,[14] Cyclafem™ 7/7/7,[14] Da-setta™ 1/35,[14] Dasetta™ 7/7/7,[14] Errin, Estro-step® Fe,[14]Femcon® Fe,[14] femhrt®,[14] femhrt® Lo,[14] Generess™ Fe,[14] Gildess® FE 1.5/30,[14] Gildess® FE 1/20,[14] Heather, Jinteli™,[14] Joli-vette, Junel® 1.5/30,[14] Junel® 1/20,[14] Junel® Fe 1.5/30,[14] Junel® Fe 1/20,[14] Leena®,[14] Lo Loes-trin™ Fe,[14] Loestrin®,[21] 1.5/30,[14] Loestrin® 21 1/20,[14] Loestrin® 24 Fe,[14] Loestrin® Fe 1.5/30,[14] Loestrin® Fe 1/20,[14] Microgestin® 1.5/30,[14]

Microgestin® 1/20,[14] Microgestin® Fe 1.5/30,[14] Microgestin® Fe 1/20,[14] Mimvey™,[6] Modicon®,[14] Necon® 0.5/35,[14] Necon® 1/35,[14] Necon® 1/50,[19] Necon® 10/11,[14] Necon® 7/7/7,[14] Norinyl® 1+35,[14] Nor-QD, Nora-BE, Norinyl® 1+50,[19] Nortrel® 0.5/35,[14] Nortrel® 1/35,[14] Nortrel® 7/7/7,[14] Ortho Micronor, Ortho-Novum® 1/35,[14] Ortho-Novum® 7/7/7,[14] Ovcon® 35,[14] Tilia™ Fe,[14] Tri-Legest™ Fe,[14] Tri-Norinyl®,[14] Wera™,[14] Wymżya™ Fe,[14] Zenchent®,[14] Zenchent Fe™,[14] Zeosa™[14])

NORGESTIMATE (nor JES ti mate) PR=X *(Estarylla™,[17] MonoNessa®,[17] Ortho-Cyclen®,[17] Ortho Tri-Cyclen®,[17] Ortho Tri-Cyclen® Lo,[17] Previfem®,[17] Sprintec®,[17] Tri-Estarylla™,[17] Tri-Previfem®,[17] Tri-Sprintec®,[17] TriNessa®[17])*

NORGESTREL (nor JES trel) PR=X *(Cryselle®-28,[15] Lo/Ovral®-28,[15] Low-Ogestrel®,[15] Ogestrel®[15])*

PROGESTERONE (proe JES ter one) PR=B *(Crinone, Endometrin, First-Progesterone VGS 100, First-Progesterone VGS 200, First-Progesterone VGS 25, First-Progesterone VGS 400, First-Progesterone VGS 50, Prometrium)*

SELECTIVE ESTROGEN RECEPTOR MODULATORS (SERMS):

CLOMIPHENE (KLOE mi fene) PR=X *(Clomid®, Serophene®)*

OSPEMIFENE (os PEM i fene) PR=X *(Osphena)*

RALOXIFENE (ral OKS i fene) PR=X *(Evista®)*

TAMOXIFEN (ta MOKS i fen) PR=D *(Soltamox™)*

TOREMIFENE (TORE em i fene) PR=D *(Fareston®)*

OTHER:

DINOPROSTONE (dye noe PROST one) PR=C *(Cervidil®, Prepidil®, Prostin E2®)*

ULIPRISTAL (ue li PRIS tal) PR=X *(Ella)*

Sex hormones, in general, are used for a variety of reasons. **Endogenous** hormones are used for conception, embryonic growth, and primary and secondary sexual traits. The agents in this category are used as replacement therapy, menopausal symptom relief, for osteoporosis, for treatment of malignancies, and as contraception. They are all derived from cholesterol.

Contraception is a very common use of these agents. They are used in many forms including injection, implantables, topical agents, and orally in oral contraceptive pills (OCP). They can be used postcoitally as well. This section of the book will emphasize the oral use of these agents.

OCPs are usually estrogen and progestin or progestin alone. The typical method of use is to be three weeks on the OCP and one week off for a "withdrawal" bleed (see Figure 7.3). One brand can be used for 12 weeks straight and 1 week off, allowing menses to occur 4 times a year, and other OCPs are also used in this way, though this has only been recently approved. OCP use is among the best choices for contraception, having only a .3% pregnancy rate when properly used, lower than any other method. Progestin-alone OCPs are not as effective as the combination pills and are used when the combination pills cannot be tolerated or when there are contraindications for their use.

Another consideration for OCP choice is choosing a monophasic, biphasic, or triphasic formulation. This terminology refers to the ratio between the estrogen component and the progestin component. In monophasic formulations, this ratio does not change. In biphasic formulations, there are 2 ratios of mixtures that change during the month. In triphasic there are 3 different ratios of estrogen to progestin components used. The main advantages of bi- and triphasic preparations are an overall smaller dose of hormones and possibly some decreased adverse effects.

Endogenous: Originating from within the body

Hypogonadism: A lack of secretion of sex hormones from the testes or ovaries

FUNCTION

Androgens are primarily used to treat reduced androgen production in men, which is either primary, due to **hypogonadism**, or secondary, for example a dysfunction of the hypothalamic-

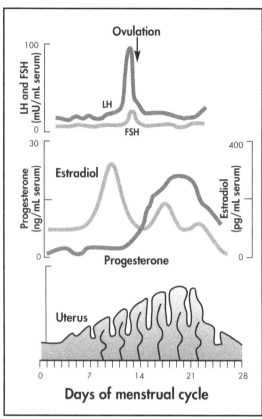

Figure 7.3 This figure shows hormone levels and thickness of uterine lining at various stages of the menstrual cycle.

cases of replacement in postmenopausal women, it is usually used with progestin, as this combination reduces the risk for endometrial cancer in long-term use. However in women who are postmenopausal due to surgical removal of the uterus, estrogen is generally used alone in order to avoid an unfavorable shift in the HDL/LDL ratio. Hormone replacement can also be beneficial in preventing osteoporosis. Combination therapy is also employed in young women (11-13 years old) who have hypogonadism.

Progestins are commonly used in contraception and to treat hormone deficiency. They are also used to treat dysfunctional uterine bleeding, dysmenorrhea, suppression of postpartum lactation, endometriosis, and malignancy of the endometrium. Megestrol is used in treating breast and endothelial carcinomas.

Selective estrogen receptor modulators act by attaching to estrogen receptors. Tamoxifen and toremifene are both used to treat estrogen receptor positive breast cancers. Tamoxifen may increase the risk of endometrial cancer, while toremifene does not increase this risk. Raloxifene is used in preventing osteoporosis in postmenopausal women. While it does reduce the incidence of breast cancer in postmenopausal women, it is currently not approved for treating it. Clomiphene stimulates the ovaries to treat infertility. Dinoprostone is used to terminate pregnancy and to promote cervical ripening when inducing labor.

MECHANISM OF ACTION

Androgens act in similar ways to other steroid hormones in that they bind nuclear receptors and stimulate synthesis of RNA and proteins. In the muscle and liver, testosterone is the main chemical that initiates this. However in other tissues, it needs to be metabolized to other chemicals before being able to exert their actions. 5-α-dihydrotestosterone (DHT) and estradiol are two of these possible active metabolites.

Antiandrogens have several mechanisms of action. Finasteride and dutasteride both inhibit the enzyme 5-α-reductase, which converts testosterone to DHT, an active metabolite. The decrease of DHT results in less androgen activa-

pituitary axis. They can also be used for their **anabolic** effects in treating osteoporosis in the elderly, severe burns, the **catabolic** effects of adrenocortical hormones, or to speed recovery from surgery or chronic disease. They can be used to treat pituitary dwarfism in prepubertal males. Danazol can be used to treat endometriosis.

Most antiandrogens are used to treat metastatic prostate cancer. There are exceptions to this, however. For example, dutasteride and finasteride are used to treat benign prostatic hypertrophy (BPH).

Mifepristone, the most common antiprogestin, is used as an abortifacient and can be used up to 49 days into pregnancy to terminate it. It is often combined with a prostaglandin-like misoprostol for this purpose.

Estrogens are primarily used for contraception, as postmenopausal hormone replacement, and for primary hypogonadism. For contraception and

Anabolism: Biological processes that primarily build up large compounds from smaller chemicals

Catabolism: Biological processes that primarily break down large storage and other chemicals, often releasing energy in the process

tion. Many of the others are straight competitive inhibitors of androgens.

The antiprogestin mifepristone acts as a straight progestin receptor antagonist with some agonist activity. It also engages in antiglucocorticoid and antiandrogenic action by blocking the negative feedback of cortisol on corticotropin release.

Estrogen acts on two main estrogen receptors: α and β. They are both receptors that affect DNA transcription into RNA and ultimately regulate protein production. The α subtype activates transcription and is much more prevalent than the repressive β subtype. They have different affinities for different domains of the DNA and are selectively activated depending on the exact structure of the activating estrogen.

Progestins act in similar ways as other steroid hormones and activate DNA transcription into RNA and proteins. They have a specific effect on several tissues. In the liver, they increase glycogen stores, probably through an insulin-like effect. In the kidneys, they compete with aldosterone and cause a decrease in sodium reabsorption. They can increase the body's temperature, though the exact mechanism is unknown. They also decrease some plasma amino acids and increase excretion of urinary nitrogen.

The exact mechanism of action for contraception is not completely understood, but it is thought that estrogen provides negative feedback on the pituitary and prevents LH and FSH release that stimulates ovulation. No ovulation means no release of the ovum so that it can be fertilized by sperm and therefore no pregnancy. Progestin thickens the cervical mucus and thereby prevents access by sperm. It also stimulates normal bleeding at the end of the menstrual cycle.

Selective estrogen receptor modulators (SERMs) act by, as their name implies, modulating the activity of estrogen receptors. This means these agents can agonize or antagonize individual receptors depending on the specific tissue where the receptor is located. For example, tamoxifen acts as an estrogen antagonist in breast cancer tissue and as a partial agonist in the uterus. Clomiphene acts as a partial estrogen agonist to interfere with negative feedback on the hypothalamus and pituitary by estrogens. This increases gonadotropin-releasing hormone, ultimately stimulating ovulation.

Dinoprostone is an endogenous prostaglandin. When used as an abortifacient, it causes uterine contractions similar to natural labor. When used during labor induction, it relaxes the cervix allowing dilation facilitating passage of the fetus through the birth canal.

DOSAGES

ABIRATERONE ACETATE, for *adults*, for prostate cancer, metastatic, castration-resistant, 1000 mg once daily.

BICALUTAMIDE, for metastatic prostate cancer, 50 mg once daily (in combination with an LHRH analogue).

CLOMIPHENE, for *female* ovulatory failure, 50 mg/d for 5 days (first course); start the regimen on or about the fifth day of cycle; dose should be increased only in those patients who do not ovulate in response to cyclic 50 mg Clomid®; a low dosage or duration of treatment course is particularly recommended if unusual sensitivity to pituitary gonadotropin is suspected, such as in patients with polycystic ovary syndrome; if ovulation does not appear to occur after the first course of therapy, a second course of 100 mg/d (two 50 mg tablets given as a single daily dose) for 5 days should be given; this course may be started as early as 30 days after the previous one after precautions are taken to exclude the presence of pregnancy; increasing the dosage or duration of therapy beyond 100 mg/d for 5 days is not recommended.

DANAZOL, for female endometriosis, initiate at 100-200 mg/d bid for mild disease; usual maintenance dose is 400 mg/d bid to achieve amenorrhea and rapid response to painful symptoms; continue therapy uninterrupted for 3-6 months and up to 9 months; for female fibrocystic breast disease, usual range is 50-200 mg/d bid. For *both men and women*, for hereditary angioedema, initiate at 200 mg 2-3 times/d;

after favorable response, decrease the dosage by 50% or less at intervals of 1-3 months or longer if the frequency of attacks dictates; if an attack occurs, increase the dosage by up to 200 mg/d.

DESOGESTREL, used only in combination with other drugs, and therefore its individual dosing is not covered here.

DINOPROSTONE, for *adults*, as an abortifacient, vaginal suppository: insert 20 mg (1 suppository) high in vagina; repeat at 3-5 hour intervals until abortion occurs; administration for longer than 2 days not advisable; for cervical ripening, endocervical gel: using catheter supplied with gel, insert 0.5 mg into the cervical canal. May repeat every 6 hours if needed up to a maximum cumulative dose of 1.5 mg/d; vaginal insert: insert 10 mg transversely into the posterior fornix of the vagina; remove at the onset of active labor or after 12 hours.

DROSPIRENONE, used only in combination with other drugs, and therefore its individual dosing is not covered here.

DUTASTERIDE, for *men*, 0.5 mg once daily.

ENZALUTAMIDE, for *adults*, for prostate cancer, metastatic, castration-resistant, 160 mg once daily.

ESTRADIOL, all dosage needs to be adjusted based upon the patient's response. For *men* with prostate cancer (androgen-dependent, inoperable, progressing), 10 mg tid for at least 3 months; for breast cancer (inoperable, progressing in appropriately selected patients), 10 mg tid for at least 3 months; for osteoporosis prophylaxis in postmenopausal females, 0.5 mg/d in a cyclic regimen (3 weeks on and 1 week off); for female hypoestrogenism (due to hypogonadism, castration, or primary ovarian failure), 1-2 mg/d; increase as necessary to control symptoms using minimal effective dose for maintenance therapy; for moderate to severe vasomotor symptoms associated with menopause, 1-2 mg/d, adjusted as necessary to limit symptoms; administration should be cyclic (3 weeks on, 1 week off).

ESTROGENS (Conjugated A/Synthetic), the lowest dose that will control symptoms should be used;

medication should be discontinued as soon as possible. For *adults*, for moderate-to-severe vasomotor symptoms, 0.45 mg/d; may be increased up to 1.25 mg/d; attempts to discontinue medication should be made at 3- to 6-month intervals; for vulvar and vaginal atrophy, 0.3 mg/d.

ESTROGENS (Conjugated B/Synthetic), the lowest dose that will control symptoms should be used; medication should be discontinued as soon as possible. For *adults*, moderate-to-severe vasomotor symptoms associated with menopause, 0.3 mg/d; may be increased up to 1.25 mg/d; attempts to discontinue medication should be made at 3-6 month intervals.

ESTROGENS (Conjugated/Equine), for *adults*, for male androgen-dependent prostate cancer palliation, 1.25-2.5 mg tid. For *women*, for prevention of postmenopausal osteoporosis, initiate at 0.3 mg/d 3 weeks on/1 week off or daily; the lowest effective dose should be used; for moderate-to-severe vasomotor symptoms associated with menopause, initiate at 0.3 mg/d, 3 weeks on/1 week off or daily; the lowest dose that will control symptoms should be used; for vulvar and vaginal atrophy, initiate at 0.3 mg/d, 3 weeks on/1 week off or daily; the lowest dose that will control symptoms should be used; medication should be discontinued as soon as possible; for abnormal acute/heavy uterine bleeding, 1.25 mg; may repeat every 4 hours for 24 hours, followed by 1.25 mg once daily for 7-10 days; for nonacute/lesser bleeding, 1.25 mg once daily for 7-10 days; for female hypogonadism, 0.3-0.625 mg/d given 3 weeks on/1 week off; dose may be increased in 6-12 month intervals; progestin treatment should be added to maintain bone mineral density once skeletal maturity is achieved; for female castration and primary ovarian failure, 1.25 mg/d given 3 weeks on/1 week off; adjust according to severity of symptoms and patient response; for maintenance, adjust to the lowest effective dose.

ESTROGENS (Esterified), for *adults*: for prostate cancer (palliation), 1.25-2.5 mg tid; for female hypogonadism, 2.5-7.5 mg of estrogen daily for 20 days followed by a 10-day rest period; administer cyclically (3 weeks on and 1 week off), for moderate to severe vasomotor symptoms associated with menopause, 1.25 mg/d administered cyclically (3 weeks on and 1 week off), for short-term use only and should be discontinued as soon as possible, re-evaluate at 3- to 6-month intervals for tapering or discontinuation of therapy; for atopic vaginitis and kraurosis vulvae, 0.3 to ≥1.25 mg/d, depending on the tissue response of the individual patient, administer cyclically, for short-term use only and should be discontinued as soon as possible, re-evaluate at 3- to 6-month intervals for tapering or discontinuation of therapy; for breast cancer (palliation), 10 mg tid for at least 3 months; for osteoporosis in postmenopausal women, initiate at 0.3 mg/d and increase to a maximum daily dose of 1.25 mg/d, initiate therapy as soon as possible after menopause, cyclically or daily, monitor patients with an intact uterus for signs of endometrial cancer, rule out malignancy if unexplained vaginal bleeding occurs; for female castration and primary ovarian failure, 1.25 mg/d, cyclically, increase/decrease dose according to severity of symptoms and patient response, for maintenance, adjust dosage to lowest level that will provide effective control.

ESTROPIPATE, for moderate to severe vasomotor symptoms associated with menopause, usual dosage range is 0.75-6 mg estropipate daily, use the lowest dose and regimen that will control symptoms, and discontinue as soon as possible, attempt to discontinue or taper medication at 3-6 month intervals; for *female* hypogonadism, 1.5-9 mg daily for the first 3 weeks, followed by a rest period of 8-10 days, use the lowest dose and regimen that will control symptoms; for *female* castration or primary ovarian failure, 1.5-9 mg/d for the first 3 weeks of a theoretical cycle, followed by a rest of 8-10 days, use the lowest dose/regimen that will control symptoms; for osteoporosis prophylaxis, 0.75 mg daily for 25 days of a 31-day cycle; for atrophic vaginitis or kraurosis vul-

vae, 0.75-6 mg daily, administer cyclically, use the lowest dose and regimen that will control symptoms, discontinue as soon as possible.

ETHINYL ESTRADIOL; ETHYNODIOL DIACETATE, These drugs are used only in combination with other drugs and therefore individual dosing is not covered here.

ETONOGESTREL, for *women*, for contraception, subdermal: Implant 1 rod in the inner side of the upper, non-dominant arm. Remove no later than 3 years after the date of insertion.

FINASTERIDE, for *men*, for benign prostatic hyperplasia (Proscar®), 5 mg/d as a single dose, clinical responses occur 3-6 months of initiation of therapy, long-term administration recommended for maximal response. For male pattern baldness (Propecia®), 1 mg/d.

FLUOXYMESTERONE, for *men*, for hypogonadism, 5-20 mg/d; for delayed puberty, 2.5-20 mg/d for 4-6 months. For *female* inoperable breast carcinoma, 10-40 mg/d in divided doses for 1-3 months.

FLUTAMIDE, for *men* for prostatic carcinoma, 250 mg tid.

HYDROXYPROGESTERONE CAPROATE, for *women*, to reduce the risk of preterm birth, for pregnant females 16 years or older, IM: 250 mg once weekly.

LEVOMEFOLATE, this drug is used only in combination with other drugs and therefore its individual dosing is not covered here.

LEVONORGESTREL, for *women*, for emergency contraception, one 0.75 mg tablet as soon as possible within 72 hours of unprotected sexual intercourse, a second 0.75 mg tablet should be taken 12 hours after the first dose, may be used at any time during menstrual cycle.

MEDROXYPROGESTERONE, for *adolescents* and *adults*, for amenorrhea, 5-10 mg/d for 5-10 days; for abnormal uterine bleeding, 5-10 mg for 5-10 days starting on day 16 or 21 of cycle. For *adults*, for accompanying cyclic estrogen therapy, postmenopausal, 5-10 mg for 12-14 consecutive days each month, starting on day 1 or day 16 of the cycle, lower doses used if given with estrogen continuously throughout cycle.

MEGESTROL, for *women*, for breast carcinoma, 40 mg qid; for endometrial carcinoma, 40-320 mg/d in divided doses; use for 2 months to determine efficacy; maximum doses used up to 800 mg/d. For *men* or *women*, for HIV-related **cachexia**, Megace®, initiate at 800 mg/d; daily doses of 400–800 mg/d were found to be clinically effective, Megace ES®, 625 mg/d.

Cachexia: Severe weight loss and weakness due to serious disease

METHYLTESTOSTERONE, for hypogonadism or delayed puberty in *males*, dose should be based on response and toleration; for androgen deficiency in males, 10-50 mg/d; for breast cancer in females, 50-200 mg/d.

MESTRANOL, used only in combination with other drugs, and therefore its individual dosing is not covered here.

MIFEPRISTONE, for *adults*, for termination of pregnancy, treatment consists of 3 office visits by the patient. Day 1, 600 mg taken as a single dose. Day 3, unless abortion has occurred (confirmed using ultrasound or clinical examination), 400 mcg. Day 14, confirm complete termination of pregnancy by ultrasound or clinical exam.

NILUTAMIDE, 300 mg daily for 30 days starting the same day or day after surgical castration, then 150 mg/d.

NORETHINDRONE, for *adolescents* and *adults*, for *women*, for contraception, 0.35 mg every day of the year starting on first day of menstruation; for amenorrhea and abnormal uterine bleeding, 5-20 mg/d for 5-10 days during the second half of the menstrual cycle; acetate salt: 2.5-10 mg/d for 5-10 days during the second half of the menstrual cycle; for endometriosis, 10 mg/d for 2 weeks; increase at increments of 5 mg/d every 2 weeks until 30 mg/d; continue for 6-9 months or until breakthrough bleeding demands temporary termination. Acetate salt, 5 mg/d for 14 days; increase at increments of 2.5 mg/d every 2 weeks up to 15 mg/d; continue for 6-9 months or until breakthrough bleeding demands temporary termination.

NORGESTIMATE, NORGESTREL, used only in combination with other drugs, and therefore individual dosing is not covered here.

OSPEMIFENE, for postmenopausal *women*, for moderate-to-severe dyspareunia, 60 mg once daily.

OXANDROLONE, for *children*, total daily dose is ≤0.1 mg/kg or ≤0.045 mg/lb. For *adults*, 2.5-20 mg in divided doses 2-4 times/d based on individual response; a course of therapy of 2-4 weeks is usually adequat;, this may be repeated intermittently as needed. For the *elderly*, 5 mg tid.

OXYMETHOLONE, for *children* and *adults*, for erythropoietic effects, 1-5 mg/kg/d in one daily dose; usual effective dose is 1-2 mg/kg/d; give for a minimum trial of 3-6 months because response may be delayed.

PROGESTERONE, for *females*, for amenorrhea, IM: 5-10 mg/d for 6-8 consecutive days; for secondary amenorrhea, 400 mg nocte for 10 days; intravaginal gel: 45 mg (4% gel) every other day for 6 doses; may increase to 90 mg (8% gel) with the same schedule; for assisted reproductive techniques (ART), intravaginal gel: 90 mg (8% gel) once daily. If pregnancy occurs, may continue treatment for 10-12 weeks; intravaginal tablet: 100 mg 2-3 times daily starting at oocyte retrieval and continuing for up to 10 weeks; for endometrial hyperplasia prevention, 200 mg nocte for 12 days sequentially per 28-day cycle; for functional uterine bleeding, IM: 5-10 mg/d for 6 doses.

RALOXIFENE, for *women*, for osteoporosis, 60 mg/d; for invasive breast cancer risk reduction, 60 mg/d for 5 years.

TAMOXIFEN, for *adults*, for breast cancer, metastatic (males and females) or adjuvant therapy (females), 20-40 mg/d; daily doses >20 mg should be given in 2 divided doses (morning and evening); for prevention (high-risk females), 20 mg/d for 5 years; for DCIS (females), 20 mg once daily for 5 years.

TESTOSTERONE, for *adolescent males* with delayed puberty or hypogonadism, please refer to adult dosing. For *adults*, for inoperable metastatic breast cancer in females, IM: 200-400 mg every 2-4 weeks; for hypogonadism or hypogonadotropic hypogonadism in males, IM: 50-400 mg every 2-4 weeks; subcutaneous pellet implantation: 150-450 mg every 3-6 months, Topical, buccal: 30 mg bid applied to the gum region above the incisor tooth; AndroGel® 1%: 50 mg applied mane to the shoulder and upper arms or abdomen; may be increased up to a maximum of 100 mg/d; AndroGel® 1.62%: 40.5 mg applied mane to the shoulder and upper arms; may be increased to a maximum of 81 mg/d; Fortesta™: 40 mg mane applied to the thighs; dosing range is 10-70 mg/d; Testim®: 5 g applied once daily (preferably in the morning) to the shoulder and upper arms; may be increased up to a maximum of 10g/d; Solution (Axiron®): 60 mg once daily; usual dose range is 30-120 mg/d apply to the axilla at the same time each morning; transdermal system (Androderm®): initiate at 4 mg/d and adjust according to testosterone serum levels; for delayed puberty in males, IM: 50-200 mg every 2-4 weeks for a limited duration; subcutaneous pellet implantation: 150-450 mg every 3-6 months.

TOREMIFENE, for *adults*, 60 mg once daily; generally continued until disease progression is observed.

ULIPRISTAL, for *women*, for emergency contraception, 30 mg as soon as possible but within 120 hours of unprotected intercourse or contraceptive failure.

▦ ADVERSE EFFECTS

Androgens have many adverse effects depending on who is taking them. In women, they can cause masculinization effects such as acne, deepening of the voice, facial hair, baldness, and muscle production. They can also cause menstrual disorders. In men, they can cause **priapism**, impotence, decreased sperm production, and **gynecomastia**. In children, these agents can cause abnormal sexual maturation and growth disturbances. In general, androgens may cause an increase in the LDL to HDL ratio, fluid retention, and edema.

The androgen receptor antagonist antiandrogens, such as bicalutamide, flutamide, and nilutamide, may cause liver problems. The adverse effects of nilutamide are worse than the other receptor antagonists. The 5-α-reductases, such as dutasteride and finasteride, may infrequently cause impotence.

The antiprogestin mifepristone may cause significant uterine bleeding and the possibility of an incomplete abortion.

Estrogens can cause headache, edema, hypertension, nausea, and vomiting. Postmenopausal uterine bleeding may occur. Long-term use can lead to **thromboembolic** effects, myocardial infarction, and increased risk of breast and endometrial cancers. Diethylstilbestrol has been shown to have numerous serious risks not only in the user but their offspring, especially daughters. It is no longer used in women who are fertile.

A higher incidence of stroke and invasive breast cancer were observed in women >75 years in a WHI substudy using conjugated equine estrogen.

Progestins cause edema and depression. The 19-nortestosterone derivatives, such as norethindrone and ethynodiol diacetate, may increase the ratio of LDL to HDL and cause thromboembolic events, **hirsutism**, acne, and weight gain.

Most adverse effects of OCPs are considered to be caused by the estrogen component; however cardiovascular effects are considered to be caused by both the estrogen and progestin components. Major side effects include depression, heavy breasts, dizziness, edema, nausea and vomiting, and headaches. Cardiovascular effects include thromboembolic events, **thrombophlebitis**, hypertension, and myocardial infarction. Smoking may increase the risk of these cardiovascular adverse effects. While OCPs may decrease the incidence of endometrial and ovarian cancer, they may induce others, such as breast or liver cancer. Lipid changes may occur. OCPs should not be used in patients with cardiovascular disease, thromboembolic disorders, estrogen-

---

Priapism: An abnormal prolonged or constant erection of the penis

Gynecomastia: An abnormal enlargement of one or two breasts in men

Thromboembolism: Blockage of a blood vessel due to a piece of a clot breaking off from another location and preventing blood flow

Hirsutism: Excessive body hair in a masculine distribution

Thrombophlebitis: Inflammation of a vein often accompanied by a blood clot

dependent cancers, liver disease, or migraine headaches.

SERMs generally increase the risks of thromboembolic events such as deep-vein thrombosis (DVT) and pulmonary embolism. Tamoxifen frequently causes hot flashes, nausea, and vomiting in addition to the less frequent effects such as menstrual irregularities and vaginal bleeding. Endometrial hyperplasia and cancer have been reported with this agent. Toremifene does not appear to increase the risk of endometrial cancer. Clomiphene may cause ovarian enlargement, hot flashes, and visual disturbances. These effects are dose-related.

RED FLAGS

An FDA advisory discusses two additional deaths after using mifepristone for abortions. Actual cause of death in these cases is being investigated.

INTERACTIONS

DRUG

Raloxifene should not be used with warfarin or cholestyramine. The latter significantly reduces absorption of raloxifene from the intestines. Raloxifene may cause prothrombin time disturbances in those taking warfarin.

HERB

ESTROGEN

- *Dang Gui* (Angelica sinensis) (B)–has been suggested to have phytoestrogen content (Miller, 1998) Level 5 evidence. However, this is still speculative. One rat study showed significant estrogenic effect (Circosta, De Pasquale *et al.*, 2006). Level 5 evidence; in vitro research showed little or no estrogen activity (Zava, Dollbaum & Blen, 1998) Level 5 evidence. Finally, a double-blind RCT showed no estrogen-like effects in postmenopausal women (Hirata, Small *et al.*, 1997) Level 1b evidence. There is some controversy, but the preponderance of evidence suggests there is no estrogen-like activity.
- *Fan Xie Ye* (Senna leaves) (B-)–caused reduced serum levels of estrogen in a small crossover study due to its intestinal motility effect (Lewis, Oakey & Heaton, 1998) Level 3b evidence.

- *Gan Cao* (Licorice) (B-)–may increase blood pressure and fluid retention when used with oral contraceptives, as shown in two case studies (de Klerk, Nieuwenhuis & Beutler, 1997) Level 4 evidence; and in an uncontrolled human study (Bernardi, D'Intino, Trevisani, Cantelli-Forti, Raggi, Turchetto *et al.*, 1994) Level 2c evidence.

ETHINYLOESTRADIOL AND DESOGESTRAL

- *Guan Ye Lian Qiao* (St. John's wort, hypericum) (D)–may induce the cytochrome P450 system and increase metabolism and reduce plasma concentration of several drugs including digoxin, desogestrel, ethinyloestradiol, cyclosporine, indinavir, theophyline, and phenprocoumon, expert opinion (Fugh-Berman, 2000) Level 5 evidence.

HORMONE REPLACEMENT THERAPY

- *Man Jing Zi* (D)–may interfere with efficacy of oral contraceptive pills, progesterone, and hormone replacement therapy due to its hormone regulation activity, expert opinion (Mills & Bone, 2000) Level 5 evidence.

ORAL CONTRACEPTIVES

- *Gan Cao* (Licorice) (B-)–may increase blood pressure and fluid retention when used with oral contraceptives; shown in two case studies (de Klerk, Nieuwenhuis & Beutler, 1997) Level 4 evidenc;, and in an uncontrolled human study (Bernardi, D'Intino, Trevisani, Cantelli-Forti, Raggi, Turchetto *et al.*, 1994) Level 2c evidence.
- *Lu Cha* (Green tea) (D)–the effect of caffeine in *Lu Cha* may be potentiated by oral contraceptives, expert opinion (Chen & Chen, 2004) Level 5 evidence.
- *Man Jing Zi* (D)–may interfere with efficacy of oral contraceptive pills, progesterone, and hormone replacement therapy due to its hormone regulation activity, expert opinion (Mills & Bone, 2000) Level 5 evidence.

ORAL CONTRACEPTIVE PILLS

- *Guan Ye Lian Qiao* (St. John's wort) (C)–hypericum caused breakthrough bleeding and unplanned pregnancies when used concomitantly with oral contraceptives (Zhou, Chan, Pan & Huang, Lee, 2004) Level 2b evidence; (Izzo & Ernst, 2009) Level 4 evidence.

PROGESTERONE

- *Gan Cao* (Licorice) (B-)–may increase blood pressure and fluid retention used with oral contraceptives; two case studies (de Klerk, Nieuwenhuis & Beutler, 1997) Level 4 evidence; and in an uncontrolled human study (Bernardi, D'Intino *et al.*, 1994) Level 2c evidence.
- *Man Jing Zi* (D)–may interfere with efficacy of oral contraceptive pills, progesterone, and hormone replacement therapy due to its hormone regulation activity, expert opinion (Mills & Bone, 2000) Level 5 evidence.

TAMOXIFEN

- *Dan Dou Chi* (Fermented soy bean) (D)–may decrease effects of tamoxifen, expert opinion (Gruenwald, Brendler & Jaenicke, 2004) Level 5 evidence.
- *Xi Yang Shen* (American ginseng) (D)–when combined with tamoxifen, cytoxan, doxorubicin, taxol, and methotrexate may increase suppression of breast cell growth as shown in an in vitro study (Duda, Zhong, Navas, Li, Toy & Alavarez, 1999) Level 5 evidence.

TESTOSTERONE

- *Bai Zhi* (D)–has an inhibitory effect on cytochrome P450 in rats, which can lead to increased plasma concentration of testosterone, diazepam, tolbutamide, nifedipine, bufuralol, and potentially other drugs (Ishi-hara, Kushida *et. al.*, 2000) Level 5 evidence.
- *Gan Cao* (Licorice) (D)–decreases endogenous testosterone levels in men and women with polycystic ovary disease; may affect testosterone supplementation, expert opinion (Gruenwald, Brendler & Jaenicke, 2004) Level 5 evidence.

INTERACTION ISSUES

A:

D: Abiraterone acetate is 99% protein bound; bicalutamide is 96% protein bound; dutasteride is 99% bound; enzalutamide is 97-98% bound; fluoxymesterone is 98% protein bound; flutamide is 94-96% bound; mifepristone is 98% protein bound; ospemifene is over 99% boun;, raloxifene is over 95% bound; tamoxifen is 99% bound; testosterone is 98% protein bound; toremifene is over 99.5% bound.

M: Abiraterone acetate is a major substrate of CYP3A4, a strong inhibitor of 1A2, 2C8, and 2D6, and a moderate inhibitor of 2C19, 2C9, and 3A4; bicalutamide is a moderate inhibitor of CYP3A4; enzalutamide is a major substrate of CYP2C8 and 3A4, a weak/moderate inducer of 2C9 and 2C19, and a strong inducer of 3A4; estradiol is a major substrate of CYP1A2 and 3A4 and a weak/moderate inducer of 3A4; estrogens (Conjugated A/Synthetic) are a major substrate and a weak/moderate inducer of CYP3A4; estrogens (Conjugated B/Synthetic) are a major substrate of CYP3A4; estrogens (Conjugated/Equine, Systemic) are a major substrate of CYP1A2 and a major substrate of and weak/moderate inducer of 3A4; estrogens (Esterified) and estropipate are a major substrate of CYP1A2 and 3A4; flutamide is major substrate of CYP1A2 and 3A4; hydroxyproges-terone caproate is a major substrate of CYP3A4, a weak/moderate inducer of 1A2 and 2B6, and a strong inducer of 2A66; levonorgestrel is a major substrate of CYP3A4; medroxyprogesterone is a major substrate and a weak/moferate inducer of CYP3A4; mifepristone is a major substrate of CYP3A4; nilutamide is a major substrate of CYP2C19; norethindrone is a major substrate of CYP3A4 and a weak/moderate inducer of 2C19; ospemifene is a major substrate of CYP2C9 and 3A4; progesterone is a major substrate of CYP2C19 and 3A4; tamoxifen is a major substrate of CYP2C9, 2D6, and 3A4 and a moderate inhibitor of 2C8; toremifene is a major substrate of CYP 3A4; ulipristal is a major substrate of CYP 3A4.

E:

Pgp: Abiraterone acetate, enzalutamide, and mifepristone inhibit Pgp; estradiol is a substrate of Pgp; progesterone, tamoxifen, and ulipristal inhibit Pgp.

TI:

The adrenal glands, located just superior to each

SECTION 4: ADRENOCORTICOSTERIOD HORMONES

CORTICOSTEROIDS:

ALCLOMETASONE (al kloe MET a sone)
PR=C *(Aclovate)*

AMCINONIDE (am SIN oh nide) PR=C

BECLOMETHASONE (be kloe METH a sone)
PR=C *(Beconase® AQ, Qnasi, QVAR®)*

BETAMETHASONE (bay ta METH a sone)
PR=C *(AlphaTrex, Celestone, Celestone Soluspan, Diprolene, Diprolene AF, Lotrisone®,38 Luxiq, Taclonex®43)*

**BUDESONIDE (byoo DES oh nide) PR=C
(Oral)/B (inhaled)** *(Entocort® EC, Pulmicort®, Pulmicort Flexhaler®, Uceris)*

CICLESONIDE (sye KLES oh nide) PR=C
(Alvesco®)

CLOBETASOL (kloe BAY ta sol) PR=C
(Clobetasol Propionate E, Clobex, Clobex Spray, Cormax Scalp Application, Olux, Olux-E, Temovate, Temovate E)

CLOCORTOLONE (kloe KOR toe lone) PR=C
(Cloderm, Cloderm Pump)

CORTICOTROPIN (kor ti koe TROE pin) PR=C
(Acthar HP)

DESONIDE (DES oh nide) PR=C *(Desonate, DesOwen, DesOwen Cream w/Cetaphil Lot, DesOwen Lot w/Cetaphil Cream, DesOwen Ointment w/Cetaphil Lot, LoKara, Verdeso)*

DESOXIMETASONE (des oks i MET a sone)
PR=C *(Topicort)*

CORTISONE (KOR ti sone) PR=C

COSYNTROPIN (koe sin TROE pin) PR=C
(Cortrosyn)

DEXAMETHASONE (deks a METH a sone)
PR=C *(Baycadron, Dexamethasone Intensol®, DexPak 6-Day, DexPak 10-Day, DexPak 13-Day)*

DIFLORASONE (dye FLOR a sone) PR=C
(ApexiCon, ApexiCon E)

FLUDROCORTISONE (floo droe KOR ti sone) PR=C *(Florinef®)*

FLUNISOLIDE (floo NISS oh lide) PR=C
(Aerospan™)

FLUOCINOLONE (floo oh SIN oh lone) PR=C
(Capex, Derma-Smoothe/FS Body, Derma-Smoothe/FS Scalp, DermOtic, Fluocinolone Acetonide Body, Fluocinolone Acetonide Scalp, Retisert®, Synalar, Synalar (Cream), Synalar (Ointment), Synalar TS, Tri-Luma®44)

FLUOCINONIDE (floo oh SIN oh nide) PR=C
(Vanos)

FLURANDRENOLIDE (flure an DREN oh lide)
PR=C *(Cordran, Cordran SP)*

FLUTICASONE (floo TIK a sone) PR=C *(Advair Diskus®,39 Advair® HFA,39 Cutivate®, Flonase®, Flovent Diskus, Flovent® HFA)*

HALCINONIDE (hal SIN oh nide) PR=C *(Halog)*

HALOBETASOL (hal oh BAY ta sol) PR=C
(Halonate, Ultravate)

HYDROCORTISONE (hye droe KOR ti sone)
PR=C *(A-Hydrocort, Alcortin® A,45 Carmol-HC®,47 Cortef, Cortisporin®,46 Cortisporin® Oint-ment,42 Cortomycin,46 Dermazene®,45 Neo-Polycin™ HC,42 Solu-Cortef, Xerese™,41)*

METHYLPREDNISOLONE (meth il pred NIS oh lone) PR=C *(A-Methapred, Depo-Medrol, Medrol, Medrol-Pak, Solu-Medrol®)*

MOMETASONE (moe MET a sone) PR=C
(Asmanex®, Dulera,40)

PREDNISOLONE (pred NISS oh lone) PR=C
(AsmalPred, AsmalPred Plus, Flo-Pred™, Millipred, Millipred DP, Millipred DP 12-Day, Orapred, Orapred ODT, Pediapred, Prelone, Veripred 20)

PREDNISONE (PRED ni sone) PR=N
(Prednisone Intensol™, Rayos)

TRIAMCINOLONE (trye am SIN oh lone)
PR=D *(Aristospan Intra-Articular, Aristospan Intralesional, Kenalog®)*

INHIBITORS OF ADRENOCORTICOIDS:

EPLERENONE *(See Chapter 6, Class 3)*

KETOCONAZOLE *(See Chapter 10, Section 5)*

METYRAPONE (me TEER a pone) PR=C
(Metopirone®)

MIFEPRISTONE *(See Section 3)*

MITOTANE (MYE toe tane) PR=C *(Lysodren®)*

SPIRONOLACTONE *(See Chapter 6, Class 3)*

kidney, secrete various hormones and can be broken down into two major parts: the outer cortex and the inner medulla. The medulla primarily synthesizes sympathomimetic hormones, especially epinephrine. The cortex is made up of three zones, each of which produces a class of hormones. The outer zona glomerulosa makes mineralocorticoids, which regulate water and salt metabolism and excretion. The most important hormone produced here is aldosterone. The middle zona fasciculata produces glucocorticoids, used in regular body metabolism and stress reactions. Cortisol is a prime example of hormones produced here. Finally, the inner zona reticularis produces adrenal androgens as discussed in the previous section. Most, but not all, of these hormones are controlled by the hypothalamus-pituitary axis, primarily accomplished through corticotropin-releasing hormone (CRH) secretion from the hypothalamus, which causes secretion of adrenocorticotropic hormone (ACTH), also known as corticotrophin. Glucocorticoids provide negative feedback to both CRH and ACTH secretion. This is summarized in Figure 7.4.

■ FUNCTION

Both glucocorticoid and mineralocorticoid hormones have numerous functions on the body. Glucocorticoids can cause **gluconeogenesis** by causing the breakdown of fats and protein and redistributing them to the liver to build glucose. They aid growth hormone in its functions. They aid in the body's stress response by causing glucose to enter the blood for energy and a hypertensive effect by enhancing vasoconstrictor action of adrenergic mediators on the small blood vessels. They reduce the immune response and increase the oxygen-carrying capacity and clotting ability of the blood by shifting immune mediators such as eosinophils, basophils, monocytes, and lymphocytes from the blood to the lymphoid tissue and shifting hemoglobin, **erythrocytes**, platelets, and polymorphonuclear lymphocytes into the blood. They also dramatically lower the inflammatory response throughout the body. They not only provide negative

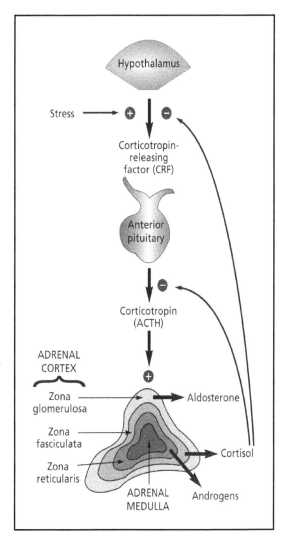

Figure 7.4: **Hypothalamus-pituitary axis** in relation to the adrenals and feedback inhibition.

feedback for cortical hormone production but they lower the secretion of thyroid hormone and stimulate the secretion of growth hormone.

Mineralocorticoids aid in the control of the body's water volume and electrolyte levels.

The glucocorticoids are particularly used in a variety of capacities and in most forms of administration including inhaled, topically applied, injected, and oral. They are used, sometimes with an exogenous mineralocorticoid, as replacement therapy to treat Addison's disease, a primary insufficiency of the adrenal

Gluconeogenesis: The formation of glucose from fatty acids and proteins rather than carbohydrates

Erythrocytes: Red blood cells

cortex. They can also be used to treat secondary, ACTH insufficiency, or tertiary, CRH deficiency. They can be used to diagnose Cushing's syndrome, a hypersecretion of glucocorticoids, by tracing whether the issue is with the pituitary or an adrenal tumor. They can be used to treat the effects of congenital adrenal hyperplasia by causing negative feedback inhibition for adrenocorticoid hormone release. One of the most common uses of glucocorticoids is in the treatment of inflammation and allergies, especially in asthmatic patients where they are used both through inhalation and orally. They are also commonly used topically to treat inflammatory skin conditions. Prednisone is used in treating acute lymphocytic leukemia (ALL), and Hodgkin's and non-Hodgkin's lymphomas.

▓ MECHANISM OF ACTION

Glucocorticoids and mineralocorticoids basically act as their endogenous counterparts would. There may be pharmacological differences in time of onset, duration of effect, and half-life, but the mechanisms of action are very similar. Corticosteroids easily transverse the cell membrane due to their **hydrophobicity**. Once in the cytoplasm of the cell they bind with a receptor and enter the nucleus, where they exert their effects by either inhibiting or stimulating gene transcription, which ultimately increases or decreases protein formation of various products. Glucocorticoid receptors are widely distributed throughout the body, but the effects differ based on the type of tissue. Mineralocorticoid receptors are primarily restricted to organs of elimination. The mechanism of action for these agents is summarized in Figure 7.5.

Inhibitors of adrenocorticoids work by one of two methods. Metyrapone and ketoconazole act by preventing the biosynthesis of corticosteroids through blocking a specific step in the synthesis of these chemicals. Amino-glutethimide does this at a very early step in steroid synthesis and can affect the synthesis of all steroid hormones. The other method of inhibition is competitive inhibition at

---

Hydrophobic: Chemicals that prefer to be in a fat- or oil-based solution rather than an aqueous solution

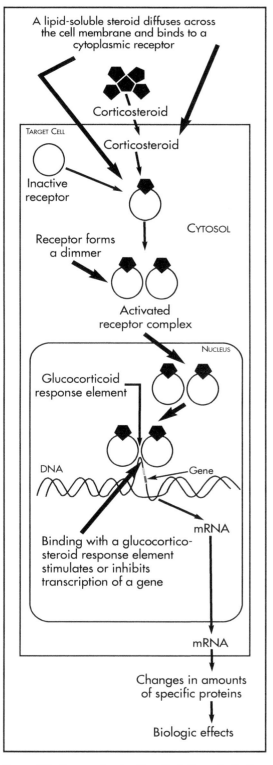

Figure 7.5: How corticosteroids affect the cell. Corticosteroids easily diffuse through the cell membrane and activate a receptor that then enters the nucleus from the cytosol. In the nucleus, it binds with DNA and either inhibits or promotes the transcription of a gene into mRNA, which is ultimately translated into a protein.

the receptor. Mifespristone, spironolactone, and eplerenone act in this fashion.

DOSAGES

ALCLOMETASONE, for *children* 1 or over, for steroid-responsive dermatoses, topical: apply thin film to affected area 2-3 times/d; do not use for >3 weeks. For *adults*, for steroid-responsive dermatoses, topical: apply a thin film to the affected area 2-3 times/d.

AMCINONIDE, for *adults*, for steroid-responsive dermatoses, topical: apply a thin film to the affected area 2-3 times/d.

BECLOMETHASONE, for asthma (titrate dose to the lowest effective dose once asthma is controlled) (QVAR®), for *children* 5-11 years, initiate at 40 mcg bid; maximum dose is 80 mcg bid. For *children* 12 or over and *adults*, for patients previously on bronchodilators only, initiate at 40-80 mcg bid; maximum dose is 320 mcg bid; for patients previously on inhaled corticosteroids, initiate at 40-160 mcg bid; maximum dose is 320 mcg bid.

BETAMETHASONE, for *children*, for inflammatory conditions, 0.0175-0.25 mg/kg/d divided every 6-8 hours or 0.5-7.5 mg/m2/d divided every 6-8 hours; IM: 0.0175-0.125 mg base/kg/d divided every 6-12 hours or 0.5-7.5 mg base/m^2/d divided every 6-12 hours; for steroid-responsive dermatoses, refer to adult dosing. For *children* over 12 and *adults*, for inflammatory conditions: 2.4-4.8 mg/d in 2-4 doses; usual range is 0.6-7.2 mg/d; IM: sodium phosphate and acetate solutions, 0.6-9 mg/d divided every 12-24 hours; for scalp psoriasis, topical foam: apply to the scalp twice daily; for rheumatoid arthritis or osteoarthritis, intrabursal, intra-articular, or intradermal: 0.25-2 mL; intralesional: for very large joints, 1-2 mL; large joints, 1 mL; medium joints, 0.5-1 mL; small joints: 0.25-0.5 mL; for steroid-responsive dermatoses, therapy should be discontinued when control is achieved; gel: apply once or twice daily; rub in gently; do not exceed 2 weeks of treatment or 50 g/wk; lotion: apply a few drops twice daily;

cream/ointment, apply once or twice daily.

BUDESONIDE, for *children* 6 yrs and older with previous therapy of bronchodilators alone, 200 mcg twice initially; may be increased up to 400 mcg bid; for patients on previous therapy of inhaled corticosteroids, 200 mcg twice initially, which may be increased up to 400 mcg bid; for patients on previous therapy of oral corticosteroids, the highest recommended dose in children is 400 mcg bid. For *adults*, previous therapy of bronchodilators alone, 200-400 mcg twice initially, which may be increased up to 400 mcg bid; for patients on previous therapy of inhaled corticosteroids, 200-400 mcg twice initially, which may be increased up to 800 mcg bid; for patients on previous therapy of oral corticosteroids, 400-800 mcg twice daily, which may be increased up to 800 mcg bid; for Crohn's disease (active), 9 mg once daily in the morning for up to 8 weeks; recurring episodes may be treated with a repeat 8-week course of treatment.

CICLESONIDE, for *children* 12 and older and *adults*, for asthma, prior therapy with bronchodilators alone, initiate at 80 mcg bid up to a maximum of 320 mcg/d; prior therapy with inhaled corticosteroids, initiate at 80 mcg bid up to a maximum of 640 mcg/d; prior therapy with oral corticosteroids, initiate at 320 mcg bid up to a maximum of 640 mcg/d.

CLOBETASOL, use in *children* under 12 is not recommended. For *children* 12 and over and *adults*, for steroid-responsive dermatoses, topical: apply bid for up to 2 weeks and a maximum dose of 50 g/wk; for steroid-responsive dermatoses of the scalp, topical foam (Olux®): apply to affected scalp bid for up to 2 weeks and a maximum dose of 50 g or 50 mL/wk; for mild-to-moderate plaque-type psoriasis of nonscalp areas, topical foam: apply to affected area bid for up to 2 weeks and a maximum dose of 50 g/wk; not to be applied to face or intertriginous areas; for moderate-to-severe plaque-type psoriasis, topical: apply bid for up to 2 weeks; maximum dose is 50 g/wk, spray: apply by spraying directly onto affected area bid and gently rubbed into skin; should not be used for longer than 4 weeks; total dose should not exceed 50 g or mL/wk; for scalp psoriasis, topical shampoo: apply thin film to dry scalp once daily, let sit for 15 minutes, then add water, lather, and rinse thoroughly.

CLOCORTOLONE, for *adults*, for steroid-responsive dermatoses, topical: apply sparingly and gently rub into affected area from 1-4 times/d.

CORTICOTROPIN, for *children*, for infantile spasms, for *children* under 2 years: IM: 75 units/m²/dose bid for 2 weeks followed by a gradual taper over a 2-week period. For all other indications, for *children* over 2 years, refer to adult dosing. For *adults*, for acute exacerbation of multiple sclerosis, IM or subcutaneous: 80-120 units/d for 2-3 weeks; for all other indications, IM or subcutaneous: 40-80 units every 24-72 hours.

CORTISONE, if possible, administer glucocorticoids before 9 AM to minimize adrenocortical suppression; dosing depends upon the condition being treated and the response of the patient. For *children*, as an anti-inflammatory or immunosuppressive, 2.5-10 mg/kg/d or 20-300 mg/m²/d in divided doses every 6-8 hours; as a physiological replacement, 0.5-0.75 mg/kg/d or 20-25 mg/m²/d in divided doses every 8 hours. For *adults*, as an anti-inflammatory or immunosuppressive, 25-300 mg/d in divided doses every 12-24 hours; as a physiologic replacement, 25-35 mg/d.

COSYNTROPIN, for *children*, for diagnostic screening of adrenocortical insufficiency, IM: for *children* 2 years and younger, 0.125 mg, for *children* over 2 years, refer to adult dosing. For *adults*, for diagnostic screening of adrenocortical insufficiency, IM: 0.25 mg.

DESONIDE, for *children* 3 months and older, for atopic dermatitis, please refer to adult dosing. For *adults*, for corticosteroid responsive dermatoses, topical: apply sparingly 2-3 times/d; for atopic dermatitis, topical foam or gel: apply sparingly bid.

DESOXIMETASONE, for *children* and *adolescents*, for corticosteroid-responsive dermatoses,

please refer to adult dosing. For *adults*, for corticosteroid-responsive dermatoses, topical: apply a thin film to affected area bid; for plaque psoriasis treatment, topical spray: apply a thin film to affected area bid.

DEXAMETHASONE, for *children*, as an anti-inflammatory immunosuppressant, 0.08-0.3 mg/kg/d or 2.5-10 mg/m²/d in divided doses every 6-12 hours; for extubation or airway edema, 0.5-2 mg/kg/d in divided doses every 6 hours beginning 24 hours prior to extubation and continuing for 4-6 doses afterwards; for physiological replacement, 0.03-0.15 mg/kg/d or 0.6-0.75 mg/m²/d in divided doses every 6-12 hours. For *adults*, as an antiemetic, prophylaxis: 10-20 mg 15-30 minutes before treatment on each treatment day, for continuous infusion regimen, 10 mg every 12 hours on each treatment day; for mildly emetogenic therapy, 4 mg every 4-6 hours; for delayed nausea/vomiting, 4-10 mg 1-2 times/d for 2-4 days or 8 mg every 12 hours for 2 days, then 4 mg every 12 hours for 2 days or 20 mg 1 hour before chemotherapy, then 10 mg 12 hours after chemotherapy, then 8 mg every 12 hours for 4 doses, then 4 mg every 12 hours for 4 doses; as an anti-inflammatory, 0.75-9 mg/d in divided doses every 6-12 hours for chemotherapy, 40 mg every day for 4 days, repeated every 4 weeks; for Cushing's syndrome, diagnostic, 1 mg at 11 PM, draw blood at 8 AM; greater accuracy for Cushing's syndrome may be achieved by the following: 0.5 mg by mouth every 6 hours for 48 hours (with 24-hour urine collection for 17-hydroxycorticosteroid excretion); for differentiation of Cushing's syndrome due to ACTH excess from Cushing's due to other causes, 2 mg qid for 48 hours (with 24-hour urine collection for 17-hydroxy-corticosteroid excretion); for multiple sclerosis (acute exacerbation), 30 mg/d for 1 week followed by 4-12 mg/d for 1 month.

DIFLORASONE, for *adults*, for corticosteroid-responsive dermatosis, topical: apply ointment sparingly 1-3 times/d; apply cream sparingly 2-4 times/d.

FLUDROCORTISONE, for *infants* and *children*,

0.05-0.1 mg/d. For *adults*, 0.1-0.2 mg/d with ranges of 0.1 mg 3 times/wk to 0.2 mg/d; for Addison's disease, initiate at 0.1 mg/d, if transient hypertension develops, reduce the dose to 0.05 mg/d; for salt-losing adrenogenital syndrome, 0.1-0.2 mg/d.

FLUNISOLIDE, for asthma, for *children* 6-15 years, 2 inhalations bid (morning and evening) up to 4 inhalations/d; for *children* 16 or over and *adults*, 2 inhalations bid (morning and evening) up to 8 inhalations/d maximum. For *children* 12 years or over and *adults*, 2 inhalations bid up to 8 inhalations/d.

FLUOCINOLONE, for *children* 3 months and over, for atopic dermatitis, topical: moisten skin and apply a thin film to affected area bid; for corticosteroid-responsive dermatoses, refer to adult dosing. For *adults*, for atopic dermatitis, apply thin film to affected area tid; for corticosteroid-responsive dermatoses, topical: apply a thin layer to affected area 2-4 times/d; for inflammatory and pruritic manifestations (dental use), topical: apply to oral lesion qid after meals and at bedtime; for scalp psoriasis, topical: massage thoroughly into wet or dampened hair/scalp, cover with shower cap; and leave on overnight (or for at least 4 hours), remove by washing hair with shampoo and rinsing thoroughly; for seborrheic dermatitis of the scalp, topical: apply no more than 1 ounce to scalp once daily, work into lather, allow to remain on scalp for approximately 5 minutes, rinse and thoroughly with water.

FLUOCINONIDE, for *children*, for itching and inflammation, refer to adult dosing; for children 12 and older, for plaque-type psoriasis, refer to adult dosing. For *adults*, for pruritus and inflammation, topical (0.05% cream): apply thin layer to affected area 2-4 times/d depending on the severity of the condition; for plaque-type psoriasis, topical (0.1% cream): apply a thin layer once or twice daily to affected areas.

FLURANDRENOLIDE, for *children*, for steroid-responsive dermatosis, topical cream: apply sparingly 1-2 times per day; topical lotion or tape: refer to adult dosing. For *adults*, for steroid-responsive dermatosis, topical cream or lotion: apply sparingly 2-3 times/d; topical tape: apply 1-2 times per day.

FLUTICASONE, for asthma, Flovent® HFA: for *children* 4-11 years, 88 mcg bid; for *children* ≥12 years, refer to adult dosing. For *adults*, for asthma, decrease to the lowest effective dose once asthma stability is achieved; Flovent® HFA: initiate at 88 mcg bid; highest recommended dose is 440 mcg bid. Oral corticosteroids, Flovent® HFA: 440 mcg bid; highest recommended dose is 880 mcg bid.

HALCINONIDE, for *children*, refer to adult dosing. For *adults*, for steroid-responsive dermatoses, topical: apply sparingly 2-3 times daily; avoid excessive application.

HYDROCORTISONE, for *infants* and *children*, as an anti-inflammatory or immunosuppressive, 2.5-10 mg/kg/d or 75-300 mg/m^2/d every 6-8 hours. For *children*, for physiological replacement, 0.5-0.75 mg/kg/d or 20-25 mg/m^2/d every 8 hours. For adolescents and *adults*, as an anti-inflammatory or immunosuppressive, 15-240 mg every 12 hours; for congenital adrenal hyperplasia, initiate at 10-20 mg/m^2/d in 3 divided doses; for physiological replacement, 500 mg to 2 g every 2-6 hours. For *adults*, for chronic adrenal corticoid insufficiency, 20-30 mg/d.

METHYLPREDNISOLONE, for *children*, as an anti-inflammatory or immunosuppressive, 0.5-1.7 mg/kg/d or 5-25 mg/m^2/d in divided doses every 6-12 hours. For *adults*, as an anti-inflammatory or immunosuppressive, 2-60 mg/d in 1-4 divided doses to start, followed by gradual reduction in dosage to the lowest possible level consistent with maintaining an adequate clinical response.

METYRAPONE, for *children*, 15 mg/kg every 4 hours for 6 doses; maximum dose is 250 mg. For *adults*, 750 mg every 4 hours for 6 doses.

MITOTANE, for *children*, 0.1-0.5 mg/kg or 1-2 g/d in divided doses increasing gradually to a maximum of 5-7 g/d. For *adults*, start at 1-6 g/d in divided doses, then increase incrementally to 8-10 g/d in 3-4 divided doses up to a maximum daily dose of 18 g.

MOMETASONE, for *children* ≥12 years and *adults* who were previously on bronchodilators or inhaled corticosteroids, initiate at 1 inhalation (220 mcg) daily up to a maximum of 2 inhalations or 440 mcg/d; may be given in the evening or in divided doses bid; oral corticosteroids, initiate at 440 mcg bid up to a maximum of 880 mcg/d; maximum effects may not be evident for 1-2 weeks or longer; dose should be adjusted to effect using the lowest possible dose.

PREDNISOLONE, for *children*, acute asthma, 1-2 mg/kg/d in divided doses 1-2 times/d for 3-5 days; as an anti-inflammatory or immunosuppressive dose, 0.1-2 mg/kg/d in divided doses 1-4 times/d; for nephrotic syndrome, initiate at (first 3 episodes) 2 mg/kg/d or 60 mg/m^2/d up to a maximum of 80 mg/d; administer in divided doses 3-4 times/d until urine is protein free for 3 consecutive days, (maximum: 28 days) followed by 1-1.5 mg/kg/ dose or 40 mg/m^2/dose given every other day for 4 weeks; for maintenance (long-term maintenance dose for frequent relapses), 0.5-1 mg/kg/dose given every other day for 3-6 months. For *adults*, usual dose range is 5-60 mg/d; for multiple sclerosis, 200 mg/d for 1 week followed by 80 mg every other day for 1 month; for rheumatoid arthritis, initiate at 5-7.5 mg/d; adjust dose as necessary.

PREDNISONE, dose depends upon condition being treated and patient response; base dosage for *infants* and *children* on severity of the disease and patient response rather than strict adherence to dosage indicated by age, weight, or body surface area; consider alternate-day therapy for long-term use, discontinuation of long-term therapy requires gradual withdrawal by tapering the dose. For *children*, as an anti-inflammatory or immu-nosuppressive dose, 0.05-2 mg/kg/d divided 1-4 times/d; for acute asthma, 1-2 mg/kg/d in divided doses 1-2 times/d for 3-5 days; alternatively (for 3-5 day "burst"), <1 year, 10 mg every 12 hours; 1-4 years, 20 mg every 12 hours, 5-13 years; 30 mg every 12 hours; >13 years, 40 mg every 12 hours; for asthma long-term therapy (alternative dosing by age), <1 year, 10 mg every other day; 1-4 years, 20 mg every other day, 5-13 years, 30 mg every other day; >13 years, 40 mg every other day; for nephrotic syndrome, initiate at (first 3 episodes) 2 mg/kg/d or 60 mg/m^2/ up to a maximum of 80 mg/d, in divided doses 3-4 times/d until urine is protein free for 3 consecutive days (maximum: 28 days) followed by 1-1.5 mg/kg/dose or 40 mg/m^2/dose given every other day for 4 weeks; maintenance dose (long-term maintenance dose for frequent relapses), 0.5-1 mg/kg/dose given every other day for 3-6 months. For *children* and *adults*, as physiological replacement, 4-5 mg/m^2/d. For *children* ≥5 years and *adults*, for asthma, moderate persistent, inhaled corticosteroid (medium dose) or inhaled corticosteroid (low-medium dose) with a long-acting bronchodilator; severe persistent, inhaled corticosteroid (high dose) and corticosteroid tablets or syrup long-term, 2 mg/kg/d, generally not to exceed 60 mg/d. For *adults*, as an immunosuppression/chemotherapy adjunct, dose range is 5-60 mg/d in divided doses 1-4 times/d; for allergic reaction (contact dermatitis), Day 1: 30 mg divided as 10 mg before breakfast, 5 mg at lunch, 5 mg at dinner, 10 mg at bedtime; Day 2: 5 mg at breakfast, 5 mg at lunch, 5 mg at dinner, 10 mg at bedtime; Day 3: 5 mg 4 times/d (with meals and at bedtime); Day 4: 5 mg tid (breakfast, lunch, bedtime); Day 5: 5 mg bid (breakfast, bedtime); Day 6: 5 mg mane; for pneumocystis carinii pneumonia (PCP): 40 mg bid for 5 days followed by 40 mg once daily for 5 days followed by 20 mg once daily for 11 days or until antimicrobial regimen is completed; for thyrotoxicosis, 60 mg/d; as chemotherapy (refer to individual protocols), dose range is 20 mg/d to 100 mg/m^2/d; for rheumatoid arthritis, use lowest possible daily dose (often ≤7.5 mg/d); for idiopathic thrombocytopenia purpura (ITP), 60 mg daily for 4-6 weeks, gradually tapered over several weeks;

for systemic lupus erythematosus (SLE), acute, 1-2 mg/kg/d in 2-3 divided doses; maintain by reducing to lowest possible dose, usually less than 1 mg/kg/d mane.

TRIAMCINOLONE, for *adults,* for acute rheumatic carditis, initiate at 20-60 mg/d; reduce dose during maintenance therapy; for acute seasonal or perennial allergic rhinitis, 8-12 mg/d; for adrenocortical insufficiency, dose range is 4-12 mg/d; for bronchial asthma, 8-16 mg/d; for dermatological disorders, contact/atopic dermatitis, initiate at 8-16 mg/d; for ophthalmic disorders, 12-40 mg/d; for rheumatic disorders, dose range is 8-16 mg/d; for SLE, initiate at 20-32 mg/d; some patients may need initial doses ≥48 mg; reduce dose during maintenance therapy; for oral inhalation in asthma, for *children* 6-12 years, 100-200 mcg 3-4 times/d or 200-400 mcg bid; maximum dose is 1200 mcg/d; for *children* over 12 years and *adults,* 200 mcg 3-4 times/d or 400 mcg bid; maximum dose is 1600 mcg/d.

ADVERSE EFFECTS

There are numerous, serious adverse effects of long-term corticosteroid use. These include loss of calcium leading to osteoporosis, decreased immunity and therefore increased infections, reduced wound healing, increased appetite, emotional issues including euphoria and depression, hypertension, whole body edema, stomach ulcers, glaucoma, hirsutism, and hypokalemia. Large doses can cause a Cushing's-like syndrome that includes **moon facies, buffalo hump,** increased body hair, acne, insomnia, increased appetite, and redistribution of body fat. Vitamin D and calcium supplementation is recommended to prevent osteoporosis. Diabetics should monitor their glucose carefully as these agents can interfere.

RED FLAGS

Hypokalemia can result from corticosteroid use. Withdrawal is a major concern with these agents. Sudden withdrawal can cause an acute adrenal insufficiency syndrome that can be lethal. Weaning from corticosteroids, even short-term use, should always be accomplished over time with a step-wise reduction under doctor supervision.

INTERACTIONS

DRUG

Many of these agents are minor substrates of some CYP isoenzymes and may have an effect on the metabolism of other drugs.

HERB

CORTICOSTEROIDS

• *Gan Cao* (Licorice) (D)–may increase the half-life of systemic corticosteroids, expert opinion (Fugh-Berman, 2000, as cited in Chen & Chen, 2004); (Gruenwald, Brendler & Jaenicke, 2004) Level 5 evidence.

• *Huang Qi* (Astragulus) (D)–may stimulate T-cell activity; may decrease the immunosuppressant effects of cyclosporine and corticosteroids, expert opinion (Miller, 1998) Level 5 evidence.

• *Lu Hui* (Aloe) (D)–can increase potassium loss due to thiazide and loop diuretics and corticosteroids, expert opinions (Blumenthal, 1998); (Gruenwald, Brendler & Jaenicke, 2004) Level 5 evidence.

• *Ma Huang* (Ephedra) (B-)–based on ephedrine content, may increase the metabolism of corticosteroids in a human study using ephedrine and not the whole herb (Brooks, Sholiton, Werk Jr, Altenau, 1977) Level 3b evidence.

• *Ren Shen* (Ginseng) (D)–may have additive effects with corticosteroids, expert opinion (Miller, 1998) Level 5 evidence.

CORTISONE

• *Gan Cao* (Licorice) (D)–may increase the half-life of systemic corticosteroids, expert opinions (Fugh-Berman, 2000, as cited in Chen & Chen); (Gruenwald, Brendler & Jaenicke, 2004) Level 5 evidence.

DEXAMETHASONE

• *Gan Cao* (Licorice) (D)–may increase half-life of systemic corticosteroids, expert opinions (Fugh-Berman, 2000); (Gruenwald, Brend-ler & Jaenicke, 2004) Level 5 evidence.

Moon facies: A rounded, puffy face caused by high doses of corticosteroids

Buffalo hump: An accumulation of fat on the back of the neck caused by high doses of glucocorticoids or Cushing's syndrome

- Kidney supplement herbs (D)–in male rats a recipe of kidney supplement herbs can treat and prevent dexamethasone-induced osteoporosis (Shen, Chen & Zhang, 1998) Level 5 evidence.
- *Ma Huang* (Ephedra) (B-)–based on ephedrine content, may increase metabolism of corticosteroids in a human study using ephedrine, not the whole herb (Brooks, Sholiton *et al.*, 1977) Level 3b evidence.

HYDROCORTISONE

- *Gan Cao* (Licorice) (D)–may increase the half-life of systemic corticosteroids, expert opinions (Fugh-Berman, 2000); (Gruenwald, Brendler & Jaenicke, 2004) Level 5 evidence.

PREDNISONE

- *Guan Ye Lian Qiao* (St. John's wort) (C)–decreases blood concentrations of this drug (Izzo & Ernst, 2009) Level 4 evidence.

INTERACTION ISSUES

A:

D: Beclomethasone is 94-96% protein bound; ciclesonide is over 99% bound; fluticasone is 99% bound; mometasone is 98-99% bound.

M: Budesonide and ciclesonide are major substrates of CYP3A4; dexamethasone is a major substrate and strong inhibitor of CYP3A4 and a weak/moderate inhibitor of 2A6, 2B6, and 2C9; flunisolide and fluticasone are major substrates of CYP3A4; hydrocortisone is a weak/moderate inducer of CYP3A4; metyrapone is a weak/moderate inducer of CYP3A4; prednisone is a weak to moderate inducer of CYP2C19 and 3A4.

E:

Pgp: Dexamethasone is a substrate of, induces, and inhibits Pgp; hydrocortisone is a substrate of Pgp.

TI:

SECTION 5: AIDS FOR REPRODUCTION

CETRORELIX (set roe REL iks) PR=X *(Cetrotide®)*

CHORIONIC GONADOTROPIN (Human) (HCG) (kor ee ON ik goe NAD oh TROE pin, HYU man) PR=X *(Novarel, Pregnyl)*

CHORIONIC GONADOTROPIN (RECOMBINANT) (kor ee ON ik goe NAD oh TROE pin ree KOM be nant) PR=X *(Ovidrel®)*

CLOMIPHENE *(See Chapter 7, Section 3)*

FOLLITROPIN ALPHA (foe li TRO pin AL fa) PR=X *(Gonal-f®; Gonal-f® RFF; Gonal-f® RFF Pen)*

FOLLITROPIN BETA (foe li TRO pin BAY ta) PR=X *(Follistim AQ)*

GANIRELIX (ga ni REL ix) PR=X

LUTROPIN ALFA (LOO troe pin AL fa) PR=X

MENOTROPINS (men oh TROE pins) PR=X *(Menopur®, Repronex®)*

UROFOLLITROPIN (yoor oh fol li TROE pin) PR=X *(Bravelle®)*

▓ FUNCTION

These agents, often among other uses, stimulate the ovaries to produce more than one egg per ovulation cycle. This increases the chance of at least one egg conceiving.

Both cetrorelix and ganirelix are adjunctive agents that inhibit premature luteinizing hormone surges in women undergoing ovarian stimulation. This allows for follicles to develop adequately before ovulation.

Chorionic gonadotropin is used to treat hypogonadotropic hypogonadism, prepubertal cryptorchidism, and spermatogenesis induction with follitropin alfa in addition to inducing ovulation.

Follitropin alpha and beta are also used to stimulate spermatogenesis in men with primary and secondary hypogonadotropic hypogonadism.

Menotropins are used for all of the above; however, spermatogenesis is an off-label use.

MECHANISM OF ACTION

These agents are similar to luteinizing hormone or follicle stimulating hormone and directly stimulate ovulation in women and production of androgen in the testes.

Cetrorelix and ganirelix act as competitive inhibitors of pituitary receptors delaying the LH surge and preventing ovulation until follicles are of an appropriate size.

DOSAGES

CETRORELIX, for *adults*, for controlled ovarian stimulation in conjunction with gonadotropins, subcutaneous single-dose regimen: 3 mg given when serum estradiol levels show appropriate stimulation response, usually stimulation day 7; if hCG is not administered within 4 days, continue at 0.25 mg/d until hCG is administered; multiple-dose regimen: 0.25 mg morning or evening of stimulation day 5 or morning of stimulation day 6; continue until hCG is administered. Not for use in women over 65.

CHORIONIC GONADOTROPIN (HUMAN), for *children*, for prepubertal cryptorchidism, IM: 4000 units 3 times/wk for 3 weeks or 5000 units every second day for 4 injections or 500 units 3 times/wk for 4-6 weeks or 15 injections of 500-1000 units given over 6 weeks; for hypogonadotropic hypogonadism in boys, IM: 500-1000 units 3 times/wk for 3 weeks followed by same dose 2 times/wk for 3 weeks or 4000 units 3 times/wk for 6-9 months, then reduce to 2000 units 3 times/wk for additional 3 months. For *adults*, to induce ovulation in women, IM: 5000-10,000 units 1 day following last dose of menotropins; to start spermatogenesis associated with hypogonadotropic hypogonadism in men, 1000-2000 units 2-3 times/wk until serum testosterone levels are normal (may require 2-3 months of ther-apy); continue to maintain testosterone levels.

CHORIONIC GONADOTROPIN (RECOMBINANT), for *adults*, for assisted reproductive technologies

(ART) and ovulation induction in females, subcutaneous: 250 mcg given 1 day following the last dose of follicle stimulating agent.

FOLLITROPIN ALPHA, for *adults*, to induce ovulation, subQ: initiate at 75 units/d; can increase by up to 37.5 units after 14 days and every 7 days afterwards up to a maximum 300 units/d; hCG is given 1 day following the last dose; for spermatogenesis induction, should begin with hCG pretreatment until serum testosterone is in normal range, then 150 units 3 times/wk with hCG 3 times/wk; continue with lowest dose needed to induce spermatogenesis; maximum 300 units 3 times/wk for up to 18 months.

FOLLITROPIN BETA, for *adults*, for ovulation induction, IM or subQ: initiate at 75 units/d for at least the first week; increase by 25-50 units at weekly intervals until follicular growth or serum estradiol levels indicate adequate response; maximum daily dose 300 units; hCG is given 1 day following the last dose; for ART in women, IM or subcutaneous: start with 150-225 units for at least the first 4 days of treatment; can be adjusted for the individual patient based upon their ovarian response up to a maximum daily dose of 600 units; for spermatogenesis induction in men, pretreatment with hCG is required, Follitropin beta therapy may be initiated after normal serum testosterone levels have been attained, subcutaneous 225 units 2 times/wk or 150 units 3 times/wk.

GANIRELIX, for *adults*, as an adjunct to controlled ovarian hyperstimulation, subQ: 250 mcg/d during the mid-to-late phase after initiating follicle stimulating hormone on day 2 or 3 of cycle; continue daily until hCG administration.

LUTROPIN ALPHA, for *adults*, for female infertility, subcutaneous 75 units daily until adequate follicular development is noted up to a maximum duration of treatment of 14 days; once adequate follicular development is evident, administer hCG to induce final follicular maturation in preparation for oocyte retrieval.

MENOTROPINS, for *adults*, for induction of ovulation using Repronex®, IM or subQ: initiate with 150 units daily for the first 5 days of treatment;

may adjust dose every 2 days or longer with 75-150 units per adjustment; maximum daily dose is 450 units for no longer than 12 days; hCG should be given 1 day following the last dose; for assisted reproductive technologies, IM or subQ: initiate with 225 units; adjustments in dose should not exceed more than 75-150 units per adjustment with at least 2 days between adjustments; the maximum daily dose should not exceed 450 units or longer than 12 days; hCG should be administered to induce final follicular maturation in preparation for oocyte retrieval.

UROFOLLITROPIN, for *adults*, for ovulation induction, IM or subcutaneous: initiate with: 150 units daily for the first 5 days of treatment; dose adjustments of no more than 75-150 units can be made with at least 2 days in between up to a maximum daily dose of 450 units for 12 days; hCG is given 1 day following the last dose; for ART, subQ: 225 units daily for the first 5 days; may be adjusted based on patient response, with no more than 75-150 units every two days or more up to a maximum daily dose of 450 units for 12 days.

ADVERSE EFFECTS

Ovarian hyperstimulation syndrome (OHSS) can occur with these agents and involves severe enlargement of an/both ovary(ies), abdominal pain, nausea, vomiting, diarrhea, scanty urine, trouble breathing and possibly ascites, pleural effusion, and thromboemboli. Menotropins and urofollitropin have been reported to cause serious pulmonary conditions and thromboembolic events not associated with OHSS.

Many of these agents have been shown to be teratogenic in animal studies.

ENDNOTES

[1] Combination of Pioglitazone and Metformin.

[2] Combination of Rosiglitazone and Metformin.

[3] Combination of Rosiglitazone and Glimepiride.

[4] Combination of Glipizide and Metformin.

[5] Combination of Glyburide and Metformin.

[6] Combination of Estradiol and Norethindrone.

[7] Combination of Estradiol and Drospirenone.

[8] Combination of Estradiol and Levonorgestrel.

[9] Combination of Estradiol and Norgestimate.

[10] Combination of Estrogens (Conjugated/Equine) and Medroxyprogesterone.

[11] Combination of Estrogens (Esterified) and Methyltestosterone.

[12] Combination of Ethinyl Estradiol and Levonorgestrel.

[13] Combination of Ethinyl Estradiol and Desogestrel.

[14] Combination of Ethinyl Estradiol and Norethindrone.

[15] Combination of Ethinyl Estradiol and Norgestrel.

[16] Combination of Ethinyl Estradiol and Ethynodiol Diacetate.

[17] Combination of Ethinyl Estradiol and Norgestimate.

[18] Combination of Ethinyl Estradiol and Drospirenone.

[19] Combination of Mestranol and Norethindrone.

[20] Advair Diskus comes in 3 varieties: 100/50, 250/50, and 500/50. The first number is the dosage of Fluticasone in mcg; the second is the dosage of Salmeterol, which is a constant 50 mcg.

[20] Combination of Metformin and Alogliptin.

[21] Combination of Metformin and Linagliptin.

[22] Combination of Metformin and Repaglinide.

[23] Combination of Metformin and Saxagliptin.

[24] Combination of Metformin and Sitagliptin.

[25] Combination of Alogliptin and Pioglitazone.

[26] Combination of Glimepiride and Pioglitazone.

[27] Combination of Glimepiride and Rosiglitazone.

[28] This is a combination of 70% Insulin Aspart Protamine, an intermediate-acting Insulin, and 30% Insulin Aspart, which is rapid acting.

[29] This is a combination of 50% Insulin Lispro Protamine, an intermediate-acting Insulin, and 50% Insulin Lispro, which is rapid acting.

[30] This is a combination of 75% Insulin Lispro Protamine, an intermediate-acting Insulin, and 25% Insulin Lispro, which is rapid acting.

[31] This is a combination of 50% Insulin NPH, an intermediate-acting Insulin, and 50 % Insulin Regular, which is short acting.

[32] This is a combination of 70% Insulin NPH, an intermediate-acting Insulin, and 30% Insulin Regular, which is short acting.

[33] Combination of Dutasteride and Tamsulosin.

[34] Combination of Estradiol and Dienogest.

[35] Combination of Ethinyl Estradiol and Etonogestrel.

[36] Combination of Ethinyl Estradiol and Norelgestromin.

[37] Combination of Ethinyl Estradiol, Drospirenone, and Levomefolate.

[38] Combination of Betamethasone and Clotrimazole.

[39] Combination of Fluticasone and Salmeterol.

[40] Combination of Mometasone and Formoterol.

[41] Combination of Acyclovir and Hydrocortisone.

[42] Combination of Hydrocortisone, Bacitracin, Neomycin, and Polymyxin B.

[43] Combination of Betamethasone and Calcipotriene.

[44] Combination of Fluocinolone, Hydroquinone, and Tretinoin.

[45] Combination of Hydrocortisone and Iodoquinol.

[46] Combination of Hydrocortisone, Neomycin, and Polymyxin B.

[47] Combination of Hydrocortisone and Urea.

[48] Combination of Sitagliptin and Simvastatin.

CHINESE MEDICAL DESCRIPTIONS

The Chinese medical explanation of the drug categories in this chapter may be found in Chapter 15 on pages 385–417.

Drugs Affecting the Respiratory System

This chapter covers four major pathologies of the lungs. These include asthma, allergic **rhinitis**, chronic obstructive pulmonary diseases, and coughs. There is a lot of overlap amongst drugs used in these areas as well as many drugs discussed in other chapters and sections. Given how important and widely used these agents are, this chapter will look at both oral and inhaled agents.

SECTION 1: AGENTS USED FOR ASTHMA

5-LIPOXYGENASE INHIBITORS:

ZILEUTON (zye LOO ton) PR=C *(Zyflo®CR)*

ANTICHOLINERGIC AGENTS:

IPRATROPIUM & TIOTROPIUM *(see Chapter 4, Section 3)*

β₂-ADRENERGIC AGONISTS *(See Chapter 4, Section 4)*

CORTICOSTEROIDS *(See Chapter 7, Section 4)*

LEUKOTRIENE RECEPTOR ANTAGONISTS:

MONTELUKAST (mon te LOO kast) PR=B *(Singulair®)*

ZAFIRLUKAST (za FIR loo kast) PR=B *(Accolate®)*

MAST CELL STABILIZERS:

CROMOLYN (KROE moe lin) PR=B *(Gastrocrom®, NasalCrom [O])*

THEOPHYLLINE DERIVATIVES:

AMINOPHYLLINE (am in OFF i lin) PR=C

DYPHYLLINE (DYE fi lin) PR=C *(Difil-G® 400,[1] Lufyllin®)*

THEOPHYLLINE (thee OFF i lin) PR=C *(Elixophyllin®, Theo-24®, Theochron®)*

Asthma affects 12-17 million people in the U.S. and is growing in prevalence. It is a disease of inflammation in the airways of the lungs. Many things may trigger this inflammation; among the most common include allergies, cold air, exercise, emotions, and viral infections. Common symptoms include wheezing, **dyspnea**, and chest tightness. It is the leading cause for hospitalization in children, and about 5,000 deaths occur annually. While there is a clear genetic component, this susceptibility does not predict the disease, as it is multifactorial, and the environment and exposures play a large role in developing asthma. In Figure 8.1, a normal bronchus is compared with one in an asthmatic patient.

▦ FUNCTION

These agents are used to treat asthma. Many of these agents have many different functions besides those that affect the respiratory system, which are explained in their own sections.

▦ MECHANISM OF ACTION

FIRST-LINE ASTHMA AGENTS:

Asthma causes temporary **bronchoconstriction** and obstruction due to three main mechanisms: smooth muscle contraction causing narrowing of airways, increased mucus secretion, and inflammation that causes swelling of the airway lining. First-line drugs try to

Rhinitis: Inflammation of the mucus membranes of the nose

Dyspnea: Shortness of breath or difficulty breathing

Bronchoconstriction: A decrease in the diameter of the lungs' bronchi causing less airflow

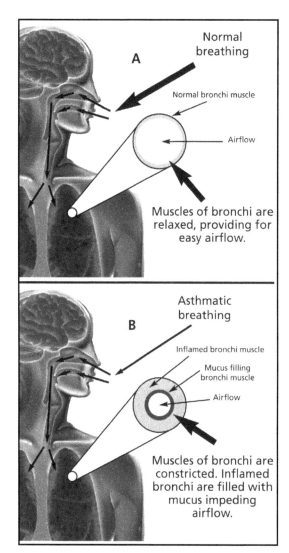

Figure 8.1: Comparing a normal bronchial tube with an asthmatic one. A: A normal bronchial tube shows relaxation of the smooth muscles and a wide open airway. B: In an asthmatic bronchial tube, the smooth muscles are contracted, the lining is inflamed and enlarged, and the lumen is filled with mucus. These add up to restricted airflow.

Adrenergic: Pertaining to nerve fibers in the SNS that react to epinephrine, norepinephrine, or dopamine neurotransmitters

Leukotrienes: Biological compounds that have a role in inflammation and allergic reactions

Chemoattractant: A chemical that influences the migration of cells

nists used in asthma treatment include albuterol and terbutaline. Long-acting agonists have a relatively slow onset and a longer duration of action. These are used to prevent attacks from occurring rather than treating acute episodes. Common long-acting agents include salmeterol and formoterol.

If the asthma is mild and intermittent, a short-acting agonist to treat acute episodes may be all that is needed. If it is persistent in any way, corticosteroid use is considered necessary. While adrenergic agonists act to relax the smooth muscle, corticosteroids act by reducing inflammation. They work by reducing the number of inflammatory cells and their activity in the lungs. This causes reduction of edema in the airways, decreases the capillary permeability, and inhibits the release of **luekotrienes**. In general, corticosteroids used for asthma control are inhaled; in severe cases, they can be taken orally. While inhaled steroids do reduce the number of systemic effects, large portions (up to 90%) are swallowed and absorbed systemically. This can be reduced dramatically by the use of a spacer and by rinsing the mouth with water after use of an inhaler. These first-line asthma treatments are summarized in Figure 8.2.

ADJUNCTIVE AGENTS FOR TREATING ASTHMA:

Leukotrienes are chemicals that are involved in many aspects of asthma. Some cause greater infiltration of immune and inflammatory cells, which can exacerbate symptoms, and others directly cause smooth muscle contraction and edema. Many leukotrienes are produced from arachidonic acid. Leukotriene receptor antagonists and 5-lipoxygenase inhibitors prevent the normal functioning of these chemicals. 5-lipoxygenase is an enzyme in mast cells, basophils, eosinophils, and neutrophils used to convert arachidonic acid to **chemoattractant** leukotrienes. 5-lipoxygenase inhibitors block this enzyme and prevent the formation of these leukotrienes. The leukotriene receptor antagonists act by reversibly binding to leukotriene receptors and thus prevent their direct

counteract these effects. Inhaled **Adrenergic** agonists directly activate β₂-adrenergic receptors that relax the smooth muscle of the airways. These agents can be short-acting or long-acting. Short-acting agonists have a rapid onset of action and are used to treat acute attacks for 4 to 6 hours. These are primary agents for acute treatment. Common short-acting ago-

CLASSIFICATION	BRONCHO-CONSTRICTIVE EPISODES	RESULTS OF PEAK FLOW OR SPIROMETRY	QUICK RELIEF OF SYMPTOMS	LONG-TERM CONTROL
Mild intermittent	Less than two per week	Near normal	Short-acting β_2 agonist	No daily medication
Mild persistent	More than two per week	Near normal	Short-acting β_2 agonist	Low-dose inhaled corticosteroids
Moderate persistent	Daily	60-80 percent of normal	Short-acting β_2 agonist	Low- to medium-dose inhaled corticosteroids and a long-acting β_2 agonist
Persistent	Continual	Less than 60 percent of normal	Short-acting β_2 agonist	High-dose inhaled corticosteroids and a long-acting β_2 agonist

Figure 8.2: First-line asthmatic agents for given classifications of asthma.

effects on the airways. These agents are used in the long-term prevention of asthma, not in the acute treatment of an episode. It is possible to reduce the amount of adrenergic agonist and corticosteroid use by adding these agents. Figure 8.3 summarizes these effects.

Mast cell stabilizers are used in the prevention of asthma attacks and are not useful for acute treatment. They work by preventing release of histamine, leukotrienes, and other chemicals of inflammation in mast cells. They are especially useful in allergy- and exercise-induced asthma.

Anticholinergic agents act by blocking vagus nerve impulses that contract airway smooth muscle and stimulate mucus secretion. They are generally used in patients that cannot tolerate adrenergic agonists.

Theophylline was one of the first asthma agents discovered and widely used. Adrenergic agonists and corticosteroid use have largely supplanted its use. It and its derivatives act by a cAMP-induced cascade that, among other effects, causes bronchodilation.

■ DOSAGES

AMINOPHYLLINE, for *children* at least 45 kg and *adults*, initiate at 380 mg/d in divided doses every 6-8 hours; may increase dose after 3 days up to a maximum dose of 928 mg/d.

CROMOLYN, for systemic mastocytosis, for *children* 2-12 years, 100 mg qid but not to exceed 40 mg/kg/d and given 1/2 hour prior to meals

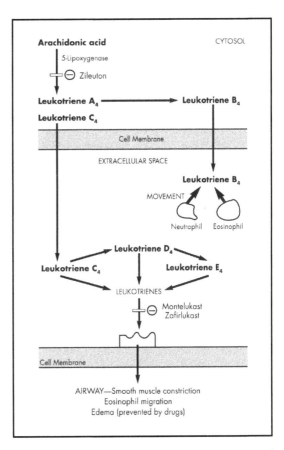

Figure 8.3: The effects of 5-Lipoxygenase inhibitors and leukotriene receptor antagonists on the airways. Physiological functioning converts arachidonic acid to a series of chemoattractant leukotrienes that brings immune cells to the area and initiates an immune response. 5-lipoxyoygenase inhibitors stop this cascade at the beginning. Other leukotrienes initiate airway smooth muscle contraction, edema, and immune cell migration after activating cell membrane receptors. Leukotriene receptor antagonists prevent these actions by blocking the receptors.

and nocte. For *children* >12 years and *adults*, 200 mg qid to be given 1/2 hour prior to meals and nocte; dose may be increased to a maximum 40 mg/kg/d. For inhalation use: for chronic control of asthma, taper frequency to the lowest effective dose. For use as a metered spray, for *children* 5-12 years, initiate at 2 inhalations qid with a usual dose of 1-2 inhalations 3-4 times/d; for *children* 12 years and over and *adults*, initiate at 2 inhalations qid with a usual dose of 2-4 inhalations 3-4 times/d. For prevention of allergen- or exercise-induced bronchospasm, use 10-15 minutes prior to exercise or allergen exposure but no longer than 1 hour before; for use as a metered spray, for *children* over 5 years and *adults*, use a single dose of 2 inhalations.

DYPHYLLINE, for *adults*, may use up to 15 mg/kg qid.

MONTELUKAST, for *children*, 6-11 months, for asthma, 4 mg (oral granules) once daily, taken in the evening; for 6-23 months, for perennial allergic rhinitis, 4 mg (oral granules) once daily; for 12-23 months, for asthma, 4 mg (oral granules) once daily, taken in the evening; for 2-5 years, for asthma or seasonal or perennial allergic rhinitis, 4 mg once daily, taken in the evening; for 6-14 years, for asthma, seasonal or perennial allergic rhinitis, one 5 mg chewable tablet/d, taken in the evening; for *children* ≥15 years and *adults*, for asthma, seasonal or perennial allergic rhinitis, 10 mg/d, taken in the evening.

THEOPHYLLINE, for oral use, use a loading dose. If no theophylline has been administered in the previous 24 hours, use 4-6 mg/kg theophylline. If theophylline has been administered in the previous 24 hours, 1/2 loading dose or 2-3 mg/kg theophylline can be given in emergencies. For bronchial asthma, doses should be initiated slowly and increased to a maintenance dose. For each of the following ages, the first dose is to be administered for the initial three days, the second for the next three days, and the third as a maintenance dose. Doses are in mg. In all cases, toxicity should be looked for and serum levels taken. For *children* <1, 0.2 x (age in weeks) + 5 for the first 6 days and 0.3 x (age in weeks) + 8 thereafter; for *children* 1-9, 16 up to a maximum of 400 mg/d, 20, 22; for *children* 9-12, 16 up to a maximum of 400 mg/d, 16 up to a maximum of 600 mg/d, 20 up to a maximum of 800 mg/d; for 12-16 years of age, 16 up to a maximum of 400 mg/d, 16 up to a maximum of 600 mg/d, 18 up to a maximum of 900 mg/d; for *adults*, 400 mg/d, 600 mg/d, 900 mg/d. The dosage may be increased in approximately 25% increments at 2-3 day intervals so long as the drug is tolerated or until the maximum dose is reached.

ZAFIRLUKAST, for *children* 5-11 years, 10 mg bid; for *children* 12 years and over and *adults*: 20 mg bid.

ZILEUTON, for *children* 12 years and over and *adults*, 600 mg qid.

ADVERSE EFFECTS

Many of these agents have diverse adverse effects. They are covered in their original sections. The following adverse effects are for drugs introduced here or for drugs introduced elsewhere but have specific adverse effects when used to treat these pathologies. In general, by inhaling these agents especially with a spacer, systemic effects are minimized if not completely eliminated.

Oropharyngeal candidiasis, commonly called thrush, can occur with the use of inhaled or systemic steroids due to locally reduced immunity.

Leukotriene receptor antagonists and 5-lipoxygenase inhibitors can cause headaches GI complaints, and rarely, **eosinophilic vasculitis** especially when concurrent corticosteroids are reduced. They also have been reported to elevate hepatic enzymes, which should be periodically monitored.

Mast cell stabilizers may cause a bitter taste and irritate the pharynx and larynx.

Eosinophils: A type of leukocyte that stains yellow-red or orange with Wright stain; they are motile phagocytes with an antiparasitic function; they also play a role in allergies

Vasculitis: Inflammation of the blood vessels

RED FLAGS

The FDA has issued a warning regarding the use of long-acting β_2-agonists (LABA), including salmeterol and formoterol. Recent studies have shown there are more asthma-related deaths in patients who use regular asthma treatments when combined with LABAs than with regular treatment alone. The warning emphasizes that LABAs should not be used for the acute treatment of asthma attacks.

Theophylline, and possibly its derivatives, has a narrow therapeutic index. An overdose may cause seizures and potentially fatal arrhythmias.

INTERACTIONS

DRUG

Zafirlukast and Zileuton are both inhibitors of cytochrome P450 and can increase warfarin levels.

Theophylline, and possibly its derivatives, interferes with many drugs and caution should be used.

HERB

THEOPHYLLINE

• *Chuan Xin Lian* (Andrographis) (D)–A rat study showed a significant increase in elimination of theophylline when combined with chuan xin lian. This suggests CYP1A2 inducement (Chien, Wu, Lee, Lin, Tsai, 2010) Level 5 evidence

• *Guan Ye Lian Qiao* (St. John's wort, hypericum) (C)–may induce the cytochrome P-450 system and increase metabolism and reduce plasma concentration of several drugs including digoxin, cyclo-sporine, theophyline, and phenprocoumon, expert opinions (Fugh-Berman, 2000) Level 5 evidence. (Izzo & Ernst, 2009) Level 4 evidence, (Hu, Yang, Ho, Chan, et al 2005) Level 2b evidence.

• *Ku Shen* (Sophora) (D)–A rat study showed

higher clearance and lowered area under the curve of theophylline when coadministered with sophora. It was speculated that this was due to inducement of several cytochrome P450 enzymes (Ueng, Tsai, Lo, Yun, 2010) Level 5 evidence.

• *Hei Hu Jiao* (Black pepper) (B-)–increased absorption kinetics of propranolol, the amount of theophylline, and increased maximum concentrations of both in a small human crossover study (Bano, Raina, Zutshi, Bedi, Johri, Sharma, 1991) Level 3b evidence.

• *Ma Huang* (Ephedra) (A)–may increase thermogenesis and weight loss when combined with methylxanthines such as theophylline and caffeine in both mice (Dulloo & Miller, 1986a) Level 5 evidence, and human studies (Dulloo & Miller, 1986b) Level 2b evidence, (Malchow-Moller, Larsen, Hey, Stokholm, Juhl, Quaade, 1981) Level 2b evidence, (Boozer, Daly, Homel, Solomon, Blanchard, Nasser, *et al.*, 2002) Level 1b evidence, (Greenway, de Jonge, Blanchard, Frisard, Smith, 2004) Level 2b evidence, (Astrup, Breum, Toubro, Hein, Quaade, 1992) Level 1b evidence.

INTERACTION ISSUES

A:

D: Montelukast and zafirlukast are over 99% protein bound.

M: Aminophylline is a major substrate of CYP1A2; montelukast is a major substrate of CYP2C9 and 3A4; theophylline is a major substrate of CYP1A2, 2E1, and 3A4; zafirlukast is a major substrate and a moderate inhibitor of CYP2C9.

E:

Pgp:

TI: Theophylline and its derivatives, including aminophylline and dyphylline, have a narrow therapeutic index.

SECTION 2: AGENTS USED FOR ALLERGIC RHINITIS

α-ADRENERGIC AGONISTS *(See Chapter 4, Section 4)*

ACRIVASTINE (AK ri vas tene) PR=B *(Semprex®-D²)*

AZELASTINE (a ZEL as tene) PR=C *(Astelin, Astepro, Optivar)*

BROMPHENIRAMINE (brome fen IR a mene) PR=C *(Anaplex® DM,³³ Bromaline® DM [O],³³ Bromdex D,³³ Bromfed® DM,³³ Bromphenex™ DM [O],³³ Brotapp [O],³² Brotapp-DM,³³ BroveX™ PEB [O],³¹ Dimaphen™ Children's Cold & Allergy [O],³¹ Dimetapp® Children's Cold & Allergy [O],³¹ Entre-B [O],³¹ J-Tan D PD [O],³² J-Tan PD [O], Lodrane® D [O],³² LoHist PEB [O],³¹ LoHist PSB [O],³² LoHist PSB DM [O],³³ Neo DM,³³ PediaHist DM,³³ Q-Tapp Cold & Allergy [O],³² Q-Tapp Cold & Cough [O],³³ Respa-BR, Resperal-DM,³³ Rynex PE; Vazobid-PD™ [O]³¹)*

CARBINOXAMINE (kar bi NOKS a mene) PR=C *(Arbinoxa, Palgic)*

CETIRIZINE (se TI ra zene) PR=B *(All Day Allergy Childrens [O], All Day Allergy [O], Cetirizine HCl Allergy Child [O], Cetirizine HCl Children's [O], Cetirizine HCl Children's Allergy [O], Cetirizine HCl Hives Relief [O], ZyrTEC-D® Allergy & Congestion [O],³⁴ ZyrTEC Allergy [O], ZyrTEC Children's Allergy [O], ZyrTEC Children's Hives Relief [O], ZyrTEC Hives Relief [O])*

CHLORPHENIRAMINE (klor fen IR a mene) PR=B *(Advil® Allergy Sinus,³⁷ Advil® Multi-Symptom Cold,³⁷ Aller-Chlor [O], Allergy [O], Allergy 4-Hour [O], Allergy Relief [O], Allergy-Time [O], Cardec™ DM [O],¹⁰ Chlor-Trimeton [O], Chlor-Trimeton Allergy [O], Chlorphen [O], Coldcough PD,³ Corfen-DM [O],¹⁰ Coricidin HBP® Cold and Flu [O],³⁶ Coricidin® HBP Cough & Cold [O],³⁷ De-Chlor DM [O],¹⁰ Dicel® Chewable [O],¹³ Dicel® DM Chewables [O],¹⁴ Dimetapp® Children's Long Acting Cough Plus Cold [O],³⁷ Ed-A-Hist™ [O],⁶ Ed A-Hist DM [O],¹⁰ Ed-Chlor-Tan; Ed-Chlortan [O], Ed ChlorPed; Ed ChlorPed D [O],⁶ Ed Chlorped Jr [O], EndaCof [O],¹⁰ Father John's® Plus [O],¹⁰ Kidkare Children's Cough/Cold [O],¹⁴ LoHist [O],⁶ LoHist-D [O],¹³ M-END DM [O],¹⁴ Maxichlor PEH [O],⁶ Maxichlor PSE [O],¹³*

Nasohist™ [O],⁶ Nasohist™ DM Pediatric [O],¹⁰ Neo DM [O],¹⁰ Neutrahist PDX [O],¹⁴ Neutrahist Pediatric [O],¹³ NoHist DM [O],¹⁰ NoHist LQ [O],⁶ Norel® SR,³⁵ Novahistine DH,³ PE-Hist-DM [O],¹⁰ Pedia Relief™ Cough-Cold [O],¹⁴ Pediatric Cough & Cold [O],¹⁴ Pharbechlor [O], Phenagil [O],⁶ Phenylhistine DH [O],¹⁵ Rescon DM [O],¹⁴ Robitussin® Children's Cough & Cold Long-Acting [O],³⁷ Scot-Tussin® DM Maximum Strength [O],³⁷ Sudafed PE® Sinus + Allergy [O],⁶ SudoGest™ Sinus & Allergy [O],¹³ Triaminic® Children's Cold & Allergy [O],⁶ Triaminic® Children's Softchews® Cough & Runny Nose [O],³⁷ Tricode® AR,¹⁵ Tusscough DHC™,³ TussiCaps®,¹² Tussionex® Pennkinetic®,¹² Virdec [O],⁶ Virdec DM [O],¹⁰ Zutripro™⁹)

CLEMASTINE (KLEM as tene) PR=B *(Dayhist Allergy 12-Hour Relief [O], Tavist Allergy [O])*

CYCLIZINE (SYE kli zene) PR=B *(Cyclivert [O])*

CYPROHEPTADINE (si proe HEP ta dene) PR=B

DESLORATADINE (des lor AT a dene) PR=C *(Clarinex®, Clarinex-D® 12-Hour,³⁸ Clarinex® Reditabs)*

DEXCHLORPHENIRAMINE (deks klor fen EER a mene) PR=B

DIMENHYDRINATE (dye men HYE dri nate) PR=B *(Dramamine [O], Driminate [O], Motion Sickness [O])*

DIPHENHYDRAMINE (dye fen HYE dra mene) PR=B *(Aceta-Gesic®,⁴⁰ Advil PM [O],²¹ Aldex® CT,³⁹ Aler-Dryl [O], Allergy [O], Allergy Relief [O], Allergy Relief Children's [O], Altaryl [O], Anti-Hist [O], Anti-Hist Allergy [O], Anti-Itch [O], Anti-Itch Maximum Strength [O], Banophen [O], Bayer® PM [O],⁴² Benadryl [O], Benadryl-D® Allergy & Sinus [O],³⁹ Benadryl-D® Children's Allergy & Sinus [O],³⁹ Benadryl Allergy [O], Benadryl® Allergy and Cold [O],⁴¹ Benadryl® Allergy and Sinus Headache [O],⁴¹ Benadryl Allergy Children's [O], Benadryl Dye-Free Allergy [O], Benadryl Itch Relief [O], Benadryl Itch Stopping [O], Benadryl Maximum Strength [O], Benadryl® Maximum Strength Severe Allergy and Sinus Headache [O],⁴¹ Cold Control PE [O],⁴¹ Complete Allergy Medication [O], Complete*

Allergy Relief [O], Dimetapp® Children's
Nighttime Cold & Congestion [O],[39] Diphen
[O], Diphenhist [O], Excedrin PM® [O],[40]
Genahist [O], Geri-Dryl [O], Goody's PM®
[O],[40] Ibuprofen PM [O],[21] Itch Relief [O],
Legatrin PM®,[40] Mapap PM [O],[40] Motrin PM
[O],[21] Nighttime Sleep Aid [O], Nytol [O],
Nytol Maximum Strength [O], One Tab™
Allergy & Sinus [O],[41] One Tab™ Cold & Flu
[O],[41] PediaCare Childrens Allergy [O],
Percogesic® Extra Strength [O],[40] Pharbedryl
[O], Q-Dryl [O], Quenalin [O], Robitussin®
Peak Cold Nighttime Multi-Symptom Cold
[O],[41] Scot-Tussin Allergy Relief [O], Siladryl
Allergy [O], Silphen Cough [O], Simply Allergy
[O], Simply Sleep [O], Sleep Tabs [O], Sominex
[O], Sominex Maximum Strength [O], Sudafed
PE® Nighttime Cold [O],[41] Sudafed PE®
Severe Cold [O],[41] Tetra-Formula Nighttime
Sleep [O], Theraflu Multi-Symptom [O],
Theraflu® Nighttime Severe Cold & Cough
[O],[41] Theraflu® Sugar-Free Nighttime Severe
Cold & Cough [O],[41] Theraflu® Warming
Relief™ Flu & Sore Throat [O],[41] Theraflu®
Warming Relief™ Nighttime Severe Cold &
Cough [O],[41] TopCare® Pain Relief PM [O],[40]
Total Allergy [O], Total Allergy Medicine [O],
Triaminic® Children's Night Time Cold &
Cough [O],[39] Triaminic Cough/Runny Nose
[O], Tylenol® Allergy Multi-Symptom
Nighttime [O],[41] Tylenol® Children's Plus Cold
and Allergy [O],[41] Tylenol® PM [O],[40] Tylenol®
Severe Allergy [O],[40] ZzzQuil [O])

DOXYLAMINE (dox IL a mene) PR=N (Aldex
AN [O], Diclegis®,[43] Doxytex, Nitetime Sleep-
Aid [O], Sleep Aid [O])

FEXOFENADINE (feks oh FEN a dene) PR=C
(Allegra-D® 12-Hour,[44] Allegra-D® 24 Hour,[44]
Allegra Allergy [O], Allegra Allergy Children's
[O])

HYDROXYZINE (hye DROKS i zene) PR=N
(Vistaril®)

LEVOCETIRIZINE (LEE vo se TI ra zene) PR=B
(Xyzal)

LORATADINE (lor AT a dene) PR=B (Alavert
[O], Alavert™ Allergy and Sinus [O],[45] Allergy
[O], Allergy Relief [O], Allergy Relief For Kids
[O], Childrens Loratadine [O], Claritin [O],
Claritin-D® 12 Hour Allergy & Congestion
[O],[45] Claritin-D® 24 Hour Allergy &
Congestion [O],[45] Claritin Reditabs [O],
Loradamed [O], Loratadine-D 12 Hour [O],[45]
Loratadine Childrens [O], Loratadine Hives
Relief [O], Triaminic Allerchews [O])

MECLIZINE (MEK li zene) PR=B (Antivert®,
Dramamine Less Drowsy [O], Medi-Meclizine
[O], Travel Sickness [O], UniVert; Vertin-32 [O])

OLOPATADINE (oh la PAT a dene) PR=C
(Pataday, Patanase, Patanol)

**PHENYLTOLOXAMINE (fen il tole LOKS a
mene) PR=C** (Norel® SR,[35] Zgesic[46])

PROMETHAZINE (proe METH a zene) PR=C
(Phenadoz™, Phenergan®, Promethazine
VC,[47] Promethegan™)

PYRILAMINE (pie RIL a mene) (Codituss DM
[O],[22] Pyril DM [O],[22] Ru-Hist-D,[23] Ru-Hist Plus
[O][22])

TRIPROLIDINE (trye PROE li dene) PR=C
(Aprodine [O],[48] Pediatex® TD[48])

CORTICOSTEROIDS (See Chapter 7, Section 4)

MAST CELL STABILIZERS (See Section 1
Above)

Allergic rhinitis is an inflammation of the nose
and sinuses caused by allergies. If it is seasonal, it
is hay fever. Symptoms include itching, sneezing,
rhinorrhea, and/or nasal congestion. Allergic
rhinitis and asthma often coexist, and the treatments for each can overlap.

FUNCTION

Antihistamines prevent the release of histamine,
a major moderator of inflammation. They generally prevent congestion. They are used in treating
allergies and inflammatory conditions. Some of
the older antihistamines have central sedating
tendencies and are used to treat insomnia. These effects are summarized in
Figure 8.4 on page 238.

Hydroxyzine, diphenhydramine, and many of
the over-the-counter antihistamines are used to
treat motion sickness and prevent nausea and
vomiting.

Desloratadine and fexofenadine are considered non-sedating antihistamines.

Rhinorrhea: Discharge of thin nasal
mucus

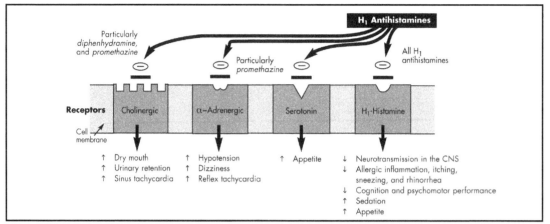

Figure 8.4: Effects of antihistamines on specific receptors and their resulting actions. All antihistamines act to block H_1 receptors while most have effects on other receptors at varying affinities.

MECHANISM OF ACTION

The first-line treatment of allergic rhinitis is the use of antihistamines and decongestants. Anti-histamines are competitive inhibitors of the H_1-receptors. This inhibition prevents release of histamine, a major mediator of inflammation. Many of the side effects of antihistamines are due to blockage of receptors other than the histamine receptors.

α-adrenergic agonists, which are often called nasal decongestants, act by causing vasoconstriction of nasal mucosa arterioles, which prevents leakage and reduces airway resistance.

Mast cell stabilizers and corticosteroids are also used infrequently and reduce the inflammatory process."

DOSAGES

ACRIVASTINE, used only in combination with other drugs, and therefore its individual dosing is not covered here.

AZELASTINE, for *children* 5-11 years, for seasonal allergic rhinitis, intranasal: 1 spray each nostril bid. For *children* 12 and older and *adults*, for seasonal allergic rhinitis, intranasal: 1-2 sprays in each nostril bid; for vasomotor rhinitis, intranasal: 2 sprays each nostril bid.

BROMPHENIRAMINE, for *children* 2-6, for allergic rhinitis, allergic symptoms, and vasomotor rhinitis, J-Tan PD: 1 mg (1 mL) every 4-6 hours up to a maximum of 6 mg/d; for children 6-12, for allergic rhinitis, allergic symp-

toms, and vasomotor rhinitis, J-Tan PD: 2 mg (2 mL) every 4-6 hours up to a maximum of 12 mg/d; LoHist-12: 1 tablet every 12 hours up to a maximum of 2 tablets/d. For *children* over 12 and *adults*, for allergic rhinitis, allergic symptoms, and vasomotor rhinitis, Bromax: 1 tablet bid; LoHist-12: 1-2 tablets every 12 hours up to a maximum of 4 tablets/d.

CARBINOXAMINE, for *children* 2-5 years, for allergic rhinitis or urticaria, 0.2-0.4 mg/kg/d divided into 3-4 doses or 1-2 mg 3-4 times/d; for *children* 6-11, for allergic rhinitis or urticaria, 2-4 mg, 3-4 times/d. For *adults*, for allergic rhinitis or urticaria, 4-8 mg 3-4 times/d.

CETIRIZINE, for *children*, for chronic urticaria and perennial allergic rhinitis, 6-12 months, 2.5 mg once daily; 12 months to <2 years, 2.5 mg once daily; may increase to 2.5 mg every 12 hours prn; 2-5 yrs, initiate at 2.5 mg once daily; may increase to 2.5 mg every 12 hours or 5 mg once daily. For *children* 6 years and older and *adults*, for chronic urticaria and perennial or seasonal allergic rhinitis, 5-10 mg once daily, depending on symptom severity. For the *elderly*, initiate at 5 mg once daily; may increase to 10 mg/d. Manufacturer recommends 5 mg/d in patients over 77 years of age.

CHLORPHENIRAMINE, for *children*, 0.35 mg/kg/d in divided doses every 4-6 hours; 2-6 years, 1 mg every 4-6 hours, not to exceed 6 mg in 24 hours; 6-12 years, 2 mg every 4-6 hours, not to exceed 12 mg/d, or sustained release 8 mg nocte. For *children* >12 years and *adults*, 4 mg every 4-6 hours, not to exceed 24 mg/d, or sustained release 8-12 mg every 8-12 hours, not to exceed 24 mg/d.

CLEMASTINE, for rhinitis or other allergic symptoms, for *infants* and *children* under 6 years, 0.05 mg/kg/d divided into 2 or 3 doses up to a maximum daily dose of 1 mg; for *children* 6-12 years, 0.5-1 mg bid, not to exceed 3 mg/d; for children 12 and older, refer to adult dosing. For *adults*, for rhinitis or allergic symptoms, 1 mg bid to 2 mg tid, not to exceed 6 mg/d.

CYCLIZINE, for *children* 6-11 years, for prevention and treatment of motion sickness, 25 mg 1 hour before travel or at onset of symptoms; repeat every 6-8 hours up to maximum of 3 tablets/d. For *children* 12 and older and *adults*, for prevention and treatment of motion sickness, 50 mg taken 30 minutes before departure; may repeat in 4-6 hours prn up to 200 mg/d.

CYPROHEPTADINE, for *children*, for allergic conditions, 0.25 mg/kg/day or 8 mg/m^2/d in 2-3 divided doses; for 2-6 years, 2 mg every 8-12 hours (not to exceed 12 mg/d); 7-14 years, 4 mg every 8-12 hours (not to exceed 16 mg/d); for migraine headaches, 4 mg 2-3 times/d. For *adults*, for allergic conditions, 4-20 mg/d divided every 8 hours not to exceed 0.5 mg/kg/d; for cluster headaches, 4 mg qid; for migraine headaches, 4-8 mg tid.

DESLORATADINE, for *children*, 6-11 months, 1 mg once daily; 12 months to 5 years, 1.25 mg once daily; 6-11 years, 2.5 mg once daily. For *children* 12 and older and *adults*, 5 mg once daily.

DEXCHLORPHENIRAMINE, for *children*, 2-5 years, 0.5 mg every 4-6 hours (do not use timed release); 6-11 years, 1 mg every 4-6 hours or 4 mg timed release nocte. For *adults*, 2 mg every 4-6 hours or 4-6 mg timed release nocte or every 8-10 hours.

DIMENHYDRINATE, for the prevention of and treatment of motion sickness, for *children* 2-5 years, 12.5-25 mg every 6-8 hours up to a maximum of 75 mg/d; for *children* 6-12 years, 25-50 mg every 6-8 hours up to a maximum of 150 mg/d; IM: 1.25 mg/kg or 37.5 mg/m^2 qid up to a maximum of 300 mg/d; for *adults*, 50-100 mg every 4-6 hours up to a maximum of 400 mg/d; IM: 50 mg every 4 hours up to a maximum of 100 mg every 4 hours.

DIPHENHYDRAMINE, for *children*, for allergic reactions or motion sickness, oral or IM: 5 mg/kg/d or 150 mg/m^2/d in divided doses every 6-8 hours; maximum 300 mg/d; for *children* 12 years and older, as a nighttime sleep aid, 50 mg nocte; as an antitussive: for *children* 2-6, 6.25 mg every 4 hours up to maximum 37.5 mg/d; for *children* 6-12, 12.5 mg every 4 hours up to maximum 75 mg/d; for *children* 12 and older, 25 mg every 4 hours up to maximum 150 mg/d; for *children*, for treatment of dystonic reactions, IM: 0.5-1 mg/kg/dose. For *adults*, for allergic reactions or motion sickness, 25-50 mg every 6-8 hours, IM: 10-50 mg per dose and up to 100 mg if needed; maximum is 400 mg/d; as an antitussive, 25 mg every 4 hours up to maximum 150 mg/d; as a nighttime sleep aid, 50 mg nocte; for dystonic reactions, IM: 50 mg in a single dose; may repeat in 20-30 minutes prn. For the *elderly*, initiate at 25 mg 2-3 times/d increasing prn.

DOXYLAMINE, for *adults*, for insomnia, one tablet 30 mins before bedtime.

FEXOFENADINE, for chronic idiopathic urticaria and seasonal allergic rhinitis, for *children* 6-11 years, 30 mg bid; for *children* 12 and over and *adults*, 60 mg bid or 180 mg once daily.

HYDROXYZINE, for *children*, for preoperative sedation, 0.6 mg/kg/dose every 6 hours; for **pruritis**, and anxiety, under 6 years, 50 mg daily in divided doses; over 6 years, 50-100 mg daily in divided doses. For *adults*, for anxiety, 25-100 mg qid up to a maximum dose of 600 mg/d; for preoperative sedation, 50-100 mg; for management of pruritus, 25 mg 3-4 times/d.

Pruritis: Itching

LEVOCETIRIZINE, for perennial allergic rhinitis, seasonal allergic rhinitis, or chronic urticaria, for *children* 6 mos. to 5 years, 1.25 mg nocte; for *children* 6-11 years, 2.5 mg nocte; for *children* 12 and older, refer to adult dosing. For *adults*, for allergic rhinitis or chronic urticaria, 5 mg nocte; 2.5 mg daily may provide adequate symptom relief in some patients.

LORATADINE, for seasonal allergic rhinitis or chronic

idiopathic urticaria, for *children* 2-5 years, 5 mg once daily; for *children* 6 or older, use adult dosing. For *adults*, for seasonal allergic rhinitis or chronic idiopathic urticaria, 10 mg/d.

MECLIZINE, for *children* over 12 years and *adults*, for motion sickness, 12.5-25 mg 1 hour before travel; repeat dose every 12-24 hours if needed; doses up to 50 mg may be needed; for vertigo, 25-100 mg/d in divided doses.

OLOPATADINE, for *children* 6-11 years, for seasonal allergic rhinitis, intranasal: 1 spray into each nostril bid. For *children* 12 and older and *adults*, for seasonal allergic rhinitis, intranasal: 2 sprays into each nostril bid.

PHENYLTOLOXAMINE, used only in combination with other drugs, and therefore its individual dosing is not covered here.

PROMETHAZINE, for *children* 2 years and over, for allergic conditions, 0.1 mg/kg/dose up to a maximum of 12.5 mg every 6 hours during the day and 0.5 mg/kg/dose up to a maximum of 25 mg, nocte prn; as an antiemetic, 0.25-1 mg/kg 4-6 times/d as needed up to a maximum of 25 mg/dose; for motion sickness, 0.5 mg/kg/dose 30 minutes to 1 hour before departure, then every 12 hours as needed up to a maximum dose of 25 mg bid; for sedation, 0.5-1 mg/kg/dose every 6 hours as needed up to a maximum of 50 mg/dose. For *adults*, for allergic conditions (including allergic reactions to blood or plasma), 25 mg nocte or 12.5 mg before meals and at bedtime; usual range is 6.25-12.5 mg tid; as an antiemetic, 12.5-25 mg every 4-6 hours as needed; for motion sickness, 25 mg 30-60 minutes before departure, then every 12 hours as needed; for sedation, 12.5-50 mg/dose.

PYRILAMINE, used only in combination with other drugs, and therefore its individual dosing is not covered here.

TRIPROLIDINE, used only in combination with other drugs, and therefore its individual dosing is not covered here.

ADVERSE EFFECTS

Antihistamines may cause sedation of various intensities depending on the agent. Caution should be used when using machinery while taking sedating antihistamines. Dry mouth and eyes are also common. Other effects include urinary retention, **tachycardia**, hypotension, vertigo, and increased appetite. Overdoses, while rare, do happen especially in children. Signs and symptoms of an overdose include hallucinations, **ataxia**, excitement, convulsions, and ultimately a deepening coma and collapse of the cardiac and respiratory systems.

RED FLAGS

An FDA alert was released regarding promethazine. This agent should not be used in patients under 2 years of age due to the potential for fatal respiratory depression.

INTERACTIONS

DRUG

Antihistamines should not be used with other CNS depressants including ethanol. MAO inhibitors should not be used concurrently as they will enhance the anticholinergic effects.

HERB

ANTIHISTAMINES
- *Bai Jiang Cao* (Dahurian patrinia herb) (Indeterminate)–has a sedative effect and may increase sedative effects of drugs (Chinese language article cited in Chen & Chen, 2004) Indeterminate level of evidence.
- *Bai Shao* (White peony root) (Indeterminate)–has a sedative and analgesic effect and may increase sedative effects of drugs (Chinese language article cited in Chen & Chen, 2004) Indeterminate level of evidence.
- *Chan Tui* (Cicada moulting) (Indeterminate)–has an inhibitory effect on the CNS potentiating sedative drugs (Chinese language article cited in Chen & Chen, 2004) Indeterminate level of evidence.
- *Jiao Gu Lan* (Gynostemma) (Indeterminate)–has sedative, hypnotic, analgesic effects and may increase sedative effects of drugs (Chinese language article cited in Chen & Chen, 2004) Indeterminate level of evidence.

Tachycardia: A rapid heart rate defined as over 100 bpms

Ataxia: Incoordination of voluntary muscles resulting in jerky movements that may affect the limbs, head, or trunk

- *Lang Dan Cao* (Gentiana) (Indeterminate)–has a sedative effect and may increase sedative effects of drugs (Chinese language article cited in Chen & Chen, 2004) Indeterminate level of evidence.
- *Niu Huang* (Cow gallstone) (Indeterminate)–has a mild sedative effect and may increase sedative effects of drugs (Chinese language article cited in Chen & Chen, 2004) Indeter-minate level of evidence.
- *Qin Jiao* (Gentiana macrophylla root) (Indeterminate)–has an inhibitory effect on the CNS potentiating sedative drugs (Chinese language article cited in Chen & Chen, 2004) Indeterminate level of evidence.
- *Shen*-calming herbs (D)–may have marked sedative and tranquilizing effects and may increase sedative effects of drugs, expert opinion (Chen & Chen, 2004) Level 5 evidence.
- *Tian Nan Xing* (Arisaema) (Indeterminate)–has a marked sedative and analgesic effect and may increase sedative effects of drugs (Chinese language article cited in Chen & Chen, 2004) Indeterminate level of evidence.
- *Wu Jia Pi* (Acanthopanax) (Indeterminate)–has a mild sedative effect and may increase sedative effects of drugs (Chinese language article cited in Chen & Chen, 2004) Indeterminate level of evidence.
- *Xi Jiao* (Rhinoceros horn) (Indeterminate)–has a sedative effect and may increase sedative effects of drugs (Chinese language article cited in Chen & Chen, 2004) Indeterminate level of evidence.
- *Zhi Zi* (Gardenia, cape jasmine fruit) (Indeterminate)–has a sedative effect and may increase sedative effects of drugs (Chinese language article cited in Chen & Chen, 2004) Indeterminate level of evidence.

FEXOFENADINE

- *Guan Ye Lian Qiao* (St. John's wort) (C)–decreases blood concentrations (Zhou, Chan, Pan, Huang & Lee, 2004) Level 2b evidence; (Izzo & Ernst, 2009) Level 4 evidence.

INTERACTIONS

A:

D: Cyproheptadine* is 96-99% protein bound; Dimenhydrinate* and Diphenhydramine are 98-99% bound; Loratadine* is 97-99% bound.

M: Chlorpheniramine is a major substrate of CYP2D6; diphenhydramine is a moderate inhibitor of CYP2D6; Loratadine* is a strong inhibitor CYP2C19 and a major substrate of 3A4; promethazine is a major substrate of CYP2B6 and 2D6.

E:

Pgp: Azelastine* inhibits Pgp; cetirizine, desloratadine, fexofenadine, and loratadine are substrates of Pgp.

TI:

SECTION 3: AGENTS USED FOR CHRONIC OBSTRUCTIVE PULMONARY DISEASE

β-ADRENERGIC AGONISTS *(See Chapter 4, Section 4)*

CORTICOSTEROIDS *(See Chapter 7, Section 4)*

ANTICHOLINERGIC AGENT:

IPRATROPIUM *(See Chapter 4, Section 3)*

Chronic obstructive pulmonary disease (COPD) is the fourth leading cause of death in the U.S., where it affects 24 million people. Symptoms include a productive cough, **dyspnea**, decreased breath sounds, and wheezing. Severe cases can lead to weight loss, pneumothorax, right heart and/or respiratory failure. Two diseases are commonly considered COPD: emphysema and chronic bronchitis. Emphysema is destruction of the lung **parenchyma,** which reduces elasticity and destroys the

Dyspnea: Shortness of breath or difficulty breathing

Parenchyma: The distinguishing or specific cells of a gland or organ supported in a connective tissue framework

Septum: A thin wall dividing two cavities or two areas of soft tissue; septa is plural

Septum: A thin wall dividing two cavities or two areas of soft tissue; septa is plural

alveolar **septa**. These cause airway collapse, secondary lung hyperinflation, and air trapping. Chronic bronchitis is caused by excessive mucus secretion, which obstructs the normal functioning of the lungs.

FUNCTION

The drugs used to treat COPD either cause bronchodilation or reduce inflammation.

MECHANISM OF ACTION

COPD drugs are primarily used as bronchodilators. β_2-adrenergic agonists are primarily used to achieve this, though anticholinergics may also be used. Moderate to severe COPD also requires corticosteroid use to reduce inflammation. Severe

COPD may need antibiotics, for episodes of exacerbations, and long-term oxygen therapy.

DOSAGES

See dosages of drugs in their original sections.

ADVERSE EFFECTS

See the adverse effects of these drugs in their original sections.

RED FLAGS

See red flags of these drugs in their original sections.

INTERACTIONS

See interactions for these drugs in their original sections.

SECTION 4: AGENTS USED TO TREAT COUGH

ANTITUSSIVES:

BENZONATATE (ben ZOE na tate) PR=C *(Tessalon®)*

EXPECTORANTS:

GUAIFENESIN (gwye FEN e sin) PR=C *(Allfen CD,[29] Allfen CDX,[29] Altarussin [O], Ambi 10PEH/400GFN [O],[25] Ambifed DM,[51] Ambifed-G [O],[27] Ambifed-G DM,[51] Bidex [O], BP 8 Cough,[51] Buckley's Chest Congestion [O], Cheracol® D [O],[26] Cheracol® Plus [O],[26] Cheratussin® DAC,[50] Codar® GF,[29] Congestac® [O],[27] Coricidin HBP® Chest Congestion and Cough [O],[26] Cough Syrup [O], Dex-Tuss,[29] Diabetic Siltussin DAS-Na [O], Diabetic Siltussin-DM DAS-Na [O],[26] Diabetic Siltussin-DM DAS-Na Maximum Strength [O],[26] Diabetic Tussin [O], Diabetic Tussin® DM [O],[26] Diabetic Tussin® DM Maximum Strength [O],[26] Diabetic Tussin Mucus Relief [O], Difil-G® 400,[49] Double Tussin DM [O],[26] Entre-Cough,[51] ExeFen-DMX,[51] ExeFen-IR, Fenesin DM IR [O],[26] Fenesin IR [O], Fenesin PE IR; Geri-Tussin [O], GoodSense Mucus Relief [O], Guaiatussin AC,[29] Guaicon DMS* *[O],[26] Iophen C-NR,[29] Iophen DM-NR [O],[26] Iophen-NR [O], J-Max [O],[25] Kolephrin® GG/DM [O],[26] Liquibid [O], Liquibid® D-R [O],[25] Liquibid® PD-R [O],[25] Liquituss GG [O], M-Clear,[29] M-Clear WC,[29] Mar-Cof® CG,[29] Maxifed [O],[27] Maxifed DMX,[51] Maxiphen DMX,[28] Medent®-PEI [O],[25] Mucinex [O], Mucinex Chest Congestion Child [O], Mucinex® Children's Multi-Symptom Cold [O],[28] Mucinex® Cold [O],[25] Mucinex® D [O],[27] Mucinex® D Maximum Strength [O],[27] Mucinex® DM [O],[26] Mucinex® DM Maximum Strength [O],[26] Mucinex For Kids [O], Mucinex® Kid's Cough [O],[26] Mucinex® Kid's Cough Mini-Melts™ [O],[26] Mucinex Maximum Strength [O], Mucosa [O], Mucus-ER [O], Mucus Relief [O], Mucus Relief Children's [O], Mucus Relief Sinus [O],[25] Mytussin® DAC,[50] Nu-COPD [O],[25] OneTab™ Congestion & Cold [O],[25] Organ-I NR [O], Q-Tussin [O], Q-Tussin DM [O],[26] Refenesen [O], Refenesen 400 [O], Refenesen™ DM [O],[26] Refenesen™ PE [O],[25] Refenesen Plus [O],[27] Rescon GG [O],[25] Robafen [O], Robafen AC,[29] Robafen CF Cough & Cold [O],[28] Robafen DM Clear [O],[26]*

Robafen DM [O],[26] Robitussin Chest Congestion [O], Robitussin® Children's Cough & Cold CF [O],[28] Robitussin Mucus+ Chest Congestion [O], Robitussin® Peak Cold Maximum Strength Multi-Symptom Cold [O],[28] Robitussin® Peak Cold Multi-Symptom Cold [O],[28] Robitussin® Peak Cold Cough + Chest Congestion DM [O],[26] Robitussin® Peak Cold Maximum Strength Cough + Chest Congestion DM [O],[26] Robitussin® Peak Cold Sugar-Free Cough + Chest Congestion DM [O],[26] Safe Tussin® DM [O],[26] Scot-Tussin Expectorant [O], Scot-Tussin® Senior [O],[26]

Silexin [O],[26] Siltussin DAS [O], Siltussin DM [O],[26] Siltussin DM DAS [O],[26] Siltussin SA [O], Sudafed PE® Non-Drying Sinus [O],[25] Triaminic® Children's Chest & Nasal Congestion [O],[25] Tricode® GF,[50] Tusicof® [O],[28] Tussin [O], Vicks® 44E [O],[26] Vicks® DayQuil® Mucus Control DM [O],[26] Vicks® Nature Fusion™ Cough & Chest Congestion [O],[26] Vicks® Pediatric Formula 44E [O],[26] Xpect [O], Yodefan-NF Chest Congestion [O], Zyncof® [O][26])

OPIATES (See Chapter 5, Section 8)

FUNCTION

The antitussives function by reducing the urge to cough. In contrast, the expectorants act by loosening mucus in the lungs for easier expulsion.

MECHANISM OF ACTION

Benzonatate acts by causing a topical anesthetic effect on respiratory stretch receptors. This reduces the initial impulse to initiate a cough. Guaifenesin is an expectorant and stimulates secretions in the respiratory tract, which increases fluid volumes and reduces viscosity of the mucus. Opiates act on the cough centers in the CNS, decreasing their sensitivity to peripheral stimuli.

DOSAGES

BENZONATATE, for *children* over 10 years and *adults*, 100 mg tid or every 4 hours up to 600 mg/d.

GUAIFENESIN, as a cough expectorant, for *children* 6 mos. to 2 years, 25-50 mg every 4 hours up to a maximum of 300 mg/d; for *children* 2-5 years, 50-100 mg every 4 hours up to a maximum of 600 mg/d; for *children* 6-11 years, 100-200 mg every 4 hours up to a maximum of 1.2 g/d; for *children* 12 years and older and *adults*, 200-400 mg every 4 hours up to a maximum of 2.4 g/d; extended release tablets: 600-1200 mg every 12 hours up to a maximum of 2.4 g/d.

ADVERSE EFFECTS

Guaifenesin may cause kidney stones when used in large quantities.

RED FLAGS

No major red flags noted.

INTERACTIONS

No interactions found.

ENDNOTES

[1] Combination of Dyphylline and Guaifenesin.

[2] Combination of Acrivastine and Pseudoephedrine.

[3] Combination of Phenylephrine, Chlorpheniramine, and Dihydrocodeine.

[4] Combination of Carbinoxamine, Pseudoephedrine, and Hydrocodone.

[5] Combination of Chlorpheniramine, Methscopolamine, and Phenylephrine.

[6] Combination of Chlorpheniramine and Phenylephrine.

[7] Combination of Phenylephrine, Chlorpheniramine, and Dihydrocodeine.

[8] Combination of Chlorpheniramine, Carbetapentane, and Phenylephrine.

[9] Combination of Chlorpheniramine, Pseudoephedrine, and Hydrocodone.

[10] Combination of Dextromethorphan, Chlorpheniramine, and Phenylephrine.

[11] Combination of Chlorpheniramine, Phenylephrine, and Phenyltoloxamine.

[12] Combination of Chlorpheniramine, and Hydrocodone.

[13] Combination of Pseudoephedrine and Chlorpheniramine.

[14] Combination of Chlorpheniramine, Pseudoephedrine, and Dextromethorphan.

[15] Combination of Codeine, Chlorpheniramine, and Pseudoephedrine.

[16] Combination of Chlorpheniramine, Pseudoephedrine, and Dihydrocodeine.

[17] Combination of Acetaminophen, Caffeine, Hydrocodone, Chlorpheniramine, and Phenylephrine.

[18] Combination of Carbetapentane, Ephedrine, Phenylephrine, and Chlorpheniramine.

[19] Combination of Carbetapentane and Chlorpheniramine.

[20] Combination of Pseudoephedrine and Dexchlorpheniramine.

[21] Combination of Diphenhydramine and Ibuprofen.

[22] Combination of Dextromethorphan, Phenylephrine, and Pyrilamine.

[23] Combination of Pyrilamine and Phenylephrine.

[24] Combination of Carbetapentane, Pyrilamine, and Phenylephrine.

[25] Combination of Guaifenesin and Phenylephrine.

[26] Combination of Dextromethorphan, an over-the-counter cough suppressant, and Guaifenesin.

[27] Combination of Guaifenesin and Pseudoephedrine.

[28] Combination of Guaifenesin, Dextromethorphan, and Phenylephrine.

[29] Combination of Codeine and Guaifenesin.

[30] Combination of Guaifenesin, Hydrocodone, and Phenylephrine.

[31] Combination of Brompheniramine and Phenylephrine.

[32] Combination of Brompheniramine and Pseudoephedrine.

[33] Combination of Brompheniramine, Pseudoephedrine, and Dextromethorphan.

[34] Combination of Cetirizine and Pseudoephedrine.

[35] Combination of Chlorpheniramine, Acetaminophen, Phenylephrine, and Phenyltoloxamine.

[36] Combination of Chlorpheniramine and Acetaminophen.

[37] Combination of Chlorpheniramine, Ibuprofen, and Pseudoephedrine.

[38] Combination of Desloratadine and Pseudoephedrine.

[39] Combination of Diphenhydramine and Phenylephrine.

[40] Combination of Diphenhydramine and Acetaminophen.

[41] Combination of Diphenhydramine, Phenylephrine, and Acetaminophen.

[42] Combination of Diphenhydramine and Aspirin.

[43] Combination of Doxylamine and Pyridoxine.

[44] Combination of Fexofenadine and Pseudoephedrine.

[45] Combination of Loratadine and Pseudoephedrine.

[46] Combination of Phenyltoloxamine and Acetaminophen.

[47] Combination of Promethazine and Phenylephrine.

[48] Combination of Triprolidine and Pseudoephedrine.

[49] Combination of Guaifenesin and Dyphylline.

[50] Combination of Guaifenesin, Pseudoephedrine, and Codeine.

[51] Combination of Guaifenesin, Pseudoephedrine, and Dextromethorphan.

■ CHINESE MEDICAL DESCRIPTIONS

The Chinese medical explanation of the drug categories in this chapter may be found in Chapter 15 on pages 385–417.

SECTION 1: AGENTS USED IN PEPTIC ULCER DISEASE

ANTACIDS

ALUMINUM HYDROXIDE (a LOO mi num hye DROKS ide) PR=B *(Acid Gone [O],[7] Acid Gone Extra Strength [O],[7] Alamag [O],[8] Alamag Plus [O],[13] Aldroxicon I [O],[13] Aldroxicon II [O],[13] Almacone® [O],[13] Almacone® Double Strength [O],[13] DermaMed [O], Gaviscon® Extra Strength [O],[7] Gaviscon® Liquid [O],[7] Gaviscon® Tablet [O],[9] Gelusil® [O],[13] Maalox® Advanced Maximum Strength [O],[13] Maalox® Advanced Regular Strength [O],[13] Mag-Al [O],[8] Mag-Al Ultimate [O],[8] Mi-Acid [O],[13] Mintox Plus [O],[13] Mylanta® Classic Maximum Strength Liquid [O],[13] Mylanta® Classic Regular Strength Liquid [O],[13] Rulox [O][13])*

CALCIUM CARBONATE (KAL see um KAR bun ate) PR=N *(Alcalak [O], Antacid [O], Antacid Extra Strength [O], Cal-Carb Forte [O], Cal-CO3S [O], Cal-Gest Antacid [O], Cal-Mint [O], Calcarb 600 [O], Calci-Chew [O], Calci-Mix [O], Calcio del Mar [O], Calcium 600 [O], Calcium Antacid [O], Calcium Antacid Extra Strength [O], Calcium Antacid Ultra Maximum Strength [O], Calcium High Potency [O], Caltrate 600 [O], Chewable Calcium [O], Florical [O], Gas Ban™ [O],[11] Maalox [O], Maalox® Advanced Maximum Strength [O],[11] Maalox Children's [O], Maalox® Junior Plus Antigas [O],[11] Mi-Acid™ Double Strength [O],[10] Mylanta® Gelcaps® [O],[10] Mylanta® Supreme [O],[10] Mylanta® Ultra [O],[10] Os-Cal [O], Oysco 500 [O], Pepcid® Complete® [O],[12] Rolaids® [O],[10] Rolaids® Extra Strength [O],[10] Titralac [O], Titralac® Plus [O],[11] Tums [O], Tums Calcium for Life Bone [O], Tums® Dual Action [O],[12] Tums E-X 750 [O], Tums Freshers [O], Tums Kids [O], Tums Lasting Effects [O], Tums Smoothies [O], Tums Ultra 1000 [O])*

MAGNESIUM HYDROXIDE (mag NEE zee um hye DROKS ide) PR=N *(Alamag [O],[8] Alamag Plus [O],[13] Aldroxicon I [O],[13] Aldroxicon II [O],[13] Almacone® Double Strength [O],[13] Almacone® [O],[13] Dulcolax Milk of Magnesia [O], Gelusil® [O],[13] Maalox® Advanced Maximum Strength [O],[13] Maalox® Advanced Regular Strength [O],[13] Mag-Al [O],[8] Mag-Al Ultimate [O],[8] Mi-Acid [O],[13] Mi-Acid™ Double Strength [O],[10] Milk of Magnesia [O], Milk of Magnesia Concentrate [O], Mintox Plus [O],[13] Mylanta® Classic Maximum Strength Liquid [O],[13] Mylanta® Classic Regular Strength Liquid [O],[13] Mylanta® Gelcaps® [O],[10] Mylanta® Supreme [O],[10] Mylanta® Ultra [O],[10] Pedia-Lax [O], Pepcid® Complete® [O],[12] Phillips'® M-O [O],[18] Rolaids® [O],[10] Rolaids® Extra Strength [O],[10] Rulox [O],[13] Tums® Dual Action [O][12])*

SODIUM BICARBONATE (SOW dee um bye KAR bun ate) (NEUT) PR=C

ANTIMICROBIAL AGENTS: *(See Chapter 10)*

AMOXICILLIN

BISMUTH *(See Section 3)*

LARITHROMYCIN

METRONIDAZOLE

TETRACYCLINE

ANTIMUSCARINIC AGENTS:

DICYCLOMINE *(See Chapter 4, Section 3)*

H$_2$-HISTAMINE ANTAGONISTS:

CIMETIDINE (sye MET i dene) PR=B *(Cimetidine Acid Reducer [O], Tagamet HB [O®])*

FAMOTIDINE (fa MOE ti dene) PR=B *(Acid Reducer [O], Acid Reducer Maximum Strength [O], Duexis®,[14] Heartburn Relief [O], Heartburn Relief Maximum Strength [O],*

...continued on the following page

SECTION 1: AGENTS USED IN PEPTIC ULCER DISEASE cont.

Pepcid, Pepcid® Complete® [O],[12] Tums® Dual Action® [O][12])

NIZATIDINE (ni ZA ti dene) PR=B (Axid®, Axid AR [O])

RANITIDINE (ra NI ti dene) PR=B (Acid Reducer [O], Acid Reducer Maximum Strength [O], Ranitidine 75 [O], Ranitidine Acid Reducer [O], Zantac®, Zantac®75 [O], Zantac® 150 Maximum Strength [O], Zantac® in NaCl®)

PROTON-PUMP INHIBITORS:

DEXLANSOPRAZOLE (deks lan SOE pra zole) PR=B (Dexilant™)

ESOMEPRAZOLE (es oh ME pray zol) PR=B (Nexium®, Nexium® IV, Vimovo™[15])

LANSOPRAZOLE (lan SOE pra zole) PR=B (First-Lansoprazole, Heartburn Relief 24 Hour [O], Omeclamox-Pak®,[1] Prevacid®, Prevacid® 24 HR, Prevacid® SoluTab™, Prevpac®[2])

OMEPRAZOLE (oh ME pray zol) PR=C (First-Ome-prazole, Omeprazole+Syrspend SF Alka, Prilosec, Prilosec OTC [O], Zegerid®,[3] Zegerid OTC™ [O][3])

PANTOPRAZOLE (pan TOE pra zole) PR=B (Protonix®)

RABEPRAZOLE (ra BE pray zole) PR=B (AcipHex®)

PROSTAGLANDINS:

MISOPROSTOL (mye soe PROST ole) PR=X (Arthrotec®,[4] Cytotec®)

MISCELLANEOUS GASTROINTESTINAL AGENTS:

CISAPRIDE (SIS a pride) PR=C (Propulsid®)

MEPENZOLATE (See Chapter 4, Section 3)

SUCRALFATE (soo KRAL fate) PR=B (Carafate®)

These agents are used to treat gastro-esophageal reflux disease (GERD) and peptic ulcer disease. Peptic ulcer disease causes an erosion of the mucosal lining of the stomach (gastric) or the first part of the small intestine (duodenal). This erosion can cause pain, usually alleviated by food or antacids, but can become life threatening if it causes a hemorrhage or perforation. While the complete pathogenesis of peptic ulcer disease is not completely understood, there are three factors that are commonly recognized. The first is an infection of *helicobacter pylori* (H. pylori), a small, difficult-to-eradicate bacteria. The second factor is increased hydrochloric acid secretion in the stomach. And the final factor is inadequate mucosal protection against the acid in the stomach. This final factor may be caused by long-term or overuse of NSAIDs. Treatment is geared towards each of these factors.

While GERD has a completely different patho-physiology, it is treated similarly to peptic ulcer disease with the exception of antibiotics. GERD is caused by reflux of acid from the stomach into the esophagus. This can cause changes in the esophagus including **esophagitis**, **strictures**, and Barrett's esophagus, a **metaplastic** condition that is precancerous. Drug treatment is geared towards reducing the acidity of the gastric secretions.

Many of these agents are also useful in treating Zollinger-Ellison syndrome. This syndrome is caused by a tumor that excessively secretes **gastrins,** which causes hypersecretion of acid leading to ulceration.

█ FUNCTION

The antimicrobials are used to eradicate the *H. pylori* infection in peptic ulcer disease. Antimuscarinic agents, histamine antagonists, proton-pump inhibitors, and prostaglandins all work to reduce the acidity of the gastric secretions. Antimuscarinic agents are used as an adjunct to other treatments and are generally used only in patients where other treatments have failed because they have extensive adverse effects. Prostaglandins are generally milder acting than the histamine antagonists and proton-pump

---

Esophagitis: Inflammation of the esophagus

Stricture: A narrowing or stenosis of a tube, duct, or hollow structure, usually consisting of a contracture or deposition of abnormal tissue

Metaplastic: Pertaining to an abnormal transformation of adult, fully differentiated tissue of one kind into a differentiated tissue of another kind; often cancerous or precancerous

Gastrins: Hormones secreted in the mucosa of the stomach that stimulate hydrochloric acid secretion

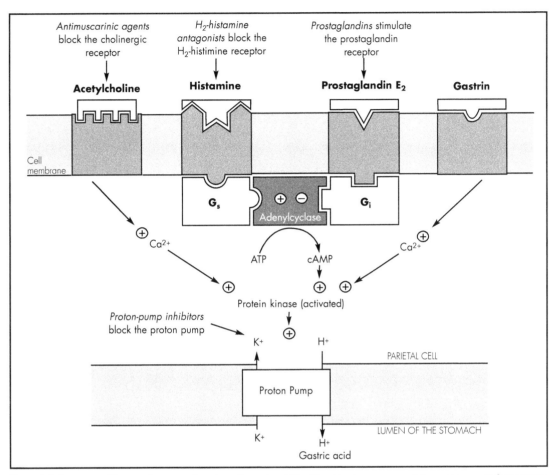

Figure 9.1: Summary of how various agents reduce stomach acidity. All act to slow or prevent the proton pump from secreting hydrogen ions into the lumen of the stomach. Antimuscarinic agents do this by blocking cholinergic receptors, which normally release calcium ions and activate protein kinase and the proton pump. H_2-histamine antagonists and prostaglandins both down regulate adenyl cyclase, lowering cAMP and protein kinase activity and ultimately decreasing proton-pump action. Proton-pump inhibitors directly block the proton pump.

inhibitors, but are especially useful in NSAID-induced ulceration.

Current treatment of peptic ulcer disease (PUD) follows either a triple-therapy or quadruple-therapy regimen for two weeks. The triple-therapy includes a proton pump inhibitor (to reduce acid), either metronidazole or amoxicillin, and clarithromycin to attack the *H. pylori*. Quadruple therapy consists of a proton-pump inhibitor, metronidazole, tetracycline, and bismuth subsalicylate.

Antacids directly, if mildly, reduce the acidity of the gastric secretions. They have been found to be more effective in treating duodenal ulcers than gastric ulcers. Calcium carbonate is also used as a calcium supplement.

Sucralfate enhances the mucosal layer and adds protection to the stomach lining. Bismuth compounds, in addition to being antimicrobial, also help to form a protective mucosal lining.

Cisapride is used in treating GERD and has been shown to increase the pressure of the lower esophageal sphincter and accelerate gastric emptying, both of which reduce reflux.

MECHANISM OF ACTION

Antacids act through a direct chemical reaction between a basic substance, the antacid, and the acidic gastric secretions. This raises the pH and reduces the acidity of the stomach contents.

Antimuscarinic agents decrease GI motility and gastric secretion.

H_2-histamine antagonists, antimuscarinic agents, and prostaglandins all act to indirectly reduce the function of the H+/K+-ATPase or proton pump which pumps hydrogen ions, the ions that cause acidity, into the stomach lumen. Antimuscarinic agents do this by blocking the normal function of cholinergic receptors, which release calcium ions that activate the proton-pump. Cyclic AMP (cAMP) can also induce proton pump action. H_2-histamine antagonists reversibly act on histamine receptors that activate adenylate cyclase, the enzyme that produces cAMP. Therefore, these antagonists prevent this normal activation and reduce the amount of cAMP and activation of the proton pump. Prostaglandins directly activate a receptor that down regulates adenylate cyclase and reduces the amount of cAMP. While these agents all indirectly reduce the action of the proton pump, proton-pump inhibitors directly and irreversibly block proper functioning of the proton pump. These effects are summarized in Figure 9.1 on page 247.

Cisapride acts by stimulating release of acetylcholine in the **myenteric plexus,** which causes an increase in pressure of the lower esophageal sphincter and accelerates gastric emptying.

Myenteric plexus: A plexus of unmyellnated nerve fibers and postganglionic autonomic cell bodies lying within the musculature of the esophagus, stomach, and intestines, it communicates with the enteric plexus

Sucralfate protects the mucosal layer by bonding with proteins in the mucosal wall and forming a complex gel that prevents mucus degradation and inhibits acid secretion. In addition, it stimulates prostaglandin secretion, mucus production, and bicarbonate release.

▪ DOSAGES

ALUMINUM HYDROXIDE, for *children*, for hyperphosphatemia, 50-150 mg/kg/d in divided doses every 4-6 hours; as a skin protectant, topical: refer to adult dosing. For *adults*, for hyperphosphatemia, initiate at 300-600 mg tid with meals; for hyperacidity, 600-1200 mg between meals and nocte; as a skin protectant, topical: apply to affected area prn; reapply at least every 12 hours.

CALCIUM CARBONATE, for *children*, for hypocalcemia (dose depends on clinical condition and serum calcium level), dose is expressed in mg of elemental calcium, 45-65 mg/kg/d in 4 divided doses; as an antacid, for *children* 2-5 years (24-47 lbs.), elemental calcium, 161 mg prn up to a maximum of 483 mg/d; for *children* 6-11 years (48-95 lbs.), elemental calcium, 322 mg prn up to a maximum of 966 mg/d. For *adults*, for hypocalcemia, 1-2 g elemental calcium or more/d in 3-4 divided doses; for dietary supplementation, 500 mg to 2 g divided 2-4 times/d; as an antacid, generally, 2-4 tablets or 5-10 mL every 2 hours, based as acid-relieving capacity of specific agent, up to a maximum of 7500 mg calcium carbonate per day; for osteoporosis, for *adults* over 51 years, 1200 mg/d.

CIMETIDINE, for *children*, 20-40 mg/kg/d in divided doses every 6 hours. For *children* over 12 years and *adults*, for heartburn, acid indigestion, or sour stomach (OTC labeling), 200 mg up to twice daily; may take 30 minutes prior to eating foods or beverages expected to cause heartburn or indigestion. For *adults*, for short-term treatment of active ulcers, 300 mg qid or 800 mg nocte or 400 mg bid for up to 8 weeks; higher doses of 1600 mg nocte for 4 weeks may be beneficial for a subpopulation of patients with larger duodenal ulcers (over 1 cm defined endoscopically) who are also heavy smokers (at least 1 pack/d); for duodenal ulcer prophylaxis, 400 mg nocte; for gastric hypersecretory conditions, 300-600 mg every 6 hours; dosage not to exceed 2.4 g/d; for gastroesophageal reflux disease, 400 mg qid or 800 mg bid for 12 weeks.

CISAPRIDE, for *children*, 0.15-0.3 mg/kg/dose 3-4 times/d up to a maximum of 10 mg/dose. For *adults*, initiate at 10 mg qid at least 15 minutes before meals and at bedtime; in some patients the dosage will need to be increased to 20 mg to obtain a satisfactory result.

DEXLANSOPRAZOLE, for *adults*, for erosive esophagitis, for short-term treatment, 60 mg once daily for up to 8 weeks; for maintenance and symptomatic relief of heartburn, 30 mg once daily for up to 6 months; for GERD, 30 mg once daily for 4 weeks.

DICYCLOMINE, for *infants* over 6 months, 5 mg/

dose 3-4 times/d. For *children*, 10 mg tid or qid. For *adults*, initiate at 20 mg qid, then increase up to 160 mg/d.

ESOMEPRAZOLE, for *adolescents* 12-17 years, for GERD, 20-40 mg once daily for up to 8 weeks. For *adults*, for erosive esophagitis (healing), initiate at 20-40 mg once daily for 4-8 weeks; if incomplete healing, may continue for an additional 4-8 weeks; maintenance dose is 20 mg once daily; for symptomatic GERD, 20 mg once daily for 4 weeks; may continue an additional 4 weeks if symptoms persist; for *H. pylori* eradication, 40 mg once daily for 10 days; requires combination therapy; for prevention of NSAID-induced gastric ulcers, 20-40 mg once daily for up to 6 months.

FAMOTIDINE, for *children*, for peptic ulcers, 1-16 years, 0.5 mg/kg/d nocte or divided twice daily up to a maximum dose of 40 mg/d; for GERD, under 3 months, 0.5 mg/kg once daily; 3-12 months, 0.5 mg/kg bid, 1-16 years; .5 mg/kg/d bid up to a maximum dose of 40 mg bid. For *children* over 12 years and *adults*, for heartburn, indigestion, or sour stomach, 10-20 mg every 12 hours; dose may be taken 15-60 minutes before eating foods known to cause heartburn. For *adults*, for duodenal ulcer, acute therapy: 40 mg/d nocte for 4-8 weeks; maintenance therapy, 20 mg/d nocte; for gastric ulcer, acute therapy: 40 mg/d nocte; for hypersecretory conditions, initiate at 20 mg every 6 hours; may increase in increments up to 160 mg every 6 hours; for GERD, 20 mg bid for 6 weeks; for esophagitis and accompanying symptoms due to GERD, 20 mg or 40 mg bid for up to 12 weeks.

HYOSCYAMINE, for *children*, for gastrointestinal disorders, using 0.125 mg/mL drops, repeat dose every 4 hours as needed: *children* <2 years, 3.4 kg, 4 drops up to a maximum of 24 drops/24 hours; 5 kg, 5 drops up to a maximum of 30 drops/24 hours; 7 kg, 6 drops up to a maximum of 36 drops/24 hours; 10 kg, 8 drops up to a maximum of 48 drops/24 hours. For *children* 2-12 years, for gastrointestinal disorders, repeat dose every 4 hours as needed: 10 kg, 0.031-0.033 mg up to a maximum

of 0.75 mg/24 hours; 20 kg, 0.0625 mg up to a maximum of 0.75 mg/24 hours; 40 kg, 0.0938 mg up to a maximum of 0.75 mg/24 hours; 50 kg, 0.125 mg up to a maximum of 0.75 mg/24 hours. For *children* >12 years and *adults*, for gastrointestinal disorders, 0.125-0.25 mg every 4 hours or as needed (before meals or food) up to a maximum of 1.5 mg/24 hours; Cysto-spaz®: 0.15-0.3 mg up to 4 times/d. For timed release: for *children* >12 years and *adults*, for gastrointestinal disorders, 0.375-0.75 mg every 12 hours up to a maximum of 1.5 mg/24 hours.

LANSOPRAZOLE, for *children* 1-11 years, for GER or erosive esophagitis, ≤30 kg, 15 mg once daily; >30 kg, 30 mg once daily. For *children* 12-17 years, for nonerosive GERD, 15 mg once daily for up to 8 weeks; for erosive esophagitis, 30 mg once daily for up to 8 weeks. For *adults*, for duodenal ulcer, short-term treatment: 15 mg once daily for 4 weeks; maintenance dose is 15 mg once daily; for gastric ulcer, short-term treatment: 30 mg once daily for up to 8 weeks; for NSAID-associated gastric ulcer (healing), 30 mg once daily for 8 weeks; controlled studies did not extend past 8 weeks of therapy; for NSAID-associated gastric ulcer (to reduce risk), 15 mg once daily for up to 12 weeks; for symptomatic GERD, short-term treatment, 15 mg once daily for up to 8 weeks; for erosive esophagitis, short-term treatment: 30 mg once daily for up to 8 weeks; continued treatment for an additional 8 weeks may be considered for recurrence or for patients that do not heal after the first 8 weeks of therapy; maintenance therapy dose is 15 mg once daily; for hypersecretory conditions, initiate at 60 mg once daily; adjust dose based upon patient response and to reduce acid secretion to <10 mEq/hour (5 mEq/hour in patients with prior gastric surgery); doses of 90 mg bid have been used,;administer doses over 120 mg/d in divided doses; for *H. pylori* eradication, dose varies with regimen; 30 mg once daily or 30 mg bid; requires combination therapy with antibiotics.

MAGNESIUM HYDROXIDE, as a laxative, liquid: for *children*, 400 mg/5 mL: 1-3 mL/kg/d; adjust to induce daily bowel movement; OTC labeling: for *children* 2-5 years, 400 mg/5 mL: 5-15 mL/d nocte or in divided doses; for children 6-11 years, 400 mg/5 mL: 15-30 mL/d or 800 mg/5 mL: 7.5-15 mL/d nocte or in divided doses; tablet: for *children* 3-5 years, 311 mg/tablet, 2 tablets/d nocte or in divided doses; for *children* 6-11 years, 311 mg/tablet: 4 tablets/d nocte or in divided doses. For *children* over 12 years and *adults*, as an antacid, 400 mg/5 mL liquid: 5-15 mL prn up to 4 times/d; 311 mg tablet: 2-4 tablets every 4 hours up to 4 times/d; as a laxative, 400 mg/5 mL liquid: 30-60 mL/d nocte or in divided doses; 800 mg/5 mL liquid: 15-30 mL/d nocte or in divided doses; 311 mg tablet: 8 tablets/d nocte or in divided doses.

METHSCOPOLAMINE, for *adults*, 2.5 mg 30 minutes before meals or food and 2.5-5 mg nocte; may increase dose to 5 mg bid.

MISOPROSTOL, for *adults*, for prevention of NSAID-induced gastric ulcers, 200 mcg qid with food; if not tolerated, may decrease dose to 100 mcg qid with food or 200 mcg bid with food; last dose of the day should be taken at bedtime.

NIZATIDINE, for *adults*, for duodenal ulcer, treatment of active ulcer, 300 mg nocte or 150 mg bid; maintenance of healed ulcer, 150 mg/d nocte; for gastric ulcer, 150 mg bid or 300 mg nocte; for GERD, 150 mg bid; for meal-induced heartburn, acid indigestion, and sour stomach, 75 mg tablet [OTC] bid,;30 to 60 minutes prior to consuming food or beverages.

OMEPRAZOLE, for *children* 2 years or older, for GERD or other acid-related disorders, <20 kg, 10 mg once daily; ≥20 kg, 20 mg once daily. For *adults*, for active duodenal ulcer, 20 mg/d for 4-8 weeks; for gastric ulcers, 40 mg/d for 4-8 weeks; for symptomatic GERD, 20 mg/d for up to 4 weeks; for erosive esophagitis, 20 mg/d for 4-8 weeks; maintenance dose is 20 mg/d for up to 12 months total therapy (including treatment period of 4-8 weeks); for *H. pylori* eradication, 20 mg once daily or 40 mg/d as single dose or in 2 divided doses; requires combination therapy with antibiotics; for pathological hypersecretory conditions, initiate at 60 mg once daily,;doses up to 120 mg tid have been administered,;administer daily doses >80 mg in divided doses; for frequent heartburn (OTC labeling), 20 mg/d for 14 days; treatment may be repeated after 4 months if needed.

PANTOPRAZOLE, for *adults*, for erosive esophagitis associated with GERD, 40 mg once daily for up to 8 weeks; an additional 8 weeks may be used in patients who have not healed after an 8-week course; maintain at 40 mg once daily; lower doses (20 mg once daily) have been used successfully in mild GERD treatment and maintenance of healing; for hypersecretory disorders (including Zollinger-Ellison), initiate at 40 mg bid; adjust based on patient needs; doses up to 240 mg/d have been administered.

RABEPRAZOLE, for *adults*, for GERD, 20 mg once daily for 4-8 weeks; maintenance is 20 mg once daily; for duodenal ulcer, 20 mg/d before breakfast for 4 weeks; for *H. pylori* eradication, 20 mg bid for 7 days, to be administered with amoxicillin 1000 mg and clarithromycin 500 mg, also given twice daily for 7 days; for hypersecretory conditions, 60 mg once daily; dose may need to be adjusted as necessary; doses as high as 100 mg once daily and 60 mg bid have been used.

RANITIDINE, for *children* 1 month to 16 years, for duodenal and gastric ulcer, 1-2 mg/kg/d divided twice daily; maximum treatment dose is 300 mg/d; maintain at 2-4 mg/kg once daily, maximum maintenance dose is 150 mg/d; for GERD and erosive esophagitis, 5-10 mg/kg/d divided twice daily; maximum for GERD is 300 mg/d, and for erosive esophagitis, it is 600 mg/d. For *children* ≥12 years, for prevention of heartburn, 75 mg 30-60 minutes before eating food or drinking beverages that cause heartburn; maximum dose is 150 mg/d, do not use for more than 14 days. For *adults*, for duodenal ulcer, 150 mg bid; or 300 mg once daily after the evening meal or at bedtime; maintenance dose is 150 mg nocte; for *H. pylori* eradication, 150 mg bid; requires combination therapy; for pathological hypersecretory conditions, 150 mg bid,;adjust dose or frequency as clinically indicated; doses of up to 6 g/d have been used; for gastric ulcer, benign, 150 mg bid; maintenance dose is 150 mg nocte; for erosive esophagitis, 150 mg qid, maintenance dose is 150 mg bid; for prevention of heartburn, 75 mg 30-60 minutes before taking food or beverages that cause heartburn; maximum dose is 150 mg in 24 hours,;do not use for more than 14 days.

SODIUM BICARBONATE, for *children*, for chronic renal failure, when plasma bicarbonate is less than 15 mEq/L, initiate at 1-3 mEq/kg/d; for distal renal tubular acidosis, 2-3 mEq/kg/d; for proximal renal tubular acidosis, initiate at 5-10 mEq/kg/d; for urine alkalinization, 1-10 mEq (84-840 mg)/kg/d in divided doses every 4-6 hours. For *adults*, for chronic renal failure, when plasma bicarbonate is less than 15 mEq/L, start with 20-36 mEq/d in divided doses and titrate to a bicarbonate level of 18-20 mEq/L; for renal tubular acidosis, distal: 0.5-2 mEq/kg/d in 4-5 divided doses; proximal, initiate at 5-10 mEq/kg/d; for urine alkalinization, initiate at 48 mEq (4 g), then 12-24 mEq (1-2 g) every 4 hours; as an antacid, 325 mg to 2 g 1-4 times/d.

SUCRALFATE, for *children*, dose not established; doses of 40-80 mg/kg/d divided every 6 hours have been used; for stomatitis (unlabeled use), 2.5-5 mL (1 g/10 mL suspension), swish and spit or swish and swallow qid. For *adults*, for stress ulcer prophylaxis, 1 g qid; for stress ulcer treatment, 1 g every 4 hours; for duodenal ulcer, 1 g qid on an empty stomach and at bedtime for 4-8 weeks, or alternatively 2 g bid; treatment is recommended for 4-8 weeks in adults; the *elderly* may require 12 weeks; maintenance for prophylaxis, 1 g bid.

ADVERSE EFFECTS

Antimuscarinic agents are used only in refractory cases given the amount of adverse effects reported at doses necessary for gastric effects. Two serious side effects include **arrhythmias** and urinary retention.

H_2-histamine antagonists are generally well tolerated with a small number of users complaining of side effects. The most common of these effects include headache, diarrhea, dizziness, and muscular pain. Some nervous system effects, such as confusion or hallucinations, occur in elderly patients or with IV administration. Cimetidine has an antiandrogen effect and may cause **gynecomastia**, **galactorrhea**, and reduced sperm count when used long term and/or in large quantities.

Prostaglandins can produce uterine contractions and are contraindicated during pregnancy. The most common side effects are nausea and diarrhea and are dose-related.

Proton-pump inhibitors have been shown to produce gastrin-secreting tumors in animals, but no evidence exists of the same occurring in humans. There have been reports of viable bacteria colonies in the stomach with the use of these agents.

RED FLAGS

Patients taking cisapride have reported serious cardiac arrhythmias including ventricular **tachycardias**, ventricular **fibrillations**, **Torsade de Pointes**, and QT prolongations.

INTERACTIONS

DRUG

Cimetidine inhibits cytochrome P450 and can slow metabolism of warfarin, diazepam, phenytoin, quinidine, carbamazepine, theophylline, and imipramine.

Cisapride should not be used with clarithromycin among other drugs as they can increase the blood levels of cisapride.

H_2-receptor antagonists should not be used with ketoconazole as the latter needs an appropriately acidic environment for absorption. Theoretically, this interaction should be true of all the agents in this category that reduce acidity.

Arrhythmia: An irregular heartbeat

Gynecomastia: An abnormal enlargement of one or two breasts in men

Galactorrhea: Abnormal production and secretion of milk from the beasts or any white discharge from the nipple

Tachycardia: A rapid heart rate defined as over 100 bpm

Fibrillation: Recurrent, abnormal muscle contraction that is not physiologically useful

Torsade de Pointes: A specific type of ventricular tachycardia characterized by rapid, irregular QRS complexes; it may end spontaneously or degenerate into ventricular fibrillation. It causes significant blood flow compromise and often causes death

Omeprazole interferes with the oxidation of warfarin, phenytoin, diazepam, and cyclosporine.

Sucralfate should not be combined with histamine antagonists or antacids as it needs an acidic environment to exert its effects. It can also affect the absorption of other drugs by binding with them.

HERB

Given that most of these drugs reduce the acidity of the stomach, herbs that are hard to digest may not be fully absorbed.

ANTACIDS
• *Ma Huang* (Ephedra) (C)–based on ephedrine content, antacids may cause ephedrine and pseudoephedrine toxicity from *Ma Huang* due to alkalinization of the urine (Brater *et al.*, 1980) Level 4 evidence.

CIMETIDINE
• *Lu Cha* (Green tea) (D)–the effect of caffeine in tea may be potentiated by cimetidine, expert opinion (Chen & Chen, 2004) Level 5 evidence.

CISAPRIDE
• *Shan Zha* (Hawthorn berry) (D)–may inhibit potassium inflow causing increased action potential in cardiac ventricular cells when used with cisapride, expert opinion (Gruenwald, Brendler & Jaenicke, 2004) Level 5 evidence.

FAMOTIDINE
• Aromatic and damp resolving herbs (D)–may increase stomach acid and peristalsis possibly antagonizing histamine-$_2$ receptor antagonists and proton-pump inhibitors, expert opinion (Chen & Chen, 2004) Level 5 evidence.

HISTAMINE-$_2$ RECEPTOR ANTAGONISTS
• Aromatic and damp resolving herbs (D)–may increase stomach acid and peristalsis possibly antagonizing histamine-$_2$ receptor antagonists and proton-pump inhibitors, expert opinion (Chen & Chen, 2004) Level 5 evidence.

LANSOPRAZOLE
• Aromatic and damp resolving herbs (D)–may increase stomach acid and peristalsis possibly antagonizing histamine-$_2$ receptor antagonists and proton-pump inhibitors, expert opinion (Chen & Chen, 2004) Level 5 evidence.

OMEPRAZOLE
• Aromatic and damp resolving herbs (D)–may increase stomach acid and peristalsis possibly antagonizing histamine-$_2$ receptor antagonists and proton-pump inhibitors, expert opinion (Chen & Chen, 2004) Level 5 evidence.
• *Bai Zhu* (White atractylodes) (D)–a component, hinesol, may potentiate omeprazole, bench research (Satoh, Nagaia & Kano, 2000) Level 5 evidence.
• *Cang Zhu* (Atractylodes) (D)–a component, hinesol, may potentiate omeprazole (Satoh, Nagaia & Kano, 2000) Level 5 evidence.
• *Guan Ye Lian Qiao* (St. John's wort) (C)–decreases blood concentrations (Izzo & Ernst, 2009) Level 2b evidence.
• *Yin Guo Ye* (Gingko) (C)–decreases blood concentrations (Izzo & Ernst, 2009) Level 2b evidence.

PROTON-PUMP INHIBITORS
• Aromatic and damp resolving herbs (D)–may increase stomach acid and peristalsis possibly antagonizing histamine-$_2$ receptor antagonists and proton-pump inhibitors, expert opinion (Chen & Chen, 2004) Level 5 evidence.

RANITIDINE
• Aromatic and damp resolving herbs (D)–may increase stomach acid and peristalsis possibly antagonizing histamine-$_2$ receptor antagonists and proton-pump inhibitors, expert opinion (Chen & Chen, 2004) Level 5 evidence.

VITAMIN

Prolonged inhibition of gastric acid can cause vitamin B_{12} depletion as acid is required for absorption.

INTERACTION ISSUES

A: Many of the agents that treat peptic ulcer disease either reduce acidity (raise pH) or coat the stomach lining. Either of these effects theoretically may impair the absorption of other agents or herbs taken at the same time. To minimize possible interactions, it may be wise to separate the use of these medications and other substances. Consider taking drugs or herbs 1 hour before or 2 hours after these agents.

D: Cisapride is 97.5 to 98% protein bound; dexlansoprazole is 96-99% protein bound; esomeprazole and lansoprazole are 97% bound; omeprazole is approximately 95% bound; pantoprazole is 98% bound; rabeprazole is approximately 96% bound.

M: Cimetidine is a moderate inhibitor of CYP1A2, 2C19, 2D6, and 3A4; cisapride is a major substrate of CYP3A4; esomeprazole is a major substrate and a moderate inhibitor of CYP2C19; lansoprazole is a major substrate of CYP2C19 and 3A4 and a weak or moderate inducer of 1A2; omeprazole is a major substrate of CYP2C19, a moderate inhibitor of 2C9 and 2C19, and a weak or moderate inducer of 1A2; pantoprazole is a major substrate of CYP2C19 and a weak or moderate inducer of 1A2; rabeprazole is a major substrate of 2C19 and 3A4 and a moderate inhibitor of 2C8.

E:

Pgp: Cimetidine and ranitidine are substrates of Pgp.

SECTION 2: ANTIEMETIC AGENTS

ANTICHOLINERGIC AGENTS:

SCOPOLAMINE, TRIMETHOBENZAMIDE (See Chapter 4, Section 3)

ANTIHISTAMINES:

MECLIZINE, PROMETHAZINE (See Chapter 8, Section 2)

ANTIPSYCHOTICS:

HALOPERIDOL, PROCHLORPERAZINE (See Chapter 5, Section 6, Class 1)

CANNABINOIDS:

DRONABINOL (droe NAB i nol) PR=C (Marinol®)

NABILONE (NA bi lone) PR=C (Cesamet™)

CORTICOSTEROIDS:

DEXAMETHASONE (See Chapter 7, Section 4)

PROKINETIC GASTROINTESTINAL AGENTS:

METOCLOPRAMIDE (met oh kloe PRA mide)

PR=B (Metozolv ODT, Reglan®)

SELECTIVE 5-HT₃ (SEROTONIN) RECEPTOR ANTAGONISTS:

DOLASETRON (dol A se tron) PR=B (Anzemet®)

GRANISETRON (gra NI se tron) PR=B (Granisol, Sancuso)

ONDANSETRON (on DAN se tron) PR=B (Zofran®, Zofran® ODT, Zuplenz®)

SUBSTANCE P/NEUROKININ 1 RECEPTOR ANTAGONIST:

APREPITANT (ap RE pi tant) PR=B (Emend®)

OTHER ANTIEMETICS:

DEXTROSE, FRUCTOSE, AND PHOSPHORIC ACID (DEKS trose, FRUK tose, & foss FOR ik AS id) PR=N (Emetrol® [O], Formula EM [O], Kalmz [O], Nausea Relief [O], Nausetrol® [O])

These agents are used to treat nausea and vomiting especially in the case of chemotherapy. Nearly 70-80% of chemotherapy patients experience nausea and vomiting, which depends on many factors including the specific chemotherapy agent, dose, route, and times of administration as well as patient factors such as age, sex, and personal tolerance.

▧ FUNCTION

In addition to other functions, these agents all reduce nausea and vomiting. Scopolamine and the antihistamines are useful for treating motion sickness. The other agents are useful for various types of chemotherapy-induced nausea and vomiting. Promethazine is useful for treating low to moderate **emetogenic** chemotherapy agents.

Antipsychotics, based on their adverse effects, are generally reserved for use when other agents fail.

Cannaboids are useful in treating moderate emetogenic agents but are generally considered second-line agents due to their adverse effects.

Corticosteroids can be useful in treating emesis from mild to moderate emetogenic agents. They are generally used in conjunction with other agents.

The selective 5-HT$_3$ (serotonin) receptor antagonists generally have a long duration of action and are useful for all types of emesis-inducing chemotherapy agents.

Prokinetic gastrointestinal agents are highly useful in treating emesis in patients who use cisplatin, which is highly emetogenic.

Substance P/Neurokinin 1 receptor antagonists are very useful in treating emesis in patients taking cisplatin. It is used in conjunction with a corticosteroid and a selective 5-HT$_3$ (serotonin) receptor antagonist.

Emetogenic: Causes nausea and vomiting

Vestibular: Pertaining to the inner ear apparati in control of body balance

Psychotropic: Can affect the mind, emotions, and behavior; pertaining to drugs used in the treatment of mental illness

▒ MECHANISM OF ACTION

There are two main areas where the impulse to nausea and vomiting are created. The first is the chemoreceptor trigger zone. This is an area of the fourth ventricle of the brain and part of the brain stem that is outside of the blood-brain barrier and is therefore sensitive to the chemistry of the cerebrospinal fluid and the blood. Adverse chemistry in either of these two fluids can cause a nausea/vomiting response.

The second area is the vomiting center located in the medulla oblongata (also just called the medulla) of the brain stem. This area oversees the physical aspects and mechanisms of vomiting. It receives input from many areas including the **vestibular** system (the main progenitor of motion sickness), the periphery, especially the pharynx and the GI tract, and higher brain stem and cortical areas of the brain.

Chemotherapy causes nausea and vomiting by directly stimulating these areas as well as potentially triggering the peripheral receptors activated through cell damage. Higher areas of the brain can also stimulate these areas and cause nausea and vomiting even before the use of chemotherapy agents in a phenomenon called anticipatory vomiting.

The cannaboids' mechanism of action is unknown but is thought not to be central given that synthetic cannaboids that are not **psychotropic** are still antiemetic.

The corticosteroids' mechanism of treating emesis is unknown but is thought to involve blocking prostaglandins.

Promethazine acts by blocking dopamine receptors in the vomiting center. Prokinetic gastrointestinal agents also work by blocking dopamine receptors as well as serotonin receptors in the chemoreceptor trigger zone.

The selective 5-HT$_3$ receptor antagonists selectively block serotonin receptors in the periphery and in the chemoreceptor trigger zone.

Substance P/Neurokinin 1 receptor antagonists act by blocking neurokinin in the brain. These agents are new, and their full activities are not completely understood.

▒ DOSAGES

APREPITANT, for *adults*, 125 mg on day 1, followed by 80 mg on days 2 and 3 in combination with a corticosteroid and 5-HT$_3$ receptor antagonist.

DEXTROSE, FRUCTOSE, AND PHOSPHORIC ACID, for *children* 2-12 years, for nausea, 5-10 mL; repeat every 15 minutes until distress subsides, up to a maximum of 5 doses. For *children* over 12 and *adults*, for nausea, 15-30 mL, repeat every 15 minutes until distress subsides, up to a maximum of 5 doses.

DOLASETRON, for *children* 2-16 years, for nausea and vomiting prophylaxis, chemotherapy-induced (initial or repeat courses), 1.8 mg/kg within 1 hour before chemotherapy up to a maximum of 100 mg/dose; for prevention of postoperative nausea and vomiting, 1.2 mg/kg within 2 hours before surgery up to a maximum of 100 mg/dose. For *adults,* for nausea and vomiting prophylaxis, chemotherapy-induced (initial or repeat courses), 100 mg single dose 1 hour prior to chemoherapy; for prevention of postoperative nausea and vomiting, 100 mg within 2 hours before surgery.

DRONABINOL, for *children* and *adults*, as an antiemetic, 5 mg/m^2 1-3 hours before chemotherapy, then 5 mg/m^2/dose every 2-4 hours after chemotherapy for a total of 4-6 doses/d; increase doses in increments of 2.5 mg/m^2 up to a maximum of 15 mg/m^2/dose. For *adults*, as an appetite stimulant, initiate at 2.5 mg bid (before lunch and dinner); increase up to a maximum of 20 mg/d.

GRANISETRON, for *adults*, for prophylaxis of chemotherapy-related emesis, 2 mg once daily up to 1 hour before chemotherapy or 1 mg bid; the first 1 mg dose should be given up to 1 hour before chemotherapy; prophylaxis of radiation-therapy-associated emesis, 2 mg once daily given 1 hour before radiation therapy.

METOCLOPRAMIDE, for *adults*, for gastroesophageal reflux, 10-15 mg/dose up to qid 30 minutes before meals or food and at bedtime; single doses of 20 mg are occasionally needed for provoking situations; treatment for over 12 weeks has not been evaluated; for diabetic gastric stasis, 10 mg 30 minutes before each meal and at bedtime; for chemotherapy-induced emesis, alternate dosing: moderate emetic risk chemotherapy: 0.5 mg/kg every 6 hours on days 2-4; low and minimal risk chemotherapy: 1-2 mg/kg every 3-4 hours; breakthrough treatment: 1-2 mg/kg every 3-4 hours or moderate emetic risk chemotherapy: 0.5 mg/kg every 6 hours or 20 mg qid on days 2-4; low and minimal risk chemotherapy: 20-40 mg every 4-6 hour;, breakthrough treatment: 20-40 mg every 4-6 hours.

NABILONE, for *adults*, 1-2 mg bid up to a maximum of 2 mg divided tid.

ONDANSETRON, for *children*, prevention of chemotherapy-induced emesis, 4-11 years, 4 mg 30 minutes before chemotherapy; repeat 4 and 8 hours after initial dose, then 4 mg every 8 hours for 1-2 days after chemotherapy completed. For *children* over 12 years and *adults*, for chemotherapy-induced emesis, for highly-emetogenic agents/single-day therapy, 24 mg given 30 minutes prior to the start of therapy; moderately emetogenic agents, 8 mg every 12 hours beginning 30 minutes before chemotherapy; continuously for 1-2 days after chemotherapy completed; for total body irradiation, 8 mg 1-2 hours before each daily fraction of radiotherapy; for single high-dose fraction radiotherapy to abdomen, 8 mg 1-2 hours before irradiation, then 8 mg every 8 hours after first dose for 1-2 days after completion of radiotherapy; for daily fractionated radiotherapy to abdomen, 8 mg 1-2 hours before irradiation, then 8 mg 8 hours after first dose for each day of radiotherapy; for postoperative nausea and vomiting: 16 mg given 1 hour prior to induction of anesthesia.

ADVERSE EFFECTS

Cannaboids have many adverse effects that limit their clinical usefulness. These include **dysphonia**, hallucinations, sedation, vertigo, and disorientation.

Prokinetic gastrointestinal agents have a variety of adverse effects from blocking dopamine including sedation, diarrhea, and **extrapyramidal symptoms**. These effects are most common in younger patients.

Promethazine causes hypotension and restlessness, and even though its antiemetic properties are increased with higher doses, so are these adverse effects. Extrapyramidal symptoms and sedation may also occur.

Selective 5-HT$_3$ receptor antagonists commonly cause headaches. Dolasetron has been reported to cause prolongation of the QT interval on ECGs and should be used with caution in patients who may be at risk.

Substance P/Neurokinin 1 receptor antagonists can cause constipation and fatigue.

Dysphonia: Any disorder affecting voice quality or the ability to produce voice

Extrapyramidal symptoms: Exhibiting movement disorders, especially postural and locomotor, resembling Parkinson's disease

▦ RED FLAGS

No red flags.

▦ INTERACTIONS

DRUG

Substance P/Neurokinin 1 receptor antagonists are metabolized by CYP3A4, and drugs needing this enzyme may have their metabolism altered. Use with warfarin may shorten its half-life.

INTERACTION ISSUES

A:

D: Aprepitant is over 95% protein bound; dronabinol is 97-99% bound.

M: Aprepitant is a major substrate, a weak or moderate inducer, and a moderate inhibitor of CYP3A4 and a strong inducer of 2C9; ondansetron is a major substrate of CYP3A4.

E:

Pgp: Ondansetron is a substrate of Pgp.

SECTION 3: ANTIDIARRHEALS

ALOSETRON (a LOE se tron) PR=B (Lotronex)

ASPIRIN (See Chapter 11, Section 1)

BISMUTH (BIZZ muth) PR=N (Bismatrol [O], Bismatrol Maximum Strength [O], Diotame [O], Helidac®,[16] Kao-Tin [O], Kola-Pectin DS [O], Peptic Relief [O], Pepto-Bismol [O], Pepto-Bismol To-Go [O], Pink Bismuth [O], Pylera™,[16] Stomach Relief [O], Stomach Relief Maximum Strength [O], Stomach Relief Plus [O])

CROFELEMER (kroe FEL e mer) PR=C (Fulyzaq)

DIFENOXIN (dye fen OKS in) PR=C (Motofe[5])

DIPHENOXYLATE (dye fen OKS i late) PR=C (Lomotil®[6])

INDOMETHACIN (See Chapter 11, Section 1)

LOPERAMIDE (loe PER a mide) PR=C (Anti-Diarrheal [O], Diamode [O], Imodium A-D [O], Imodium® Multi-Symptom Relief [O],[17] Loperamide A-D [O])

OPIUM TINCTURE (See Chapter 5, Section 7)

POLYCARBOPHIL (pol i KAR boe fil) PR=N (Fiber Laxative [O], Fiber-Lax [O], FiberCon [O], FiberGen [O], Konsyl Fiber [O])

PSYLLIUM (SIL i yum) PR=N (Dietary Fiber Laxative [O], Evac [O], Fiber Therapy [O], Geri-Mucil [O], Konsyl [O], Konsyl-D [O], Laxmar [O], Laxmar Natural Vegetable Laxative [O], Metamucil MultiHealth Fiber [O], Natural Fiber Therapy [O], Natural Psyllium Seed [O], Natural Vegetable Fiber [O], Reguloid [O], Sorbulax [O])

▦ FUNCTION

There are three main types of antidiarrheals: antimotility agents, adsorbents, and agents that modify fluid and electrolyte transport. Antimotility agents decrease peristalsis and slow the action of the intestines. These include difenoxin, diphenoxylate, and opium tincture.

Psyllium is an adsorbent. These agents can also be used as laxatives.

Agents that modify fluid and electrolyte transport include aspirin and indomethacin.

Alosetron is specifically for women with severe diarrhea or predominant irritable bowel syndrome

(IBS) that has failed to respond to other therapies.

▦ MECHANISM OF ACTION

Antimotility agents decrease peristalsis and slow the action of the intestines by activating presynaptic opioid receptors in the **enteric nervous system,** which inhibits acetylcholine release.

Adsorbents act by absorbing intestinal toxins or microorganisms and/or by protecting or coating the mucosa. When used as a laxative, this is a bulkifying agent.

Agents that modify fluid and electrolyte transport, in all probability, act by inhibition of prostaglandin synthesis.

Enteric nervous system: A semiautonomous system of nerves located within the digestive system; while a separate system from the CNS and ANS, it can still receive modifying input from these systems. Two plexuses primarily constitute this system: the submucosal nerve plexus and the myenteric nerve plexus.

Alosetron selectively antagonizes a subtype of serotonin predominant on enteric neurons. Normally, these neurons regulate visceral pain, colonic transport, and GI secretions. Blocking these receptors therefore reduce pain, abdominal discomfort, urgency, and diarrhea.

DOSAGES

ALOSETRON, for *adults*, for irritable bowel syndrome (IBS) in women, initiate at 0.5 mg bid for 4 weeks, with or without food; if tolerated, may be increased after 4 weeks to 1 mg bid.

BISMUTH, for *children* over 12 and adults, for treatment of nonspecific diarrhea and to control and relieve traveler's diarrhea, 524 mg every 30 minutes to 1 hour prn up to a maximum of 8 doses/d; for *Helicobacter pylori* eradication, 524 mg qid with meals and at bedtime with combination therapy.

CROFELEMER, for *adults*, for diarrhea, noninfectious, associated with antiretroviral therapy for HIV/AIDS, 125 mg bid.

DIFENOXIN, DIPHENOXYLATE, used only in combination with other drugs, and, therefore, individual dosing is not covered here.

LOPERAMIDE, for acute diarrhea, initiate at during the first day; for *children* 2-5 years or 13-20 kg, 1 mg tid; for *children* 6-8 years or 20-30 kg, 2 mg bid; for *children* 8-12 years or over 30 kg, 2 mg tid; to maintain, 0.1 mg/kg after each loose stool up to a maximum of the first day's dose; for traveler's diarrhea: for *children* 6-8 years, 2 mg after first loose bowel movement (BM), followed by 1 mg after each subsequent BM up to a maximum of 4 mg/d; for *children* 9-11 years, 2 mg after first loose BM, followed by 1 mg after each subsequent BM up to a maximum of 6 mg/d. For *children* 12 and over and *adults*, for acute diarrhea, initiate at 4 mg, followed by 2 mg after each loose BM, up to a maximum of 16 mg/d; for chronic diarrhea, initiate in the same manner as for acute diarrhea and slowly titrate downward to the minimum required to control symptoms; for traveler's diarrhea, initiate at 4 mg after first loose BM, followed by 2 mg after each subsequent BM, up to a maximum of 8 mg/d.

POLYCARBOPHIL, for *children* 6-12 years, for constipation or diarrhea, 625 mg 1-4 times/d. For children 12 years and older and *adults*, for constipation or diarrhea, 1250 mg 1-4 times/d.

PSYLLIUM, for *children* 6-11 years, approximately 1/2 adult dosage; for *children* over 12 and *adults*, take 1 dose up to 3 times/d; all doses should be followed with 8 oz. of water or liquid. For capsules, a dose is 4 capsules. For powder, a dose is 1 rounded tablespoonful. For tablets, a dose is 1 tablet. For wafers, a dose is equal to 2 wafers.

ADVERSE EFFECTS

Antimotility agents can cause fatigue, abdominal cramping, and dizziness.

Adsorbents can cause constipation especially when taken without enough fluids.

Alosetron has two boxed warnings in the cases of constipation and colitis. Serious complications of constipation have been infrequently reported, and this agent should be discontinued immediately if constipation develops. Acute ischemic colitis has been reported.

RED FLAGS

Antimotility agents may cause **toxic megacolon** and should not be used in young children or in patients with severe colitis.

INTERACTIONS

DRUG

Adsorbents can interfere with the absorption of other drugs and should be administered at least 2 hours before or after other drugs.

HERB

These agents are designed to alter the functioning of the small and large intestines and could therefore affect the absorption of herbs. These agents should be administered at least 2 hours before or after to minimize interactions.

Toxic megacolon: A severe complication of several conditions with a large dilation of the colon and possible bacterial overgrowth. Rupture of the colon is a possibility and has 50% mortality. Emergency treatment is necessary and can prevent sepsis, shock, and possible death.

258 | INTEGRATIVE PHARMACOLOGY

- *Guan Ye Lian Qiao* (St. John's wort) (C)–decreases blood concentrations (Izzo & Ernst, 2009) Level 4 evidence.

INTERACTION ISSUES

A:

D:

M: Alosetron is a major substrate of CYP1A2.

E: Many of the agents in this category can affect gastric motility. These effects theoretically may decrease fecal excretion; however, they are most often used to restore normal function and may not cause an interaction.

Pgp: Loperamide is a substrate of Pgp.

SECTION 4: LAXATIVES

BISACODYL (bis a KOE dil) PR=B *(Bisac-Evac [O], Bisacodyl EC [O], Bisacodyl Laxative [O], Biscolax [O], Correct [O], Ducodyl [O], Dulcolax [O], Ex-Lax Ultra [O], Fleet Bisacodyl [O], Fleet Laxative [O], Gentle Laxative [O], HalfLytely® & Bisacodyl,[19] Laxative [O], Magic Bullets [O], Stimulant Laxative [O], Women's Laxative [O])*

CASTOR OIL (KAS tor oyl) PR=X

DOCUSATE (DOK yoo sate) PR=N *(Colace [O], D.O.S. [O], Diocto [O], Doc-Q-Lax [O],[21] DocQLace [O], Docu [O], Docu Soft [O], Docuprene [O], Docusil [O], DocuSol Mini [O], DOK [O], Dok™ Plus [O],[21] Dulcolax Stool Softener [O], Enemeez Mini [O], Enemeez Plus [O], Geri-Stool [O],[21] Kao-Tin [O], KS Stool Softener [O], Laxa Basic [O], Pedia-Lax [O], Peri-Colace® [O],[21] Promolaxin [O], Senexon®-S [O],[21] Senna Plus [O],[21] SennaLax-S [O],[21] Senokot-S® [O],[21] SenoSol™-SS [O,[21] Silace [O], Sof-Lax [O], Stool Softener [O], Stool Softener Laxative DC [O], Sur-Q-Lax [O], Vacuant Mini-Enema [O])*

GLYCERIN (GLIS er in) PR=C *(Aqua Glycolic Shampoo/Body [O], Aquanil Skin Cleanser [O], Fleet Liquid Glycerin Supplement [O], Glycerin (Adult) [O], Glycerin (Pediatric) [O], Introl, Pedia-Lax [O], Sani-Supp Adult [O], Sani-Supp Pediatric [O], Wibi [O])*

LACTULOSE (LAK tyoo lose) PR=B *(Constulose®, Enulose®, Generlac, Kristalose™)*

MAGNESIUM CITRATE (mag NEE zhum SIT rate) PR=C *(Citroma [O])*

MAGNESIUM HYDROXIDE *(See Section 1)*

METHYLCELLULOSE (METH il SEL yoo lose) PR=N *(Citrucel [O], Citrucel FiberShake [O], Soluble Fiber Therapy [O])*

MINERAL OIL (MIN er al oyl) PR=N *(Ala-Bath [O], Ca-meo Oil [O], Fleet Oil [O], Mapo Bath [O], Min-O-Ear [O], Nutraderm [O], Phillips'® M-O [O][18])*

POLYETHYLENE GLYCOL (pol i ETH i leen GLY kol) PR=C *(Colyte®, GaviLAX [O], GaviLyte™ C, GaviLyte™ G, GaviLyte™ N, GoLYTELY®, GlycoLax [O], HalfLytely® and Bisacodyl,[19] HealthyLax [O], MiraLax [O], MoviPrep®, NuLYTELY®, Suclear™,[20] TriLyte®)*

PSYLLIUM *(See Previous Section)*

SENNA (SEN na) PR=C *(Doc-Q-Lax [O],[21] Dok™ Plus [O],[21] Ex-Lax [O], Ex-Lax Maximum Strength [O], Geri-kot [O], Geri-Stool [O],[21] GoodSense Senna Laxative [O], Natural Senna Laxative [O], Perdiem Overnight Relief [O], Peri-Colace® [O],[21] Senexon [O], Senexon®-S [O],[21] Senna-Gen [O], Senna-GRX [O], Senna-Lax [O], Senna-Tabs [O], Senna-Time [O], Senna Lax [O], Senna Laxative [O], Senna Maximum Strength [O], Senna Plus [O],[21] Senna Smooth [O], SennaCon [O], SennaLax-S [O],[21] Senno [O], Senokot [O], Senokot-S® [O],[21] Senokot To Go [O], Senokot XTRA [O], SenoSol™ SS [O][21])*

SODIUM PHOSPHATES (SOW dee um FOS fates) PR=C *(Fleet® Enema [O], Fleet® Enema Extra® [O], Fleet® Pedia-Lax™ Enema [O], LaCrosse Complete [O], OsmoPrep®, Visicol®)*

SODIUM PICOSULFATE, MAGNESIUM OXIDE, & CITRIC ACID (SOW dee um pye ko SUL fate, mag NEE zhum OKS ide, & SI trik AS id) PR=B *(Prepopik™)*

SODIUM SULFATE, POTASSIUM SULFATE, AND MAGNESIUM SULFATE (SOW dee um SUL fate, poe TASS ee um SUL fate, & mag NEE zhum SUL fate) PR=C *(Suclear™,[20] Suprep® Bowel Prep Kit)*

SORBITOL (SOR bi tole) PR=C *(Ora-Sweet SF [O])*

WHEAT DEXTRIN (WEET DEKS trin) PR=N
(Benefiber [O], Benefiber Drink Mix [O],

Benefiber for Children [O], Benefiber Plus Calcium [O])

FUNCTION

Laxatives cause the movement of stool, usually in order to treat constipation. They fall into three categories: irritants and stimulants, bulking agents, and stool softeners.

MECHANISM OF ACTION

Irritants and stimulants act by either irritating the GI tract and increasing peristalsis or by directly stimulating colonic activity.

Bulking agents, such as psyllium, are fiber and other indigestible foods that form a gel in the intestines by absorbing water and causing intestinal distension. This stimulates peristalsis.

Agents such as polyethylene glycol and lactulose are actually osmotic, causing water to stay in the intestines with similar effects as bulking agents.

Stool softeners are what the name implies: they soften the stool by **emulsifying** with the stool. This allows for easier passage of the stool.

DOSAGES

BISACODYL, for relief of constipation, for *children* over 6 years, 5-10 mg (0.3 mg/kg) nocte or before breakfast; for *adults*, 5-15 mg as single dose and up to 30 mg when complete evacuation of bowel is required.

CASTOR OIL, for *children* 2-11 years, for bowel evacuation or constipation, 5-15 mL as a single dose. For *children* over 12 and *adults*, for bowel evacuation or constipation, 15-60 mL as a single dose.

DOCUSATE, as a stool softener, for *infants* and *children* under 3 years, 10-40 mg/d in 1-4 divided doses; for *children* 3-5 years, 20-60 mg/d in 1-4 divided doses; for *children* 6-12 years, 40-150 mg/d in 1-4 divided doses; for *children* over 12 and *adults*, 50-500 mg/d in 1-4 divided doses.

GLYCERIN, for *children* 2 to under 6 years, for constipation, rectal: one pediatric suppository once daily prn or as directed. For *children* over 6 years and *adults*, for constipation, rectal: one adult suppository once daily prn or as directed; for *children* over 2 and *adults*, for dry mouth, apply a 1-inch strip directly to tongue and oral cavity prn.

LACTULOSE, for *infants*, for prevention of portal systemic encephalopathy (PSE), 2.5-10 mL/d divided 3-4 times/d; adjust dosage to produce 2-3 stools/d. For older *children*, for prevention of portal systemic encephalopathy (PSE), daily dose of 40-90 mL divided 3-4 times/d; if initial dose causes diarrhea, then reduce it immediately, adjust dosage to produce 2-3 stools/d. For *children*, for constipation, 5 g/d (7.5 mL) after breakfast. For *adults*, for constipation, 15-30 mL/d increased to 60 mL/d in 1-2 divided doses if necessary; for acute PSE, 20-30 g (30-45 mL) every 1-2 hours to induce rapid laxation, adjust dosage daily to produce 2-3 soft stools, doses of 30-45 mL may be given hourly to cause rapid laxation, then reduce to recommended dose; usual daily dose is 60-100 g (90-150 mL) daily.

MAGNESIUM CITRATE, as a laxative, for *children* 2-6 years, 60-90 mL given once or in divided doses up to a maximum of 90 mL/d; for *children* 6-12 years, 90-210 mL given once or in divided doses; for *children* over 12 and *adults*, 195-300 mL given once or in divided doses.

METHYLCELLULOSE, for *children* 6-11 years, for constipation, caplet: 1 caplet up to a maximum of 6 caplets/d; powder: 1 g in 8 oz. of cold water; may increase prn up to tid. For *children* over 12 and *adults*, for constipation, caplet: 2 caplets up to a maximum of 12 caplets/d; powder: 2 g in 8 oz. of cold water; may increase prn up to tid.

MINERAL OIL, for constipation, for *children* 1 or older, for disimpaction, 15-30 mL per year of age up to a maximum of 240 mL/d; maintain at 1-3 mL/kg/d and adjust to induce daily BM for

Emulsify: To disperse a liquid into another liquid

1-2 months. For *children* 12 years and older and *adults*, for constipation, 15-45 mL/d.

POLYETHYLENE GLYCOL, for *children* ≥6 months, for bowel cleansing prior to GI exam, 25-40 mL/kg/hour for 4-10 hours (until rectal effluent is clear); ideally, patients should fast for 3-4 hours prior to administration; absolutely no solid food for at least 2 hours before the solution is give;, patients <2 years should be monitored closely. For *adults*, for bowel cleansing prior to GI exam, 240 mL (8 oz.) every 10 minutes until 4 L are consumed or the rectal effluent is clear; rapid drinking of each portion is preferred to drinking small amounts continuously; ideally, patients should fast for 3-4 hours prior to administration; absolutely no solid food for at least 2 hours before the solution is given.

SENNA, for constipation, for *children* 2-6 years, sennosides: initiate at 3.75 mg once daily up to a maximum of 7.5 mg bid, 33.3 mg/mL; senna concentrate: 5-10 mL up to twice daily; for *children* 6-12 years, sennosides: initiate at 8.6 mg once daily up to a maximum of 25 mg bid, 33.3 mg/mL; senna concentrate: 10-30 mL up to twice daily. For *children* 12 years or older and *adults*, for bowel evacuation, sennosides: 130 mg between 2-4 PM the afternoon of the day prior to procedure; for constipation, sennosides: 15 mg once daily up to a maximum of 35-50 mg bid.

SODIUM PHOSPHATES, as a laxative, for *children* 5-9 years, 7.5 mL as a single dose; for *children* 10-11 years, 15 mL as a single dose. For *children* 12 and older and *adults*, as a laxative, 15 mL as a single dose, up to a maximum of 45 ml as a single daily dose; for bowel cleansing prior to colonoscopy, Visicol®: evening before colonoscopy take 3 tablets every 15 minutes for 6 doses, then 2 additional tablets in 15 minutes; 3-5 hours prior to colonoscopy take 3 tablets every 15 minutes for 6 doses, then 2 additional tablets in 15 minutes; OsmoPrep®: evening before colonoscopy take 4 tablets every 15 minutes for 5 doses; 3-5 hours prior

to colonoscopy take 4 tablets every 15 minutes for 3 doses.

SODIUM PICOSULFATE, MAGNESIUM OXIDE, and CITRIC ACID, for *adults*, for bowel cleansing, 150 mL the evening before the colonoscopy (5 PM-9 PM), followed by a second 150 mL dose approximately 5 hours before the procedure.

SODIUM SULFATE, POTASSIUM SULFATE, & MAGNESIUM SULFATE, for *adults*, for bowel cleansing prior to GI exam, evening before colonoscopy: drink the entire contents of 1 bottle diluted to a final volume of 480 mL, then drink 960 ml of water over the next hour; morning of the colonoscopy (10-12 hours after the evening dose): repeat entire process with the second bottle; complete at least 2 hours before the procedure.

SORBITOL, for *children* 2-11 years, as a laxative, 2 mL/kg as 70% solution. For *children* 12 years and older and *adults*, as a laxative, 30-150 ml as 70% solution.

WHEAT DEXTRIN, guidelines for laxative dosing are not readily available.

ADVERSE EFFECTS

No adverse effects observed.

RED FLAGS

No major red flags noted.

INTERACTIONS

DRUG

Laxatives can alter the regular kinetics of drug absorption by altering the transit time of substances in the intestines. This can affect almost any other drug. Whether or not this effect is significant depends on individual drugs.

HERB

These agents are designed to alter the functioning of the small and large intestines and could therefore affect the absorption of herbs. These agents should be administered either 4 hours before or 2 hours after to minimize interactions.

LAXATIVES

- Downward-draining herbs (D)–such as *Da Huang* (Rhubarb root), *Mang Xiao* (Sodium sulfate, mirabilite), *Fan Xie Ye* (Senna leaves), and so on, should be used with caution with laxatives as they can act synergistically and cause excessive diarrhea, dehydration, and electrolyte imbalance, expert opinon (Chen & Chen, 2004) Level 5 evidence.
- *Gan Cao* (Licorice) (D)–theoretically may lead to increased potassium loss when used with laxatives, expert opinion (Gruenwald, Brendler & Jaenicke, 2004) Level 5 evidence.

INTERACTION ISSUES

A:

D:

M:

E: Many of the agents in this category can affect gastric motility. These effects theoretically may increase fecal excretion; however, they are most often used to restore normal function and may not cause an interaction.

SECTION 5: MISCELLANEOUS DRUGS OF THE GASTROINTESTINAL SYSTEM

CHLOROPHYLL (KLOR oh fil) PR=N *(Derifil [O])*

LINACLOTIDE (lin AK loe tide) PR=C *(Linzess)*

LUBIPROSTONE (loo bi PROS tone) PR=C *(Amitiza)*

ANTIFLATULANTS:

SIMETHICONE (sye METH i kone) PR=N *(Alamag Plus [O],[13] Aldroxicon I [O],[13] Aldroxicon II [O],[13] Almacone® [O],[13] Almacone® Double Strength [O],[13] Bicarsim [O], Bicarsim Forte [O], Equalizer Gas Relief [O], Gas Ban™ [O],[11] Gas Free Extra Strength [O], Gas Relief Extra Strength [O], Gas Relief Ultra Strength [O], Gas-X [O], Gas-X Children's [O], Gas-X Extra Strength [O], Gas-X Infant Drops [O], Gas-X Ultra Strength [O], GasAid [O], Gelusil® [O],[13] Imodium® Multi-Symptom Relief [O],[17] Infants Gas Relief [O], Infants Simethicone [O], Maalox® Advanced Maximum Strength [O],[11] Maalox® Advanced Regular Strength [O],[13] Maalox® Junior Plus Antigas [O],[11] Mi-Acid [O],[13] Mi-Acid Gas Relief [O], Mintox Plus [O],[13] Mylanta® Classic Maximum Strength Liquid [O],[13] Mylanta® Classic Regular Strength Liquid [O],[13] Mytab Gas [O], Mytab Gas Maximum Strength [O], Phazyme [O], Rulox [O],[13] Simeped [O], Titralac® Plus [O][11])*

FUNCTION

Chlorophyll controls fecal odors especially in the case of colostomies or ileostomies. Linaclotide and Lubiprostone treat chronic idiopathic constipation (CIC) and irritable bowel syndrome with constipation. Antiflatulants reduce gas in the gastrointestinal tract relieving discomfort.

MECHANISM OF ACTION

Linaclotide and lubiprostone increase chloride and/or bicarbonate secretion into the intestinal lumen. More intestinal fluid decreases transit time helping to move stool.

Antiflatulants work by decreasing the surface tension of gas bubbles. By doing this, they reduce the size and stability of bubbles in the tract and reduce pain from stretch receptors.

DOSAGES

CHLOROPHYLL, for *children* 12 years and older and *adults*, for control of odors, 100-200 mg/d in divided doses; may increase to 300 mg/d if odor is uncontrolled.

LINACLOTIDE, for *adults*, for chronic idiopathic constipation (CIC), 145 mcg once daily; for irritable bowel syndrome with constipation, 290 mcg once daily.

LUBIPROSTONE, for *adults*, for chronic idiopathic constipation (CIC), 24 mcg bid; for *females* 18 and older, for irritable bowel syndrome with constipation, 8 mcg bid.

SIMETHICONE, for flatulence or bloating, for *infants* and *children* under 2 years or 11 kg, 20 mg qid prn; for *children* over 2 years or 11 kg, 40 mg qid prn; for *children* 12 years or older and *adults*, 40-360 mg after meals and at bedtime prn.

INTERACTION ISSUES

A:

D:

M:

E:

Pgp:

■ ENDNOTES

1 Combination of Omeprazole, Clarithromycin, and Amoxicillin.

2 Combination of Amoxicillin, Lansoprazole, and Clarithromycin.

3 Combination of Omeprazole and Sodium Bicarbonate.

4 Combination of Diclofenac and Misoprostol.

5 Motofen contains Difenoxin in addition to Atropine and is used in treating diarrhea.

6 Combination of Atropine and Diphenoxylate.

7 Combination of Aluminum Hydroxide and Magnesium Carbonate.

8 Combination of Aluminum Hydroxide and Magnesium Hydroxide.

9 Combination of Aluminum Hydroxide and Magnesium Trisilicate.

10 Combination of Calcium Carbonate and Magnesium Hydroxide.

11 Combination of Calcium Carbonate and Simethicone.

12 Combination of Calcium Carbonate, Famotidine, and Magnesium Hydroxide.

13 Combination of Aluminum Hydroxide, Magnesium Hydroxide, and Simethicone.

14 Combination of Famotidine and Ibuprofen.

15 Combination of Esomeprazole and Naproxen.

16 Combination of Bismuth, Metronidazole, and Tetracycline.

17 Combination of Loperamide and Simethicone.

18 Combination of Magnesium Hydroxide and Mineral Oil.

19 Combination of Polyethylene Glycol-Electrolyte Solution and Bisacodyl.

20 Combination of Polyethylene Glycol-Electrolyte Solution, and Sodium Sulfate, Potassium Sulfate and Magnesium Sulfate.

21 Combination of Senna and Docusate.

■ CHINESE MEDICAL DESCRIPTIONS

The Chinese medical explanation of the drug categories in this chapter may be found in Chapter 15 on pages 385–417.

Antimicrobial Agents

This chapter covers a wide variety of clinical agents including antibiotics to treat bacteria, antivirals, antiprotozoals, anthelminthils, and antifungals. The one thing all of these agents have in common is that they selectively kill or destroy an organism or disease without killing the host. In other words, each of these agents works by exploiting a characteristic inherent in the pathology that is not present in the host. Sometimes this works very well, in that the host is minimally affected by the agent, and sometimes not so specifically, as in the case when an agent would kill the host if the dosage is high enough.

Many factors are involved with choosing an agent to treat an infection. These include identifying the infecting organism, location of the infection, types of infections using Gram staining, whether an agent is -cidal or -static, the MIC and MBC, patient factors, the spectra of the agents, drug resistance, prophylaxis, and complications.

IDENTIFICATION OF THE INFECTING ORGANISM

Different antimicrobial agents have different effectiveness against different organisms. In other words, one agent may be great against a specific organism but minimally effective against another similar organism. Because of this, determining the infecting organism is very important in selecting the correct agent.

One of the main methods of identifying bacteria is by applying a Gram stain. This is a **histological** stain that shows if there are **lipopolysaccharides** surrounding the cell wall of the bacteria. If so, the stain is negative, if not, it is positive. Generally, Gram-negative bacteria are more difficult to treat than Gram-positive bacteria.

In general, it is better to determine the specific pathogen rather than its category. This can be done through several methods including culturing the organism and histologically determining its species, direct microscopy, detection of host responses to the organism, and DNA or RNA determination. These methods, however, take time, and therapy often needs to be initiated before complete identification is determined.

When treatment needs to be initiated prior to identification of the pathogen, many factors are considered including the location of infection (both where on the host and where in the world and in what environment the host was when infected), age and sex of the host, whether the infection is community or hospital acquired, and whether the host is immunocompromised. By taking all of this into account, the prescribing doctor should have a good idea of which organism is involved and be able to give an educated guess as to which agent would be best.

Histology: The science dealing with the microscopic identification of cells, microbes, and tissues

Lipopolysaccharides: Chemical compounds consisting of fat and multiple sugars

SUSCEPTIBILITY OF THE INFECTIVE ORGANISM

Even if the specific organism is known, its susceptibility to various agents may not be. It may have acquired resistance to specific drugs, for example, (explained below). Traditionally, susceptibility was determined by culturing and then applying tests to large quantities of the organism. In pharmacological testing, scientists would often test various concentrations of antibiotics and look at colony growth. For clinical applications, susceptibility is generally tested by applying small paper disks soaked in antibiotics to Petri dishes inoculated with organisms and determining how large the "halo" or circle around the disk was without growth of the organism. The larger the halo the more effective the antibiotic. The downside of this testing is that it takes time, which may be in short supply if the patient is seriously ill or may become so.

The pharmacological tests help determine some important numbers for antimicrobial agents. These two numbers are the minimum inhibitory concentration (MIC) and the minimum bactericidal concentration (MBC). Before explaining these two numbers we need to define the two terms. Antibiotics can do one of two things: they can either prevent further growth of an organism or they can kill live organisms. The first class of drugs is called bacteriostatic agents. These agents do not decrease the colony count of bacteria, but prevent it from getting larger. This allows the body's natural defenses to kill what already exists and mop up. Bactericidal drugs, on the other hand, actually kill what is there, leaving just the mop up to the host's immune system. Getting back to the MIC and MBC, the MIC is the minimum concentration of an agent at which bacterial growth stops, while MBC is the minimal concentration of an agent at which bacteria are killed. Technically, MBC is the minimal concentration of an agent at which only 0.1% of a bacteria colony is still living. It is important to realize that an agent may be bacteriostatic to one organism and bactericidal to another organism.

SITE OF INFECTION

The site of infection is of concern when deciding on treatment. Blood flow is a consideration. If the site has poor blood flow, the antibiotic will not reach the relevant tissues, or a larger dose is necessary to assure that it will reach the site of infection. Other areas may prevent easy flow of antibiotics to the infection site. These may include the prostate, the vitreous body of the eye, and, due to the blood-brain barrier (BBB), the entire central nervous system. Aspects of the drug that may help determine if it penetrates the BBB include how lipophilic the agent is, its molecular weight, and how protein bound the agent is. **Lipophilic** drugs can more easily cross the BBB. A lower molecular weight and a low degree of protein binding also enhance an agent's ability to cross the BBB.

Lipophilic: The opposite of hydrophilic, these are chemicals that prefer to be in a fat- or oil-based solution rather than an aqueous solution

PATIENT FACTORS

Various inherent factors can effect how well a patient responds to antimicrobial treatment. These include the state of their immune system, renal or hepatic impairment, poor perfusion, age, or whether the patient is pregnant or lactating. Whether an antibiotic is bacteriostatic or bactericidal, an intact immune system is still necessary to eliminate the remnants of infection and clean up cellular debris. In immunocompromised patients, higher concentrations of agents may be required. These patients may have such conditions as alcoholism, diabetes, HIV, or may be taking immunosuppressive drugs such as after an organ transplant. The kidneys are the main route of elimination for most of these agents; therefore renal impairment may increase blood levels of these agents possibly to toxic levels. By the same token, hepatic impairment may affect those drugs concentrated or eliminated by the liver. If a patient has poor perfusion to an area of the body, that area is more likely to become infected and is much more difficult to treat. This can happen in the lower limbs of diabetic patients.

While the concentration of antibiotics in breast milk is low, it may still be enough to cause problems in an infant.

All antibiotics cross the placenta and can affect the fetus. While adverse effects in the fetus are rare, there are some serious concerns with individual agents. These include problems with the teeth and inhibition of bone growth with the use of tetracyclines. Antithelminthics are **embryotoxic** and **teratogenic**. Aminoglycosides are **ototoxic**.

DRUG RESISTANCE

Drug resistance is defined as when bacteria's growth is not inhibited by the maximal dose of an antibiotic tolerated by the host. Some bacteria are naturally resistant to certain antibiotics. A problem arises, however, when bacteria that are normally susceptible to a certain antibiotic suddenly becoms resistant. Acquired drug resistance can take many forms depending on the organism and the method of action of the antibiotic. They involve a change in DNA that has spontaneously mutated or has been acquired from another bacteria. Drug resistant bacteria are generally more virulent and more difficult to treat than their non-resistant cousins.

There are many things that can be done to minimize resistance. First, only use antibiotics when indicated. These agents are often prescribed when they have been shown to have no effectiveness, for example in the case of a cold, which is viral. Second, treat for the full course. No antibiotic kills all of the bacteria in an infection, but it is important to kill enough so the patient's immune system can finish off the infection. Remember, in general, the last of the infection is going to be the most resistant of the organisms. Leaving a large colony that the body has trouble finishing off means that when they grow back a portion probably is going to be resistant. Take antibiotics as prescribed, at the proper dose and given intervals in order to maintain the appropriate MIC or MBC. Do not take with antacids as they can decrease the effectiveness of antibiotics by 50-90%. Reserve the best antibiotics for resistant cases so organisms do not build resistance to them. Avoid long-term use. Identify the causative organism and best antibiotic to use.

Embryotoxic: A substance that causes detrimental effects in embryos

Teratogen: A substance that causes congenital defects in fetuses

Ototoxic: Having a harmful effect on the ear or Cranial Nerve VIII

OTHER FACTORS

Cost is a factor in making clinical decisions. If more than one agent is effective, it is appropriate to choose the least expensive option. This can become quite complicated in cases where one agent may be inexpensive but, say, only 80-90% as effective as a vastly more costly alternative.

Another factor that is sometimes considered when prescribing antibiotics is the generation to which it belongs. Many antibiotic classes have been around for a very long time, up to around 100 years. Many generations of similar antibiotics have been devised. More bacteria may be resistent to older antibiotics but not to newer generations. Some later-generation antibiotics are reserved for specific types of infections or when other treatments have failed in order to preserve their efficacy over time. Generally, older generations of antibiotics are less expensive than newer ones.

Prophylactic use of antibiotics can be useful in certain situations. These situations include prevention of streptococcal infections in patients with a history of rheumatic fever, prevention of infection in patients with artificial implanted devices undergoing dental work, prevention of TB or meningitis in people who are in close contact with infected patients, before a surgery that has a high chance of causing infection such as bowel surgery, and using agents in the mother before birth to protect the baby from becoming infected with HIV.

TYPES OF BACTERIA AND ANTIBIOTIC AGENTS

There are many types of bacteria encountered in medical settings. These can be broken down into 9 major types. These include Gram-positive and -negative *cocci*, Gram-positive *bacilli*, Gram-negative rods, **anaerobic** organisms, spirochetes, mycoplasma, chlamydia, and other.

There are 7 major groups of antibiotics. These include penicillins, cephalosporins, tetracyclines, aminoglycosides, macrolides, fluoroquinolones, and other.

Antibiotic agents can be considered to be narrow spectrum, expanded spectrum, or broad spectrum in their effects. Narrow spectrum agents only act on a single or limited group of microorganisms. Extended spectrum agents describe those agents that are effective against Gram positive organisms and a significant number of Gram negative organisms. Broad spectrum agents are effective against a wide variety of organisms. While broad spectrum agents may be useful in infections where the exact bacteria is unknown, they affect so many bacteria that they can reduce beneficial organisms and cause a **superinfection**, for example an infection of *Candida albicans*, also known as thrush.

Antibiotic drugs are often referred to as drugs of first choice for a specific organism. This means that these agents should be tried before any other. When referred to as an agent of second choice, it means that agent should be used only after first- choice agents have failed to resolve the infection. These second-choice drugs can replace first-choice drugs or be added to first choice drugs.

Anaerobic: Able to grow and function without oxygen

Superinfection: An infection that develops during antimicrobial treatment of another infection

Urticaria: Skin condition consisting of wheals, usually the result of hypersensitivity; commonly called hives

Anaphylaxis: A severe and occasionally fatal hypersensitivity/allergic reaction to an antigen; symptoms often include respiratory distress, vascular collapse, and severe skin rashes

COMBINATIONS OF ANTIMICROBIAL DRUGS

In general, it is best practice to use the one agent that has been shown to be most specific for treating the infection. This minimizes the chances of superinfection, toxicity, and drug resistance. However, there are situations where combination therapy is advantageous.

While rare, certain combinations of drugs are synergistic. These include using β-lactams and aminoglycosides. Also special situations may require drug combinations. These include treating tuberculosis and infections of unknown origin. Caution needs to be taken when combining drugs, however. Some agents act on growing colonies; therefore, in general, agents that are bacteriostatic should not be combined with bactericidal agents.

COMPLICATIONS OF ANTIBIOTIC THERAPY

While there are numerous adverse effects of individual agents that will be covered in their respective sections, there are also general concepts of complications. Hypersensitivity reactions can be life-threatening allergic reactions to individual agents and can range from **urticaria** to closing of the airways to complete **anaphylaxis**. Some agents, at high serum levels, can be toxic to the host, not just the microorganism. And, as mentioned earlier, superinfections are a concern. Superinfections are generally difficult to treat.

TYPES OF ANTIMICROBIALS

Antimicrobial agents can be classified in many ways. They can be classified by their chemical structure as is the case with β-lactams or aminoglycosides, by their activity against particular types of organisms as in antibiotics, antivirals, antifungals and so on, or agents can be identified by their mechanism of action. Common classifications based on an agent's mechanism of action include cell wall synthesis inhibitors, inhibitors of metabolism, inhibitors of protein synthesis, inhibitors of nucleic acid function or synthesis, and inhibitors of cell membrane function. Many of these classifications will be used in the sections in this chapter.

SECTION 1: INHIBITORS OF CELL WALL SYNTHESIS

CARBAPENAMS: *These agents are all injected and not covered in this book.*

CEPHALOSPORINS:

FIRST GENERATION:

CEFADROXIL (sef a DROKS il) PR=B

CEPHALEXIN (sef a LEKS in) PR=B *(Keflex®)*

SECOND GENERATION:

CEFACLOR (SEF a klor) PR=B

CEFPROZIL (sef PROE zil) PR=B

CEFUROXIME (se fyoor OKS eme) PR=B *(Ceftin®, Zinacef®, Zinacef® in D5W, Zinacef® in Sterile Water)*

THIRD GENERATION:

CEFDINIR (SEF di ner) PR=B

CEFDITOREN (sef de TOR en) PR=B *(Spectracef)*

CEFIXIME (sef IKS eme) PR=B *(Suplax®)*

CEFPODOXIME (sef pode OKS eme) PR=B

CEFTIBUTEN (sef TYE byoo ten) PR=B *(Cledax®)*

FOURTH GENERATION: *There are drugs that are considered fourth and fifth generation cephalosporin;, however they are all injected and not covered here.*

MONOBACTAMS: *The only agent in this category is injected and not covered in this book.*

PENICILLINS:

AMOXICILLIN (a moks i SIL in) PR=B *(Amoclan,[1] Augmentin®,[1] Augmentin ES-600®,[1] Augmentin XR®, Moxatag, Omeclamox-Pak®,[20] Prevpac®,[2] Trimox®, Wymox)*

AMPICILLIN (am pi SIL in) PR=B

DICLOXACILLIN (dye kloks a SIL in) PR=B

PENICILLIN V (pen i SIL in five) PR=B

PENICILLIN G BENZATHINE (pen i SIL in jee BENZ a thene) PR=B *(Bicillin® C-R,[21] Bicillin® C-R 900/300,[21] Bicillin® L-A)*

PENICILLIN G PROCAINE (pen i SIL in jee PROE kane) PR=B *(Bicillin® C-R,[21] Bicillin® C-R 900/300[21])*

OTHER ANTIBIOTICS:

AZTREONAM (AZ tree oh nam) PR=B *(Azactam, Azactam in Dextrose, Cayston®)*

BACITRACIN (bas i TRAY sin) PR=C *(AK-Poly-Bac™,[27] BACiiM, Cortisporin® Ointment,[29] Neo-Polycin™,[28] Neo-Polycin™ HC,[29] Neosporin® + Pain Relief Ointment [O],[30] Neosporin® Neo To Go® [O][28] Neosporin® Topical [O],[28] Polycin™,[27] Polysporin® [O],[27] Tri Biozene [O][30])*

CYCLOSERINE (sye kloe SER ene) PR=C *(Seromycin®)*

FOSFOMYCIN (fos foe MYE sin) PR=B *(Monurol™)*

POLYMYXIN B (pol i MIKS in BEE) PR=B

VANCOMYCIN (van koe MYE sin) PR=B *(Vancocin®)*

β-LACTAMASE INHIBITORS:

CLAVULANATE POTASSIUM (klav YOO lan ate poe TASS ee um) PR=B *(Amoclan,[1] Augmentin®,[1] Augmentin ES-600®,[1] Augmentin XR®[1])*

▨ FUNCTION

These agents are used to treat bacterial infections. With the exception of β-lactamase inhibitors, they all work by attacking the cell walls of bacteria. Human cells do not have cell walls and therefore are not targeted by these agents. In fact, the penicillins are considered among the most effective antibiotics and least toxic of any drug because of this selectivity, at least when allergic reactions are not considered.

Drug resistance in organisms formerly susceptible to cell wall synthesis inhibitors often takes the form of β-lactamase. This enzyme actually breaks down β-lactam antibiotics. β-lactamase inhibitors are adjuvants to β-lactam antibiotics that inhibit the enzymatic degradation of these antibiotics. They have no clinical function when used without β-lactam antibiotics. While most antibiotics in this section are β-lactam antibiotics, clavulanate is primarily combined with Amoxicillin.

▨ MECHANISM OF ACTION

Penicillins interfere with the last step of bacterial cell wall synthesis. This results in exposure of the cell membrane, which may be **lysed** by osmotic pressures or **autolysis**. They are bactericidal but require fast-growing colonies to be most effective. Penicillins also attach to proteins known as penicillin-binding proteins (PBPs). These proteins are involved with cell wall synthesis and the maintenance of bacteria's **morphology**. Therefore, penicillins may also cause structural changes in susceptible bacteria. These changes may also increase lysis. Some bacteria, especially Gram-positive cocci, create autolysins to help remodel the cell wall. The presence of penicillin in these organisms may cause lysis of the cell wall in addition to inhibition of its synthesis. The spectrum of bacteria penicillins effect is determined by the ability for the agent to get past the cell wall into the space between the wall and the cell membrane and bind with PBPs. Factors that help determine this are the agent's size, charge, and hydrophobicity. In general, these agents are effective against Gram-positive organisms.

Lysis: Destruction of a cell or molecule through the action of an agent

Autolysis: Destruction of a cell as a result of enzymes or proteins produced by/in the same organism

Morphology: The study of the size and shape of a specimen

While Gram-negative bacteria are more difficult for the penicillin to penetrate; many have porins, enzymes that allow transmembrane entry, or allow access by penicillins. Penicillins are not effective against mycobacteria, protozoa, fungi, and viruses. Individual agents have various spectra of use.

Penicillin V is a broad spectrum agent useful in treating Gram-positive and -negative cocci, Gram-positive bacilli, spirochetes, and many anaerobic organisms. Dicloxacillin is an anti-staphylococcal agent. Amoxicillin and ampicillin are extended spectrum agents and are useful in treating Gram-negative rods and, in the case of ampicillin, Listeria monocytogenes. There is extensive resistance to these two agents so they are often prescribed with an additional β-lactamase inhibitor. Carbenicillin is called an antipseudomonal penicillin and is useful in treating Gram-negative rods. Figure 10.1 compares Gram-positive and Gram-negative cell walls.

Cephalosporins have similar mechanisms of action as penicillins but are more resistant to β-lactamases. However, other mechanisms of resistance are just as effective. First-generation cephalosporins are most effective against Gram-positive cocci, with the exception of MRSA, and Gram-negative rods. Second-generation cephalosporins are more effective against Gram-negative organisms but less effective against Gram-positive organisms. Third-generation cephalosporins are very effective against Gram-negative bacilli but less effective against Gram-positive organisms than first-generation agents.

β-lactamase inhibitors help protect antibiotics that have β-lactam rings from being degraded by β-lactamase. This enzyme binds to the β-lactam rings and inactivates the antibiotic. β-lactamase inhibitors bind and inactivate β-lactamase allowing the antibiotic to work without this form of resistance.

The other antibiotics in this section all work by affecting the cell wall through slightly different mechanisms from the cephalosporins and penicillins. Vancomycin is particularly useful as an agent for treating MRSA and MRSE. See Figure 10.2 on page 271.

▦ DOSAGES

Below are the common dosages for each agent. Specific agents may use different doses, and the doses below should not be considered definitive.

AMOXICILLIN, for *children* 3 months or less, 10-15 mg/kg/d bid. For *children* over 3 months and less than 40 kg, 20-50 mg/kg/d in divided doses every 8-12 hours. For *adults*, 250-500 mg every 8 hours or 500-875 mg bid.

AMPICILLIN, for *infants* and *children*, 50-100 mg/kg/d in doses divided every 6 hours up to a maximum 2-4 g/d. For *adults*, 250-500 mg every 6 hours.

AZTREONAM, for susceptible infections, IM: for *children* over 1 month, for mild-to-moderate infections, 30 mg/kg every 8 hours; moderate-to-severe infections, 30 mg/kg every 6-8 hours to a maximum 120 mg/kg/d or 8 g/d; for *Pseudomonas aeruginosa* infection in cystic fibrosis, nebulizer inhalation: for *children* 7 years and older, 75 mg tid for 28 days. For *adults*, for urinary tract infection, IM: 500 mg to 1 g every 8-12 hours; for moderately severe systemic infections, IM: 1 g every 8-12 hours; for *Pseudomonas aeruginosa* infection in cystic fibrosis, nebulizer inhalation: 75 mg tid for 28 days.

BACITRACIN, for *adults*, for antibiotic-associated colitis, 25,000 units qid for 7-10 days.

CEFADROXIL, for *children*, 15 mg/kg/d bid up to a maximum 2 g/d. For *adults*, .5-1 g/d bid.

CEFACLOR, for *children* over 1 month, 20-40 mg/kg/d divided every 8-12 hours to a maximum dose of 1 g/d. For *adults*, 250-500 mg every 8 hours.

CEFDINIR, for *children* 6 months to 12 years, 7 mg/kg/dose bid or 14 mg/kg/dose once daily to a maximum 600 mg/d. For *adolescents* and *adults*, 300 mg bid or 600 mg once daily.

CEFDITOREN, for *children* 12 years and older and *adults*, for acute bacterial exacerbation of chronic bronchitis, 400 mg bid for 10 days; for community-acquired pneumonia, 400 mg bid; for pharyngitis, tonsillitis, or uncomplicated skin or skin structure infections, 200 mg bid for 10 days.

CEFIXIME, *children* 6 months and older, 8-20 mg/kg/d divided every 12-24 hours to maximum 400 mg/d. For *children* over 50 kg or over 12 and *adults*, 400 mg/d divided every 12-24 hrs.

CEFPODOXIME, for *children* 2 months to 12 years, 10 mg/kg/d divided every 12 hours up to a maximum dose of 800 mg/d. For *children* 12 years and over and *adults*, 100-400 mg every 12 hours.

CEFPROZIL, for *infants* and *children* over 6 months to 12 years, 7.5-15 mg/kg/d divided every 12 hours. For *children* over 12 years and *adults*, 250-500 mg every 12 hours or 500 mg/d.

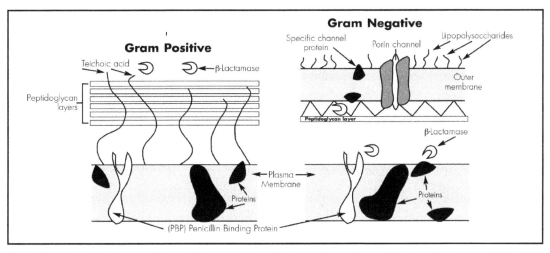

Figure 10.1: Comparing Gram-positive and Gram-negative cell bacteria. Notice the peptidoglycan layers that build the thick cell wall of Gram-positive bacteria. This is what is stained with Gram stain. In contrast, the Gram-negative bacteria have a much thinner cell wall with an outer membrane with lipopolysaccharide structures. It is this outer membrane that prevents Gram staining and makes it more difficult for antibiotics to penetrate.

CEFTIBUTEN, for *children* 6 months to under 12 years, for susceptible infections, 9 mg/kg/d for 10 days up to a maximum daily dose of 400 mg. For *children* 12 years and older and *adults*, for susceptible infections, 400 mg once daily for 10 days.

CEPHALEXIN, for *children* over 1 year, 25-100 mg/kg/d every 6-8 hours up to a maximum of 4 g/d. For *adults*, 250-1000 mg every 6 hours up to a maximum of 4 g/d.

CEFUROXIME, for *children* under 13 years, 10-15 mg/kg/d bid. For *children* 13 years or older and *adults*, 250-500 mg bid.

CYCLOSERINE, for *children*, for tuberculosis, 5-10 mg/kg/d bid up to 1000 mg/d for 18-24 months. For *adults*, for tuberculosis, initiate at 250 mg every 12 hours for 14 days, then administer 250 mg to 500 mg/d bid for 18-24 months; maximum daily dose is 1 g.

DICLOXACILLIN, for *children* under 40 kg, 12.5-100 mg/kg/d divided every 6 hours. For *children* over 40 kg, 125-250 mg every 6 hours. For *adults*, 125-1000 mg every 6 hours.

FOSFOMYCIN, for *adults*, for uncomplicated UTI in women, single dose of 3 g in 4 oz. of water.

PENICILLIN G BENZATHINE, for *children*, IM: usual dose range is 25,000-50,000 units/kg as a single dose up to a maximum of 2.4 million units. FoM: usual dose range is 1.2-2.4 million units as a single dose.

PENICILLIN G PROCAINE, for *infants* and *children*, for susceptible infections, 25,000-50,000 units/kg/d in divided doses 1-2 times/d up to a maximum 4.8 million units/d. For *adults*, for post-exposure prophylaxis inhalational anthrax, IM: 1,200,000 units every 12 hours for 60 days. Use over 2 weeks may incur additional risk of adverse reactions; for treatment of cutaneous anthrax, IM: 600,000-1,200,000 units/d.

PENICILLIN V, for *children* under 12, 25-50 mg/kg/ d in divided doses every 6-8 hours to a maximum dose of 3 g/d. For *children* 12 and over and *adults*, 125-500 mg every 6-8 hours.

POLYMYXIN B, for *adults*, for systemic infections, IM: 25,000-30,000 units/kg/d divided every 4-6 hours; for topical irri-

gation or topical solution, 500,000 units/L of normal saline; topical irrigation not to exceed 2 million units/d.

VANCOMYCIN, for pseudomembranous colitis produced by *C. difficile*, for *neonates*, 10 mg/kg/d in divided doses; for *children*, 40 mg/kg/d in divided doses, added to fluids; for *adults*, 125 mg qid for 10 days.

ADVERSE EFFECTS

Penicillins are considered among the safest drugs in the pharmacopeia, though adverse effects do occur. These include diarrhea due to disruption of the GI tract's natural flora, nephritis, neurotoxicity especially in epileptic patients, and eosinophilia. Decreased **agglutination** may occur in some patients especially those susceptible to hemorrhage or those on anticoagulants.

Cephalosporins are not generally coherent in their adverse effects. Those allergic to penicillins should not use cephalosporins as there is a significant cross-sensitivity.

Vancomycin has serious adverse effects. These include fever and chills. Ototoxicity can damage hearing in patients taking another antibiotic such as an aminoglycoside with this agent and in patients with renal failure. Nephrotoxicity may also occur when combined with other antibiotics.

RED FLAGS

Hypersensitivity reactions in patients taking penicillin can be life threatening and are thought to occur at some level in about 5% of patients taking these agents.

INTERACTIONS

HERB

AMOXICILLIN

- *Huang Qin* (Scutellaria) (D)–constituent of *Huang Qin*, baicalin, was found to potentiate β-lactam antibiotics even restoring effectiveness in β-lactam resistant *Staph. aureua* and methicillin-resistant *Staph. aureus* (MRSA) (Liu, Durham & Richards, 2000) Level 5 evidence.

AMPICILLIN

- *Huang Qin* (Scutellaria) (D)–constituent of

Agglutination: The aggregation or clumping of cells due to interaction with antibodies called agglutinins

	Gram (+) Cocci	Gram (–) Cocci	Gram (+) bacilli	Gram (–) rods	Anaerobics	Spirochetes	Mycoplasma Chlamydia Other
PENICILLINS: Amoxicillin			Listeria monocytogenes	E. coli H. influenza Proteus mirabilis Salmonella typhi			
Ampicillin			Listeria monocytogenes	E. coli H. influenza Proteus mirabilis Salmonella typhi			
Carbenicillin				Enterobacter species E. coli H. influenza Proteus mirabilis Proteus (indole positive) Pseudomonas aerugunosa			
Dicloxacillin	Staph. aureus Staph epidermidis						
Penicillin V	Strep. pneumoniae Strep. pyogenes Strep. viridans group	Neisseria gonorrhoeae Neisseria meningitidis	Bacillus anthracis Corynebacterium diphtheriae		Clostridium perfringens	Treponema pertenue (Yaws) Treponema pallidum (Syphilis)	
CEPHALOSPORINS: 1st generation:	Staph. aureus Staph epidermidis Strep. pneumoniae Strep. pyogenes Anaerobic streptococci			E. coli Klebsiella pneumoniae Proteus mirabilis			
2nd generation:	Strep. pneumoniae Strep. pyogenes Anaerobic streptococci	Neisseria gonorrhoeae		Enterobactor aerogenes E. coli H. influenza Klebsiella pneumoniae Proteus mirabilis			
3rd generation:		Neisseria gonorrhoeae		Enterobactor aerogenes E. coli H. influenza Klebsiella pneumoniae Proteus mirabilis Pseudomonas aerugunosa			
OTHER ANTIBIOTICS: Cycloserine							Mycobacterium
Fosfomycin	Enterococci			E. coli			
Vancomycin	Staph. aureus Staph epidermidis Strep. Groups A, B, C Strep. pneumoniae Enterococcus faecalis		Listeria monocytogenes		Clostridium species		Actinomyces

Figure 10.2: Antibiotic spectra.

Huang Qin, baicalin, was found to potentiate β-lactam antibiotics even restoring effectiveness in β-lactam resistant *Staph. aureua* and methicillin-resistant *Staph. aureus* (MRSA) (Liu, Durham & Richards, 2000) Level 5 evidence.

ANTIBIOTICS
• *Ci Wu Jia* (Acanthopanax root) (D)–was shown to increase the effectiveness of antibiotics, possibly by increasing T-lymphocyte activity (Brinker, 1995) Level 5 evidence.

BETA-LACTAM ANTIBIOTICS
• *Huang Qin* (Scutellaria) (D)–constituent of *Huang Qin*, baicalin, was found to potentiate β-lactam antibiotics even restoring effectiveness in β-lactam resistant *Staph. aureua* and

methicillin-resistant *Staph. aureus* (MRSA) (Liu, Durham & Richards, 2000) Level 5 evidence.

VANCOMYCIN
• *Da Suan* (Garlic) (D)–fresh *Da Suan* reduced the minimum inhibitory concentration for vancomycin-resistant enterococci (Abascal & Yarnell, 2002) Level 5 evidence.

INTERACTION ISSUES

A:

D: Dicloxacillin is 96% protein bound.

M: Dicloxacillin is a weak or moderate inducer of CYP3A4.

E:

Pgp:

SECTION 2: PROTEIN SYNTHESIS INHIBITORS

AMINOGLYCOSIDES:

GENTAMICIN (jen ta MYE sin) PR=D

NEOMYCIN (nee oh MYE sin) PR=D *(Neo-Fradin™)*

TOBRAMYCIN (toe bra MYE sin) PR=D *(Tobi®, Tobi® Podhaler®)*

MACROLIDES/KETOLIDES:

AZITHROMYCIN (az ith roe MYE sin) PR=B *(Zithromax®, Zithromax® Tri-Pak, Zithromax® Z-Pak, Zmax™)*

CLARITHROMYCIN (kla RITH roe mye sin) PR=C *(Biaxin®, Biaxin® XL, Biaxin® XL Pac, Omeclamox-Pak®,[20] Prevpac®[2])*

ERYTHROMYCIN (er ith roe MYE sin) PR=B *(Akne-Mycin, E.E.S.® 400, E.E.S.® Granules, E.S.P.®,[22] Ery, Ery-Tab®, EryPed® 200, EryPed® 400, Erythrocin Lactobionate, Erythrocin Stearate, PCE®)*

FIDAXOMICIN (fye DAX oh mye sin) PR=B *(Dificid™)*

TELITHROMYCIN (tel ith roe MYE sin) PR=C *(Ketek®)*

TETRACYCLINES:

DEMECLOCYCLINE (dem e kloe SYE klene) PR=D

DOXYCYCLINE (doks i SYE klene) PR=D *(Adoxa™, AdoxaT™ Pak 1/100, Adoxa™ Pak 1/150, Adoxa™ Pak 2/100, Alodox Convenience, Avidoxy, Doryx®, Doxy 100®, Monodox®, Morgidox, Ocudox, Oracea™, Oraxyl, Vibramycin®)*

MINOCYCLINE (mi noe SYE klene) PR=D *(Dynacin®, Minocin®, Solodyn™)*

TETRACYCLINE (tet ra SYE klene) PR=D

OTHERS:

CLINDAMYCIN (klin da MYE sin) PR=B *(Cleocin®, Cleocin-T®, Cleocin in D5W®, Cleocin Phosphate®, Clindacin Pac, Clindacin-P, Clindagel®, ClindaMax™, Evoclin™)*

LINEZOLID (li NE zoh lid) PR=C *(Lincocin®)*

▮ FUNCTION

These agents are used to treat bacterial infections. They do this by attacking bacterial ribosomes, which are different than human ribosomes. Recall that ribosomes are the protein "factory" in the cell that converts mRNA into proteins. Unfortunately, mitochondria, the "power plant" of human cells that creates ATP, are thought to have been derived from bacterial cells. Their ribosomes are similar enough to bacterial ribosomes that some of these agents can affect the host's cells if given in large enough doses.

Although neomycin is listed above as an oral aminoglycoside, due to toxicities, its use is primarily topical with the exception of its prophylactic use before bowel surgery. All other aminoglycosides are injectable only.

▮ MECHANISM OF ACTION

Tetracyclines are broad-spectrum, bacteriostatic antibiotics that reversibly bind to the 30S subunit of bacterial ribosomes and block the access of tRNA preventing translation and protein synthesis. This is summarized in Figure 10.3.

Like tetracyclines, aminoglycosides bind to the 30S portion of the ribosome. However, their action is different. These agents distort the shape of the ribosome and prevent proper initiation of protein synthesis as well as causing mRNA misreading, which in turn causes mutations and premature termination of the amino acid chain. They are particularly effective in combinations with β-lactam antibiotics as the later breaks down the cell wall and allows greater penetration of the aminoglycosides.

Macrolides, and the very similar ketolides, work by binding to the 50S subunit of bacterial ribosomes and preventing the translocation of the tRNA carrying the growing amino acid chain from moving from one spot in the ribosome to the other. This prevents further synthesis of the amino acid chain. There may be other effects that contribute to their effectiveness, but these are poorly understood. These agents are considered

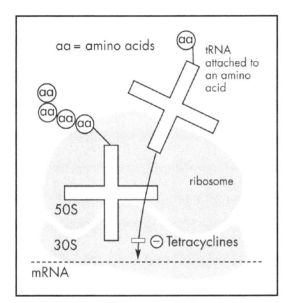

Figure 10.3: Tetracyclines prevent binding of the second transfer RNA-amino acid complex from binding to the 30S subunit of a bacterial ribosome and thus terminating protein synthesis.

to be bacteriostatic but may be bactericidal at higher doses.

Clindamycin has the same mechanism of action as the macrolides.

Linezolid prevents the formation of the entire bacterial ribosome by binding to the 50S subunit.

DOSAGES

The dosages below are the common dosages for each agent. Specific agents may use different doses, and the doses below should not be considered definitive.

AZITHROMYCIN, for *children* 6 months and older, 5-12 mg/kg given once daily to a maximum 500 mg/d or 30 mg/kg as a single dose up to a maximum of 1500 mg. For *adolescents* 16 years or older and *adults*, 250-600 mg once daily or 1-2 g as a single dose.

CLARITHROMYCIN, for *children* 6 months or older, 7.5-15 mg/kg every 12 hours up to a maximum of 500 mg/dose. For *adults*, 250-500 mg every 12 hours or 1000 mg once daily for 7-14 days.

CLINDAMYCIN, for *infants* and *children*, 8-20 mg/kg/d as hydrochloride; 8-25 mg/kg/d as palmitate in 3-4 divided doses; minimum

dose of palmitate is 37.5 mg tid. For *adults*, 150-450 mg every 6-8 hours; maximum dose is 1.8 g/d.

DEMECLOCYCLINE, for *children* 8 years or older, 8-12 mg/kg/d divided every 6-12 hours. For *adults*, 150 mg qid or 300 mg bid.

DOXYCYCLINE, for *children* 8 years or older (<45 kg), 2-5 mg/kg/d in 1-2 divided doses, not to exceed 200 mg/d. For *children* over 8 years (over 45 kg) and *adults*, 100-200 mg/d in 1-2 divided doses.

ERYTHROMYCIN, due to differences in absorption, 400 mg erythromycin ethylsuccinate produces the same serum levels as 250 mg erythromycin base, sterate, or estolate. For *infants* and *children*, base, 30-50 mg/kg/d in 2-4 divided doses, not to exceed 2 g/d; estolate, 30-50 mg/kg/d in 2-4 divided doses, not to exceed 2 g/d; ethylsuccinate, 30-50 mg/kg/d in 2-4 divided doses, not to exceed 3.2 g/d; sterate, 30-50 mg/kg/d in 2-4 divided doses, not to exceed 2 g/d. For *adults*, base, 250-500 mg every 6-12 hours; ethylsuccinate, 400-800 mg every 6-12 hours.

FIDAXOMICIN, for *adults*, for treatment of diarrhea due to *Clostridium* difficile, 200 mg bid for 10 days.

LINCOMYCIN, for *children* over 1 month, for susceptible infections, IM: 10 mg/kg every 12-24 hours. For *adults*, for susceptible infections, IM: 600 mg every 12-24 hours.

LINEZOLID, for *preterm neonates* (<34 weeks gestational age), for VRE infections, 10 mg/kg every 12 hours; *neonates* with a suboptimal clinical response can be advanced to 10 mg/kg every 8 hours; by day 7 of life, all neonates should receive 10 mg/kg every 8 hours. For *infants* (excluding preterm *neonates* <1 week) and *children* under 5, for uncomplicated skin and skin structure infections, 10 mg/kg every 8 hours for 10-14 days. For *children* 5-11, for uncomplicated skin or skin structure infections, 10 mg/kg every 12 hours for 10-14 days. For *infants* and *children* over 11 years, for VRE infections, 10 mg/kg every 8 hours for 14-28 days; for nosocomial pneumonia, complicated skin and skin structure infections, and community acquired pneumonia including concurrent bacteremia, 10 mg/kg every 8 hours for 10-14 days. For *children* 12-18 years, for uncomplicated skin and skin structure infections, 600 mg every 12 hours for 10-14 days. For *children* over 12 years and *adults*, for VRE infections, 600 mg every 12 hours for 14-28 days; for nosocomial pneumonia, complicated skin and skin structure infections, and community acquired pneumonia including concurrent bacteremia, 600 mg every 12 hours for 10-14 days. For *adults*, for uncomplicated skin and skin structure infections, 400 mg every 12 hours for 10-14 days.

MINOCYCLINE, for *children* over 8, initiate at 4 mg/kg, followed by 2 mg/kg every 12 hours. For *adults*, initiate at 200 mg, followed by 100 mg every 12 hours to maximum 400 mg/d.

GENTAMICIN, for *children* and *adults*, for skin infections, topical: apply 3-4 times/d to affected area.

NEOMYCIN, for *children*, for preoperative intestinal antisepsis, 90 mg/kg/d divided every 4 hours for 2 days, or 25 mg/kg at 1 PM, 2 PM, and 11 PM on the day preceding surgery as an adjunct to mechanical cleansing of the intestine and in combination with erythromycin base; for hepatic encephalopathy, 50-100 mg/kg/d in divided doses every 6-8 hours or 2.5-7 g/m²/d divided every 4-6 hours for 5-6 days not to exceed 12 g/d. For *adults*, for preoperative intestinal antisepsis, 1 g each hour for 4 doses, then 1 g every 4 hours for 5 doses, or 1 g at 1 PM, 2 PM, and 11 PM on day preceding surgery as an adjunct to mechanical cleansing of the bowel and oral erythromycin, or 6 g/d divided every 4 hours for 2-3 days; for hepatic encephalopathy, 500-2000 mg every 6-8 hours or 4-12 g/d divided every 4-6 hours for 5-6 days; for chronic hepatic insufficiency, 4 g/d for an indefinite period.

RIFAXIMIN, for *children* 12 and older and *adults*, for travelers' diarrhea, 200 mg tid for 3 days.

TELITHROMYCIN, for *adults*, for community-acquired pneumonia, 800 mg once daily for 7-10 days.

TETRACYCLINE, for *children* over 8 years, 25-50

	Gram (+) Cocci	Gram (−) Cocci	Gram (+) bacilli	Gram (−) rods	Anaerobics	Spirochetes	Mycoplasma	Chlamydia	Other
AMINOGLYCOSIDES:	Enterococcus species Strep. agalactiae			Brucella species Francisella tularensis (Tularemia) Klebsiella species Pseudomonas aerugunosa Yersinia pestis					
MACROLIDES:	Staph. aureus Strep. pneumoniae Strep. pyogenes	Moraxella catarrhalis Neisseria gonor- rhoeae	Corynebacterium diphtheriae	Bordetella pertussis Campylobacter jejuni Hemophilus influenzae Legionella pneumophilia (Legionnaires' Disease)		Treponema pallidum (Syphilis)	Mycoplasma pneumonia Ureaplasma urealyticum	Chlamydia pneumonia Chlamydia psittaci Chlamydia trachomatis	
TETRACYCLINES:			Bacillus anthracis	Brucella species Vibro cholerae (Chlorea) Yersinia pestis	Clostridium perfringens Clostridium tetani	Borelia burgdorferi (Lyme disease) Leptospira interrogans	Mycoplasma pneumonia	Chlamydia species	Rickettsia ricketsii (Rocky Mtn. Spotted Fever)
OTHERS: **CLINDAMYCIN:**	non-enteroccal species				Bacteroides fragilis Clostridium perfringens				
LINEZOLID:	Enteroccus faecalis VRE Enterococcus faecium Staph epidermidis Staph. haemolyticus Strep. pneumoniae Veridans group streptococci		Corynebacterium species Listeria monocytogenes						

Figure 10.4: Antibiotic spectra.

mg/kg/d in divided doses every 6 hours. For *adults*, 250-500 mg every 6 hours.

TOBRAMYCIN, for *children* 6 years and older and *adults*, for cystic fibrosis, inhalation: 300 mg every 12 hours in repeated cycles of 28 days on drug followed by 28 days off.

ADVERSE EFFECTS

Tetracyclines cause numerous adverse effects including discoloration and **hypoplasia** of the teeth and temporary stunting of growth in growing children and **phototoxicity,** which can result in a severe sunburn after sun exposure. Overgrowths of *Candida*, resistant *Staph* in the intestines, and *Clostridium difficile* have been reported. Gastric discomfort is common, and these agents should be taken with foods other than dairy. Dizziness, nausea, and vomiting may occur, especially with minocycline and doxycycline. Benign, intracranial hypertension with such symptoms as headache and blurred vision caused by pseudotumor cerebri may, rarely, occur in adults. Except for doxycycline, these agents are contraindicated in cases of renal impairment. Other contraindications for all agents include pregnant or breast-feeding women and in children under 8.

In oral use, many of the following adverse effects of aminoglycosides are minimized by short-term use. Most are prominent in injection administration. These include ototoxicity, both in the forms of possibly permanent hearing loss and vertigo and loss of balance, nephrotoxicity, and neuromuscular paralysis. Neomycin may cause contact dermatitis when applied topically.

Macrolides and ketolides commonly cause GI distress. **Cholestatic** jaundice can occur with erythromycin, as can ototoxicity at high doses. Erythromycin, telithromycin, and azithromycin should be used with caution in patients with liver dysfunction. Telithromycin should be prescribed with caution in patients with renal compromise and may worsen myasthenia gravis.

Adverse effects of clindamycin include skin rashes. A potentially fatal effect is pseudomembranous colitis caused by overgrowth of *Clostridium difficile*. Caution should be used when giving this drug to hepatic- and renal-impaired patients.

Linezolid is generally well tolerated with some reports of GI disturbances, nausea, diarrhea, headaches, and rash. In about 2% of patients on the drug longer than 2 weeks, a reversible **thrombocytopenia** occurred.

RED FLAGS

Tetracyclines have been shown to cause fatal hepatotoxicity in pregnant woman on high doses. This is worse if they have **pyelonephritis**.

Short-term clarithromycin use in patients with stable coronary artery disease may cause significantly higher cardiovascular mortality.

After five case reports of liver damage resulting in four deaths and a liver transplant, the Food and Drug Administration has changed label requirements regarding the potential for serious hepatic toxicity associated with the use of telithromycin.

An FDA alert was issued regarding linezolid after a study showed an increased mortality rate in patients with catheters. Linezolid is not approved for the treatment of catheter-related blood-stream infections, catheter-site infections, or for the treatment of infections caused by Gram-negative bacteria. The FDA is further considering the study mentioned.

INTERACTIONS

DRUG

The ototoxicity of aminoglycosides is more likely when combined with other ototoxic drugs such as furosemide, bumetanide, ethacrynic acid, or cisplatin.

Erythromycin, telithromycin, and clarithromycin may inhibit the metabolism of many drugs in the liver. These include astemizole, carbamazepine, cyclosporine, terfenadine, theophylline, valproate, and warfarin. These drugs

---

Hypoplasia: An incomplete or underdeveloped organ or tissue usually due to a reduced number of cells

Phototoxic: A substance that causes a rapidly developing, nonimmune reaction of the skin when exposed to light

Cholestatis: An interruption in the flow of bile at any point in the biliary system from liver to duodenum

Thrombocytopenia: A decreased number of platelets in the blood

Pyelonephritis: A fever inducing infection of the kidney

may cause an increase in digoxin levels due to elimination of intestinal flora that helps inactivate digoxin.

HERB

AMINOGLYCOSIDES

- *Dong Chong Xia Cao* (Cordyceps) (D)–may reduce nephrotoxicity from aminoglycosides in rats (Zhu, Halpern & Jones, 1998) Level 5 evidence.
- (D) One study showed that injection of both *Lu Han Cao* (Pyrola) and *Huang Qi* (Astragulus) in guinea pigs prevented ototoxicity and nephrotoxicity of aminoglycosides (Chen & Chen, 2004) Level 5 evidence.

ANTIBIOTICS

- *Ci Wu Jia* (Acanthopanax root) (D)–was shown to increase the effectiveness of antibiotics, possibly by increasing T-lymphocyte activity (Brinker, 1995) Level 5 evidence.

ERYTHROMYCIN

- *Ci Wu Jia* (Acanthopanax root) (B-)–may increase the efficacy of erythromycin and kanamycin antibiotics in treating *Shigella* dysentery and *Proteus* entercolitis as shown in a human clinical study (Vereshchagin, Geskina & Bukhteeva, 1982) Level 3b evidence.

- *Guan Ye Lian Qiao* (St. John's wort) (C)–A review of case reports shows *Guan Ye Lian Qiao* decreases blood concentrations of erythromycin (Izzo & Ernst, 2009) Level 3a evidence.

TETRACYCLINE

- *Hei Hu Jiao* (Indeterminate)–may cause increase in blood levels of rifampin, sulphadiazine, tetracycline, and pentobarbital (unobtainable article as cited in Brinker, 2001) Indeterminate level of evidence.
- *Rou Gui* (Cinnamon bark) (D)–may reduce absorption of tetracycline, expert opinion (Brinker, 2001) Level 5 evidence.

INTERACTION ISSUES

A:

D:

M: Clarithromycin is a major substrate and strong inhibitor of CYP3A4; erythromycin is a major substrate and moderate inhibitor of CYP3A4; telithromycin is a major substrate and strong inhibitor of CYP3A4; tetracycline is a major substrate and moderate inhibitor of CYP3A4.

E:

Pgp: Azithromycin and clarithromycin inhibit Pgp; erythromycin is a substrate of and inhibits Pgp.

SECTION 3: DNA AND RNA SYNTHESIS INHIBITORS AND URINARY TRACT ANTISEPTICS

FLUOROQUINOLONES:

FIRST GENERATION: DISCONTINUED

SECOND GENERATION:

CIPROFLOXACIN (sip roe FLOKS a sin) PR=C
(Cipro®, Cipro® HC,[24] Cipro® in D5W, Cipro® XR, Ciprodex®[23])

NORFLOXACIN (nor FLOKS a sin) PR=C
(Noroxin®)

OFLOXACIN (oh FLOKS a sin) PR=C

THIRD GENERATION:

LEVOFLOXACIN (lee voe FLOKS a sin) PR=C
(Levaquin®)

MOXIFLOXACIN (moxs i FLOKS a sin) PR=C
(Avelox®, Avelox® ABC Pack)

Moxifloxacin is placed as a third-generation agent. Some literature states that this is actually a fourth-generation agent. Given its antibiotic spectrum of action, the authors believe it should be included as a third-generation agent.

FOURTH GENERATION:

GEMIFLOXACIN (je mi FLOKS a sin) PR=C
(Factive®)

INHIBITORS OF FOLATE SYNTHESIS:

SULFONAMIDES:

SULFACETAMIDE (sul fa SEE ta mide) PR=C
(AVAR, AVAR LS, AVAR-e, AVAR-e Green, AVAR-e LS, BP 10-1, BP Cleansing Wash, Clarifoam EF, Claris, Clenia, Klaron, Mexar Wash, Ovace Plus, Ovace Plus Wash, Ovace Wash, Prascion, Prascion FC, Prascion RA, Rosanil, SSS 10-4; SSS 10-5, Seb-Prev, Seb-Prev Wash, SulfaCleanse 8/4, Sumadan; Sumaxin, Sumaxin TS, Zencia)

SULFADIAZINE (sul fa DYE a zene) PR=C

SULFADOXINE (sul fa DOKS ene) PR=C

SULFAMETHOXAZOLE (sul fa meth OKS a zole) PR=C *(Bactrim™,[6] Bactrim™ DS,[6] Septra® DS[6])*

SULFISOXAZOLE (sul fi SOKS a zole) PR=C *(Pediazole®[3])*

INHIBITORS OF FOLATE REDUCTION:

TRIMETHOPRIM (trye METH oh prim) PR=C *(Bactrim™,[6] Bactrim™ DS,[6] Polytrim®,[25] Primsol®, Septra® DS[6])*

URINARY TRACT ANTISEPTICS:

METHENAMINE (meth EN a mene) PR=C *(Hiprex®, Hyophen™,[26] Phosphasal™,[7] Prosed® IDS,[26] Urelle®,[7] Urex®, Uribel™,[7] Urimar-T,[7] Uroqid-Acid® No. 2,[8] Uta®[7])*

NITROFURANTOIN (nye troe fyoor AN toyn) PR=B *(Furadantin®, Macrobid®, Macrodantin®)*

MISCELLANEOUS:

RIFAXIMIN (rif AX i min) PR=C *(Xifaxan™)*

Many of these agents are used to treat urinary tract infections (UTIs). Abut 80% of uncomplicated upper and lower UTIs are caused by *Escherichia coli*. The second most common pathogen is *Staphylococcus saprophyticus*. Other common causes are *Klebsiella pneumoniae* and *Proteus mirabilis*.

FUNCTION

With the exception of methenamine, these agents are used to treat bacterial infections by preventing DNA synthesis.

The flouroquinolones generally are broader spectrum and more efficient than most other antibiotics and have enjoyed widespread use. Unfortunately, because of this use, resistance is beginning to emerge.

Fluoroquinolones are broken down into four generations. First-generation quinolones, which are discontinued, achieve minimal levels in the blood. Second-generation agents have better systemic activity and increased Gram-negative action. Third-generation agents have better activity towards Gram-positive bacteria and atypical pathogens. And finally, fourth-generation agents add action against anaerobes.

Sulfonamides are also known as sulfa drugs and, except for penicillin, are among the oldest of the antibiotics. Until the mid-1970s, they were mainly used in developing countries, as they had fallen out of favor in the developed countries. At that time, the combination of trimethoprim and sulfamethoxazole was introduced and ushered in new uses for the sulfa drugs especially for urinary tract infections.

The urinary tract antiseptics act primarily in the bladder to treat UTIs. Nitrofurantoin is not commonly used due to its narrow spectrum of action and its toxicity.

MECHANISM OF ACTION

Each agent in this category acts by preventing synthesis of DNA, the basic building block of genes, and/or RNA, the molecules used to translate DNA into proteins and enzymes. Fluoroquinolones have a different mechanism for preventing DNA synthesis than the other agents. The other dugs act by preventing the formation of folic acid or folate, a B vitamin. Folic acid, or more specifically, its active form of tetrahydrofolic acid, is important to purine and pyrimidine synthesis as well as amino acid synthesis and red blood cell maturation. Purines and pyrimidines are part of the molecular structure of DNA and RNA.

Flouroquinolones enter the bacterium through porins in the outer membrane by using **passive dif-**

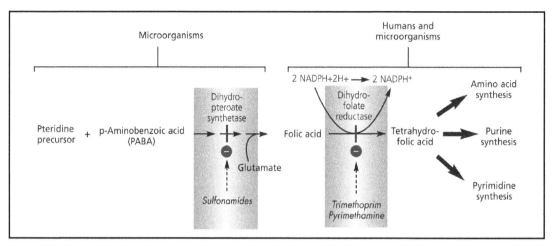

Figure 10.5: How antibiotics can interfere with folic acid synthesis and their ultimate use. Sulfonamides interfere with folic acid synthesis by inhibiting dihydropteroate synthetase. Inhibitors of folate reduction (trimethoprim and pyrimethamine) inhibit the enzyme dihydrofolate reductase and prevent synthesis of various DNA, RNA, and amino acid constituents.

Passive diffusion: The movement of small molecules across a cell membrane without the need for energy

Analog: A drug or other chemical that is similar in structure or constituents to another but differs in effects

fusion. They target bacterial DNA and prevent two enzymes, DNA gyrase (topoisomerase II and topoisomerase IV) from aiding in DNA reproduction and cell division. Ultimately, these drugs prevent reproduction by damaging the DNA. The dominant mechanism between these two inhibited enzymes is dependent on the individual organism. These drugs are bactericidal.

Sulfonamides are **analogues** of PABA, a precursor of folic acid synthesis. They compete with PABA as a substrate for dihydropteroate synthetase, an enzyme that converts a pteridine precursor and PABA into folic acid. Therefore sulfonamides prevent the synthesis of folic acid. These agents are bacteriostatic.

The inhibitors of folate reduction prevent the synthesis of the active form of folic acid, tetrahydrofolic acid. These agents act to block the enzyme dihydrofolate reductase, which converts folic acid to tetrahydrofolic acid. While this enzyme is present in both mammals and bacteria, these agents have a much higher affinity for the bacterial enzyme than the mammalian one, which allows for its safe use as an antibiotic. These agents are bacteriostatic. Figure 10.5 summarizes the mechanisms of action of both sulfa drugs and inhibitors of folate reduction.

Co-trimoxazole, a combination of trimetho-prim and sulfamethoxazole, acts on the same pathway but at different places. This allows for a synergistic effect.

Methenamine works by being transformed to formaldehyde in acidic environments. In vivo, that occurs only in the bladder where the levels of methenamine are concentrated and the pH is low enough to cause this conversion. Formaldehyde is bactericidal and does not cause resistance.

Nitrofurantoin acts by damaging DNA but its activity is greatest in acidic urine. It is bacteriostatic.

DOSAGES

The dosages below are the common dosages for each agent. Specific agents may use different doses, and the doses below should not be considered definitive.

CIPROFLOXACIN, for *children*, 10-15 mg/kg/d bid; maximum dose is 1.5 g/d. For *adults*, 250-750 mg every 12 hours.

GEMIFLOXACIN, for *adults*, 320 mg once daily.

LEVOFLOXACIN, for adults, 250-500 mg every 24 hours; for severe or complicated infections, 750 mg every 24 hours.

METHENAMINE, for *children*, 2-6 years, mandelate: 50-75 mg/kg/d in 3-4 doses or 0.25 g/30 lb qid. For *children* 6-12 years, hippurate: 0.5-1 g bid; mandelate: 50-75 mg/kg/d in 3-4 doses or 0.5 g qid. For *children* over 12 years and *adults*, hippurate, 0.5-1 g bid; mandelate: 1 g qid after meals and at bedtime.

MOXIFLOXACIN, for *adults*, 400 mg every 24 hours.

NITROFURANTOIN, for *children* over 1 month, 5-7 mg/kg/d in divided doses every 6 hours; maximum dose is 400 mg/d; for UTI prophylaxis (chronic), 1-2 mg/kg/d in divided doses every 12-24 hours; maximum dose 100 mg/d. For *adults*, 50-100 mg every 6 hours; macrocrystal/monohydrate: 100 mg bid; for UTI prophylaxis, 50-100 mg nocte.

NORFLOXACIN, for *adults*, 400 mg every 12 hours up to a maximum of 800 mg/d.

OFLOXACIN, for *adults*, 200-400 mg every 12 hours.

SULFACETAMIDE, for *children* 12 years and older and *adults*, for acne, topical: apply thin film to affected area bid; for seborrheic dermatitis, cleansing gel or wash: wash affected areas bid for 8-10 days; shampoo: wash hair at least twice weekly; for secondary cutaneous bacterial infections, cleansing gel or wash: apply to affected areas daily for 8-10 days.

SULFADIAZINE, for *infants* 1-12 months, for asymptomatic meningococcal carriers, 500 mg once daily for 2 days. For *children* over 2 months, for congenital toxoplasmosis, 25-50 mg/kg qid. For *children* 1-12 years, for asymptomatic meningococcal carriers, 500 mg bid for 2 days. For *adults*, for asymptomatic men-ingococcal carriers, 1 g bid for 2 days.

SULFADOXINE, used only in combination with other drugs, and therefore its individual dosing is not covered here.

SULFAMETHOXAZOLE, used only in combination with other drugs, and therefore its individual dosing is not covered here.

SULFISOXAZOLE, used only in combination with other drugs, and therefore its individual dosing is not covered here.

TRIMETHOPRIM, for *children*, 4 mg/kg/d in divided doses every 12 hours. For *adults*, 100 mg every 12 hours or 200 mg every 24 hours for 10 days; longer treatment periods may be necessary for prostatitis (*i.e.*, 4-16 weeks); in the treatment of *Pneumocystis carinii*, dose may be as high as 15-20 mg/kg/d in 3-4 divided doses.

ADVERSE EFFECTS

The most common adverse effects of fluoroquinolones are gastrointestinal and include diarrhea, nausea and vomiting. They may also

	Gram (+) Cocci	Gram (−) Cocci	Gram (+) bacilli	Gram (−) rods	Anaerobics	Spirochetes	Mycoplasma	Chlamydia	Other
FLUOROQUINOLONES: Second Generation:		Neisseria gonorrhoeae	Bacillus anthracis (Anthrax)	Enterobacteriaceae species Escherichia coli Pseudomonas aerugunosa Klebsiella pneumoniae Proteus mirabilis Serratia marcescens Shigella Hemophilius influenzae Legionella pneumophilia (Legionnaires' Disease)			Mycoplasma pneumonia	Chlamydia pneumonia	Mycobacterium tuberculosis
Third Generation:	Strep. pneumoniae	Neisseria gonorrhoeae		Escherichia coli Pseudomonas aerugunosa	Bacteroides fragilis			Chlamydia species	
SULFONAMIDES:	Strep. pneumoniae		Nocardia asteroide	Hemophilius influenzae Escherichia coli UTIs Shigella					Toxoplasma gondii Pneumocystis carinii
Co-trimoxazole (Combination of trimethoprim & sulfamethoxazole)			Listeria monocytogenes	Hemophilius influenzae Legionella pneumophilia (Legionnaires' Disease) Escherichia coli Proteus mirabilis Salmonella typhi Shigella					Pneumocystis carinii
URINARY TRACT ANTISEPTICS:	Staph. saprophyticus			Escherichia coli Klebsiella pneumoniae					

Figure 10.6: Antibiotic spectra.

cause headache, dizziness, light-headedness, and **phototoxicity**. The use of fluoroquinolones should be avoided in pregnant or nursing mothers and in children under 18 because they may cause articular cartilage erosion. There have been infrequent reports of ruptured tendons in adults.

Sulfonamides have many adverse effects. Nephrotoxicity due to **crystalluria** can occur especially when adequate amounts of liquid are not consumed at the same time as the medication. Sulfisoxazole and sulfamethoxazole are less likely to cause this as they are more soluble at urinary pH. Hypersensitivity reactions are fairly common and can be as benign as a rash or as life threatening as **angioedema** or Stevens-Johnson syndrome. Serious blood reactions may occur including **granulocytopenia**; **thrombocytopenia**; or, in patients with glucose 6-phosphate dehydrogenase deficiency, **hemolytic anemia**.

Co-trimoxazole commonly causes skin rashes, which may be severe in the elderly. Other adverse effects include nausea and vomiting, **glossitis**, and stomachache. Serious blood disorders, such as **megaloblastic anemia**, **leukopenia**, or thrombocytopenia may occur but can be treated by coadministration of folinic acid, which protects the patient but does not enter the bacteria. Because of the presence of sulfamethoxazole, hemolytic anemia may occur in patients with glucose 6-phosphate dehydrogenase deficiency.

The major adverse effects of methenamine are GI disturbances. At high doses, it may cause **albuminuria**, **hematuria**, and rashes. It is contraindicated in patients with renal insufficiency.

Nitrofurantoin may cause GI distress, acute pneumonitis, or neurologic problems. Its adverse effects limit the clinical usefulness of this agent.

Phototoxic: A substance that causes a rapidly developing, nonimmune reaction of skin exposed to light

Crystalluria: The presence of crystals in the urine

Angioedema: Large circumscribed area of subcutaneous edema of sudden onset frequently caused by an allergic reaction

Granulocytopenia: An abnormal blood condition where there is a decrease in the number of granulocytes, white blood cells with granules in their cytoplasm

Thrombocytopenia: A decreased number of platelets in the blood

Hemolytic anemia: An anemia, or loss of hemoglobin, characterized by red blood cell destruction

Glossitis: Inflammation of the tongue

Megaloblastic anemia: A blood disorder characterized by the production and proliferation of immature, large, and dysfunctional red blood cells, usually associated with pernicious anemia and folic acid deficiency

Leukopenia: A decreased number of white blood cells in the blood; defined as fewer than 5,000 cells per cubic millimeter

Albuminuria: Abnormal presence of albumin and possibly other proteins in the urine

Hematuria: Abnormal presence of blood in the urine

◼ RED FLAGS

Moxifloxacin may prolong the QT interval and should not be used in patients who are prone to arrhythmias or who are taking medication for arrhythmias.

Sulfonamides may cause life-threatening hypersensitivity reactions such as angioedema or Stevens-Johnson syndrome. Serious blood reactions may occur including granulocytopenia; thrombocytopenia; or, in patients with glucose 6-phosphate dehydrogenase deficiency, hemolytic anemia. Infants under two months old and late-term pregnant women should not take these drugs.

Co-trimoxazole may cause serious blood disorders, such as megaloblastic anemia, leukopenia, or thrombocytopenia.

◼ INTERACTIONS

DRUG

The ingestion of fluoroquinolones with sucralfate; antacids with aluminum or magnesium; or supplements containing zinc, iron, or calcium may interfere with absorption. Cimetidine interferes with the elimination of fluoroquinolones. Third- and fourth-generation fluoroquinolones may raise serum levels of warfarin, caffeine, and cyclosporine.

Ciprofloxacin and ofloxacin interfere with the metabolism of theophylline, may increase serum levels, and may cause seizures.

Due to displacement from protein-binding sites, the following drugs may have raised serum levels when combined with sulfonamides: tolbutamide, warfarin, bishydroxycoumarin, and methotrexate. Sulfa drugs should not be mixed with methenamine.

Co-trimoxazole may cause an increase in prothrombin times in patients taking warfarin. It may reduce the metabolism of phenytoin and hence increase its half-life. Methotrexate serum levels may increase due to displacement from albumin.

HERB

ANTIBIOTICS

- *Ci Wu Jia* (Acanthopanax root) (D)–was shown to increase the effectiveness of antibiotics, possibly by increasing T-lymphocyte activity (Brinker, 1995) Level 5 evidence.

CIPROFLOXACIN

- *Di Yu* (Sanguisorba, burnet root) (D)–has been shown in rats to reduce absorption and disposition of ciprofloxacin. The authors concluded that appropriate time should pass between administration of ciprofloxacin and *Di Yu* (Zhu & Wong & Li, 1999a) Level 5 evidence.
- *Pu Gong Ying* (Dandelion) (D)–reduced peak plasma concentration and slowed elimination of ciprofloxacin but did not change area under the curve in a study of rats (Zhu, Wong & Li, 1999b) Level 5 evidence.
- *Xiao Hui Xiang* (Fennel seed) (D)–has been shown in rats to alter absorption and disposition of ciprofloxacin (Chinese language study cited in Chen & Chen, 2004) Level 5 evidence.
- *Yu Jin* (Turmeric) (D)–A rabbit study showed significant decrease in elimination of norfloxacin when combined with *Yu Jin* (Pavithra, Prakash & Jayakumar, 2009). Level 5 evidence.

SULFADIAZINE

- *Ban Lan Gen, Da Qing Ye* (Isatis root and leaves, indigo woad root and leaves) (D)–those allergic to sulfonylureas and sulfonamides may also be allergic to *Ban Lan Gen*, expert opinion (Chen & Chen, 2004) Level 5 evidence.
- *Hei Hu Jiao* (Indeterminate)–may cause increase in blood levels of rifampin, sulphadiazine, tetracycline, and pentobarbital (unobtainable article as cited in Brinker, 2001) Indeterminate level of evidence.
- *Qing Dai* (Indigo) (D)–those allergic to sulfonylureas and sulfonamides may also be allergic to *Qing Dai*, expert opinion (Chen & Chen, 2004) Level 5 evidence.

SULFAMETHOXAZOLE, SULFISOXAZOLE, AND SULFONAMIDE ANTIBIOTICS

- *Ban Lan Gen* (Isatis root, indigo woad root); *Da Qing Ye* (Isatis leaves, indigo woad leaves) (D)–those allergic to sulfonylureas and sulfonamides may also be allergic to *Ban Lan Gen*, expert opinion (Chen & Chen, 2004) Level 5 evidence.
- *Qing Dai* (Indigo) (D)–those allergic to sulfonylureas and sulfonamides may also be allergic to *Qing Dai*, expert opinion (Chen & Chen, 2004) Level 5 evidence.

INTERACTION ISSUES

A:

D:

M: Ciprofloxacin is a strong inhibitor of CYP1A2; norfloxacin is a strong inhibitor of CYP1A2 and a moderate inhibitor of 3A4; sulfadiazine is a major substrate and strong inhibitor of CYP2C9; trimethoprim is a major substrate of CYP2C9 and 3A4 and a moderate inhibitor of both 2C8 and 2C9.

E:

Pgp: Ciprofloxacin is a substrate of Pgp.

SECTION 4: ANTIMYCOBACTERIAL DRUGS

AMINOSALICYLIC ACID (a mee noe sal i SIL ik AS id) PR=C *(Paser®)*

BEDAQUILINE (bed AK wi lene) PR=C *(Sirturo®)*

CAPREOMYCIN (kap ree oh MYE sin) PR=C *(Capastat® Sulfate)*

CYCLOSERINE *(See Section 1 above)*

DAPSONE (DAP sone) PR=C

ETHAMBUTOL (e THAM byoo tole) PR=C *(Myambutol®)*

ETHIONAMIDE (e thye on AM ide) PR=C *(Trecator®)*

ISONIAZID (eye soe NYE a zid) PR=C *(IsonaRif™,[11] Rifamate®,[11] Rifater®)*

PYRAZINAMIDE (peer a ZIN a mide) PR=C *(Rifater®[10])*

RIFABUTIN (rif a BYOO tin) PR=B *(Mycobutin®)*

RIFAMPIN (RIF am pin) PR=C *(IsonaRif™, Rifadin®, Rifamate®,[11] Rifater®[10])*

RIFAPENTINE (RIF a pen tene) PR=C *(Priftin®)*

FUNCTION

Mycobacteria are difficult to treat, requiring doses of multiple drugs over many months if not years. They are rod-shaped bacteria that are difficult to Gram stain, but once stained they cannot be destained by acidic solvents and are therefore called acid-fast. The number one infectious cause of death in the world is from tuberculosis (TB).

Mycobacterium tuberculosis causes serious infections of the genitourinary tract, skeleton, and meninges in addition to the well-known lung infection. It is thought to infect one-third of the world's population, with 30 million cases of active disease, 8 million new cases a year, and 2 million deaths annually. Resistant strains are common.

There are many first-line drugs used to treat TB: ethambutol, isoniazid, pyraziamide, and rifampin. Second-line drugs could be less effective, more toxic, or have not been studied as extensively as first-line drugs. The following second-line drugs are used when first-line drugs are not tolerated or in the case of resistant strains: aminosalicylic acid, or aspirin (see Chapter 6, Section 9), is used rarely; capreomycin, cycloserine, ethionamide, fluoroquinolones (see previous section), macrolides (see Section 2 above), rifabutin, and rifapentine more commonly.

Another mycobacterial disease is leprosy, caused by mycobacterium leprae. This is a disease of the skin, peripheral nerves, and mucous membranes. While rare in the United States, over 1 million individuals are infected worldwide, with about 70% in India. Dapsone and rifampin are used to treat it. Clofazimine is also recommended by the World Health Organization to treat leprosy; it is discontinued in the U.S., however, and therefore not covered in this book.

Treatment of mycobacteria almost always consists of multiple-drug therapy. This is because of the difficulty in treating the infection as well as how quickly resistance develops with single-agent therapy.

Aminosalicylic acid is used to treat TB as an adjunctive agent in combination with other drugs. It is also used to treat Crohn's disease.

MECHANISM OF ACTION

Aminosalicylic acid and dapsone are structurally similar to the sulfonamides and act in a similar way as a PABA antagonist, which inhibits folate synthesis. It is bacteriostatic.

Ethambutol inhibits arabinosyl transferase, an enzyme crucial for producing the mycobacterial cell wall. It is bacteriostatic.

Ethionamide is a structural analog of isoniazid, but is not thought to act in the same way. It is thought to inhibit protein synthesis.

Isoniazid acts by preventing the synthesis of mycolic acid, a component found in mycobacterial cell walls. It can be both bacteriostatic, for bacilli in the stationary phase, and bactericidal, in rapidly dividing organisms.

The mechanism of action of pyrazinamide is not known. It is bactericidal to actively dividing organisms.

Rifampin, rifabutin, and rifapentine act by inhibiting RNA synthesis by inhibiting bacterial DNA-dependent RNA polymerase. These drugs are bactericidal.

	Gram (+) Cocci	Gram (–) Cocci	Gram (+) bacilli	Gram (–) rods	Anaerobics	Spirochetes	Mycoplasma	Chlamydia	Other
Amniosalicylic acid Dapsone									Mycobacterium tuberculosis Mycobacterium leprae (leprosy) Pneumocystis jiroveci
Ethambutol									Mycobacterium tuberculosis Mycobacterium kansasii
Isoniazid									Mycobacterium tuberculosis Mycobacterium kansasii
Pyrazinamide									Mycobacterium tuberculosis
Rifabutin									Mycobacterium avium-intracellulare
Rifampin	Staph. epidermidis	Neisseria meningitidis		Hemophilius influenzae					Mycobacterium tuberculosis Mycobacterium kansasii
Rifapentine									Mycobacterium tuberculosis

Figure 10.7: Antibiotic spectra.

▦ DOSAGES

AMINOSALICYLIC ACID, for *children*, for tuberculosis, 200-300 mg/kg/d in 3-4 equally divided doses. For *adults*, for tuberculosis, 150 mg/kg/d in 2-3 equally divided doses.

BEDAQUILINE, for *adults*, for multidrug-resistant pulmonary tuberculosis (TB), should be used with 3 or more drugs to treat TB; weeks 1-2: 400 mg once daily; weeks 3-24: 200 mg 3 times weekly, spacing doses at least 48 hours apart.

CAPREOMYCIN, for *adults*, for tuberculosis, IM: 1 g/d up to a maximum of 20 mg/kg/d, for 60-120 days, followed by 1 g 2-3 times/wk or 15 mg/kg/d for 2-4 months, followed by 15 mg/kg up to a maximum of 1 g 2-3 times/wk.

DAPSONE, for *children*, for leprosy, 1-2 mg/kg/d, up to a maximum of 100 mg/d. For *adults*, for leprosy, 50-100 mg/d for 3-10 years; for dermatitis herpetiformis, start at 50 mg/d, increase to 300 mg/d or higher to achieve full control, and reduce dose to minimum level as soon as possible.

ETHAMBUTOL, for treatment of tuberculosis used as part of a multidrug regimen. For *children*, 15-20 mg/kg/d up to a maximum of 1 g/d. For *adults*, 15-25 mg/kg; 40-55 kg: 800 mg; 56-75 kg: 1200 mg; 76-90 kg: 1600 mg (maximum dose regardless of weight).

ETHIONAMIDE, for *children*, 15-20 mg/kg/d in 2-3 divided doses, not to exceed 1 g/d. For *adults*, 15-20 mg/kg/d; initiate dose at 250 mg/d for 1-2 days, then increase to 250 mg bid for 1-2 days, with gradual increases to highest tolerated dose; average adult dose is 750 mg/d; maximum is 1 g/d in 3-4 divided doses.

ISONIAZID, for *infants* and *children*, for treatment of latent TB infection (LTBI), 10-20 mg/kg/d in 1-2 divided doses up to a maximum of 300 mg/d; for 20-40 mg/kg, up to a maximum of 900 mg/dose twice weekly for 9 months; for treatment of active TB infection, 10-15 mg/kg/d in 1-2 divided doses up to a maximum of 300 mg/d. For *adults*, for treatment of LTBI, 300 mg/d or 900 mg twice weekly for 6-9 months in patients who do not have HIV infection; 9 months is optimal, 6 months may be considered to reduce costs of therapy, and 9 months in patients who have HIV infection; extend to 12 months of therapy if interruptions in treatment occur; for treatment of active TB infection (drug susceptible), 5 mg/kg/d given daily (usual dose is 300 mg/d); 10 mg/ kg/d in 1-2 divided doses in patients with disseminated disease.

PYRAZINAMIDE, used as part of a multidrug regimen, treatment regimens consist of an initial 2-month phase followed by a continuation phase of 4 or 7 additional months; frequency of dosing may differ depending on phase of therapy. For *children*, 15-30 mg/kg/d up to a maximum of 2 g/d. For *adults* (dosing is based on lean body weight), 15-30 mg/kg/d; 40-55 kg: 1000 mg; 56-75 kg: 1500 mg; 76-90 kg: 2000 mg (maximum dose regardless of weight).

RIFABUTIN, for *children* over 1 year, for prophylaxis, 5 mg/kg/d; higher dosages have been used in limited trials; for treatment (unlabeled use), initial phase (2 weeks to 2 months), 10-20 mg/kg daily up to a maximum of 300 mg; second phase, 10-20 mg/kg daily up to a maximum of 300 mg or twice weekly. For *adults*, for prophylaxis, 300 mg once daily (alone or in combination with azithromycin); for treatment (unlabeled use), initial phase, 5 mg/kg daily up to a maximum of 300 mg; second phase, 5 mg/kg daily or twice weekly.

RIFAMPIN, for *infants* under 1 month, for meningococcal meningitis prophylaxis, 10 mg/kg/d in divided doses every 12 hours for 2 days. For *infants* 1 month or over and *children*, for meningococcal meningitis prophylaxis, 20 mg/kg/d in divided doses every 12 hours for 2 days up to a maximum of 600 mg/dose. For *infants* and *children* under 12, for tuberculosis therapy (drug susceptible), 10-20 mg/kg/d usually as a single dose; maximum dose is 600 mg/d; for latent tuberculosis infection (LTBI), 10-20 mg/kg/d up to a maximum of 600 mg/d for 6 month. For *adults*, for tuberculosis therapy (drug susceptible), 10 mg/kg/d up to a maximum of 600 mg/d; for LTBI, 10 mg/kg/d up to a maximum of 600 mg/d for 4 months.

RIFAPENTINE, should not be used alone; initial phase should include a 3-4-drug regimen. For *adults*, intensive phase (initial 2 months) of short-term therapy, 600 mg (four 150 mg tablets) given twice weekly (with an interval of not less than 72 hours between doses); following the intensive phase, treatment should continue with 600 mg once weekly for 4 months in combination with INH or appropriate agent for susceptible organisms.

ADVERSE EFFECTS

Aminosalicylic acid may cause **vasculitis, pericarditis**, hepatitis, encephalopathy, GI disturbances, and hemotoxicity.

Dapsone may cause **methemoglobinemia**, peripheral neuropathy, and the possibility of developing **erythema nodosum leprosum.** Hemolysis may occur in patients with glucose 6-phosphate dehydrogenase deficiency.

Ethambutol may cause optic **neuritis** with such symptoms as decreased visual acuity and the inability to discriminate between red and green. Because of this, visual acuity should be tested regularly. It may also exacerbate an attack of gout.

Ethionamide may cause GI upset, liver issues, peripheral neuropathies, and optic neuritis. Coadministration of pyridoxine (vitamin B6) may decrease the neurological effects.

Isoniazid has a relatively low incidence of adverse effects that, except for hypersensitivity reactions, are dose and duration related. The most common adverse effect is peripheral neuritis manifesting as **paresthesias**. These can be reversed with co-administration of pyridoxine (vitamin B6). Isoniazid can cause pyridoxine deficiency in the infants of breast-feeding mothers, who

should always supplement this vitamin. Other adverse effects include convulsions in patients prone to seizures, mental abnormalities, and optic neuritis.

The adverse effects of rifampin are generally minor and include nausea and vomiting, fever, and a rash. Jaundice may occur, and caution should be taken in patients with chronic liver disease, alcoholics, and the elderly.

Rifabutin commonly causes a rash, discoloration of the urine, **neutropenia**, and **leukopenia**. GI complaints, hepatic enzyme disturbances, anemia, and thrombocytopenia may also occur. Rifapentine has similar adverse effects.

Pyrazinamide may rarely cause an attack of gout. Other adverse effects include nausea, hepatitis, **hyperuricemia**, rash, and joint pain.

RED FLAGS

Isoniazid has, rarely, caused fatal hepatitis. The incidence increases with the age of the patient, consumption of alcohol or use of rifampin.

Between 1 and 5 percent of patients taking isoniazid, rifampin, and pyrazinamide may have liver dysfunction.

INTERACTIONS

DRUG

Isoniazid can increase the serum levels of phenytoin by inhibiting cytochrome P450, which metabolizes phenytoin.

Rifampin, rifabutin, and rifapentine are strong inducers of CYP3A4 and other subsets of CYP and can increase the metabolism of clofibrate, digitoxin, ketoconazole, oral contraceptive pills, corticosteroids, quinidine, propranolol, sulfonylureas, and warfarin. Rifabutin is often used instead of rifampin in HIV patients taking protease inhibitors or non-nucleoside reverse transcriptase inhibitors as rifabutin does not increase the metabolism of these agents.

HERB

ANTIBIOTICS

- *Ci Wu Jia* (Acanthopanax root) (D)–was shown to increase the effectiveness of antibi-

---

Vasculitis: Inflammation of the blood vessels

Pericarditis: Inflammation and/or infection of the pericardium

Methemoglobinemia: The presence in the blood of methemoglobin, a form of hemoglobin that cannot bind and transport oxygen

Erythema nodosum leprosum: A systemic inflammatory complication of leprosy that manifests as painful papules or nodules that may pustulate and ulcer and may produce, among many manifestations, fever and arthritis

Neuritis: Inflammation of a nerve

Paresthesia: Numbness and tingling

Neutropenia: A reduction in the number of neutrophils, one type of immune cell, in the blood

Leukopenia: A decreased number of white blood cells in the blood; defined as fewer than 5,000 cells per cubic millimeter

Hyperuricemia: A condition of increased uric acid in the blood; associated with gout

otics, possibly by increasing T-lymphocyte activity (Brinker, 1995) Level 5 evidence.

RIFAMPIN

• *Hei Hu Jiao* (Indeterminate)–may cause increase in blood levels of rifampicin, sulphadiazine, tetracycline, and pentobarbital (unobtainable article as cited in Brinker, 2001) Indeterminate level of evidence.

INTERACTION ISSUES

A:

D: Bedaquiline is approximately 100% protein bound; rifapentine is approximately 98% bound.

M: Bedaquiline is a major substrate of CUP3A4; dapsone is a major substrate of CYP2C9 and 3A4; isoniazid is a major substrate, a moderate inhibitor, and a weak or moderate inducer of CYP2E1; a moderate inhibitor of 2A6 and 2D6; and a strong inhibitor of 2C19; rifabutin is a major substrate and strong inducer of CYP3A4; rifampin is a strong inducer of CYP1A2, 2B6, 2C19, 2C8, 2C9, and 3A4; rifapentine is a strong inducer of CYP2C8, 2C9, and 3A4.

E:

Pgp: Rifampin is a substrate and inducer of Pgp.

SECTION 5: ANTIFUNGAL DRUGS

BUTENAFINE (byoo TEN a fene) PR=C *(Lotrimin® UltraTM [O], Mentax®)*

CICLOPIROX (sye KLOE PERE oks) PR=C *(Ciclodan, Ciclodan Cream, Ciclodan Solution, Ciclopirox Treatment, CNL8 Nail, Loprox, Pedipirox-4 Nail, Penlac)*

FLUCYTOSINE (floo SYE toe sene) PR=C *(Ancobon®)*

GENTIAN VIOLET (JEN shun VYE oh let) PR=C

GRISEOFULVIN (gri see oh FUL vin) PR=X *(Grifulvin® V, Gris-PEG®)*

NAFTIFINE (NAF ti fene) PR=B *(Naftin)*

NYSTATIN (nye STAT in) PR=C *(Bio-Statin®, Nyamyc™, Nystop®, Pedi-Dri®, Pediaderm AF Complete)*

TERBINAFINE (TER bin a fene) PR=B *(Lamisil®, Lamisil Advanced [O], Lamisil AT® [O], Lamisil AT Jock Itch [O], Lamisil AT Spray [O], Lamisil Spray, Terbinex)*

TOLNAFTATE (tole NAF tate) PR=N *(Anti-Fungal [O], Antifungal [O], Athlete's Foot Spray [O], Dr G's Clear Nail [O], Fungi-Guard [O], Fungoid-D [O], Jock Itch Spray [O], Lamisil AF Defense [O], Medi-First Anti-Fungal [O], Mycocide Clinical NS [O], Podactin [O], Tinactin [O], Tinactin Deodorant [O], Tinactin Jock Itch [O], Tinamar [O], Tinaspore [O], Tolnaftate Antifungal [O])*

UNDECYLENIC ACID and DERIVATIVES (un de sil EN ik AS id) PR=N *(Fungi-Nail® [O])*

AZOLES:

BUTOCONAZOLE (byoo toe KON a zole) PR=C *(Gynazole-1®)*

CLOTRIMAZOLE (kloe TRIM a zole) PR=C *(Clotrimazole 3 Day [O], Clotrimazole Anti-Fungal [O], Desenex [O], Gyne-Lotrimin [O], Gyne-Lotrimin 3 [O], Lotrimin AF [O], Lotrimin AF For Her [O], Lotrisone®12)*

ECONAZOLE (e KONE a zole) PR=C

FLUCONAZOLE (floo KOE na zole) PR=D *(Diflucan®)*

ITRACONAZOLE (i tra KOE na zole) PR=C *(Onmel, (Onmel, Sporanox®, Sporanox® Pulsepa)*

KETOCONAZOLE (kee toe KOE na zole) PR=C *(Extina, Ketodan, Nizoral®, Nizoral® A-D [O], Xolegel®)*

MICONAZOLE (mi KON a zole) PR=C *(Aloe Vesta Antifungal [O], Antifungal [O], Azolen Tincture [O], Baza Antifungal [O], Carrington Antifungal [O], Critic-Aid Clear AF [O], Cruex Prescription Strength [O], DermaFungal [O], Desenex [O], Desenex Jock Itch [O], Desenex Spray [O], Fungoid Tincture [O], Lotrimin AF [O], Lotrimin AF Deodorant Powder [O], Lotrimin AF Jock Itch Powder [O], Lotrimin AF Powder [O], Micaderm [O], Micatin [O],*

...continued on the following page

SECTION 5: ANTIFUNGAL DRUGS cont.

Miconazole 3; Miconazole 3 Combo Pack [O], Miconazole 7 [O], Micro Guard [O], Miranel AF [O], Mitrazol [O], Oravig, Podactin [O], Remedy Antifungal [O], Secura Antifungal [O], Secura Antifungal Extra Thick [O], Soothe & Cool INZO Antifungal [O], Triple Paste AF [O], Vagistat-3 [O], Vusion®,[31] Zeasorb-AF [O])

OXICONAZOLE (oks i KON a zole) PR=B
(Oxistat®)

POSACONAZOLE (poe sa KON a zole) PR=C
(Noxafil®)

SERTACONAZOLE (ser ta KON a zole) PR=C
(Ertaczo)

SULCONAZOLE (sul KON a zole) PR=C
(Exelderm®)

TERCONAZOLE (ter KONE a zole) PR=C
(Terazol® 3, Terazol® 7, Zazole)

TIOCONAZOLE (tye oh KONE a zole) PR=C
(Monistat 1 [O], Vagistat-1 [O])

VORICONAZOLE (vor i KOE na zole) PR=D
(VFEND®)

Diseases caused by fungi are called mycoses. Fungi are different from bacteria. They are eukaryotic, meaning they have a "real" nucleus as opposed to the prokaryotic bacteria. They have rigid cell walls made of chitin as opposed to the peptidoglycan cell walls of bacteria. Fungal membranes contain ergosterol rather than cholesterol in mammalian cell membranes. Each of these characteristics is a useful target for antifungal agents. Antibiotics generally do a poor job of treating mycoses, and antifungal drugs are pretty useless in treating bacterial infections.

There are many common fungal infections including candida. They are often named for the location of the infection, for example *tinea pedis* for a fungal infection of the foot also known as athlete's foot, *tinea caput* for a head infection, *tinea cruris* for a groin infection (commonly called "jock itch"), and so on. In the last several decades, fungal infections have become more common for a number of reasons including the increase of immunosuppressive therapy following organ transplants, chemotherapy for malignancies and other tumors, and the advent of HIV and AIDS. Candidemia has become the fourth most common cause of septicemia, a life-threatening condition where there is an infection of the blood.

In that same time frame, however, there have been more numerous and more effective treatment agents. This section will discuss many of these agents.

■ FUNCTION

Fluconazole is used prophylactically to prevent fungal infections in bone marrow transplant patients. Ketoconazole is also used to treat prostate cancer.

Griseofulvin has been largely replaced by terbinafine for many reasons including shorter duration of application, more drug interactions, and that it is fungistatic rather than fungicidal.

Nystatin is not taken systemically due to its toxicity. It is used topically and orally only as a "swish and spit" agent to treat oral candidiasis, in which case it is not absorbed from the GI tract in significant amounts.

Posaconazole is used in the prophylaxis of aspergillus and candida infections in the severely immunocompromised. It also treats oropharyngeal candidiasis and can be used when itraconazole and/or fluconazole have not been successful.

■ MECHANISM OF ACTION

The azole antifungal agents, which include clotrimazole, fluconazole, itraconazole, ketoconazole, posaconazole, and voriconazole, have the same mechanism of action. They inhibit C-14 α-demethylase, a cytochrome P450 enzyme that is involved with transforming lanosterol to ergosterol, a vital component of the fungal cell membrane. This is summarized in Figure 10.8. Ketoconazole, the first agent in the azole group, is not as specific as the other agents. It inhibits

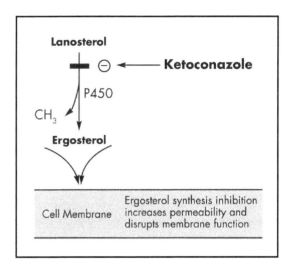

Figure 10.8: Azoles block the enzyme C-14 α-demethylase preventing ergosterol, a integral part of fungi's cell wall, from being produced.

human steroid synthesis and decreases levels of testosterone and cortisol. This is the mechanism of its usefulness for treating prostate cancer.

Flucytosine (5-FC) enters the fungal cell through a cytosine-specific permease not found in mammalian cells. From there it is metabolized to 5-flurodeoxyuridine 5-monophosphate (5-FdUMP) which inhibits the enzyme thymidine synthetase, necessary to create thymidylic acid, which is essential for DNA. 5-FdUMP is further metabolized into a substance that is incorporated into fungal RNA and disrupts nucleic acid and protein synthesis. This is summarized in Figure 10.9.

Griseofulvin acts by preventing **mitosis** by disrupting the mitotic spindle.

Terbinafine works to inhibit the synthesis of ergosterol by inhibiting the enzyme squalene epoxidase. This enzyme converts squalene to ergosterol. It is fungicidal.

ANTIMICROBIAL SPECTRA

CLOTRIMAZOLE is used in treating candidiases, dermatophytoses, and superficial mycoses.

FLUCONAZOLE is the drug of choice for treating *Cryptococcus neoformans* and is useful in treating candidemia and coccidioido-mycosis.

FLUCYTOSINE is fungistatic and is useful in treating chromoblastomycosis with itraconazole

and candidiasis and cryptococcosis with amphotericin B, an injectable antifungal agent.

ITRACONAZOLE is the drug of first choice for blastomycosis, aspergillosis, sporotrichosis, paracoccidiodomycosis, and histoplasmosis.

KETOCONAZOLE is not as commonly used as itraconazole because of the latter's broader spectrum and fewer side effects. Ketoconazole is still used however, and is useful in treating histoplasma, blastomyces, candida, and coccidioides.

TERBINAFINE is useful in treating dermatophytes, *Candida albicans,* and **onychomyces**.

VORICONAZOLE treats aspergillosis, cedosporium apiospermum, and fusarium species.

DOSAGES

The dosages below are the common dosages for each agent. Specific uses may use different doses and the doses below should not be considered definitive.

BUTENAFINE, for *children* 12 years and older and *adults,* for tinea corporis or cruris, Lotrimin® Ultra™: apply once daily for 2 weeks to affected area and surrounding skin; for tinea

Mitosis: A type of cell division that results in two identical daughter cells

Onychomycosis: A fungal infection of a nail; plural: onychomycoses

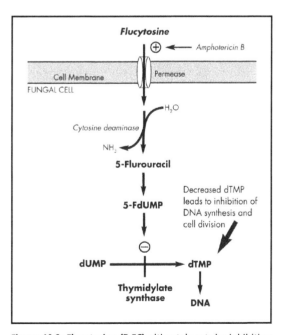

Figure 10.9: Flucytosine (5-FC) ultimately acts by inhibiting thymidylate synthase, which catalyzes the production of a vital substance, dTMP, necessary for proper DNA synthesis.

versi-color, Mentax®: apply once daily for 2 weeks to affected area and surrounding skin; for tinea pedis, Lotrimin® Ultra™: apply to affected skin between and around the toes bid for 1 week or once daily for 4 weeks.

BUTOCONAZOLE, for *adults*, for vulvovaginal candidiasis, intravaginal: insert 1 applicatorful (~5 g) intravaginally as a single dose; treatment may need to be extended for up to 6 days in pregnant women (use in pregnancy during 2nd or 3rd trimester only).

CICLOPIROX, for *children* 10 years and older (for cream and suspension) or 16 years and older (for gel) and adults, for tinea pedis or corporis, topical cream or suspension: apply bid, gently massage into affected areas; gel: apply bid, gently massage into affected areas and surrounding skin; for tinea cruris or versicolor or cutaneous candidiasis, topical cream or suspension, apply bid, gently massage into affected areas; for onychomycosis of the fingernails and toenails, topical lacquer: apply to adjacent skin and affected nails daily; remove with alcohol every 7 days; for seborrheic dermatitis of the scalp, topical gel, apply bid, gently massage into affected areas and surrounding skin; shampoo: apply ~5 mL to wet hair; lather, and leave in place approximately 3 minutes; rinse; may use up to 10 mL for longer hair; repeat twice weekly for 4 weeks; allow a minimum of 3 days between applications.

CLOTRIMAZOLE, for *children* over 3 years and *adults*, for prophylaxis, 10 mg troche dissolved tid for the duration of chemotherapy or until steroids are reduced to maintenance levels; for treatment, 10 mg **troche** dissolved slowly 5 times/d for 14 consecutive days.

ECONAZOLE, for *children* and *adults*, for tinea pedis, cover affected areas once daily for 1 month; for tinea cruris, corporis, or versicolor, cover affected areas once daily for 2 weeks; for cutaneous candidiasis, apply bid for 2 weeks.

FLUCONAZOLE, for *neonates* in the first 2 weeks of life, especially *premature neonates*, same dose as older children every 72 hours; for *children*, loading dose is 6-12 mg/kg; maintenance is 3-12 mg/kg/d; duration and dosage depends on severity of infection. For *adults*, 200-400 mg/d; duration and dosage depends on severity of infection.

FLUCYTOSINE, for *children* and *adults*, 50-150 mg/kg/d in divided doses every 6 hours.

GENTIAN VIOLET, for *children* and *adults*, for superficial skin or mucocutaneous infection, topical: apply to affected area 1-2 times daily.

GRISEOFULVIN, for *children* over 2 years, microsize: 10-20 mg/kg/d in single or 2 divided doses; for the treatment of tinea capitis, higher dosages (20-25 mg/kg/d for 8-12 weeks) have been recommended by some authors; ultramicrosize: 5-10 mg/kg/d in single or 2 divided doses for the treatment of tinea capitis, higher dosages (15 mg/kg/d for 8-12 weeks) have been recommended by some authors. For *adults*, microsize: 500-1000 mg/d in single or divided doses; ultramicrosize: 330-375 mg/d in single or divided doses doses up to 750 mg/d have been used for infections more difficult to eradicate such as tinea unguium.

ITRACONAZOLE, for *children*, efficacy and safety have not been established, a small number of patients 3-16 years of age have been treated with 100 mg/d for systemic fungal infections with no serious adverse effects reported. For *adults*, 100-400 mg/d, doses over 200 mg/d are given in 2 divided doses, length of therapy varies from 1 day to over 6 months depending on the condition and mycological response.

KETOCONAZOLE, for *children* of 2 or more years, 3.3-6.6 mg/kg/d as a single dose for 1-2 weeks for candidiasis, for at least 4 weeks in recalcitrant dermatophyte infections, and for up to 6 months for other systemic mycoses. For *adults*, 200-400 mg/d as a single daily dose for durations as stated above.

MICONAZOLE, for *adults*, for oropharyngeal candidiasis, buccal tablet: 50 mg applied to the upper gum region once daily for 14 days.

NAFTIFINE, for *adults*, for tinea corporis, cruris, or pedis, topical cream: apply once daily to

---

Troche: A small tablet containing a drug and a flavored base that dissolves in the mouth releasing the drug

affected area and surrounding skin for up to 2 weeks (1%) or up to 4 weeks (2%); gel: apply bid to affected area and surrounding skin for up to 4 weeks.

NYSTATIN, for *premature infants*, for oral candidiasis (swish and swallow), 100,000 units qid. For *infants*, for oral candidiasis (swish and swallow), 200,000 units qid or 100,000 units to each side of mouth qid. For *children* and *adults*, for oral candidiasis (swish and swallow), 400,000-600,000 units qid. For *children* and *adults*, when used as a powder for compounding, 1/8 teaspoon (500,000 units) to equal approximately 1/2 cup water qid.

OXICONAZOLE, for *children* 12 and older and adults, for tinea corporis or cruris, topical cream or lotion: apply to affected areas 1-2 times daily for 2 weeks; for tinea pedis, topical cream or lotion: apply to affected areas 1-2 times daily for 1 month; for tinea versicolor, topical cream: apply to affected areas once daily for 2 weeks.

POSACONAZOLE, for *children* 13 or older and *adults*, for prophylaxis of aspergillus and candida species, 200 mg tid; for oropharyngeal candidiasis, initiate at 100 mg bid for 1 day; maintain at 100 mg once daily for 13 days; for treating refractory oropharyngeal candidiasis, 400 mg bid; for treating refractory invasive fungal infections, 800 mg/d in divided doses.

SERTACONAZOLE, for *children* 12 and older and *adults*, for tinea pedis, topical: apply between toes and to surrounding healthy skin bid for 4 weeks.

SULCONAZOLE, for *adults*, for tinea infection, topical: apply a small amount to the affected area and gently massage once or twice daily (tinea pedis apply bid) for 3 weeks (tinea cruris, corporis, or versicolor) to 4 weeks (tinea pedis).

SULFANILAMIDE, for *adults*, for vulvovaginitis due to *Candida albicans*, intravaginal: insert one applicatorful intravaginally 1-2 times daily for 30 days.

TERBINAFINE, for *children*, 10-20 kg: 62.5 mg/d; 20-40 kg: 125 mg/d; >40 kg: 250 mg/d. For *adults*, for superficial mycoses, fingernail: 250

mg/d for up to 6 weeks; toenail: 250 mg/d for 12 weeks; doses may be given in two divided doses; for systemic mycosis, 250-500 mg/d for up to 16 months.

TERCONAZOLE, for *adults*, for vulvovaginal candidiasis, intravaginal: Terazol® 3 (0.8%) vaginal cream: insert 1 applicatorful intravaginally nocte for 3 consecutive days; Terazol® 3 vaginal suppository: insert 1 suppository intravaginally nocte for 3 consecutive days; Terazol® 7 (0.4%) vaginal cream: 1 applicatorful intravaginally nocte 7 consecutive days.

TIOCONAZOLE, for *adults*, for vulvovaginal candidiasis, vaginal: insert 1 applicatorful in vagina nocte as a single dose.

TOLNAFTATE, for *children* 2 years and older and *adults*, for tinea infection, topical: spray aerosol or apply 1-3 drops of solution or a small amount of cream or powder and rub into the affected areas bid.

UNDECYLENIC ACID AND DERIVATIVES, for *children* 2 years and older and adults, for tinea and superficial dermatophyte infections, topical: apply bid to affected area for 4 weeks.

VORICONAZOLE, for *children* under 12, dosage not established. For *children* 12 years or over and *adults*, 100-300 mg every 12 hours.

ADVERSE EFFECTS

Azoles should not be given to pregnant women.

Fluconazole may cause nausea and vomiting, rashes, and, rarely, hepatitis.

Flucytosine commonly causes GI disturbances. It may cause reversible **neutropenia**, **thrombocytopenia**, and occasional bone marrow depression and should be used with caution in patients undergoing radiation therapy or chemotherapy to depress bone marrow. Reversible liver dysfunction and liver enzyme derangement may occur. Severe **enterocolitis** may occur.

Griseofulvin may eaxcerabate intermittent **porphyria**. It should not be taken with alcohol as it will prolong its effects.

Neutropenia: A reduction in the number of neutrophils, one type of immune cell, in the blood

Thrombocytopenia: A decreased number of platelets in the blood

Enterocolitis: An inflammatory condition of both the small and large intestines

Porphyria: A group of inherited disorders characterized by accumulation of porphyrins, intermediaries of hemoglobin production

Itraconazole may cause nausea and vomiting, **hypokalemia**, hypertension, edema, headache, and a rash, especially in immuno-compromised patients.

Hypokalemia: Too little potassium in the blood

Gynecomastia: An abnormal enlargement of one or two breasts in men

Ketoconazole has many adverse effects including dose-dependent GI disturbances, **gynecomastia**, decreased libido, impotence, and menstrual difficulties. Transient liver enzyme derangements may also occur.

Posaconazole frequently causes diarrhea and other GI disturbances. Other adverse effects include headache and hypokalemia. A rash, neutropenia, anemia, thrombocytopenia, and liver function test disturbances may also occur. QT prolongation may occur in up to 4% of users.

Terbinafine causes GI discomfort, headache, rash, taste and visual disturbances, and possibly transient liver enzyme derangement. Rarely, this agent may cause neutropenia and hepatotoxicity.

Voriconazole has similar adverse effects as other azoles including nausea and vomiting and rashes. It also causes visual disturbances after a dose of the drug.

▓ RED FLAGS

Ketoconazole-caused hepatitis rarely occurs, but use of the agent should be stopped immediately if hepatitis symptoms occur.

▓ INTERACTIONS

DRUG

The azole drugs can inhibit cytochrome P450 and cause serum increases of cyclosporine, phenytoin, tolbutamide, and warfarin. Rifampin and its analogs may shorten the duration of the effects of azoles. Rather than using these, itraconazole also inhibits the metabolism of oral anticoagulants, statins, and quinidine.

Griseofulvin can induce CYP activity and can increase the metabolism of many drugs including anticoagulants.

The absorption of ketoconazole may be inhibited by drugs that reduce stomach acidity. These include H2-receptor blockers, antacids, sucralfate, and proton-pump inhibitors. It should not be used with amphotericin B.

Posaconazole is a moderate inhibitor of CYP3A4 and may interfere with many agents: calcium channel blockers (especially felodipine, nifedipine, and verapamil), cimetidine, cyclosporine, benzodiazepines, ergot derivatives, glipizide, lovastatin and simvastatin, mirtazapine, nateglinide, nefazodone, PDE-5 inhibitors, phenytoin, rifabutin, sirolimus, tacrolimus, venlafaxine, vinblastine, and vincristine.

Serum levels of terbinafine may be affected by other drugs. Rifampin decreases blood levels, while cimetidine increases blood levels of terbinafine.

HERB

AZOLE ANTIFUNGALS, KETOCONAZOLE

• *Qing Hao* (Artemesia, sweet wormwood herb) (D)–a metabolite of *Qing Hao* may interfere with the effectiveness of verapamil specifically, calcium channel blockers in general, as well as bufuralol and azole antifungals due to activation of CYP2D6 and competitive inhibition at CYP3A4 and possibly CYP3A5 (Grace, Skanchy & Aguilar, 1999) Level 5 evidence.

VORICONAZOLE

• *Guan Ye Lian Qiao* (St. John's wort) (C) decreases blood concentrations (Izzo & Ernst 2009) Level 2b evidence.

INTERACTION ISSUES

A:

D: Ciclopirox is 94-98% protein bound; itraconazole is 99.8% protein bound; ketoconazole is 93-96% bound; posaconazole is over 98% bound; terbinafine is over 99% bound.

M: Clotrimazole is a moderate inhibitor of CYP3A4; fluconazole is a strong inhibitor of CYP2C9 and 2C19 and a moderate inhibitor of 3A4; griseofulvin is a weak or moderate inducer of CYP1A2, 2C9, and 3A4; itraconazole is a major substrate and strong inhibitor of CYP3A4; ketoconazole is a major substrate and strong inhibitor of CYP3A4 as well as a strong inhibitor of 1A2 and 2C9 and a moderate inhibitor of 2A6, 2C19, and 2D6; miconazole is a moderate inhibitor of CYP2C9, 2C19, 2D6, and 3A4; posaconazole is a strong inhibitor of CYP3A4; terbinafine is a strong inhibitor of CYP2D6 and a weak or moderate inducer of

3A4; voriconazole is a major substrate and moderate inhibitor of CYP2C9 and 2C19 and a strong inhibitor of 3A4.

E:

Pgp: Itraconazole and ketoconazole inhibit Pgp. One drug that is not included in the previous list because it is not available in the U.S. is artemesinin. This has recently been used extensively to control malaria in various parts of the world because it is inexpensive and effective. It is derived from the Chinese herb *Qing Hao*, *Artemesia annua*.

SECTION 6: ANTIPROTOZOAL DRUGS

ARTEMETHER (ar TEM e ther) PR=C
(Coartem®32)

ATOVAQUONE (a TOE va kwone) PR=C
(Malarone®,13 Mepron®)

CHLOROQUINE (KLOR oh kwin) PR=N
(Aralen®)

EFLORNITHINE (ee FLOR ni thene) PR=C
(Vaniqa®)

HYDROXYCHLOROQUINE (hye droks ee KLOR oh kwin) PR=N *(Plaquenil®)*

IODOQUINOL (eye oh doe KWIN ole) PR=N
(Alcortin® A, Dermazene®, Yodoxin®)

LUMEFANTRINE (loo me FAN trene) PR=C
(Coartem®32)

MEFLOQUINE (ME floe kwin) PR=B

METRONIDAZOLE (me troe NI da zole) PR=B
(Flagyl ER®, Flagyl ER®, Metro®)

NITAZOXANIDE (nye ta ZOX a nide) PR=B
(Alinia)

PAROMOMYCIN (par oh moe MYE sin) PR=N
(Humatin®)

PENTAMIDINE (pen TAM i dene) PR=C
(Nebupent, Pentam)

PRIMAQUINE (PRIM a kwene) PR=N

PROGUANIL (pro GWA nil) PR=C
(Malarone®13)

PYRIMETHAMINE (peer i METH a mene) PR=C
(Daraprim®)

QUINIDINE *(See Chapter 6, Class 6)*

QUININE (KWYE nine) PR=C *(Qualaquin)*

TINIDAZOLE (tye NI da zole) PR=C
(Tindamax™)

FUNCTION

Protozoa are single celled, eukaryotic animals. To be eukaryotic is to have a true nucleus as opposed to the prokaryotic bacteria. Because protozoa are closer to human than bacteria, it is harder to get an agent that specifically targets the pathogen. Protozoa often enter dormant states when outside a host and become active when introduced to a host. They are very difficult to treat in their dormant state and not that easy to treat in their active state either, requiring multiple drugs over significant periods of time to eradicate. Several major protozoal infections are discussed below including which agents are used to treat them.

Entamoeba histolytica causes amebiasis or amebic dysentery. Symptoms include anything from no symptoms to full dysentery. It is transmitted through the fecal-oral route. Treatment needs to be aimed at the asymptomatic carriers just as much as patients in the full throes of the disease to prevent further contamination and infection. The life cycle of *E. histolytica* begins with ingestion of the dormant cyst. Upon entering the intestine the active trophozites are released and multiply. They may invade and ulcerate the large intestinal mucosa or continue to feed on the large intestinal bacterial flora. As they are carried towards the rectum, they return to their dormant cyst form and enter the feces. A systemic infection may occur if enough trophozites invade the colon wall, often colonizing in the liver and forming an abscess. A summary of this is in Figure 10.10.

Agents used to treat amebiasis are considered to act in the lumen of the intestine, treat systemic infection, or be mixed and do both.

Sporozoites: Any cells resulting from the sexual union of spores during the life cycle of certain protozoa known as sporozoans

Merozoites: Any organisms resulting from the asexual reproduction phase of the life cycle of certain protozoa known as sporozoans

Erythrocytes: Red blood cells

Metronidazole is the treatment of first choice. It is a mixed agent. Luminal agents include iodoquinol, a mixed agent, and paromomycin, a luminal agent. These agents should be used when an asymptomatic infection is occurring. Tetracycline can be used to destroy the luminal bacteria that *E. histolytica* feed upon. Chloroquine is used to treat systemic infection in conjunction with metronidazole. Tinidazole is another mixed agent.

Malaria is caused by four species of the genus *Plasmodium*: falciparum, vivax, malariae, and ovale. It can range from the relatively mild *P. vivax* to the lethal *P. falciparum*. The life cycle begins when a bite from an infected mosquito injects plasmodium **sporozoites** into the blood. They enter the liver and form cyst-like structures of thousands of **merozoites**. These merozoites ultimately invade a red blood cell as trophozoites and feed on hemoglobin. These multiply, become merozoites, and burst the **erythrocyte** and either infect other red blood cells or become a gameto-

cyte, a cell capable of reproduction, that is ingested by a mosquito, reinitiating the cycle. Agents act at different parts of this life cycle. The cycle and the various agents that work at different points are summarized in Figure 10.11.

Primaquine is used to treat malarias that are outside of the erythrocyte. It can destroy all four species and their gametocytes. Because it is not useful in treating erythocytic forms, it is often combined with an agent that can.

Chloroquine, mefloquine, quinine, and quinidine are erythrocytic agents. Chloroquine is the drug of choice in treating erythrocytic *P. falciparum*. Mefloquine appears effective in multi-resistant *P. falciparum*. Pyrimethamine can destroy malaria in the blood as well as a spore in the belly of the mosquito.

Giardia lamblia is the most common intestinal parasite in the U.S. It is usually contracted by drinking contaminated water and is either asymptomatic or causes severe diarrhea, which can be very serious in immune-compromised individuals. It is treated with metronidazole.

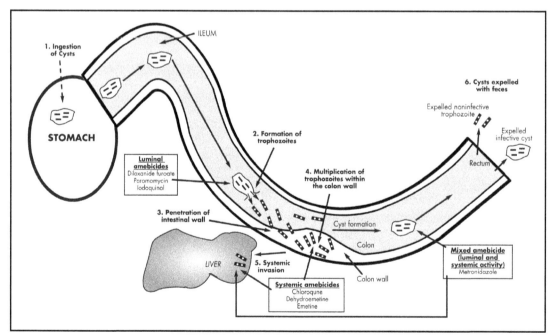

Figure 10.10: The life cycle of *Entamoeba histolytica* and where antiprotozoals can attack it. 1: Ingestion of the inactive cysts. 2: Activation of the dormant cysts into trophozoites in the intestinal lumen. Luminal amebicides act here. 3: These may penetrate the intestinal wall. 4: Trophozoites replicate in the colon wall. Systemic amebicides can attack at this step. 5: After replication, systemic invasion, especially of the liver, may occur. Mixed amebicides can work at many of these steps. 6: Trophozoites that remain in the lumen can form inactive cysts that are passed through the stool and can infect others.

Atovaquone is used to treat mild-to-moderate *Pneumocystis carinii* pneumonia (PCP) in patients who are intolerant to co-trimoxazole treatment and prophylaxis of *Toxoplasma gondii* encephalitis. When added to proguanil, it can be used to treat *P. falciparum*.

Chloroquine can be used to treat rheumatoid arthritis and discoid lupus erythematosus due to its anti-inflammatory action.

MECHANISM OF ACTION

Atovaquone's action is not understood but may inhibit electron transport in mitochondria.

Chloroquine, hydroxychloroquine, quinine, quinidine, and mefloquine work, at least as part of their action, by inhibiting the parasite's ability to convert heme from the hemoglobin into a form that is harmless to the parasite. Accumulation of heme leads to oxidative damage and ultimately lysis of both the erythrocyte and parasite.

This is summarized in Figure 10.12 on page 294.

The mechanism of action of iodoquinol is unknown.

Metronidazole acts as an electron acceptor forming cytotoxic compounds that bind to various proteins and DNA, ultimately causing cell death.

Paromomycin works in two ways. It kills many of the intestinal flora. It also works directly by causing a leaky cell membrane and ultimately cell death.

The mechanism of action of primaquine is not completely understood but is believed to be metabolized to oxidants that disrupt the mitochondria and bind to DNA.

Tinidazole acts by damaging DNA, preventing further synthesis of DNA, and ultimately causing death of the cell.

ANTIMICROBIAL SPECTRA

CHLOROQUINE is used to treat *E. histolytica*

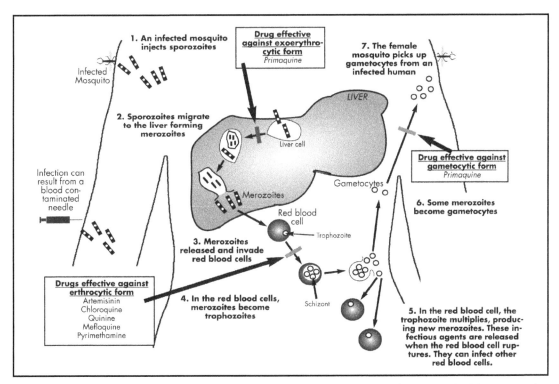

Figure 10.11: The life cycle of *Plasmodium* and how antiprotozoals may attack. 1: An infected mosquito injects sporozoites into the blood. 2: Sporozoites migrate to the liver, where they form merozoites. Primaquine acts here. 3. After replication, merozoites are released and invade red blood cells (RBCs). Drugs effective against the erythrocytic form act at this step. 4: Merozoites become trophozoites in the RBCs. 5: In the RBCs, trophozoites reproduce and form merozoites, which are released when the RBC ruptures and can then infect other RBCs. 6: Some merozoites become gametocytes. 7: Gametocytes can be picked up by female mosquitos, and the sexual cycle begins and forms sporozoites. Primaquine also works here.

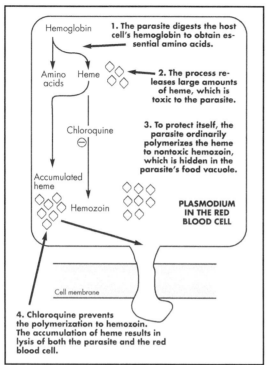

Figure 10.12: Part of the *Plasmodium* life cycle and how chloroquine, hydroxychloroquine, quinine, quinidine, and mefloquine act on the parasite. 1: The parasite eats the hemoglobin in the host's cell for its amino acid content. 2: Heme, a highly oxidant complex, is released and is toxic to the parasite. 3: Normally, to protect itself, the parasite converts heme into hemozoin and is quarantined in a vacuole in its cytosol. 4: The agents above prevent the production of hemozoin; the heme therefore results in the lysis of the parasite and red blood cell.

and malaria, especially *P. falciparum*. It is less effective against *P. vivax*.

METRONIDAZOLE is used in treating *E. histolytica*, *Giardia lamblia*, *Trichomonas vaginalis*, anaerobic cocci, and Gram-negative bacilli and is the drug of choice in treating *Clostridium difficile*.

PAROMOMYCIN is useful as a luminal agent in treating *E. histolytica* and tapeworm as well as an alternative agent for cryptosporidiosis.

PYRIMETHAMINE is useful in treating *P. falciparum* when used alone. When used with a sulfonamide (see Section 3 above), it is also useful against *P. malariae* and *Toxoplasma gondii*.

TINIDAZOLE is useful in treating *T. vaginalis*, *G. lamblia*, and intestinal amebiasis and liver abscess caused by *E. histolytica*.

DOSAGES

ARTEMETHER, used only in combination with other drugs, and therefore its individual dosing is not covered here.

ATOVAQUONE, for *adolescents* over 13 and *adults*, for prevention of PCP, 1500 mg once daily with food; for treatment of mild-to-moderate PCP, 750 mg bid with food for 21 days.

CHLOROQUINE, for *children*, for suppression or prophylaxis of malaria, administer 5 mg base/kg/wk on the same day each week (not to exceed 300 mg base/dose); begin 1-2 weeks prior to exposure; continue for 4-6 weeks after leaving endemic area; if suppressive therapy is not begun prior to exposure, double the initial loading dose to 10 mg base/kg and administer in 2 divided doses 6 hours apart, followed by the usual dosage regimen; for acute attack, 10 mg/kg (base) on day 1, followed by 5 mg/kg (base) 6 hours later and 5 mg/kg (base) on days 2 and 3; for extraintestinal amebiasis, 10 mg/kg (base) once daily for 2-3 weeks (up to 300 mg base/d). For *adults*, for suppression or prophylaxis of malaria, 500 mg/wk (300 mg base) on the same day each week; begin 1-2 weeks prior to exposure; continue for 4-6 weeks after leaving endemic area; if suppressive therapy is not begun prior to exposure, double the initial loading dose to 1 g (600 mg base) and administer in 2 divided doses 6 hours apart, followed by the usual dosage regimen; for acute attack, 1 g (600 mg base) on day 1, with 500 mg (300 mg base) 6 hours later, followed by 500 mg (300 mg base) on days 2 and 3; for extraintestinal amebiasis, 1 g/d (600 mg base) for 2 days followed by 500 mg/d (300 mg base) for at least 2-3 weeks.

EFLORNITHINE, for *children* 12 years and older and *adults*, for unwanted facial hair in females, topical: apply thin layer of cream to affected areas of face and areas under the chin bid; at least 8 hours apart.

HYDROXYCHLOROQUINE, for *children*, for chemoprophylaxis of malaria, 5 mg/kg (base) once weekly; should not exceed the recommended adult dose; begin 2 weeks before exposure; continue for 4-6 weeks after leaving endemic area; if suppressive therapy is not begun prior to the exposure, double the initial dose and give in 2 doses, 6 hours apart; for acute attack, 10 mg/kg (base) initial dose, followed by 5 mg/kg at 6, 24, and 48 hours; for JRA or SLE, 3-5 mg/kg/d divided 1-2 times/d; avoid exceeding 7 mg/kg/d. For *adults*, for chemoprophylaxis of malaria, 310 mg base weekly on same day each week; begin 2 weeks before exposure; continue for 4-6 weeks after leaving endemic area; if suppressive therapy is not begun prior to the exposure, double the initial dose and give in 2 doses, 6 hours apart; for acute attack, 620 mg first dose day 1; 310 mg in 6 hours day 1; 310 mg in 1 dose day 2; and 310 mg in 1 dose on day 3; for rheumatoid arthritis, 310-465 mg/d to start, taken with food or milk; increase dose until optimum response level is reached, usually after 4-12 weeks dose should be reduced by 1/2 and a maintenance dose of 155-310 mg/d given; for lupus erythematosus, 310 mg every day or twice daily for several weeks depending on response; 155-310 mg/d for prolonged maintenance therapy.

IODOQUINOL, for *children*, 30-40 mg/kg/d up to a maximum of 650 mg tid for 20 days, not to exceed 1.95 g/d. For *adults*, 650 mg tid after meals for 20 days, not to exceed 1.95 g/d.

MEFLOQUINE, for *children* 6 months and older and >5 kg, for malaria treatment, 20-25 mg/kg in 2 divided doses 6-8 hours apart; maximum dose is 1250 mg; take with food and an ample amount of water; if clinical improvement is not seen within 48-72 hours, an alternative therapy should be used for retreatment; for malaria prophylaxis, 5 mg/kg/once weekly; maximum dose is 250 mg; starting 1 week before arrival in endemic area; continuing weekly during travel and for 4 weeks after leaving endemic area; take with food and an ample amount of water. For

adults, for malaria treatment (mild to moderate infection), 5 tablets (1250 mg) as a single dose, take with food and at least 8 oz. of water; if clinical improvement is not seen within 48-72 hours, an alternative therapy should be used for retreatment; for malaria prophylaxis, 1 tablet (250 mg) weekly starting 1 week before arrival in endemic area; continuing weekly during travel and for 4 weeks after leaving endemic area; take with food and at least 8 oz of water.

METRONIDAZOLE, for *infants* and *children*, for amebiasis, 35-50 mg/kg/d in divided doses every 8 hours for 10 days; for trichomoniasis, 15-30 mg/kg/d in divided doses every 8 hours for 7 days; for anaerobic infections, 15-35 mg/kg/d in divided doses every 8 hours; for *Clostridium difficile* (antibiotic-associated colitis), 20 mg/kg/d divided every 6 hours; maximum dose is 2 g/d. For *adults*, for anaerobic infections (diverticulitis, intra-abdominal, peritonitis, cholangitis, or abscess), 500 mg every 6-8 hours, not to exceed 4 g/d; for amebiasis, 500-750 mg every 8 hours for 5-10 days; for antibiotic-associated pseudomembranous colitis, 250-500 mg 3-4 times/d for 10-14 days; for giardiasis, 500 mg bid for 5-7 days; for *Helicobacter pylori* eradication, 250-500 mg with meals and at bedtime for 14 days; requires combination therapy with at least one other antibiotic and an acid-suppressing agent (proton-pump inhibitor or H_2 blocker); for bacterial vaginosis or vaginitis due to *Gardnerella;* or *Mobiluncus,* 500 mg bid (regular release) or 750 mg once daily (extended release tablet) for 7 days; for trichomoniasis, 250 mg every 8 hours for 7 days or 375 mg bid for 7 days or 2 g as a single dose. For the *elderly,* use lower end of adult dose recommendations; do not administer as a single dose.

NITAZOXANIDE, for diarrhea from *Cryptosporidium parvum* or *Giardia lamblia*: for *children* 1-3 years, 100 mg every 12 hours for 3 days; for *children* 4-11 years, 200 mg every 12 hours for 3 days; for *children* 12 and older and *adults*, 500 mg every 12 hours for 3 days.

PAROMOMYCIN, for *children*, for tapeworm (fish, dog, bovine, porcine), 11 mg/kg every 15 minutes for 4 doses. For *children* and *adults*, for intestinal amebiasis, 25-35 mg/kg/d in 3 divided doses for 5-10 days; for *Dientamoeba fragilis*, 25-30 mg/kg/d in 3 divided doses for 7 days; for dwarf tapeworm, 45 mg/kg/dose/d for 5-7 days. For *adults*, for tapeworm (fish, dog, bovine, porcine), 1 g every 15 minutes for 4 doses; for hepatic coma, 4 g/d in 2-4 divided doses for 5-6 days.

PENTAMIDINE, to treat PCP, for *children* over months, IM: 4 mg/kg once daily for 14-21 days; for *adults*, inhalation for prevention: 300 mg every 4 weeks; IM: 4 mg/kg once daily for 14-21 days.

PRIMAQUINE, dosage expressed as mg of base (15 mg base=26.3 mg primaquine phosphate). For *children*, for treatment of malaria (decrease risk of delayed primary attacks and prevent relapse), 0.3 mg base/kg/d once daily for 14 days (not to exceed 15 mg/d) or 0.9 mg base/kg once weekly for 8 weeks (not to exceed 45 mg base/week). For *adults*, for treatment of malaria (decrease risk of delayed primary attacks and prevent relapse), 15 mg/d (base) once daily for 14 days or 45 mg base once weekly for 8 weeks.

PROGUANIL, used only in combination with other drugs, and therefore its individual dosing is not covered here.

PYRIMETHAMINE, for *children*, for malaria chemoprophylaxis (for areas where chloroquine-resistant *P. falciparum* exists), begin prophylaxis 2 weeks before entering endemic area, 0.5 mg/kg once weekly, not to exceed 25 mg/dose; for <4 years: 6.25 mg once weekly; 4-10 years: 12.5 mg once weekly; for toxoplasmosis, loading dose of 2 mg/kg/d divided into 2 equal daily doses for 1-3 days; up to a maximum of 100 mg/d, followed by 1 mg/kg/d divided into 2 doses for 4 weeks; maximum of 25 mg/d. For *children* over 10 and *adults*, for malaria chemoprophylaxis (for areas where chloroquine-resistant *P. falciparum* exists), begin prophylaxis 2 weeks before entering endemic area, 25 mg once weekly; dosage should be continued for all age groups for at least 6-10 weeks after leaving endemic areas.

QUININE, for *children*, for treatment of chloroquine-resistant malaria, 25-30 mg/kg/d in divided doses every 8 hours for 3-7 days with tetracycline (consider risk versus benefit in *children* under 8 years); for babesiosis, 25 mg/kg/d divided every 8 hours for 7 days. For *adults*, for treatment of chloroquine-resistant malaria, 650 mg every 8 hours for 3-7 days with tetracycline; for suppression of malaria, 325 mg bid continued for 6 weeks after exposure; for babesiosis, 650 mg every 6-8 hours for 7 days; for leg cramps, 200-300 mg nocte.

TINIDAZOLE, for *children* over 3, for intestinal amebiasis, 50 mg/kg/d for 3 days; maximum dose 2 g/d; for liver abscess amebiasis, 50 mg/kg/d for 3-5 days; maximum dose 2 g/d; for giardiasis, 50 mg/kg as a single dose; maximum dose 2 g. For *adults*, for intestinal amebiasis, 2 g/d for 3 days; for liver abscess amebiasis, 2 g/d for 3-5 days; for giardiasis, 2 g as a single dose; for trichomoniasis, 2 g as a single dose; sexual partners should be treated at the same time.

◼ ADVERSE EFFECTS

Because protozoa are closer to human than bacteria, it is harder to get an agent that specifically targets the pathogen, and most of these agents have substantial toxicities and adverse effects. Almost all should be avoided during pregnancy. The adverse effects are particularly detrimental to cells that show high metabolism such as neurons, bone marrow stem cells, renal tubular, and intestinal cells.

Atovaquone commonly causes headache, fever, insomnia, anxiety, rash, GI upset, and a cough.

Chloroquine and hydroxychloroquine have minimal adverse effects at typical doses but can cause GI upset, **pruritis**, blurring of vision, and headaches at higher doses. Chronic use may cause discoloration of mucous membranes and nailbeds.

It should be used with caution in patients with liver dysfunction, severe GI problems, neurologic or blood disorders. It is contraindicated in patients with psoriasis or **porphyria**.

Iodoquinol can cause a rash, diarrhea, peripheral neuropathy that is dose-related, and, rarely, optic **neuritis**. This agent should not be used long term.

Mefloquine, at high doses, may cause nausea and vomiting, dizziness, disorientation, hallucinations, and depression.

Metronidazole can cause GI disturbances, a metallic taste, oral candidiasis, and rarely neurological problems such as dizziness, vertigo, and peripheral neuropathy. It can cause a strong reaction to alcohol, and they should not be mixed.

Paromomycin causes GI distress and diarrhea.

Primaquine has a relatively low incidence of adverse effects. **Hemolytic anemia** can occur in patients with glucose-6-phosphate dehydrogenase deficiency. Large doses may induce GI discomfort especially when combined with chloroquine. It may cause **methemoglobinemia**. **Granulocytopenia** and **agranulocytosis** rarely occur, however, patients with lupus or arthritis are more prone to it, and this agent can aggravate these conditions.

Quinidine commonly causes GI upset, lightheadedness, and electrocardiogram abnormalities. May cause angina, palpitations, and either initiate or exacerbate an arrhythmia.

Quinine and quinidine may cause **cinchonism**, a syndrome causing nausea and vomiting, tinnitus, and vertigo. These are reversible, and therapy does not need to be suspended.

Tinidazole can cause GI upset, metallic taste, transient peripheral neuropathy, and candida overgrowth.

RED FLAGS

Chloroquine may cause electrocardiogram abnormalities.

Quinidine very rarely may cause cardiovascular conditions such as tachycardias, fibrillations, and arrhythmias.

Use of quinine should cease in case of a positive **Coomb's test** for hemolytic anemia.

INTERACTIONS

DRUG

Chloroquine may exacerbate dermatitis caused by gold or phenylbutazone.

Mefloquine may cause electrocardiogram abnormalities when combined with quinidine.

INTERACTION ISSUES

A:

D: Artemether is 95% protein bound, atovaquone is over 99% protein bound; lumefantrine is 99.7% bound; mefloquine is approxiamately 98% bound; nitazoxanide is rapidly metabolized to its active metabolite, tizoxanide, which is over 99% bound.

M: Chloroquine is a major substrate of CYP2D6 and 3A4 and a moderate inhibitor of 2D6; mefloquine is a major substrate of CYP3A4; metronidazole is a moderate inhibitor of CYP3A4; pentamidine is a major substrate of CYP2C19; Pprimaquine is a major substrate of CYP3A4 and a strong inhibitor and a weak or moderate inducer of 1A2; pyrimethamine is a moderate inhibitor of CYP2C9; quinine is a major substrate of CYP3A4 and a moderate inhibitor of 2C8, 2C9, and 2D6.

E:

Pgp: Mefloquine inhibits Pgp; quinine is a substrate and inhibitor of Pgp.

Pruritis: Itching

Porphyria: A group of inherited disorders characterized by accumulation of porphyrins, intermediaries of hemoglobin production

Neuritis: Inflammation of a nerve

Hemolytic anemia: An anemia, or loss of hemoglobin, characterized by red blood cell destruction

Methemoglobinemia: The presence in the blood of methemoglobin, a form of hemoglobin that cannot bind and transport oxygen

Granulocytopenia: An abnormal blood condition where there is a decrease in the number of granulocytes, white blood cells with granules in their cytoplasm

Agranulocytosis: The extreme reduction in the number of leukocytes or white blood cells in the blood

Cinchonism: A condition characterized by deafness, headache, tinnitus, and cerebral congestion

Coomb's test: A test for antibodies damaging red blood cells, may indicate many blood diseases

SECTION 7: ANTHELMINTHIC DRUGS

BENZIMIDAZOLES:

ALBENDAZOLE (al BEN da zole) PR=C
(Albenza®)

MEBENDAZOLE (me BEN da zole) PR=C

OTHERS:

IVERMECTIN (eye ver MEK tin) PR=C

(Stromectol®)

PRAZIQUANTEL (pray zi KWON tel) PR=B
(Biltricide®)

PYRANTEL PAMOATE (pi RAN tel PAM oh ate) PR=C *(Pamix [O], Pin-X [O], Reeses Pinworm Medicine [O])*

There are three major classes of helminths, or worms, that infect humans: nematodes; by far the most common; trematodes; and cestodes. Worldwide, helminth infections are quite common. The most common helminth infection, the *Nematode ascaris,* infects about 30% of the world's population, or almost 1.5 billion people.

FUNCTION

Nematodes are elongated round worms that have a complete digestive system including a mouth and anus unlike any of the other categories of worms. They can cause infections of the intestines, blood, and tissues. Ivermectin, mebendazole, and, as a secondary agent, piperazine are used to treat these infections. Figure 10.13 on page 299 shows other worm infections and common therapies for each.

Praziquantel is useful in treating trematodes, flukes that are leaf-shaped flatworms. Figure 10.14 on page 300 shows common trematode infections and their treatment.

Cestodes are "true tapeworms" that are flat, have a segmented body, and generally attach to the host's intestines. The drug of choice for most cestodes infections is niclosamide. This agent is not available in the United States. Albendazole is often use, either as a first choice agent in some infections or as a replacement for niclosamide in others. A summary of cestode infections and their treatment is in Figure 10.15 on page 301.

MECHANISM OF ACTION

The main subclass of anthelmintic agents is the benzimidazoles. These include albendazole and mebendazole. This subclass acts by disrupting assembly of microtubules, cellular building blocks used to form the cytoskeleton and help provide transportation of objects in the cell's cytoplasm. They also decrease uptake of glucose.

Ivermectin works by binding to glutamate-gated chlorine ion channel receptors, resulting in too much chlorine entering the cell and changing the normal voltage difference along the cell membrane to be much more negative. This prevents an action potential from starting and causes paralysis.

Piperazine works by blocking the effects of acetylcholine at neuromuscular junctions. This prevents normal contraction and causes paralysis.

Praziquantel acts by increasing the permeability of the cell membrane to calcium. Extra calcium causes muscular contraction and paralysis of the parasite.

ANTIMICROBIAL SPECTRA

ALBENDAZOLE treats cestodal infestations including *Taenia solium* larvae and *Echinococcus granulosis* (hydatid disease).

IVERMECTIN is the drug of choice for treating *Onchocerca volvulus* (river blindness), larva migrans in the skin, and strongyloides.

MEBENDAZOLE is effective in treating *Trichuris trichuria* (whipworm), *Enterobius vermicularis* (pinworm), *Necator americanus* and *Ancylostoma duodenale* (both hookworms), and *Ascariasis lumbricoides* (roundworm).

PIPERAZINE is useful in treating *Ascariasis lumbricoides* (roundworm) and *Enterobius vermicularis* (pinworm).

PRAZIQUANTEL is used to treat trematode infections and some cestode infections similar to cysticercosis. It is the agent of first choice for treating all forms of schistosomiasis and other trematode infections.

◼ DOSAGES

ALBENDAZOLE, for *children* and *adults*, for neurocysticercosis, under 60 kg: 7.5 mg/kg/d bid; up to a maximum of 800 mg/d, for 8-30 days; 60 kg or over: 400 mg bid for 8-30 days; for

hydatid, under 60 kg: 7.5 mg/kg/d bid to a maximum 800 mg/d; 60 kg or over: 400 mg bid; administer dose for three 28-day cycles with a 14-day drug-free interval in between.

IVERMECTIN, for *children* 15 kg and over and *adults*, for strongyloidiasis, 200 mcg/kg as a single dose; for onchocerciasis, 150 mcg/kg as a single dose; retreatment may be required every 3-12 months until the adult worms die.

MEBENDAZOLE, for *children* and *adults*, for pinworms, 100 mg single dose; may need to

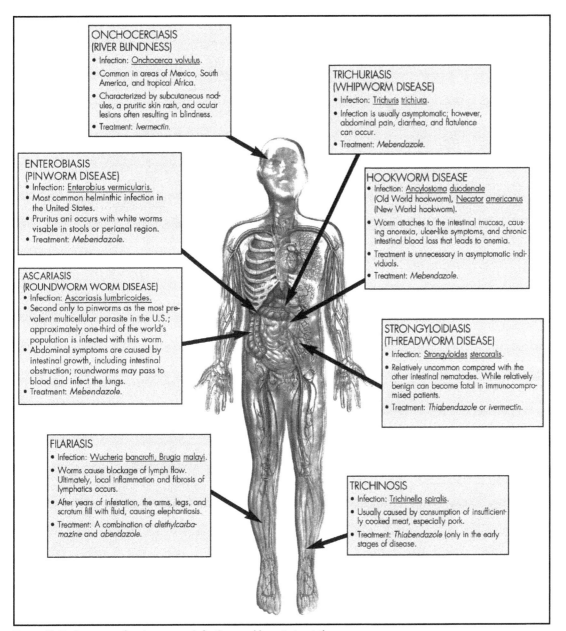

ONCHOCERCIASIS (RIVER BLINDNESS)
- Infection: Onchocerca volvulus.
- Common in areas of Mexico, South America, and tropical Africa.
- Characterized by subcutaneous nodules, a pruritic skin rash, and ocular lesions often resulting in blindness.
- Treatment: *Ivermectin.*

TRICHURIASIS (WHIPWORM DISEASE)
- Infection: Trichuris trichiura.
- Infection is usually asymptomatic; however, abdominal pain, diarrhea, and flatulence can occur.
- Treatment: *Mebendazole.*

ENTEROBIASIS (PINWORM DISEASE)
- Infection: Enterobius vermicularis.
- Most common helminthic infection in the United States.
- Pruritus ani occurs with white worms visable in stools or perianal region.
- Treatment: *Mebendazole.*

HOOKWORM DISEASE
- Infection: Ancylostoma duodenale (Old World hookworm), Necator americanus (New World hookworm).
- Worm attaches to the intestinal mucosa, causing anorexia, ulcer-like symptoms, and chronic intestinal blood loss that leads to anemia.
- Treatment is unnecessary in asymptomatic individuals.
- Treatment: *Mebendazole.*

ASCARIASIS (ROUNDWORM WORM DISEASE)
- Infection: Ascariasis lumbricoides.
- Second only to pinworms as the most prevalent multicellular parasite in the U.S.; approximately one-third of the world's population is infected with this worm.
- Abdominal symptoms are caused by intestinal growth, including intestinal obstruction; roundworms may pass to blood and infect the lungs.
- Treatment: *Mebendazole.*

STRONGYLOIDIASIS (THREADWORM DISEASE)
- Infection: Strongyloides stercoralis.
- Relatively uncommon compared with the other intestinal nematodes. While relatively benign can become fatal in immunocompromised patients.
- Treatment: *Thiabendazole* or *ivermectin.*

FILARIASIS
- Infection: Wucheria bancrofti, Brugia malayi.
- Worms cause blockage of lymph flow. Ultimately, local inflammation and fibrosis of lymphatics occurs.
- After years of infestation, the arms, legs, and scrotum fill with fluid, causing elephantiasis.
- Treatment: A combination of *diethylcarbamazine* and *abendazole.*

TRICHINOSIS
- Infection: Trichinella spiralis.
- Usually caused by consumption of insufficiently cooked meat, especially pork.
- Treatment: *Thiabendazole* (only in the early stages of disease.

Figure 10.13: Summary of various worm infections and how to treat them.

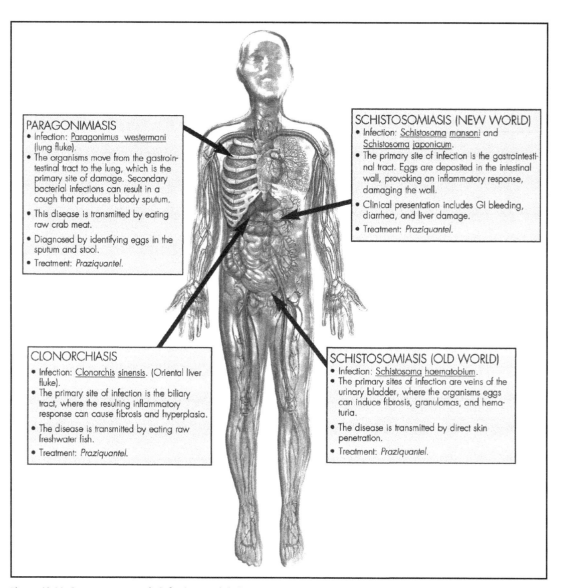

PARAGONIMIASIS
- Infection: <u>Paragonimus westermani</u> (lung fluke).
- The organisms move from the gastrointestinal tract to the lung, which is the primary site of damage. Secondary bacterial infections can result in a cough that produces bloody sputum.
- This disease is transmitted by eating raw crab meat.
- Diagnosed by identifying eggs in the sputum and stool.
- Treatment: *Praziquantel*.

SCHISTOSOMIASIS (NEW WORLD)
- Infection: <u>Schistosoma mansoni</u> and <u>Schistosoma japonicum</u>.
- The primary site of infection is the gastrointestinal tract. Eggs are deposited in the intestinal wall, provoking an inflammatory response, damaging the wall.
- Clinical presentation includes GI bleeding, diarrhea, and liver damage.
- Treatment: *Praziquantel*.

CLONORCHIASIS
- Infection: <u>Clonorchis sinensis</u>. (Oriental liver fluke).
- The primary site of infection is the biliary tract, where the resulting inflammatory response can cause fibrosis and hyperplasia.
- The disease is transmitted by eating raw freshwater fish.
- Treatment: *Praziquantel*.

SCHISTOSOMIASIS (OLD WORLD)
- Infection: <u>Schistosoma haematobium</u>.
- The primary sites of infection are veins of the urinary bladder, where the organisms eggs can induce fibrosis, granulomas, and hematuria.
- The disease is transmitted by direct skin penetration.
- Treatment: *Praziquantel*.

Figure 10.14: Common trematode infections and their treatments.

repeat after 2 weeks; treatment should include family members in close contact with patient; for whipworms, roundworms, hookworms, 1 tablet bid, morning and evening on 3 consecutive days; if patient is not cured within 3-4 weeks, a second course of treatment may be administered; for capillariasis, 200 mg bid for 20 days.

PRAZIQUANTEL, for *children* 4 years and older and *adults*, for schistosomiasis, 20 mg/kg/dose 2-3 times/d for 1 day at 4-6 hour intervals.

PYRANTEL PAMOATE, for *children* 2 years and older and *adults*, for *Enterobius vermicularis* (pinworm), 11 mg/kg administered as a single dose up to a maximum dose of 1 g.

ADVERSE EFFECTS

The benzimidazoles, albendazole, and mebendazole are contraindicated during pregnancy as is ivermectin. While not contraindicated, praziquantel should be used with caution in pregnant or breast-feeding women.

Albendazole, when used for the short term as in the treatment of nematodes, has minimal adverse effects, which include headache and nausea. Treatment of hydatid disease can last 3

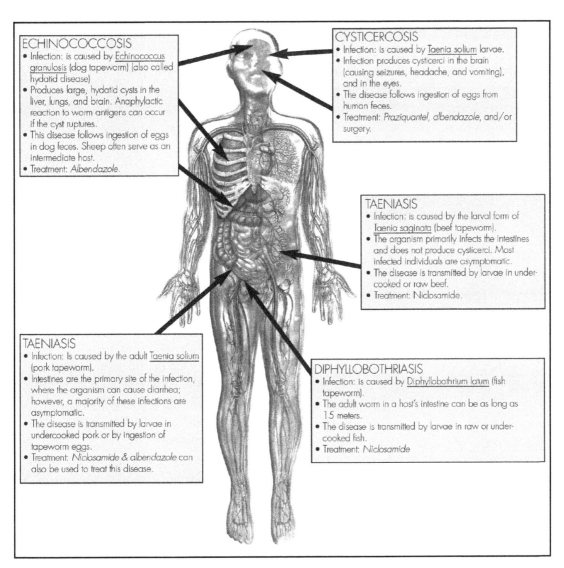

ECHINOCOCCOSIS
- Infection: is caused by <u>Echinococcus granulosis</u> (dog tapeworm) (also called hydatid disease)
- Produces large, hydatid cysts in the liver, lungs, and brain. Anaphylactic reaction to worm antigens can occur if the cyst ruptures.
- This disease follows ingestion of eggs in dog feces. Sheep often serve as an intermediate host.
- Treatment: *Albendazole.*

CYSTICERCOSIS
- Infection: is caused by <u>Taenia solium</u> larvae.
- Infection produces cysticerci in the brain (causing seizures, headache, and vomiting), and in the eyes.
- The disease follows ingestion of eggs from human feces.
- Treatment: *Praziquantel, albendazole,* and/or surgery.

TAENIASIS
- Infection: is caused by the larval form of <u>Taenia saginata</u> (beef tapeworm).
- The organism primarily infects the intestines and does not produce cysticerci. Most infected individuals are asymptomatic.
- The disease is transmitted by larvae in under-cooked or raw beef.
- Treatment: *Niclosamide.*

TAENIASIS
- Infection: Is caused by the adult <u>Taenia solium</u> (pork tapeworm).
- Intestines are the primary site of the infection, where the organism can cause diarrhea; however, a majority of these infections are asymptomatic.
- The disease is transmitted by larvae in undercooked pork or by ingestion of tapeworm eggs.
- Treatment: *Niclosamide & albendazole* can also be used to treat this disease.

DIPHYLLOBOTHRIASIS
- Infection: is caused by <u>Diphyllobothrium latum</u> (fish tapeworm).
- The adult worm in a host's intestine can be as long as 15 meters.
- The disease is transmitted by larvae in raw or under-cooked fish.
- Treatment: *Niclosamide*

Figure 10.15: Summary of cestode infection and its treatment.

months and has a risk of liver toxicity and, rarely, **agranulocytosis** or **pancytopenia**. Dying parasites, when this agent is used to treat neurocysticercosis, can cause an inflammatory response as well as headache, vomiting, fever, convulsions, and mental changes. This agent should not be used in children under 2 years of age.

Ivermectin is contraindicated in patients with meningitis as this condition makes the blood-brain barrier (BBB) more permeable and may cause serious CNS effects. Normally this agent does not transverse the BBB. Killing of the prelarval form of some worms may cause fever, head-ache, dizziness, somnolence, and hypotension.

Mebendazole has minimal adverse effects; however, patients may complain of abdominal pain and diarrhea.

Praziquantel commonly causes drowsiness, dizziness, malaise, GI upset, and **anorexia**.

RED FLAGS

Praziquantel is contraindicated in treating ocular cysticercosis as it may damage the eye.

Agranulocytosis: The extreme reduction in the number of leukocytes, or white blood cells, in the blood

Pancytopenia: A great reduction in the number of red blood cells, white blood cells, and platelets

Anorexia: Lack or loss of appetite

INTERACTIONS

DRUG

Piperazine and pyrantel pamoate should not be used together as they have antagonistic modes of action.

Praziquantel has been reported to have interactions with dexamethosone, phenytoin, and carbamazepine due to increased metabolism.

Cimetidine's effect of inhibiting cytochrome P450 may cause increased levels of praziquantel.

INTERACTION ISSUES

A:

D: Mebendazole is 90-95% protein bound.

M: Praziquantel is a major substrate of CYP3A4.

E:

Pgp: Ivermectin is a substrate of Pgp.

SECTION 8: ANTIVIRAL AGENTS

ACYCLOVIR (ay SYE kloe vir) PR=C *(Xerese™, Zovirax®)*

AMANTADINE *(See Chapter 5, Section 1)*

BOCEPREVIR (boe SE pre vir) PR=B *(Victrelis®)*

DOCOSANOL (doe KOE san ole) PR=N *(Abreva [O])*

FAMCICLOVIR (fam SYE kloe vir) PR=B *(Famvir®)*

GANCICLOVIR (gan SYE kloe vir) PR=C *(Cytovene®, Vitrasert®)*

MARAVIROC (ma RAV i rock) PR=B *(Selzentry™)*

OSELTAMIVIR (oh sel TAM i vir) PR=C *(Tamiflu®)*

PENCICLOVIR (pen SYE kloe vir) PR=B *(Denavir)*

RIBAVIRIN (rye ba VYE rin) PR=X *(Copegus®, Rebetol®, RibaPak®, ibasphere™, Virazole®)*

RIMANTADINE (ri MAN ta dene) PR=C *(Flumadine®)*

TELAPREVIR (tel A pre vir) PR=B *(Incivek™)*

VALACYCLOVIR (val ay SYE kloe vir) PR=B *(Valtrex®)*

VALGANCICLOVIR (val gan SYE kloh vir) PR=C *(Valcyte™)*

ZANAMIVIR (za NA mi vir) PR=C *(Relenza® Diskhaler)*

INTEGRASE INHIBITORS:

DOLUTEGRAVIR (doe loo TEG ra vir) PR=B *(Tivicay®)*

ELVITEGRAVIR (el vi TEG ra vir) PR=B *(Stribild™[33])*

RALTEGRAVIR (ral TEG ra vir) PR=C *(Isentress®)*

NUCLEOSIDE REVERSE TRANSCRIPTASE INHIBITORS (NRTIS):

ABACAVIR (a BAK a vir) PR=C *(Epzicom™,[14] Trizivir®,[15] Ziagen®)*

DIDANOSINE (ddI) (dye DAN oh sene) PR=B *(Videx®, Videx® EC)*

EMTRICITABINE (em trye SYE ta bene) PR=B *(Atripla™,[16] Complera™,[34] Emtriva®, Stribild™,[33] Truvada®[17])*

ENTECAVIR (en TE ka vir) PR=C *(Baraclude®)*

LAMIVUDINE (3TC) (la MI vyoo dene) PR=C *(Combivir®,[18] Epivir®, Epivir-HBV®, Epzicom™,[14] Trizivir®[15])*

STAVUDINE (d4T) (STAV yoo dene) PR=C *(Zerit®)*

TELBIVUDINE (tel BI vyoo dene) PR=B *(Tyzeka™)*

ZIDOVUDINE (AZT) (zye DOE vyoo dene) PR=C *(Combivir®,[18] Retrovir®, Trizivir®[15])*

NUCLEOTIDE REVERSE TRANSCRIPTASE INHIBITORS:

ADEFOVIR (a DEF o vir) PR=C *(Hepsera™)*

TENOFOVIR (te NOE fo vir) PR=B *(Atripla®,[16] Complera™,[34] Stribild™,[33] Truvada®,[17] Viread®)*

NON-NUCLEOSIDE REVERSE TRANSCRIPTASE INHIBITORS (NNRTIS):

DELAVIRDINE (de la VIR dene) PR=C *(Rescriptor®)*

EFAVIRENZ (e FAV e renz) PR=C *(Atripla™,[16] Sustiva®)*

ETRAVIRINE (et ra VIR ene) PR=B *(Intelence®)*

NEVIRAPINE (ne VYE ra pene) PR=B *(Viramune®, Viramune XR®)*

RILPIVIRINE (ril pi VIR ene) PR=B *(Complera™,[34] Edurant®)*

PROTEASE INHIBITORS:

ATAZANAVIR (at a za NA vir) PR=B *(Reyataz®)*

DARUNAVIR (dar OO na vir) PR=C *(Prezista™)*

FOSAMPRENAVIR (FOS am pren a vir) PR=C *(Lexiva®)*

INDINAVIR (in DIN a vir) PR=C *(Crixivan®)*

LOPINAVIR (loe PIN a vir) PR=C *(Kaletra®[19])*

NELFINAVIR (nel FIN a vir) PR=B *(Viracept®)*

RITONAVIR (ri TOE na vir) PR=B *(Kaletra®,[19] Norvir®)*

SAQUINAVIR (sa KWIN a vir) PR=B *(Invirase®)*

TIPRANAVIR (tip RA na vir) PR=C *(Aptivus®)*

Treating viruses has many difficulties. Since viruses are intracellular parasites, the first hurdle a would-be antiviral agent has to overcome is how to get into an infected human cell. They do not have their own cell walls or membranes, usual targets of other drugs against microorganisms. They generally use the host's reproductive machinery for most of its reproduction, so it is difficult to target specific viral reproductive processes. Unlike bacteria, viral symptoms usually appear late in the infection after most of the reproduction is accomplished. This means antiviral drugs have fewer targets to act upon.

Given these constraints antivirals are often used to prevent infection or treat specific infections. In other words, most viruses are not affected by these agents.

Viruses have an interesting life cycle that is dependent on hijacking a host cell's internal machinery in order to reproduce. This cycle begins when a viral **capsid** comes into contact with a potential host cell. It is then absorbed, losing its coat to expose either viral DNA or RNA. This drives transcription, the replication of mRNA or messenger RNA, and translation, converting mRNA into proteins. Ultimately enough material is produced, and DNA or RNA as well as some proteins are once again packaged into capsids and released, often killing the host cell in the process. Figure 10.16 on the next page shows a summary of this process. While this is a good general life cycle, there are many variations, and this should be viewed as a simplification.

FUNCTION

Among diseases commonly treated by antiviral drugs are viral infections of the respiratory tract, including influenzae A and B*

*Influenza is a very confusing disease. There is a bacteria called *Haemophilus influenzae*. Then there are the classes of viruses that are members of the orthomyxovirus family: influenza Group A, B, or C. When one talks about the "flu," they are talking about an influenza A or B viral infection. Group C influenza viruses generally only cause mild respiratory infections. *H. influenzae* causes meningitis, and upper respiratory tract infections such as otitis media, sinusitis, and epiglottitis.

and respiratory syncytial virus (RSV); hepatic infections, herpes; cytomegalovirus; and human immuno-deficiency virus.

Agents such as oseltamivir that treat orthomyxoviruses, specifically influenzae type A and B viruses, treat the neuraminidase inhibitors. Amantidine and rimantadine are useful in treating influenza type A infections.

Amantidine is also useful in treating Parkinson's disease as discussed in Chapter 5, Section 1.

Ribavarin is a broad-spectrum antiviral useful in treating RSV, hanta virus, and Lassa fever as well as hepatitis C when used with interferon.

Capsid: The layer of protein encapsulating a virus

Of the various types of hepatites, only 2 are aided by antiviral therapy: B and C. Hepatitis B virus (HBV) can be treated with lamivudine. Hepatitis C virus (HCV) is treated by a combination of ribavarin and the injection-only interferon -α. Adefovir, entecavir, and telbivudine are also used to treat hepatitis B virus.

Lamivudine is also used to treat HIV.

There are five common herpesviruses: Herpes

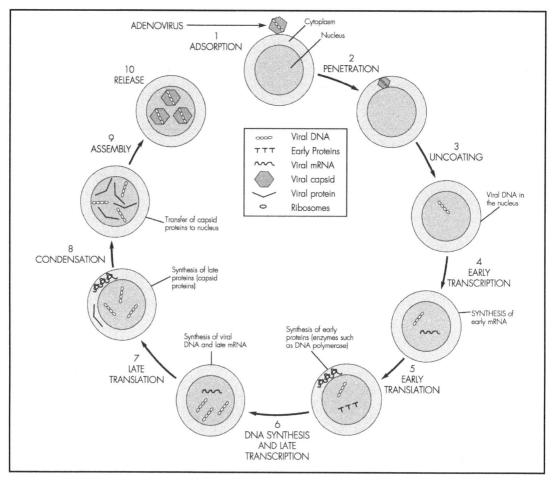

Figure 10.16: The general life cycle of a virus.

simplex type 1 and 2 (HSV-1 and HSV-2), varicella-zoster virus (VZV), cytomegalovirus (CMV), and Epstein-Barr virus (EBV). Acyclovir and valacyclovir act on all five of these. Famciclovir acts on the HSVs and VZV. Ganciclovir and valganciclovir act on CMV.

The first treatment for HIV/AIDS was in 1987. Since then, the entire life cycle of a new class of viruses, retroviruses, was discovered, and highly effective drugs and drug regimens have, in developed countries, made HIV a disease of management rather than death. In developing countries it is still a leading cause of death because of the expense of the drug regimen, with estimates that over 50% of the populations of some countries in Africa are infected. It is also said to be rampant in other areas of the world such as the former Soviet Union and many Asian countries including China, India, and many Southeast Asian countries, though statistics, due to political reasons, are hard to come by.

The current regimen for treating HIV is called highly active antiretroviral therapy (HAART). It recommends two nucleoside or nucleotide reverse transcriptase inhibitors (NRTIs) and either a protease inhibitor (PI) or a non-nucleoside reverse transcriptase inhibitor (NNRTI). The exact agents depend on the **genotype** or **phenotype** of the virus, the **viral load**, patient factors, disease symptoms, concurrent illnesses, drug interactions, and patient compliance. Combination therapy minimizes the chances of resistance developing in this rapidly mutating virus. This is summarized in Figure 10.17.

Genotype: The complete genetic makeup of an organism

Phenotype: The complete observable characteristics of an organism regardless of its genetics

Viral load: The level of viral RNA present in the blood plasma

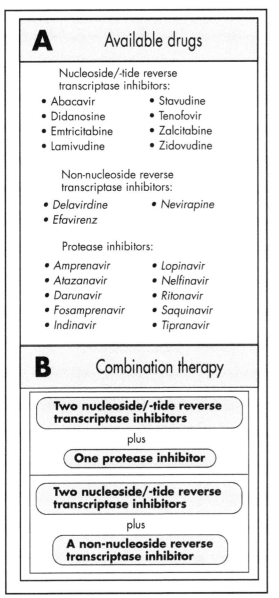

A   Available drugs

Nucleoside/-tide reverse
transcriptase inhibitors:
- Abacavir
- Didanosine
- Emtricitabine
- Lamivudine
- Stavudine
- Tenofovir
- Zalcitabine
- Zidovudine

Non-nucleoside reverse
transcriptase inhibitors:
- Delavirdine
- Efavirenz
- Nevirapine

Protease inhibitors:
- Amprenavir
- Atazanavir
- Darunavir
- Fosamprenavir
- Indinavir
- Lopinavir
- Nelfinavir
- Ritonavir
- Saquinavir
- Tipranavir

B   Combination therapy

Two nucleoside/-tide reverse
transcriptase inhibitors

plus

One protease inhibitor

Two nucleoside/-tide reverse
transcriptase inhibitors

plus

A non-nucleoside reverse
transcriptase inhibitor

Figure 10.17: Drugs available for the treatment of human immunodeficiency virus (HIV) and acquired immunodeficiency syndrome (AIDS). A: These are the available agents and the class they belong in. B: Shows the combinations of drug classes that constitute highly active antiretroviral therapy (HAART).

Zidovudine is used to prevent transmission of HIV from mother to child during birth. Nevirapine has recently been shown to have a similar effect and may be a substitute for this purpose.

Maraviroc, a very recently approved drug, represents a new drug class for treating HIV and AIDS. It is currently approved for use in HIV infections resistant to multiple antiviral drugs.

■ MECHANISM OF ACTION

Nucleoside and nucleotide reverse transcriptase inhibitors (NRTIs) act by creating an **analog** of a normal constituent of RNA. These have a greater affinity for viral reverse transcriptase than host DNA polymerases. Reverse transcriptase is an enzyme necessary to convert double-stranded RNA into DNA so that the host cell's normal DNA replication mechanisms can be utilized. When the analogs of normal RNA are incorporated into the elongating chain of DNA, it prevents further elongation of the chain and stops viral DNA and RNA reproduction. Without this, viral reproduction is unsuccessful.

> **Analog:** A drug or other chemical that is similar in structure or constituents to another but differs in effects

> **Virions:** A rudimentary viral particle that includes a capsid, protein sheath, and a central nucleoid

Non-nucleoside reverse transcriptase inhibitors act by binding to HIV-1 reverse transcriptase near its active site and inhibiting its action. They are synergistic with NRTIs.

Protease inhibitors act by inhibiting aspartyl protease. This enzyme is responsible for cleaving the viral polyprotein, which contains many proteins necessary for the proper functioning and reproduction of HIV including reverse transcriptase, protease, integrase, and several structural proteins. When the enzyme is inhibited these proteins are not able to be in their active states. This prevents the maturation of viral particles and produces noninfective **virions**. The protease inhibitors work on both HIV-1 and HIV-2. They have at least a thousand fold greater affinity for HIV aspartyl protease as comparable to human enzymes.

Figure 10.18 on the next page summarizes these 3 classes of HIV drugs and places them in the context of the HIV life cycle. Maraviroc is the first of a new class of drugs known as CCR5 co-receptor blockers or antagonists. The CCR5 co-receptor on the CD-4 T-cell helps the virus enter the immune cells. By blocking the co-receptor it prevents the HIV from entering the cell. Approximately 50-60% of HIV type 1 patients

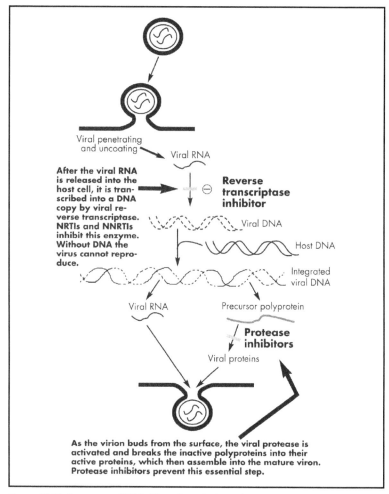

After the viral RNA is released into the host cell, it is transcribed into a DNA copy by viral reverse transcriptase. NRTIs and NNRTIs inhibit this enzyme. Without DNA the virus cannot reproduce.

Viral penetrating and uncoating

Viral RNA

Reverse transcriptase inhibitor

Viral DNA

Host DNA

Integrated viral DNA

Viral RNA

Precursor polyprotein

Protease inhibitors

Viral proteins

As the virion buds from the surface, the viral protease is activated and breaks the inactive polyproteins into their active proteins, which then assemble into the mature viron. Protease inhibitors prevent this essential step.

Figure 10.18: Summary of HIV's life cycle and where drugs act on it.

Pinocytosis: A method of absorption for a cell where it indents and encloses an external area and internalizes it

Pro-analog: A drug or other chemical that after metabolism is similar in structure or constituents to another but differs in effects

the virus by **pinocytosis** and the virus begins to shed its membrane exposing its genes to the host cell. The M2 ion channels help create a more acidic environment that facilitates this uncoating, a necessary step in the virus's life cycle.

All of the herpesvirus agents, acyclovir, valacyclovir, famciclovir, ganciclovir, and valganciclovir, act in similar ways. They all inhibit DNA polymerase, an enzyme necessary for the normal DNA and RNA reproduction of these viruses. They inhibit it by either being a direct analog or a **pro-analog** of a normal DNA constituent that gets incorporated into the growing DNA chain but prevents further elongation of the chain.

Lamivudine is a competitive inhibitor of HBV DNA polymerase, the necessary enzyme for DNA reproduction, at levels well below those necessary to disrupt human DNA polymerase. It also inhibits HIV reverse transcriptase, an enzyme necessary to convert double-stranded RNA into DNA so that the host cell's normal DNA replication mechanisms can be utilized. Adefovir and entecavir act in a similar way in that they are DNA constituents that are incorporated into DNA and prevent further DNA reproduction of HBV.

Oseltamivir, a neuraminidase inhibitor, acts on influenzae type A and B viruses. These viruses place a specific enzyme, a neuraminidase, into the host's cell membrane in order to facilitate newly reproduced virions to exit the cell. This agent specifically inhibits this enzyme and prevents the virion from exiting. They accumulate at the internal surface of the infected cell.

Ribavarin's mode of action is understood in relation to how it treats influenza viruses. It acts by inhibiting GTP formation, preventing mRNA capping and blocking RNA-dependent RNA polymerase. Capping of the mRNA is a necessary step in mRNA production. RNA-dependent RNA polymerase is a necessary enzyme in reproducing mRNA; blocking it prevents reproduction.

■ **DOSAGES**

ABACAVIR, for *children*, 3 months to 16 years, 8

who have not responded to other treatments have the CCR5 co-receptor.

Integrase inhibitors are a relatively new class of anti-HIV drugs. Integrase is a viral enzyme necessary for retroviral DNA to integrate into the host cell's chromosomes. By inhibiting it, these drugs prevent translation into mRNA (preventing protein synthesis) and RNA transcription (preventing RNA genomes in new viral particles).

The adamantine derivatives, amantidine and rimantidine, are inhibitors of viral uncoating. They block the viral membrane protein M2, an ion channel necessary for fusion of the viral membrane with the host cell's membrane. Uncoating happens after the host cell absorbs

mg/kg body weight bid to a maximum 300 mg bid combined with other antiretroviral agents. For *adults*, 300 mg bid or 600 mg once daily combined with other antiretroviral agents.

ACYCLOVIR, for *children*, for genital HSV, initial episode, 40-80 mg/kg/d in 3-4 doses for 5-10 days up to maximum 1 g/d. For *children* 2 years and over and 40 kg or less, for varicella-zoster (chicken pox), begin treatment within the first 24 hours of rash onset, 20 mg/kg/dose (up to 800 mg) qid for 5 days. For *children* over 40 kg and *adults*, for varicella-zoster (chicken pox), begin treatment within the first 24 hours of rash onset, 800 mg/dose qid for 5 days. For *adults*, for genital HSV, initial episode, 200 mg every 4 hours while awake (5 times/d) for 10 days (per manufacturer's labeling); 400 mg tid for 5-10 days has also been reported; for recurrence, 200 mg every 4 hours while awake (5 times/d) for 5 days (per manufacturer's labeling; begin at earliest signs of disease;, 400 mg tid for 5 days has also been reported; for chronic suppression, 400 mg bid or 200 mg 3-5 times/d for up to 12 months followed by reevaluation (per manufacturer's labeling); 400-1200 mg/d in 2-3 divided doses has also been reported; for herpes zoster (shingles), 800 mg every 4 hours (5 times/d) for 7-10 days; for mucocutaneous HSV in the immunocompromised, 400 mg 5 times a day for 7-14 days; for prevention of HSV reactivation in HIV-positive patients, use only when recurrences are frequent or severe, 200 mg tid or 400 mg bid.

ADEFOVIR, for *adults*, 10 mg once daily.

ATAZANAVIR, for *adolescents* 16 and over and *adults*, for antiretroviral-naive patients, 400 mg once daily; administer with food; for antiretroviral-experienced patients, 300 mg once daily plus ritonavir 100 mg once daily; administer with food.

BOCEPREVIR, for *adults*, for treatment of chronic hepatitis C (CHC), 800 mg tid (in combination with peginterferon alfa and ribavirin).

DARUNAVIR, for *adults*, 600 mg bid with meals.

DELAVIRDINE, for *adolescents* 16 and older and *adults*, 400 mg tid.

DIDANOSINE, for *children* 2 weeks to 8 months, for treatment of HIV infection, administer on an empty stomach; 100 mg/m^2 bid is recommended by the manufacturer; 50 mg/m^2 may be considered in *infants* 2 weeks to 4 months. For *children* over 8 months, for treatment of HIV infection, administer on an empty stomach 120 mg/m^2 bid; usual dosing range is 90-150 mg/m^2 bid; patients with CNS disease may require higher dose. For *adolescents* and *adults*, for treatment of HIV infection, administer on an empty stomach; dosing based on patient weight: under 60 kg 125 mg bid or 250 mg once daily; over 60 kg 200 mg bid or 400 mg once daily. For delayed-release capsule (Videx® EC), under 60 kg, 250 mg once daily; over 60 kg, 400 mg once daily.

DOCOSANOL, for *children* 12 years and older and *adults*, for herpes simplex of the face or lips, topical: apply 5 times/d to affected area of face or lips, starting at first sign of cold sore or fever blister and continuing until healed.

DOLUTEGRAVIR, for *adults* and *children* 12 years or older and over 40 kg, 50 mg once daily.

EFAVIRENZ, dosing at bedtime is recommended to limit central nervous system effects; not to be used as single-agent therapy. For *children* 3 years and over, dose is based on body weight: 10-15 kg, 200 mg once daily; 15-20 kg, 250 mg once daily; 20-25 kg, 300 mg once daily; 25 to under 32.5 kg, 350 mg once daily; 32.5 to under 40 kg: 400 mg once daily; 40 kg or over, 600 mg once daily. For *adults*, 600 mg once daily.

ELVITEGRAVIR, used only in combination with other drugs.

EMTRICITABINE, for *children* 3 months to 17 years, capsule: for *children* over 33 kg, 200 mg once daily; solution: 6 mg/kg once daily up to a maximum 240 mg/d. For *adults*, capsule; 200 mg once daily; solution: 240 mg once daily.

ENTECAVIR, for *adolescents* 16 or over and *adults*, for the nucleoside-treatment naïve, 0.5 mg daily; for lamivudine-resistant viremia (or known lamivudine-resistant mutations), 1 mg/d.

ETRAVIRINE, for treatment of HIV-1 infection, for *children* 6 to under 18 years, 16 kg and over to under 20 kg, 100 mg bid; 20 kg to under 25 kg, 125 mg bid; 25 kg to under 30 kg, 150 mg bid; 30 kg and over, 200 mg bid; for *adults*, 200 mg bid.

FAMCICLOVIR, for *adults*, for acute herpes zoster, 500 mg every 8 hours for 7 days; initiate within 72 hours of rash onset; for recurrent genital herpes simplex in immunocompetent patients, initiate at 1000 mg bid for 1 day; initiate within 6 hours of symptoms/lesions\; continue with 250 mg bid for up to 1 year; for recurrent herpes labialis (cold sores), 1500 mg as a single dose; initiate therapy at first sign or symptom such as tingling, burning, or itching; for recurrent mucocutaneous/genital herpes simplex in HIV patients, 500 mg bid for 7 days.

FOSAMPRENAVIR, for *adults*, for HIV infection, in antiretroviral-therapy-naive patients, 1400 mg bid.

GANCICLOVIR, for CMV retinitis, 1000 mg tid with food or 500 mg 6 times/d with food; for prevention of CMV disease in patients with advanced HIV infection and normal renal function, 1000 mg tid with food; for prevention of CMV disease in transplant patients, same initial and maintenance dose as CMV retinitis except duration of initial course is 7-14 days; duration of maintenance therapy is dependent on clinical condition and degree of immunosuppression.

INDINAVIR, for *adults*, 800 mg every 8 hours.

LAMIVUDINE, for HIV, for *infants* 1-3 months, 4 mg/kg bid; for *infants* and *children* 3 months to 16 years, 4 mg/kg bid up to a maximum of 150 mg bid; for *children* 16 years and older and *adults*, 150 mg bid or 300 mg once daily.

LOPINAVIR, used only in combination with other drugs, and therefore its individual dosing is not covered here.

MARAVIROC, dosage is dependent on what other medications are prescribed with it. When given with strong CYP3A inhibitors (with or without CYP3A inducers) including protease inhibitors (except tipranavir/ritonavir), delavirdine, ketoconazole, itraconazole, and/or clarithromycin, 150 mg bid; with NRTIs, tipranavir/ritonavir, nevirapine, and other drugs that are not strong CYP3A inhibitors or CYP3A inducers, 300 mg bid; with CYP3A inducers including efavirenz, rifampin, carbamazepine, phenobarbital, and phenytoin (without a strong CYP3A inhibitor), 600 mg bid.

NELFINAVIR, for *children* 2-13 years, 45-55 mg/kg bid or 25-35 mg/kg tid up to a maximum of 2500 mg/d; all doses should be taken with a meal. For *adults*, 750 mg tid with meals or 1250 mg bid with meals in combination with other antiretroviral therapies.

NEVIRAPINE, for *children* 2 months to under 8 years, initiate at 4 mg/kg once daily for 14 days; increase to 7 mg/kg every 12 hours if no rash or other adverse effects occur; maximum dose is 200 mg every 12 hours. For *children* 8 and older, initiate at 4 mg/kg once daily for 14 days; increase to 4 mg/kg every 12 hours if no rash or other adverse effects occur; maximum 200 mg every 12 hours. For *adults*, initiate at 200 mg once daily for 14 days; maintenance dose is 200 mg bid (in combination with an additional antiretroviral agent). If patient experiences a rash during the 14-day lead-in period, do not increase dose until the rash resolves; discontinue if severe rash or rash with constitutional symptoms is noted. For prevention of maternal-fetal HIV transmission in women with no prior antiretroviral therapy (AIDS information guidelines), *mother*: 200 mg as a single dose at onset of labor; may be combined with zidovudine; *Infant*: 2 mg/kg as single dose at age 48-72 hours. if maternal dose was given under 1 hour prior to delivery, administer 2 mg/kg dose as soon as possible after birth; repeat at 48-72 hours. May combine with zidovudine.

OSELTAMIVIR, initiate treatment within 2 days of onset of symptoms; duration of treatment is 5 days. For *children*: 1-12 years, under 15 kg, 30 mg bid; over 15 kg to under 23 kg, 45 mg bid;

over 23 kg to under 40 kg, 60 mg bid; over 40 kg, 75 mg bid. For *adolescents* 13 or older and *adults*, 75 mg bid. For prophylaxis, initiate treatment within 2 days of contact with an infected individual; duration of treatment is 10 days; for *children* 1-12 years, 15 kg or over, 30 mg bid; over 15 kg to under 23 kg, 45 mg bid; over 23 kg to less than 40 kg, 60 mg bid; over 40 kg, 75 mg bid; for *adolescents* 13 years or older and *adults*, 75 mg once daily.

PENCICLOVIR, for *children* 12 years and older and *adults*, for herpes simplex labialis (cold sores), topical: apply cream at the first sign or symptom of cold sore and every 2 hours during waking hours for 4 days.

RALTEGRAVIR, for *children* 2-12 years, chewable tablets: 0 to 13 kg, 75 mg bid; 14 to 19 kg, 100 mg bid, 20 to 27 kg, 150 mg bid; 28 to 39 kg, 200 mg bid; 40 kg or over, 300 mg bid. For *adults* and *children* 6 years and older and over 25 kg, film-coated tablets: 400 mg bid.

RIBAVIRIN, for *children* 3 years or older, for chronic hepatitis C (combined with interferon alfa-2b), 7.5 mg/kg bid (morning/evening); dosing recommendations: 25-36 kg, 400 mg/d (200 mg morning and evening); 37-49 kg: 600 mg/d (200 mg morning and two 200 mg capsules evening), 50-61 kg: 800 mg/d (two 200 mg capsules morning and evening), over 61 kg: use adult dosing; duration of therapy is 48 weeks in pediatric patients with genotype 1 and 24 weeks in patients with genotype 2 or 3; discontinue treatment in any patient if HCV-RNA is not below the limit of detection of the assay after 24 weeks therapy. For *adults* using the oral capsule (Rebetol®, Ribasphere™), for chronic hepatitis C (combined with interferon alfa-2b), 75 kg or less: 400 mg morning, then 600 mg evening; over 75 kg: 600 mg morning, then 600 mg evening; for chronic hepatitis C (combined with peginterferon alfa-2b), 400 mg bid; dur-ation of therapy 1 year; after 24 weeks treatment, if serum HCV-RNA is not below limit of detection of the assay, consider discontinuation. For *adults* using oral tablet (Copegus® combined with peginterferon

alfa-2b), for chronic hepatitis C, monoinfection, genotype 1 or 4, 75 kg or less: 500 mg/d bid for 48 weeks; over 75 kg: 600 mg/d bid for 48 weeks; for monoinfection, genotype 2 or 3, 400 mg/d bid for 24 weeks; for coinfection with HIV, 400 mg/d bid for 48 weeks.

RILPIVIRINE, for *adults*, for treatment of HIV-1 infection, 25 mg once daily.

RIMANTADINE, for *children* 1-10 years or under 40 kg, for prophylaxis, 2.5 mg/kg/d bid; maximum is 150 mg/d. For *children* over 10 and *adults*, for prophylaxis, 100 mg bid. For *adults*, for treatment, 100 mg bid. For the *elderly*, for prophylaxis, 100 mg/d in nursing home patients or all elderly patients who may experience adverse effects using the adult dose; for treatment, 100 mg once daily in patients 65 or older.

RITONAVIR, for *children* over 1 month, 350-400 mg/m^2 bid up to maximum 600 mg bid; initiate at 250 mg/m^2 bid; increase dose upward every 2-3 days by 50 mg/m^2 bid. For *adults*, 600 mg bid; dose escalation tends to avoid nausea that many patients experience upon initiation of full dosing; increase dose as follows: 300 mg bid for 1 day, 400 mg bid for 2 days, 500 mg bid for 1 day, then 600 mg bid.

SAQUINAVIR, for *children* 16 years or older and *adults*, Fortovase® and Invirase® are not bioequivalent and should not be used interchangeably. Use only Fortovase® to initiate therapy: 1200 mg (six 200 mg capsules) tid or 1600 mg bid within 2 hours after a meal combined with a nucleoside analog.

STAVUDINE, for *newborns*, 0.5 mg/kg every 12 hours. For *children* over 14 days and under 30 kg, 1 mg/kg every 12 hours; over 30 kg, use adult dosing. For *adults* over 60 kg, 40 mg every 12 hours; under 60 kg, 30 mg every 12 hours.

TELAPREVIR, for *adults*, for treatment of chronic hepatitis C (CHC), 750 mg tid (in combination with peginterferon alfa and ribavirin).

TELBIVUDINE, for *adolescents* 16 years and over and *adults*, 600 mg once daily.

TENOFOVIR, for HIV infection, for *children* 2 to

under 12 years, 8 mg/kg once daily up to a maximum of 300 mg once daily, in combination with other antiretrovirals; for *children* 12 years and older and *adults*, 300 mg once daily, in combination with other antiretrovirals; for hepatitis B infection, for *children* 12 years and older and *adults*, 300 mg once daily.

TIPRANAVIR, for *adults*, 500 mg bid with a high-fat meal.

VALACYCLOVIR, for *adolescents* and *adults*, for herpes labialis (cold sores), 2 g bid for 1 day (separate doses by 12 hours). For *adults*, for herpes zoster (shingles), 1 g tid for 7 days; for genital herpes, initial episode, 1 g bid for 10 days; for recurrent episodes, 500 mg bid for 3 days; for reduction of transmission, 500 mg once daily; for suppressive therapy, 1000 mg once daily (500 mg once daily in patients with less than 9 recurrences per year); for suppression in HIV-infected patients (CD4 ≥100 cells/mm^3), 500 mg bid.

VALGANCICLOVIR, for *adults*, for CMV retinitis, initiate at 900 mg bid for 21 days (with food); maintain at a recommended dose of 900 mg once daily (with food); for prevention of CMV disease following transplantation, 900 mg once daily (with food) beginning within 10 days of transplantation; continue therapy until 100 days post-transplantation.

ZANAMIVIR, for influenzae A and B, for *children* 5 and older and *adults*, for prophylaxis in the household setting, two inhalations (10 mg) once daily for 10 days; for *adolescents* and *adults*, for prophylaxis of a community outbreak, two inhalations (10 mg) once daily for 28 days, beginning within 5 days of outbreak; for *children* 7 years and older and *adults*, for treatment, two inhalations (10 mg total) bid for 5 day;, doses on first day should be separated by at least 2 hours and on subsequent days by approximately 12 hours; begin within 2 days of signs or symptoms; longer treatment may be considered for

patients who remain severely ill after 5 days.

ZIDOVUDINE, for prevention of maternal-fetal HIV transmission: for *neonates*, dosing should begin 8-12 hours after birth and continue for the first 6 weeks of life; for *full-term infants*, 2 mg/kg every 6 hours; for *infants* over 30 weeks and under 35 weeks gestation at birth, 2 mg/kg every 12 hours; at 2 weeks of age, advance to 2 mg/kg every 8 hours; for *infants* under 30 weeks gestation at birth, 2 mg/kg every 12 hours; at 4 weeks advance to 2 mg/kg every 8 hours; maternal: 100 mg 5 times/d or 200 mg tid or 300 mg bid; begin at 14-34 weeks gestation and continue until start of labor. For *children* 6 weeks to 12 years for treatment of HIV infection, 160 mg/m^2/dose every 8 hours up to a maximum of 200 mg every 8 hours. For *adults*, 300 mg bid or 200 mg tid.

ADVERSE EFFECTS

HIV protease inhibitors commonly cause nausea and vomiting, **paresthesias**, and diarrhea. Glucose and lipid metabolism may occur resulting in diabetes, **hypertriglyceridemia**, and hypercholesterolemia. Long-term use may cause fat redistribution that includes loss of fat from the extremities, accumulation in the abdomen and the lower part of the neck ("buffalo hump"), and enlarged breasts.

Abacavir commonly causes GI disturbances, headache, and dizziness. More rarely, it can cause **drug fever**, malaise and a rash.

Acyclovir can cause headache, diarrhea, nausea, and vomiting. At high doses, renal dysfunction may occur.

Adefovir and entecavir should be used with caution in patients with renal dysfunction. Patients who have terminated entecavir should be monitored for several months because of the possibility of severe hepatitis.

Amprenavir can cause nausea and vomiting, diarrhea, paresthesias, fatigue, and headaches.

Atazanavir may cause jaundice and slow the heart rate.

Darunavir commonly causes GI disturbances, **nasopharyngitis**, and **neutropenia**.

Paresthesias: Numbness and tingling

Hypertriglyceridemia: Abnormally high amounts of triglycerides in the blood

---

Drug fever: A fever associated with the use of a drug. This can be caused by an immune reaction, the inherent effects of the drug, or a complication.

Nasopharyngitis: Inflammation or infection of the nose and throat

---

Neutropenia: A reduction in the number of neutrophils, one type of immune cell, in the blood

Delavirdine can cause a rash, nausea, dizziness, and headache.

Didanosine and stavudine can cause peripheral neuropathy at high doses.

Nearly one-half of those on efavirenz had dizziness, headache, vivid dreams, and loss of concentration, but these adverse effects usually resolved within weeks. Developing a rash is also very common. Women should not become pregnant while taking this agent.

Emtricitabine can cause headache, diarrhea, rash, nausea, and hyperpigmentation of the palms and soles. It may cause lactic **acidosis**, **hepatomegaly**, and fatty liver. HBV patients may see a worsening of the condition when this agent is withdrawn.

Famciclovir can cause headaches and nausea. Animal studies have shown an increased incidence of **adenocarcinomas** and testicular toxicity.

Fosamprenavir commonly causes headache, fatigue, rash, and GI disturbances.

Ganciclovir and valganciclovir can cause GI upset and severe, dose-dependent neutropenia. They have been shown to be carcinogenic, **embryotoxic**, and **teratogenic** in animals.

Indinavir is generally well tolerated but can cause headache and GI disturbances. It also causes **nephrolithiasis**, which can be minimized by drinking adequate water, and **hyperbilirubinemia**. The fat redistribution of protease inhibitors is particularly bothersome with this agent.

Lamivudine rarely causes headache and dizziness.

Lopinavir is generally well tolerated, with GI issues being the most common adverse effect.

Maraviroc had the following common adverse effects: cough, fever, upper respiratory tract infections, rash, musculoskeletal symptoms, abdominal pain, and dizziness. It can possibly increase risk of myocardial infarction and is hepatotoxic.

Nelfinavir commonly causes diarrhea which can be controlled by loperamide.

Nevirapine can cause headache, fever, rash, and elevated liver enzymes. **Stevens-Johnson syndrome** and toxic epidermal necrolysis have also

been reported. These serious epidermal reactions can be minimized by using a half-dose for 14 days prior to increasing to a full dose.

Oseltamivir commonly causes GI discomfort, which can be alleviated by taking it with food.

Ribavarin has been reported to cause elevated bilirubin and dose-dependent transient anemia. It is contraindicated for use during pregnancy.

Rimantidine can cause gastrointestinal intolerance and should be used with caution in pregnant and breast-feeding women.

Ritonavir may cause nausea and vomiting, diarrhea, **asthenia**, headache, and **circumoral** paresthesia.

Saquinavir can cause fatigue, headache, diarrhea, nausea, and other GI disturbances. Elevated liver enzymes have been reported especially in patients with hepatitis B or C.

Telbivudine can cause fatigue, headache, diarrhea, nausea, and other GI disturbances. Elevated liver enzymes have been reported.

Tenofovir commonly causes nausea, vomiting and diarrhea.

Tipranavir causes diarrhea, nausea, and transaminase increases.

Valacyclovir can cause GI distress and thrombotic **thrombocytopenia** purpura in AIDS patients.

Zidovudine commonly causes headaches. At high doses, this agent is toxic to bone marrow and may cause severe anemia and **leukopenia**. Seizures have been reported when taken by patients with advanced AIDS.

▨ RED FLAGS

With the exception of lamivudine and abacavir, NRTIs have been associated with potentially fatal liver conditions characterized by lactic acidosis,

Acidosis: Abnormal increase in hydrogen ions in the body

Hepatomegaly: Abnormal enlargement of the liver

Adenocarcinoma: A cancer stemming from the epithelium of a gland

Embryotoxic: A substance that causes detrimental effects in embryos

Teratogen: A substance that causes congenital defects in fetuses

Nephrolithiasis: A disorder of calculi or stones, in the kidney

Hyperbilirubinemia: A condition of too much of the bile pigment bilirubin in the blood

Stevens-Johnson syndrome: A serious, often fatal inflammatory disease, potentially caused by an allergic reaction to a drug. Symptoms include fever, skin lesions, and mucous membrane ulcers.

Asthenia: The lack or loss of strength or energy; weakness; debility

Circumoral: Around the mouth

Thrombocytopenia: A decreased number of platelets in the blood

Stomatitis: An inflammation and/or infection of the mouth

Leukopenia: A decreased number of white blood cells in the blood; defined as fewer than 5,000 cells per cubic millimeter

hepatomegaly, and steatosis, fatty transformation.

When taking abacavir, sensitized individuals are never reintroduced because of rapid, severe, and fatal reactions.

Didanosine and zalcitabine may cause fatal pancreatitis, and serum amylase should be monitored on a regular basis. This effect can be exacerbated by using pentamidine with zalcitabine.

Maraviroc is hepatotoxic.

Nevirapine has caused fatal liver pathology, and liver enzymes should be monitored closely for the first 6 months of therapy.

The FDA has required a new black box warning for tipranavir. There have been 14 reports of tipranavir coadministered with ritonavir causing intracranial hemorrhage. Of these, 8 reports involved fatalities. Other medications and conditions were also involved and may have caused the hemorrhage.

INTERACTIONS

DRUG

HIV protease inhibitors are strong inhibitors of CYP. Because this may cause toxic levels, the following drugs should not be used at the same time: midazolam, triazolam, warfarin, and fentanyl. Strong inducers of CYP may cause failure of HIV protease inhibitor; therefore, the following drugs should not be combined: rifampin, barbiturates, and carbamazepine. Quinidine and the ergot derivatives are also contraindicated.

Delavirdine inhibits CYP metabolism and significantly increases levels of saquinavir and indinavir. Plasma levels of delavirdine are increased by fluoxetine and ketoconazole, while phenytoin, phenobarbital, and carbamazepine decrease plasma levels.

Didanosine should not be used with zalcitabine due to similar toxicities and adverse effects.

Efavirenz is a modest inducer of CY, and the dose of indinavir may need to be increased when coadministered.

Maraviroc has numerous drug-drug interactions that are taken into account when determining dosing. See dosing above for more specific information.

Nevirapine is an inducer of CYP3A4 and can increase the metabolism of oral contraceptives, ketoconazole, methadone, metronidazole, quinidine, theophylline, and warfarin. It should not be used with saquinavir.

Saquinavir should not be taken with the following: rifabutin, nevirapine, efavirenz, and other enzyme inducers. These agents could enhance the metabolism of saquinavir and lower its levels.

Zalcitabine should not be used with lamivudine.

Zidovudine should not be taken with probenecid, acetaminophen, loazepam, indomethacin, and cimetidine as they can potentiate the toxic effects by competing with the glucoronylation process. Since zidovudine acts by the same pathways as staudine and ribavarin, they should not be coadministered.

HERB

ACYCLOVIR

- *Huang Qi* (Astragulus) (D)–potentiates acyclovir's antiviral effects against herpes in mice (Upton, 1999) Level 5 evidence.

INDINAVIR

- *Guan Ye Lian Qiao* (St. John's wort) (B-)–was found to decrease the effectiveness of indinavir in a small human study (Piscitelli, Burstein, Chaitt, Alfaro & Falloon, 2000) Level 2c evidence. (Zhou, Chan, Pan, Huang & Lee, 2004) Level 3b evidence.
- *Guan Ye Lian Qiao* (St. John's wort, hypericum) (D)–may induce the cytochrome P450 system and increase metabolism and reduce plasma concentration of several drugs including digoxin, desogestrel, ethinyloestradiol, cyclosporine, indinavir, theophyline, and phenprocoumon, expert opinion (Fugh-Berman, 2000) Level 5 evidence.

MARAVIROC

- *Guan Ye Lian Qiao* (St. John's Wort, hypericum) (D)–concomitant use of maraviroc and St. John's wort is not recommended as it may substantially decrease maraviroc concentrations and may result in suboptimal levels of maraviroc and lead to loss action and possible resistance to maraviroc, expert opinion (Pfizer Labs, 2007) Level 5 evidence.

NEVIRAPINE

• *Guan Ye Lian Qiao* (St. John's wort) (C)–decreases blood concentrations. (Zhou, Chan, Pan, Huang & Lee, 2004) Level 3b evidence.

RALTEGRAVIR

• *Ren Shen* (Ginseng) (C)–a case study showed raised plasma levels of raltegravir 30 days after starting *ren shen* supplementation that tapered off after stopping supplementation (Mateo-Carrasco, Gálvez-Contreras, Fernández-Ginés, Nguyen, 2012) Level 4 evidence.

RITONAVIR

• *Guan Ye Lian Qiao* (St. John's wort) (C)–decreases blood concentrations. (Izzo & Ernst, 2009) Level 2b evidence.

SAQUINAVIR

• *Da Suan* (Garlic) (C)–decreased the area under the plasma concentration-time curve (AUC) and maximum plasma concentration of saquinavir (Hu, Yang, Ho, Chan *et. al.* 2005) Level 2b evidence.

PROTEASE INHIBITORS

• *Da Suan* (Garlic) (D)–may induce increased metabolism of protease inhibitors by inducing cytochrome P450 3A4. Human studies on individual protease inhibitors showed no interference except when large doses of *Da Suan* were used in combination with saquinavir in a small human study (Piscitelli, Burstein, Welden *et. al.,* 2002) Level 3b evidence.

• *Guan Ye Lian Qiao* (St. John's wort, hypericum) (D)–may interfere with metabolism of HIV protease inhibitors, and concurrent use is contraindicated, expert opinion (Howland & Mycek, 2006) Level 5 evidence.

INTERACTION ISSUES

A:

D: Delavirdine is approximately 98% protein bound; darunavir is approximately 95% bound; efavirenz is over 99% bound, etravirine is 99.9% bound; lopinavir is 98-99% bound; nelfinavir is over 98% bound; rilpivirine is 99.7% bound; ritonavir is 98-99% bound; saquinavir is approximately 98% bound; tyipranavir is over 99% bound.

M: Atazanavir, boceprevir, and darunavir are major substrates and strong inhibitors of CYP3A4; delavirdine is a major substrate of CYP3A4 and a strong inhibitor of 2C9, 2C19, 2D6, and 3A4; efavirenz is a major substrate of CYP2B6 and 3A4, a moderate inhibitor of 2C9, 2C19, and 3A4, a weak or moderate inducer of 2B6, and a strong inducer of 3A4; etravirine is a major substrate and a moderate inhibitor of CYP2C9 and 2C19 and a major substrate and strong inducer of 3A4; fosamprenavir and indinavir are major substrates and strong inhibitors of CYP3A4; maraviroc is a major substrate of CYP3A4; nelfinavir is a major substrate of CYP2C19 and 3A4 and a strong inhibitor of 3A4; nevirapine is a major substrate of CYP3A4 and a strong inducer of 2B6 and 3A4; rilpivirine is a major substrate of CYP3A4; ritonavir is a major substrate of CYP3A4, a strong inhibitor 2C8, 2D6, and 3A4, and a weak or moderate inducer of 1A2, 2C9, and 3A4; saquinavir and telaprevir are major substrates and strong inhibitors of CYP3A4; tipranavir is a major substrate of CYP3A4 and a strong inhibitor of 2D6.

E:

Pgp: Boceprevir is a substrate and inhibitor of Pgp; darunavir inhibits Pgp; fosamprenavir, indinavir, and maraviroc are substrates of Pgp; nelfinavir, ritonavir, saquinavir, and telaprevir are substrates and inhibitors of Pgp; tenofovir induces Pgp; tipranavir induces PgP.

ENDNOTES

1 Combination of Amoxicillin and Clavulanate Potassium.

2 Combination of Amoxicillin, Lansoprazole, and Clarithromycin.

3 Combination of Erythromycin and Sulfisoxazole.

4 Combination of Bismuth, Metronidazole, and Tetracycline.

5 Combination of Pyrimethamine and Sulfadoxine.

6 Combination of Sulfamethoxazole and Trimethoprim.

7 Combination of Hyoscyamine, Methenamine, Sodium Biphosphate, Phenyl Salicylate, and Methylene Blue.

8 Combination of Methenamine and Sodium Acid Phosphate.

9 Folate and folic acid basically mean the same thing with folate being a salt of folic acid. For the purposes of this book, they will be used interchangeably.

10 Combination of Isoniazid, Rifampin, and Pyrazinamide.

11 Combination of Isoniazid and Rifampin.

12 Combnation of Betamethasone and Clotrimazole.

13 Combination of Atovaquone and Proguanil.

14 Combination of Abacavir and Lamivudine.

15 Combination of Abacavir, Lamivudine, and Zidovudine.

16 Combination of Efavirenz, Emtricitabine, and Tenofovir.

17 Combination of Emtricitabine and Tenofovir.

18 Combination of Lamivudine and Zidovudine.

19 Combination of Lopinavir and Ritonavir. Lopinavir is a protease inhibitor, just like ritonavir. It is only used in combination with ritonavir, never alone.

20 Combination of Amoxicillin, Omeprazole, and Clarithromycin

21 Combination of Penicillin G Benzathine and Penicillin G Procaine.

22 Combination of Erythromycin and Sulfisoxazole.

23 Combination of Ciprofloxacin and Dexamethasone.

24 Combination of Ciprofloxacin and Hydrocortisone.

25 Combination of Trimethoprim and Polymyxin B.

26 Combination of Methenamine, Phenyl Salicylate, Methylene Blue, Benzoic Acid, and Hyoscyamine.

27 Combination of Bacitracin and Polymyxin B.

28 Combination of Bacitracin, Neomycin, and Polymyxin B

29 Combination of Bacitracin, Neomycin, Polymyxin B, and Hydrocortisone.

30 Combination of Bacitracin, Neomycin, Polymyxin B, and Pramoxine.

31 Combination of Miconazole and Zinc Oxide.

32 Combination of Artemether and Lumefantrine.

33 Combination of Emtricitabine, Elvitegravir, Cobicistat, and Tenofovir

■ CHINESE MEDICAL DESCRIPTIONS

The Chinese medical explanation of the drug categories in this chapter may be found in Chapter 15 on pages 410-412.

Anticancer Agents

Cancer, it is estimated, will be diagnosed in 25% of the U.S. population. There are 1.3 million new cases diagnosed per year. Of those, 65% will survive past five years. That makes cancer the second-largest cause of death in the U.S. It is defined as a disease where there is unregulated cell growth with the potential for invasion of other tissues. Chemotherapy is used on approximately 70% of diagnosed cancers. Only about 10% of cases are resolved with chemotherapy alone with the rest using it to slow progression of the disease or as an adjunct to surgery or radiation therapy.

Although not possible in many cases, the goal in cancer treatment is a cure, defined as surviving the five-year point after diagnosis. Other treatment goals include disease control and palliation. Disease control is an attempt to both prolong and increase quality of life. When a cancer is beyond either cure or control, palliation becomes the goal, which is an attempt to relieve symptoms and improve quality of life where prolonging it is not likely.

Ideally, anticancer or antineoplastic agents would act only on cancer cells. While there are a number of new agents in testing that attempt to achieve this, most do not select between host cells and cancer cells. Many, but not all, attack all quickly reproducing cells, which minimizes harm to most cells in the body. Normally rapidly reproducing cells in the body include mouth mucosa, bone marrow, hair, and GI mucosa, which explains many side effects of anticancer agents. Most often, chemotherapy is used after a tumor is "debulked" by surgery or radiation therapy or when the **neoplasms** are disseminated. When used after surgery, it is called adjuvant chemotherapy. An attempt to shrink a tumor before surgery is called neoadjuvant chemotherapy.

Often more than one agent is used to treat cancer. These are often agents with no overlapping of effects and are used at full strength. Sometimes overlapping chemotherapy agents are used but at reduced dosages. Advantages of combining agents include providing maximal cell killing with tolerable toxicity, effectiveness against a broader range of cells and in heterogenous tumors, and possibly delaying development of resistance in cell lines.

As mentioned, chemotherapy agents work on rapidly growing cells. Technically this means cells in the G_0 phase are generally not susceptible to many anticancer agents. Those that work during a particular phase of the cell cycle are said to be cell-cycle specific (see Figure 11.1). Those that are not are called cell-cycle nonspecific and are useful against tumors with a low percentage of replicating cells.

Generally, tumors grow very rapidly initially and then slow. This is due to a lack of both oxygen and nutrients from a lack of vascularization and blood flow. Debulking a tumor can cause any remaining cells to become replicating and therefore more susceptible to chemotherapy.

Common problems with chemotherapy include resistance to the agents and toxicity. Resistance can be inherent to a specific type of cancer cell (such as in melanomas) or acquired through suboptimal drug levels. The best way to avoid resistance is to utilize short-term, intensive, and intermittent chemotherapy and to use multiple agents. One way multidrug resistance is created is through selection of cells expressing a gene producing P-glycoprotein (Pgp). Pgp is a transmembrane protein that uses adenosine triphosphate (ATP) to power the pumping of drugs from the inside to the outside of a particular cell. The end result is that not enough of an agent is available intracellularly to exert its effect.

Neoplasm: Any abnormal growth of new tissue, whether benign or malignant

315

Stomatitis: An inflammation and/or infection of the mouth

Alopecia: Partial or complete hair loss

Mutagen: An agent (environmental or physical) that causes, induces, or increases the rate of genetic mutation

Common toxicities involve the destruction of normal rapidly replicating cells in the body such as buccal mucosa, bone marrow, gastrointestinal mucosa, and hair follicles. This leads to common adverse effects such as severe vomiting, **stomatitis**, bone marrow suppression, and **alopecia**. Of course, specific agents have inherent toxic effects, which are explained under each of the sections in this chapter. There are methods to reduce adverse effects such as using antiemetic agents or cytoprotectant agents, perfusing a tumor locally as opposed to

systemically, or removing some bone marrow before the treatment and replacing it after.

Another problem with chemotherapy is that most agents are **mutagens**. Treatment-induced tumors are relatively common and may arise 10 years or more after the original cure. Alkylating agents are particularly prone to these tumors.

Cancer is not a monochromatic disease. In other words, most cancers have very little in common with one another. Therefore one agent will not work for every type of cancer. While all the agents in this chapter are antineoplastic, they are effective usually only on a handful of cancers.

SECTION 1: ALKYLATING AGENTS

BENDAMUSTINE (ben da MUS tene) PR=D (*Treanda®*)

BUSULFAN (byoo SUL fan) PR=D (*Busulfex®, Myleran®*)

CARBOPLATIN (KAR boe pla tin) PR=D

CARMUSTINE (kar MUS tene) PR=D (*BiCNU®, Gliadel Wafer®*)

CHLORAMBUCIL (klor AM byoo sil) PR=D (*Leukeran®*)

CISPLATIN (SIS pla tin) PR=D

CYCLOPHOSPHAMIDE (sye kloe FOS fa mide) PR=D

DACARBAZINE (da KAR ba zene) PR=C

ESTRAMUSTINE (es tra MUS tene) PR=N (*Emcyt®*)

IFOSFAMIDE (eye FOSS fa mide) PR=D (*Ifex®*)

LOMUSTINE (loe MUS tene) PR=D (*CeeNU®*)

MECHLORETHAMINE (me klor ETH a mene) PR=D (*Mustargen®*)

MELPHALAN (MEL fa lan) PR=D (*Alkeran®*)

OXALIPLATIN (ox AL i pla tin) PR=D (*Eloxatin®*)

PROCARBAZINE (proe KAR ba zene) PR=D (*Matulane®*)

STREPTOZOCIN (strep toe ZOE sin) PR=D (*Zanosar®*)

TEMOZOLOMIDE (te moe ZOE loe mide) PR=D (*Temodar®*)

THIOTEPA (thye oh TEP a) PR=D

Alkylating agents kill cells by covalently bonding to various cell constituents. DNA alkylation is most useful for tumor cytotoxicity. While they can be useful for both cycling and resting cells, they are most effective against rapidly dividing cells. All are mutagenic and carcinogenic and can increase the risk of secondary malignancies.

▓ FUNCTION

Bendamustine is used to treat many cancers including non-Hodgkin's lymphoma and chronic lymphocytic leukemia (CLL).

Busulfan is used to treat chronic granulocytic

leukemia.

Chlorambucil is used to treat multiple myeloma and chronic lymphocytic leukemia (CLL).

Carboplatin is primarily used in advanced ovarian cancers; however, it is used off label for treating various other cancers including bladder, breast, cervical, endometrial, esophageal, head and neck, Hodgkin's and non-Hodgkin's lymphoma, mesotheliomas, melanoma, small and nonsmall cell lung cancer, sarcomas, testicular, thymic, and unknown primary adenocarcinomas.

Carmustine is primarily used for brain tumors, Hodgkin's and non-Hodgkin's lymphoma, multiple myeloma, and gliomas, glioblastoma multiforme as well as off label for mycosis fungoides and stem cell or bone marrow transplants.

Cisplatin is primarily used in advanced bladder cancer, metastatic ovarian and testicular cancers, and off label in treating cervical, endometrial, head and neck, mesotheliomas, small cell and nonsmall cell lung cancers.

Cyclophosphamide can be used in a wide variety of cancers including Burkitt lymphoma and breast cancer as well as other diseases such as nephritic syndrome and intractable rheumatoid arthritis.

Dacarbazine is used to treat melanoma and Hodgkin's lymphoma but can also treat soft-tissue sarcomas, islet cell tumors, pheochromocytomas, and some carcinomas of the thyroid off label.

Estramustine is used in prostate cancer. Ifosfamide is used to treat testicular cancer but is also used off label for cervical, Hodgkin's and non-Hodgkin's lymphoma, Ewing sarcoma, osteosarcoma, and soft-tissue sarcoma cancers. Lomustine is used primarily in treating brain cancers given its ability to enter the CNS.

Mechlorethamine treats Hodgkin's and non-Hodgkin's lymphoma and pleaural or other malignant effusions. It can be used as an intercavity injection for treatment of a metastatic tumor. It is also used off label topically to treat mycoses fungsoides.

Melphalan is used to treat multiple myeloma and chronic lymphocytic leukemia (CLL).

Oxaliplatin is used to treat colorectal cancer and off label for esophageal, gastric, hepatobiliary, non-Hodgkin's lymphoma, ovarian, pancreatic, and testicular cancers.

Streptozocin is used on label for metastatic pancreatic islet cell carcinoma, off label for adrenal carcinoma.

Temozolomide is used to treat treatment-resistant gliomas and **anaplastic** astrocytomas in the brain.

Thiotepa is used to treat bladder cancer, palliation for breast or ovarian cancer, and for controlling effusions caused by metastatic cancers.

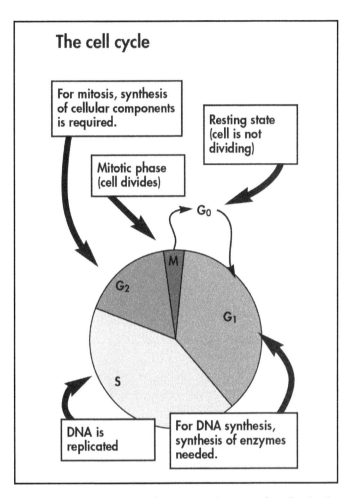

Figure 11.1 The cell cycle This figure shows the stages of a cell cycle. The G_0 phase is the resting state. Different cells will spend different amounts of time in the various stages. Many chemotherapy agents act on cells during specific stages.

MECHANISM OF ACTION

Alkylating agents act by adding a chemical side group to various molecules in the cell but especially DNA. An alkylation means to add a chemical group to another molecule.

Bendamustine, busulfan, chlorambucil, and melphalan inhibit DNA replication and RNA transcription by alkylating DNA.

Carboplatin, cisplatin, ifosfamide, mechlorethamine, oxaliplatin, streptozocin, and thiotepa cause crosslinking within strands of DNA and prevent its proper functioning.

Carmustine causes crosslinking in RNA as well as DNA and may inhibit enzyme reactions due to alkylation of amino acids in proteins.

Anaplasia: A condition where a cell changes its structure into a less differentiated, more primitive form; generally seen in malignancies

Cyclophosphamide is first converted to its active form by CYP. In its active form, it reacts with DNA and prevents normal DNA replication. The exact mechanism of action of estramustine is unknown, but its effects on prostate cancer are thought to occur solely by its estrogenic effect.

Lomustine acts by alkylating DNA and preventing its reproduction as well as the synthesis of RNA and proteins. The exact action of procarbazine is unknown but is thought to involve alkylation of DNA.

Temozolomide adds a methyl group to DNA and inhibits the DNA repair enzyme O6-guanine-DNA-alkyltransferase. It can cross the blood-brain barrier. Dacarbazine also methylates DNA.

DOSAGES

BENDAMUSTINE, for *adults*, for chronic lymphocytic leukemia (CLL), IV: 100 mg/m^2 over 30 minutes on days 1 and 2 of a 28-day treatment cycle for up to 6 cycles; for non-Hodgkin's refractory indolent B-cell lymphomas, IV: 120 mg/m^2 over 60 minutes on days 1 and 2 of a 21-day treatment cycle for up to 8 cycles.

BUSULFAN, for *children*, for remission induction of CML, 0.06-0.12 mg/kg/d or 1.8-4.6 mg/m^2/d; adjust dosage to maintain leukocyte count above 40,000/mm^3; reduce dosage by 50% if the leukocyte count reaches 30,000-40,000/mm^3; discontinue drug if counts fall to 20,000/mm^3 or lower; as a BMT marrow-ablative conditioning regimen, 1 mg/kg/dose (ideal body weight) every 6 hours for 16 doses. For *adults*, for remission induction of CML, 4-8 mg/d (may be as high as 12 mg/d); usual maintenance doses are 1-4 mg/d to 2 mg/wk to maintain WBC 10,000-20,000 cells/mm^3; as a BMT marrow-ablative conditioning regimen, 1 mg/kg/dose (ideal body weight) every 6 hours for 16 doses; for polycythemia vera (unlabeled use), 2-6 mg/d.

CARBOPLATIN, for *adults*, for advanced ovarian cancer, IV: 360 mg/m^2 every 4 weeks alone or 300 mg/m^2 every 4 weeks in combination with cyclophosphamide.

CARMUSTINE, for *adults*, for brain tumors, Hodgkin's and non-Hodgkin's lymphoma, or multiple myeloma, IV: 150-200 mg/m^2 every 6 weeks or 75-100 mg/m^2/d for 2 days every 6 weeks; for recurrent glioblastoma multiforme or newly diagnosed high-grade malignant glioma, implantation: 8 wafers placed in the resection cavity; total dose of 61.6 mg; if necessary due to size and/or shape restrictions of the resected area, fewer wafers can be used.

CHLORAMBUCIL, for *adults*, 0.1-0.2 mg/kg/d or 3-6 mg/m^2/d for 3-6 weeks, then adjust dose based on blood counts, or 0.4 mg/kg increased 0.1 mg/kg biweekly or monthly, or 14 mg/m^2/d for 5 days repeated every 21-28 days.

CISPLATIN, for *adults*, pretreatment hydration with 1-2 L of IV fluid is recommended; for advanced bladder cancer, IV: 50-70 mg/m^2 every 3-4 weeks; for metastatic ovarian cancer, IV: 100 mg/m^2 every 4 weeks; with other agents, 75-100 mg/m^2 every 4 weeks; for metastatic testicular cancer, IV: 20 mg/m^2/d for 5 days repeated every 3 weeks.

CYCLOPHOSPHAMIDE, for *children* and *adults*, 50-100 mg/m^2/d as continuous therapy or 400-1000 mg/m^2 in divided doses over 4-5 days as intermittent therapy; for nephrotic syndrome, 2-3 mg/kg/d every day for up to 12 weeks when corticosteroids are unsuccessful.

DACARBAZINE, for *children*, for Hodgkin's disease in combination chemotherapy, IV: 375 mg/m^2/dose days 1 and 15 every 4 weeks. For *adults*, for Hodgkin's disease in combination chemotherapy, IV: 375 mg/m^2/dose days 1 and 15 every 4 weeks; for metastatic melanoma, IV: 250 mg/m^2/dose days 1-5 every 3 weeks.

ESTRAMUSTINE, for *adults*, for prostate cancer, 10-16 mg/kg/d (14 mg/kg/d is most common) or 140 mg qid.

IFOSFAMIDE, for *adults*, to prevent bladder toxicity, should be given with the urinary protector mesna and hydration of at least 2 L of oral or IV fluid per day; for testicular cancer, IV: as part of combination chemotherapy and with mesna, 1200 mg/m^2/d for 5 days every 3 weeks or after hematologic recovery.

LOMUSTINE, for *children*, 75-150 mg/m^2 as a single dose every 6 weeks; subsequent doses readjusted after initial treatment based on platelet and leukocyte counts. For *adults*, 100-130 mg/m^2 as a single dose every 6 weeks; readjust after initial treatment based on platelet and leukocyte counts; for patients with compromised marrow function, initiate at 100 mg/m^2 as a single dose every 6 weeks; repeat courses to be administered only after adequate recovery.

MECHLORETHAMINE, for *adults*, for lymphoma, IV: 0.4 mg/kg as a single dose or in divided doses of 0.1 mg/kg/d (for 4 days) or 0.2 mg/kg/d (for 2 days) per treatment course; for intracavitary injection of metastatic tumors, 0.4 mg/kg as a single dose.

MELPHALAN, adjust dose to patient response and weekly blood counts. For *adults*, for multiple myeloma (multiple regimens have been employed), response is gradual; may require repeated courses; 6mg/d for 2-3 weeks initially, followed by up to 4 weeks rest, then maintenance dose 2 mg/d as hematologic recovery begins or 10 mg daily for 7-10 days, institute after WBC are more than 4000 cells/mcL and platelets over 100,000 cells/mcL (~4-8 weeks) and adjust to hematologic response or 0.15 mg/kg/d for 7 days, with a 2-6 week rest followed by a maintenance dose of 0.05 mg/kg/d or lower as hematologic recovery begins or 0.25 mg/kg/d for 4 days (or 0.2 mg/kg/d for 5 days); repeat at 4-6 week intervals as ANC and platelet counts return to normal; for ovarian carcinoma, 0.2 mg/kg/d for 5 days; repeat each 4-5 weeks.

OXALIPLATIN, for *adults*, for advanced colorectal cancer, IV: 85 mg/m^2 every 2 weeks until disease progression or unacceptable toxicity; should be used in combination with fluorouracil/leucovorin.

PROCARBAZINE, for *children*, for BMT aplastic anemia conditioning regimen, 12.5 mg/kg/d every other day for 4 doses; for Hodgkin's disease, 100 mg/m^2/d for 14 days, repeated every 4 weeks; for neuroblastoma and medulloblastoma; doses as high as 100-200 mg/m^2/d once daily have been used. For *adults*, initiate at 2-4 mg/kg/d in single or divided doses for 7 days, then increase to 4-6 mg/kg/d until response is obtained or leukocyte count decreases to under 4000/mm^3 or platelet count decreases to under 100,000/mm^3; maintenance dose is 1-2 mg/kg/d.

STREPTOZOCIN, for *adults*, for metastatic pancreatic islet cell carcinoma, IV: daily schedule: 500 mg/m^2/d for 5 consecutive days every 6 weeks until maximum benefit or unacceptable toxicity; weekly schedule: 1000 mg/m^2 once weekly; if therapeutic response not achieved after 2 weeks, may escalate to a maximum 1500 mg/m^2 per week.

TEMOZOLOMIDE, for *adults*, for anaplastic astrocytoma, initiate at 150 mg/m^2/d for 5 days; repeat every 28 days; subsequent doses of 100-200 mg/m^2/d for 5 days per treatment cycle; based upon hematologic tolerance, this monthly cycle regimen may be preceded by a 6-7 week regimen of 75 mg/m^2/d. For glioblastoma multiforme, concomitant phase, 75 mg/m^2/d for 42 days with radiotherapy.

THIOTEPA, for *adults*, for bladder cancer, intravesical: 60 mg in 30-60 mL retained for 2 hours once weekly for 4 weeks; for ovarian or breast cancer, IV: 0.3-0.4 mg/kg by rapid IV administration every 1-4 weeks; for effusions, intracavitary: 0.6-0.8 mg/kg.

ADVERSE EFFECTS

Common adverse effects of anticancer agents include severe vomiting, stomatitis, anorexia, diarrhea, and hair loss. Many suppress bone marrow. Treatment-induced neoplasms can occur many years after treatment. While this can happen with almost any agent, it is most prominent with alkylating agents.

Alkylating agents are mutagenic and carcinogenic and can lead to a second cancer.

Busulfan can cause pulmonary **fibrosis**.

Cisplatin is among the most emetogenic chemotherapy agents.

Cyclophosphamide can cause hemor-

Fibrosis: An abnormal proliferation of fibrous connective tissue

Cystitis: Inflammation and/or infection of the urinary bladder and ureters

Gynecomastia: An abnormal enlargement of one or two breasts in men

rhagic **cystitis,** which can lead to bladder fibrosis. It can also cause amenorrhea, testicular atrophy, and sterility. About 25% of patients develop venoocclusive disease of the liver.

Estramustine commonly causes **gynecomastia** and breast tenderness.

Ifosfamide can have bladder toxicity and should always be administered with plenty of fluids, either orally or IV, and a bladder protectant such as mesna.

Lomustine may cause renal toxicity and pulmonary fibrosis with prolonged use.

▧ RED FLAGS

Estramustine very commonly causes cardiac impairments including ischemic heart disease, thromboembolism, and cardiac decompensation.

▧ INTERACTIONS

HERB

CYCLOPHOSPHAMIDE

- *Gan Jiang/Sheng Jiang* (Ginger) (D)–using an acetone extract of an active ingredient in ginger, 6-gingerol, prevented vomiting in suncus (Yamahara *et al.,* 1989) Level 5 evidence.
- *Huang Lian* (Coptis root) (D)–berberine, a constituent of *Huang Lian*, was shown to prevent cyclophosphamide-induced cystitis in rats (Xu & Malavé, 2001) Level 5 evidence.
- *Huang Qi* (Astragulus) (D)–may increase

immune response and decrease immunosuppressant effects of cyclophosphamide in mice (Zhao, Mancini *et al.,* 1990) Level 5 evidence.

- *Xi Yang Shen* (American ginseng) (D)–when combined with tamoxifen, cyclophosphamide, doxorubicin, taxol, and methotrexate, may increase suppression of breast cell growth as shown in an in vitro study (Duda, Zhong, Navas *et al.,* 1999) Level 5 evidence.

PROCARBAZINE

- *Ma Huang* (Ephedra) (D)–based on ephedrine content, may increase sympathomimetic activity of sympathomimetic drugs such as furazolidone and procarbazine, expert opinion (Gruenwald, Brendler & Jaenicke, 2004) Level 5 evidence.

INTERACTION ISSUES

A:

D: Bendamustine is 94-96% protein bound; chlorambucil is approximately 99% bound.

M: Busulfan is a major substrate of CYP3A4; cyclophosphamide is a major substrate of CYP2B6 and a weak or moderate inducer of 2B6 and 2C9; dacarbazine is a major substrate of CYP1A2 and 2E1; ifosfamide is a major substrate of CYP2A6, 2C19, and 3A4 and a weak or moderate inducer of 2C9; thiotepa is a strong inhibitor of CYP2B6.

E:

Pgp: Bendamustine is a substrate of Pgp.

SECTION 2: ANTIMETABOLITES

CAPECITABINE (cape SITE a bene) PR=D *(Xeloda®)*

CLADRIBINE (KLA dri bene) PR=D

CLOFARABINE (klo FARE a bene) PR=D *(Clolar®)*

CYTARABINE (sye TARE a bene) PR=D *(DepoCyt®)*

FLOXURIDINE (floks YOOR i dene) PR=D

FLUDARABINE (floo DARE a bene) PR=D *(Fludara®)*

FLUOROURACIL (flure oh YOOR a sil) PR=X

(Carac™, Efudex®, Fluoroplex®)

GEMCITABINE (jem SITE a bene) PR=D *(Gemzar®)*

HYDROXYUREA *(See Chapter 6, Section 13)*

MERCAPTOPURINE (6-MP) (mer kap toe PYOOR ene) PR=D *(Purinethol®)*

METHOTREXATE (MTX) (meth oh TREKS ate) PR=X *(Rheumatrex®, Trexall™)*

NELARABINE (nel AY re bene) PR=D *(Arranon®)*

PEMETREXED (pem e TREKS ed) PR=D

(Alimta®)

PENTOSTATIN *(See next section)*

PRALATREXATE (pral a TREX ate) PR=D
(Folotyn)

**THIOGUANINE (6-TG) (thye oh GWAH nene)
PR=D** *(Tabloid®)*

Antimetabolites are structurally similar to endogenous cellular compounds. Usually they interfere with DNA or RNA synthesis and are maximally effective in the S phase of cell growth and are therefore cell-cycle specific.

FUNCTION

Capecitabine is used in breast cancer resistant to first-line drugs and also in colorectal cancer. Cladribine treats hairy cell leukemia and, off label, acute myeloid leukemia (AML); chronic lymphocytic leukemia (CLL); non-Hodgkin's lymphoma; Waldenström's macroglobulinemia; and Langerhans cell histiocytosis.

Clofarabine is used to treat acute lymphoblastic leukemia (ALL) in children and adults 21 years and younger. Off label it is used to treat ALL in adults older than 21 years and acute myeloid leukemia (AML) in adults 60 years and older.

Cytarabine comes in two forms: conventional and liposomal. Conventional form treats acute myeloid leukemia (AML), acute lymphocytic leukemia (ALL), chronic myelocytic leukemia (CML), and meningeal leukemia. Off label, it is used for acute promyelocytic leukemia (APL), primary central nervous system lymphoma, chronic lymphocytic leukemia (CLL), and both Hodgkin's and non-Hodgkin's lymphomas. Its liposomal form is used intrathecally to treat lymphomatous meningitis.

Floxuridine is used to manage hepatic metastases of colorectal and gastric cancers.

Fludarabine is used to treat B-cell chronic lymphocytic leukemia (CLL); off label for non-Hodgkin's lymphoma, acute myeloid leukemia (AML), relapsed acute lymphocytic leukemia (ALL), AML in pediatric patients, and Waldenström's macroglobulinemia.

Fluorouracil is used topically to treat actinic or solar keratoses and superficial basal cell carcinomas (BCC). Mercaptopurine is useful in treating acute lymphocytic leukemia (ALL) and Crohn's disease. Methotrexate, in combination with other drugs, is useful in treating acute lymphocytic leukemia (ALL); choriocarcinoma; Bur-kitt lymphoma in children; and breast, head, and neck cancers. In smaller doses, it can be effective for some inflammatory diseases such as rheumatoid arthritis, severe psoriasis, and Crohn's disease.

Gemcitabine treats breast, non-small-cell lung, ovarian, and pancreatic cancers. Off label it can be used for bladder, cervical, head and neck, hepatobiliary, renal cell, small cell lung, and testicular cancers; Hodgkin's and non-Hodgkin's lymphomas; Ewing's, osteo-, soft tissue, and uterine sarcoma;, and mesotheliomas.

Nelarabine is used to treat T-cell acute lymphoblastic leukemia (ALL) and T-cell lymphoblastic lymphoma.

Pemetrexed is used to treat malignant pleural mesothelioma and nonsquamous nonsmall cell lung cancer. Off label, it is used to treat bladder, cervical, ovarian, and thymic cancers and pleural mesothelioma.

Pralatrexate treats peripheral T-cell lymphoma (PTCL) on label and cutaneous T-cell lymphomas and Sézary syndrome off label.

Thioguanine is used to treat acute non-lymphocytic leukemia.

MECHANISM OF ACTION

Antimetabolites, through differing mechanisms, all prevent RNA or DNA synthesis by preventing their constituents from being formed or by more directly interfering with their synthesis. Below are how individual agents in this class work.

Capecitabine acts by inhibiting thymidylate synthase, an enzyme necessary to convert deoxy-UMP to deoxy-TMP, which is necessary for DNA synthesis and cell growth.

Cladribine incorporates into DNA and causes breakage of the DNA strand and subsequent shutdown of DNA synthesis and repair.

Cytarabine, a pyrimidine analog, is incorporated into DNA and inhibits DNA polymerase resulting in decreased DNA synthesis and repair.

Both floxuridine and flurouracil act similarly as a pyrimidine antagonist that inhibits DNA and RNA synthesis and methylation of deoxyuridylic acid to thymidylic acid.

Mercaptopurine prevents the formation of adenosine monophosphate (AMP), necessary for RNA and DNA reproduction. It also forms TGMP, which gets incorporated into RNA and DNA and creates nonfunctional RNA and DNA.

Methotrexate acts by inhibiting dihydrofolate reductase (DHFR), an enzyme that converts ingested folic acid into the active form of tetrahydofolate (FH4). This coenzyme is necessary for producing the nucleotides adenine (A), guanine (G), and thymidine (T) and the amino acids methionine and serine. Ultimately, the lack of these chemicals results in cell death due to reduced DNA, RNA, and protein synthesis.

Pemetrexed and pralatrexate are antifolates that prevent synthesis of DNA and RNA.

Thioguanine prevents synthesis of the purine ring of adenine (A) and guanine (G) and prevents conversion of GMP to GDP. It can also be incorporated into DNA and RNA.

▌ DOSAGES

CAPECITABINE, for *adults*, 1250 mg/m^2 bid for 2 weeks every 21-28 days; as adjuvant therapy for Dukes' C colon cancer, recommended for a total of 24 weeks (8 cycles of 2 weeks of drug administration and a 1-week rest period).

CLADRIBINE, for *adults*, for hairy cell leukemia, IV: 0.09 mg/kg/d continuous infusion for 7 days for 1 cycle.

CLOFARABINE, for *children* 1 year and older, for acute lymphoblastic leukemia (ALL), IV: 52 mg/m^2/d days 1 through 5; repeat every 2-6 weeks; subsequent cycles should begin at least 14 days from day 1 of the previous administra-

tion. For *adults* 21 years and younger, for acute lymphoblastic leukemia (ALL), IV: 52 mg/m^2/d days 1 through 5; repeat every 2-6 weeks; subsequent cycles should begin at least 14 days from day 1 of the previous administration.

CYTARABINE, for *children* and *adults*, for acute myeloid leukemia (AML), IV: 100 or 200 mg/m^2/d continuous infusion for 7 days.

FLOXURIDINE, for *adults*, for colorectal or gastric metastases, intra-arterial: 0.1-0.6 mg/kg/d continuous intra-arterial administration for 14 days, then heparinized saline for 14 days.

FLUDARABINE, for *adults*, for chronic lymphocytic leukemia (CLL), IV: 25 mg/m^2/d for 5 days every 28 days.

FLUOROURACIL, for *adults*, for actinic keratosis, topical: Carac™: apply thin film to lesions once daily for up to 4 weeks as tolerated; Efudex®: apply to lesions bid for 2-4 weeks; complete healing may not be evident for 1-2 months following treatment; Fluoroplex®: apply to lesions bid for 2-6 weeks; for superficial basal cell carcinoma, topical, Efudex® 5%: apply to affected lesions bid for 3-6 weeks; treatment may continue up to 10-12 weeks.

GEMCITABINE, for *adults*, for metastatic breast cancer, IV: 1250 mg/m^2 days 1 and 8; repeat every 21 days combined with paclitaxel; for non-small-cell lung cancer, IV: 1000 or 1250 mg/m^2 on days 1, 8, and 15; repeat every 28 days; for advanced ovarian cancer, IV: 1000 mg/m^2 days 1 and 8; repeat every 21 days combined with carboplatin; for pancreatic cancer, IV: initiate at 1000 mg/m^2 over 30 minutes once weekly for 7 weeks, then 1-week rest, then once weekly for 3 weeks out of every 4.

MERCAPTOPURINE, for *children*, for acute lymphoblastic leukemia (ALL), initiate at 2.5-5 mg/kg/d or 70-100 mg/m^2/d once daily; maintain at 1.5-2.5 mg/kg/d or 50-75 mg/m^2/d once daily. For *adults*, for ALL, initiate at 2.5-5 mg/kg/d (100-200 mg); maintain at 1.5-2.5 mg/kg/d or 80-100 mg/m^2/day once daily.

METHOTREXATE, for *children*, for dermatomyositis, 15-20 mg/m^2/week single dose once weekly or 0.3-1 mg/kg once weekly; for juvenile rheumatoid arthritis, 10 mg/m^2 once weekly, then 5-15 mg/m^2/wk single dose or as 3 divided doses 12 hours apart; antineoplastic dosage range is 7.5-30 mg/m^2/wk or every 2 weeks. For *adults*, for trophoblastic neoplasms, 15-30 mg/d for 5 days; repeat in 7 days for 3-5 courses; for head and neck cancer, 25-50 mg/m^2 once weekly; for mycosis fungoides (cutaneous T-cell lymphoma), 5-50 mg once weekly or 15-37.5 mg twice weekly; for rheumatoid arthritis, 7.5 mg once weekly or 2.5 mg every 12 hours for 3 doses/wk, not to exceed 20 mg/wk; for psoriasis, 2.5-5 mg every 12 hours for 3 doses given weekly, or 10-25 mg once weekly. For the *elderly*, for rheumatoid arthritis/psoriasis, initiate at 5-7.5 mg/wk, not to exceed 20 mg/wk.

NELARABINE, for T-cell acute lymphoblastic leukemia (ALL) or T-cell lymphoblastic lymphoma, IV: 650 mg/m^2 for *children* or 1500 mg/m^2 for *adults* on days 1, 3, and 5; repeat every 21 days until transplant, disease progression, or excessive toxicity.

PEMETREXED, for *adults,* for malignant pleural mesothelioma, IV: 500 mg/m^2 day 1 of each 21-day cycle combined with cisplatin; for non-small-cell lung cancer, IV: initiate at 500 mg/m^2 on day 1 of each 21-day cycle in combination with cisplatin; maintain at 500 mg/m^2 on day 1 of each 21-day cycle as a single agent.

PRALATREXATE, for *adults*, for peripheral T-cell lymphoma (PTCL), IV: 30 mg/m^2 once weekly for 6 weeks of a 7-week treatment cycle; continue until disease progression or excessive toxicity.

THIOGUANINE, total daily dose can be given at one time. For *infants* and *children* under 3 years, combination drug therapy for acute nonlymphocytic leukemia, 1.65 mg/kg bid for 4 days. For *children* and *adults*, 2-3 mg/kg/d calculated to nearest 20 mg or 75-200 mg/m^2/d in 1-2 divided doses for 5-7 days or until remission is attained.

ADVERSE EFFECTS

Common adverse effects of anticancer agents include severe vomiting, stomatitis, anorexia, diarrhea, and hair loss. Many suppress the bone marrow. Treatment-induced neoplasms can occur many years after treatment.

Capecitabine may cause severe ulceration of the mouth and GI mucosa, along with anorexia. It should be used cautiously in patients with renal or liver impairment. It is contraindicated in patients who are hypersensitive to fluorouracil or women who are pregnant or lactating.

Mercaptopurine and thioguanine can cause nausea and diarrhea, and liver toxicity has been reported.

Methotrexate, in addition to the common adverse effects above, may cause **erythema**, rash, and urticaria; rare complications may include renal damage, liver fibrosis or cirrhosis, and pulmonary toxicity. This agent should be avoided in pregnant women due to the potential for fetal death and/or congenital abnormalities.

> Erythema: Redness or inflammation of the skin

INTERACTIONS

DRUG

When using capecitabine with coumarin or phenytoin, levels of anticoagulation and drug concentrations should be monitored.

HERB

METHOTREXATE

- *Xi Yang Shen* (American ginseng) (D)–when combined with tamoxifen, cytoxan, doxorubicin, taxol, and methotrexate may increase suppression of breast cell growth as shown in an in vitro study (Duda, Zhong, Navas, Li, Toy & Alavarez, 1999) Level 5 evidence.

INTERACTION ISSUES

A:

D:

M: Capecitabine, floxuridine, and fluorouracil are strong inhibitors of CYP2C9.

E:

Pgp: Methotrexate is a substrate of Pgp.

SECTION 3: ANTIBIOTICS

BLEOMYCIN (blee oh MYE sin) PR=D

DACTINOMYCIN (dak ti noe MYE sin) PR=D
(Cosmegen)

IDARUBICIN (eye da ROO bi sin) PR=D
(Idamycin® PFS)

MITOMYCIN (mye toe MYE sin) PR=N
(Mitosol)

PENTOSTATIN (pen toe STAT in) PR=D
(Nipent®)

Antibiotics interfere with DNA, either through intercalation, production of free radicals, or inhibition of enzymes, causing cytotoxicity. They are cell-cycle nonspecific.

FUNCTION

Bleomycin is used to treat squamous cell carcinomas of the head and neck, penis, cervix, or vulva; testicular carcinoma; and Hodgkin's and non-Hodgkin's lymphoma. It is also used off label to treat ovarian germ cell cancers.

Dactinomycin is used to treat Wilms' tumor, childhood rhabdomyosarcoma, Ewing's sarcoma, metastatic testicular tumors, gestational trophoblastic neoplasm, and regional perfusion. Off label it is used to treat ovarian cancer and osteo- and soft-tissue sarcomas.

Idarubicin treats acute myeloid leukemia (AML) on label and acute lymphocytic leukemia (ALL) off label.

Mitomycin is used to treat adenocarcinoma of the stomach or pancreas. Off label it is used for treating anal carcinoma and bladder, cervical, esophageal, gastric, and non-small-cell lung cancers (NSCLC).

Pentostatin treats hairy cell leukemia. Off label it is used to treat T-cell lymphoma, chronic lymphocytic leukemia (CLL), and acute and chronic graft-versus-host-disease (GVHD).

MECHANISM OF ACTION

Bleomycin works by inhibiting DNA synthesis and binding DNA to cause breaks in their strands. See Figure 11.2. To a lesser degree, it also inhibits RNA and protein synthesis.

Dactinomycin acts by binding to DNA between guanine and cytosine base pairs and prevents DNA, RNA, and protein synthesis.

Idarubicin also works by getting between base pairs and preventing DNA and RNA synthesis.

Mitomycin creates cross-links within DNA and therefore inhibits DNA and RNA synthesis.

Pentostatin reduces synthesis of purines (one of the two types of bases in DNA) and therefore inhibits DNA synthesis and can cause cell death.

DOSAGES

BLEOMYCIN, for *adults*, for malignant pleural effusion, intrapleural: 60 units as a single instillation. Pulmonary toxicity is also relatively common in those using bleomycin. Lifetime dose of over 400 units increases this risk and it is more common in the *elderly*.

DACTINOMYCIN, for *children* over 6 months, for Wilms's tumor, rhabdomyosarcoma, Ewing's sarcoma, IV: 15 mcg/kg/d for 5 days. For *adults*, for testicular cancer, IV: 1000 mcg/m^2 on day 1 as part of a combined chemotherapy regimen; for gestational trophoblastic neoplasm, IV: 12 mcg/kg/d for 5 days alone or 500 mcg days 1 and 2 as part of combined chemotherapy; for Wilms's tumor, Ewing's sarcoma, or rhabdomyosarcoma, IV: 15 mcg/kg/d for 5 days; for regional perfusion, for lower extremity or pelvis, 50 mcg/kg; upper extremity, 35 mcg/kg.

IDARUBICIN, for *adults*, for acute myeloid leukemia (AML), IV: 12 mg/m^2/d for 3 days to induce, 10-12 mg/m^2/d for 2 days to consolidate.

MITOMYCIN, for *adults*, for stomach or pancreas adenocarcinoma, IV: 20 mg/m^2 every 6-8 weeks.

PENTOSTATIN, for *adults*, for hairy cell leukemia, IV: 4 mg/m^2 every 2 weeks.

ADVERSE EFFECTS

Common adverse effects of anticancer agents

include severe vomiting, stomatitis, anorexia, diarrhea, and hair loss. Many suppress bone marrow. Treatment-induced neoplasms can occur many years after treatment.

Bleomycin can cause a reaction in about 1% of lymphoma patients resulting in hypotension, mental confusion, fever, chills, and wheezing. This usually occurs after the first or second dose.

Dactinomycin is a hazardous agent. Precautions when handling or disposing are important. Experienced chemotherapy physicians should supervise its administration.

Idarubicin can cause heart failure, arrhythmias, or cardiomyopathies. Risks for these increase in those with preexisting cardiac conditions.

INTERACTIONS

INTERACTION ISSUES

A:

D: Idarubicin is 94-97% protein bound.

M:.

E:

Pgp: Idarubicin and mitomycin are substrates of Pgp.

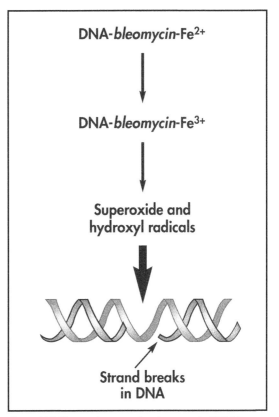

Figure 11.2 Bleomycin acts to break a strand of DNA by creating free radicals.

SECTION 4: MICROTUBULE INHIBITORS

ADO-TRASTUZUMAB EMTANSINE (a do tras TU zoo mab em TAN sene) PR=D *(Kadcyla)*

CABAZITAXEL (ca baz i TAKS el) PR=D *(Jevtana®)*

DOCETAXEL (doe se TAKS el) PR=D *(Docefrez, Taxotere)*

ERIBULIN (er i BUE lin) PR=D *(Halaven™)*

IXABEPILONE (ix ab EP i lone) PR=D *(Ixempra Kit)*

PACLITAXEL (pac li TAKS el) PR=D

VINBLASTINE (vin BLAS tene) PR=D

VINCRISTINE (vin KRIS tene) PR=D *(Vincasar PFS)*

VINCRISTINE (LIPOSOMAL) (vin KRIS teen lye po SO mal) PR=D

VINORELBINE (vi NOR el bene) PR=D *(Navelbine®)*

Microtubules make up part of the cytoskeleton (the support structure for cells) providing a basis for movement of structures in the cytoplasm. This is extremely important in eukaryotic cell division as it supports the even partitioning of chromosomes between the two daughter cells. These agents disrupt this function.

FUNCTION

Ado-Trastuzumab Emtansine is used to treat HER2 positive breast cancer where the patient has previously received trastuzumab and ataxane.

Cabazitaxel treats prostate cancer.

Docetaxel is used to treat breast cancer, non-small-cell lung cancer, and prostate cancer. Off label it is used to treat bladder, ovarian, cervical, esophageal, small-cell lung cancers, and soft-tissue and Ewing's sarcomas.

Eribulin is used to treat breast cancer in patients who have had at least two prior anti-cancer chemotherapy regimens.

Ixabepilone is primarily used to treat breast cancer but can also be used to treat endometrial cancer off label.

Paclitaxel is used to treat non-small-cell lung, breast, and ovarian cancer, and AIDS-related Kaposi's sarcoma (KS).

Vinblastine treats Hodgkin's and non-Hodgkin's lymphoma, testicular and breast cancers, mycosis fungoides, Kaposi's sarcoma, histiocytosis (Letterer-Siwe disease), and choriocarcinoma. Off label, it treats bladder, non-small-cell lung, and ovarian cancers; melanoma; and soft-tissue sarcomas.

Vincristine treats lymphocytic leukemia (ALL), Hodgkin's and non-Hodgkin's lymphomas, Wilms's tumor, neuroblastoma, and rhabdomyosarcoma. Off label, it treats central nervous system tumors, chronic lymphocytic leukemia (CLL), Ewing's sarcoma, gestational trophoblastic tumors, multiple myeloma, ovarian germ cell tumors, retinoblastoma, small-cell lung cancer (SCLC) and advanced thymoma.

Vincristine (Liposomal) is used to treat relapsed Philadelphia chromosome-negative (Ph-) acute lymphoblastic leukemia (ALL) when the disease has endured two or more therapy protocols.

Vinorelbine treats non-small-cell lung cancer (NSCLC) on label and breast, cervical, relapsed ovarian, salivary gland, and small-cell lung cancers; relapsed or refractory Hodgkin's lymphoma; pleural mesothelioma; and advanced soft-tissue sarcoma off label.

MECHANISM OF ACTION

Microtubules are used in a variety of cellular functions including cell movement, mitosis, and intracellular transport. Microtubule inhibitors generally work by inhibiting the microtubules used during mitosis of the cell and prevent the ability of the cell to divide.

Vinca (a plant) derived alkaloids prevent the proper functioning of microtubules and disordered cell division.

Paclitaxel and docetaxel work in almost the opposite manner to vinca alkaloids in that they cause the microtubules to become overly stable thus freezing cell division in metaphase. This prevents normal cell division, as shown in Figure 11.3 on the next page.

Ado-Trastuzumab Emtansine attaches an antimicrotubule agent with an antibody that targets HER2. This allows for targeted delivery of the active agent directly to the tumor.

DOSAGES

ADO-TRASTUZUMAB EMTANSINE, for *adults*, for HER2 positive breast cancer, IV: 3.6 mg/kg every 3 weeks until disease progression or unacceptable toxicity; maximum dose 3.6 mg/kg.

CABAZITAXE, for *adults*, for prostate cancer, IV: 25 mg/m^2 once per 3 weeks with prednisone.

DOCETAXEL, for *adults*, for breast cancer, IV: 60-100 mg/m^2 every 3 weeks as a single agent; for non-small-cell lung cancer, IV: 75 mg/m^2 every 3 weeks as single agent or with cisplatin; for prostate cancer, IV: 75 mg/m^2 every 3 weeks with prednisone; for gastric adenocarcinoma, IV: 75 mg/m^2 every 3 weeks with cisplatin and fluorouracil; for head and neck cancer, IV: 75 mg/m^2 every 3 weeks with cisplatin and fluorouracil for 3-4 cycles, followed by radiation therapy.

ERIBULIN, for *adults*, for breast cancer, IV: 1.4 mg/m^2 on days 1 and 8 of a 21-day cycle.

IXABEPILONE, for *adults*, for breast cancer, IV: 40 mg/m^2 to maximum 88 mg over 3 hours every 3 weeks.

PACLITAXEL, for *adults*, for ovarian carcinoma, IV: 135-175 mg/m^2 over 3 hours every 3 weeks or 135 mg/m^2 over 24 hours every 3 weeks or 50-80 mg/m^2 over 1-3 hours weekly or 1.4-4 mg/m^2/d continuous infusion for 14 days every 4 weeks; for breast cancer, IV: 175-250 mg/m^2 over 3 hours every 3 weeks or 50-80 mg/m^2 weekly or 1.4-4 mg/m^2/d continuous infusion for 14 days every 4 weeks; for non-small-cell lung carcinoma, IV: 135 mg/m^2 over 24 hours every 3 weeks; for AIDS-related Kaposi's sarcoma, IV: 135 mg/m^2 over 3 hours every 3 weeks or 100 mg/m^2 over 3 hours every 2 weeks.

VINBLASTINE, for *children*, for Hodgkin's disease, IV: initiate with 6 mg/m^2, not administered less than every 7 days; for Letterer-Siwe disease, IV: initiate with 6.5 mg/m^2, not administered less than every 7 days; for testicular cancer, IV: initiate with 3 mg/m^2, not administered less than every 7 days. For *adults*, as typical doses for

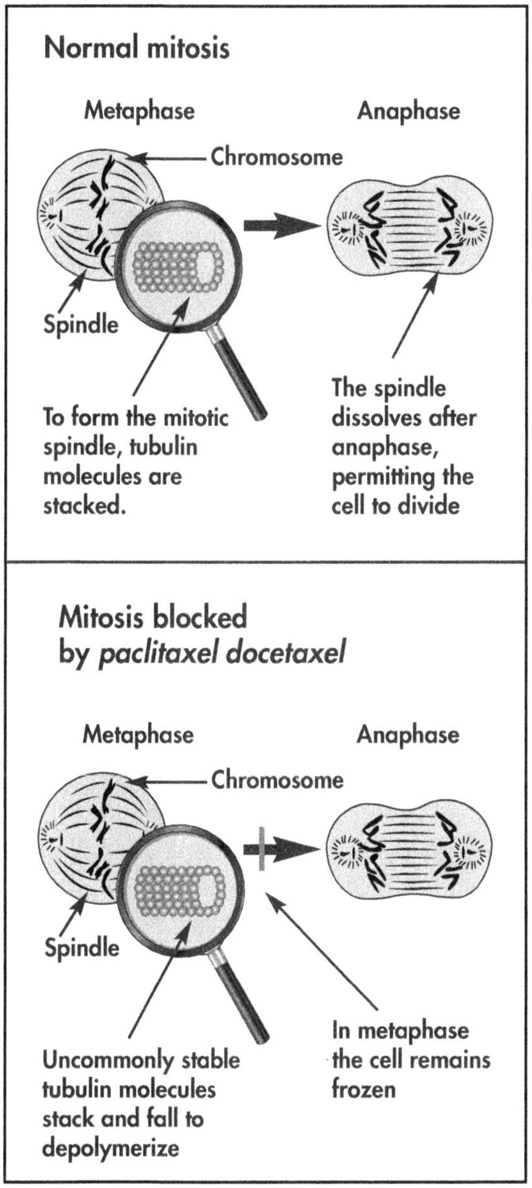

Figure 11.3 This figure shows normal mitosis versus that stabilized by paclitaxel or docetaxel.

treating neoplastic diseases, IV: initiate with 3.7 mg/m^2; adjust dose every 7 days based on white blood cell (WBC) response up to 5.5 mg/m^2 for the second dose, 7.4 mg/m^2 for the third dose, 9.25 mg/m^2 for the fourth, and 11.1 mg/m^2 for the fifth, not to be administered less frequently than every 7 days; usual range is 5.5-7.4 mg/m^2 every 7 days to a maximum 18.5 mg/m^2.

VINCRISTINE, for *children*, the following are recommended doses and can be changed for specific cancers: children 10 kg or under, 0.05 mg/kg/dose once weekly; children over 10 kg: 1.5-2 mg/m^2; frequency varies depending on specific protocols. For *adults*, general dosing is IV: 1.4 mg/m^2; frequency varies depending on specific protocols.

VINCRISTINE (LIPOSOMAL), for *adults*, acute lymphoblastic leukemia (ALL), IV: 2.25 mg/m^2 once every 7 days.

VINORELBINE, for *adults*, for non-small-cell lung cancer (NSCLC), IV: 30 mg/m^2 every 7 days or 25-30 mg/m^2 every 7 days with cisplatin.

ADVERSE EFFECTS

Common adverse effects of anticancer agents include severe vomiting, stomatitis, anorexia, diarrhea, and hair loss. Many suppress bone marrow. Treatment-induced neoplasms can occur many years after treatment.

Ado-Trastuzumab Emtansine may cause left ventricular ejection fraction reductions and hepatotoxicity.

Docetaxel can cause severe fluid retention resulting in pleural effusion, ascites, edema, cardiac tamponade, and resting dyspnea.

Ixabepilone can cause hepatic impairment and death caused by neutropenia.

Vinorelbine can cause severe granulocytopenia according to a boxed warning.

INTERACTIONS

HERB

ANTIMICROTUBULE DRUGS

- *Bai Xian Pi* (Dictamnus, dense fruit pittany root bark) (D)–a constituent, obacunone, may potentiate microtubule inhibitors such as vincristine, vinblastine, and taxol. Bench research (Jung, Sok *et al.,* 2000) Level 5 evidence.

- *Yin Guo Ye* (Gingko) (D)–a study using in vitro hepatocytes demonstrated inhibition of metabolism of paclitaxel when combined with gingko. This interaction may result in elevated levels of this anticancer agent when used concomitantly (Etheridge, Kroll & Mathews, 2009) Level 5 evidence.

INTERACTION ISSUES

A:

D: Docetaxel is approximately 94-97% protein bound; Paclitaxel is 89-98% bound, vinblastine is 99% bound.

M: Ado-Trastuzumab emtansine, cabazitaxel, docetaxel, and ixabepilone are major substrates of CYP3A4; paclitaxel is a major substrate of CYP2C8 and 3A4 and a weak or moderate inducer of 3A4; vinblastine, vincristine, vincristine (liposomal), and vinorelbine are major substrates of CYP3A4.

E:

Pgp: Docetaxel, paclitaxel, vincristine, and vincristine (Liposomal) are substrates of Pgp; vinblastine is a substrate and inducer of Pgp.

SECTION 5: STEROID HORMONES AND THEIR ANTAGONISTS

ANASTROZOLE (an AS troe zole) PR=X *(Arimidex®)*

BICALUTAMIDE *(See Chapter 7, Section 3)*

ESTROGENS *(See Chapter 7, Section 3)*

EXEMESTANE (ex e MES tane) PR=X *(Aromasin®)*

FLUTAMIDE *(See Chapter 7, Section 3)*

LETROZOLE (LET roe zole) PR=X *(Femara®)*

MEGESTROL *(See Chapter 7, Section 3)*

MIFEPRISTONE *(See Chapter 7, Section 3)*

NILUTAMIDE *(See Chapter 7, Section 3)*

PREDNISONE *(See Chapter 7, Section 4)*

TAMOXIFEN *(See Chapter 7, Section 3)*

TOREMIFENE *(See Chapter 7, Section 3)*

FUNCTION

Most of these agents are used to treat cancers of the sex organs: breast, ovarian, endometrial, testicular, prostate, and so on.

The aromatase inhibitors, anastrozole, letrozole, and exemestane, decrease estrogen and are used to treat hormone- dependent breast cancer.

MECHANISM OF ACTION

Steroid hormones and their antagonists work on tumors by either providing a specific hormone or by blocking certain hormone(s). Some tumors are hormone-responsive which means that the presence of a specific hormone can treat the tumor. Some are hormone-dependent where the tumor will regress if a specific hormone is removed. And there are tumors that are both hormone-respondent and hormone-dependent.

The aromatase inhibitors, anastrozole, letrozole, and exemestane, act by preventing synthesis of estrogen from andro-stenedione in the liver, fat, muscle, skin, and breast tissue. This is especially useful in post-menopausal women. Anastrozole and letrozole have many advantages over other antiestrogen agents including their increased potency, their selectivity, fewer side effects, and the fact they do not contribute to endometrial cancer. Figure 11.4 shows how these agents prevent breast cancer.

DOSAGES

ANASTROZOLE, for *adults*, for breast cancer, 1 mg once daily.

EXEMESTANE, for *adults*, 25 mg once daily.

LETROZOLE, for *adults*, for breast cancer, 2.5 mg once daily.

ADVERSE EFFECTS

Common adverse effects of anticancer agents include severe vomiting, stomatitis, anorexia, diarrhea, and hair loss. Many suppress the bone marrow. Treatment-induced neoplasms can occur many years after treatment.

INTERACTIONS

INTERACTION ISSUES

A:

D:

M: Exemestane is a major substrate and a weak or moderate inducer of CYP3A4; letrozole is a strong inhibitor of CYP2A6.

E:

Pgp:

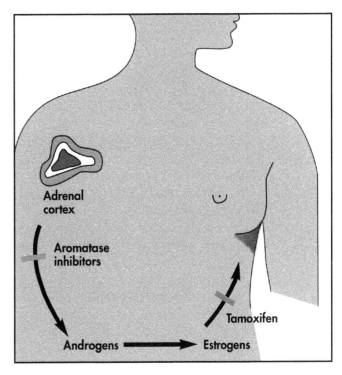

Figure 11.4 Aromatase inhibitors work to treat estrogen-dependent tumors by blocking formation of pre-estrogenic androgens. Tamoxifen acts by blocking the effects of estrogens.

SECTION 6: MONOCLONAL ANTIBODIES

BEVACIZUMAB (be vuh SIZ uh mab) PR=C *(Avastin®)*

BRENTUXIMAB VEDOTIN (bren TUX i mab ve DOE tin) PR=D *(Adcetris™)*

CETUXIMAB (se TUK see mab) PR=C *(Erbitux®)*

IBRITUMOMAB (ib ri TYOO mo mab) PR=D *(Zevalin In-111, Zevalin Y-90)*

IPILIMUMAB (ip i LIM u mab) *(Yervoy®)* **PR=C**

OFATUMUMAB (oh fa TOOM yoo mab) PR=C *(Arzerra™)*

PANITUMUMAB (pan i TOOM yoo mab) PR=C *(Vectibix®)*

PERTUZUMAB (per TU zoo mab) PR=D *(Perjeta)*

RITUXIMAB (ri TUK si mab) PR=C *(Rituxan)*

TOSITUMOMAB and IODINE I 131 TOSITUMO-MAB (toe si TYOO mo mab) PR=D *(Bexxar®)*

TRASTUZUMAB (tras TU zoo mab) PR=D *(Herceptin®)*

Monoclonal antibodies are a quite recent class of anticancer agents used to target specific kinds of cancer.

FUNCTION

Bevacizumab is used to treat colorectal, nonsquamous, non-small-cell lung and renal cell cancers and gliobastomas. Off label it is used to treat breast, recurrent cervical, and ovarian cancers as well as soft-tissue sarcomas and age-related macular degeneration (AMD).

Brentuximab vedotin is used to treat Hodgkin's lymphoma after failing at least two prior chemotherapy regimens and systemic anaplastic large-cell lymphoma (sALCL) after failing at least one chemotherapy regimen.

Cetuximab is used to treat KRAS mutation-negative (wild-type), EGFR-expressing colorectal cancer and squamous cell cancer of the head and neck. Off label it is used to treat EGFR-expressing advanced non-small-cell lung cancer (NSCLC), squamous cell skin cancer, and the neurological symptoms of chordoma.

Ibritumomab is used to treat non-Hodgkin's lymphoma.

Ipilimumab treats melanoma.

Ofatumumab treats refractory chronic lymphocytic leukemia (CLL).

Panitumumab is used to treat KRAS mutation-negative colorectal cancer. Off label it is used to treat KRAS positive colorectal cancer in combination with other agents.

Pertuzumab treats HER2 positive breast cancer in combination with trastuzumab and docetaxel.

Rituximab is used to treat various subtypes of non-Hodgin's lymphoma, chronic lymphocytic leukemia (CLL), rheumatoid arthritis, granulomatosis with polyangiitis (GPA) also known as Wegener's granulomatosis, and microscopic polyangiitis (MPA). Off label it is used to treat various types of lymphomas and lymphoproliferative disorders, Waldenström's macroglobulinemia, autoimmune hemolytic anemia in children, chronic immune thrombocytopenia (ITP), refractory pemphigus vulgaris, chronic graft-versus-host disease (GVHD), lupus nephritis, thrombotic thrombocytopenic purpura-hemolytic uremic syndrome, resistant idiopathic membranous nephropathy, and refractory nephrotic syndrome in children.

Tositumomab is used to treat refractory non-Hodgkin's lymphoma (NHL), with progression during or after rituximab treatment.

Trastuzumab treats HER2 positive breast cancer and HER2 gastric or gastroesophageal junction adenocarcinoma.

MECHANISM OF ACTION

The basic mechanism of action of all monoclonal antibodies is that the drug is designed to hook to a very specific binding site. Sometimes this means delivering an active drug as a payload to a particular site. Other times the binding causes a direct inhibition on a process.

Bevacizumab binds to vascular endothelial growth factor inhibiting angiogenesis. Without more blood vessels, tumor growth is retarded.

Brentuximab vedotin is a complex of a monoclonal antibody, an antimicrotubule agent, and an enzyme that forms a permanent bond. What this does is bind to tubules within the cell preventing reproduction of the cell and apoptosis.

Cetuximab binds with epidermal growth factor receptor (EGFR) inhibiting cell growth, increasing apoptosis, and decreasing vascularization.

Ibritumomab is a monoclonal delivery system that delivers a radioactive isotope to B lymphocytes.

Ipilimumab binds with cytotoxic T-lymphocytes and activates them. It is thought that this causes a T-cell response against tumors.

Ofatumumab and rituximab bind with B lymphocytes and cause cell lysis.

Panitumumab also binds with EGFR and inhibits cell survival, growth, and proliferation.

Pertuzumab and trastuzumab target the extracellular human epidermal growth factor receptor 2 protein (HER2) inhibiting cell growth and initiating apoptosis.

Tositumomab is an antibody that attaches to B lymphocytes and can have direct functions to induce apoptosis or cytotoxicity. Iodine I[131] tositumomab is where this antibody is attached to radioactive iodine and can cause radiation-induced cell death.

DOSAGES

BEVACIZUMAB, for *adults,* for colorectal cancer, 5 mg/kg every 2 weeks or 7.5 mg/kg every 3 weeks with fluoropyrimidine-irinotecan- or fluoropyrimidine-oxaliplatin-based regimen; for glioblastoma, 10 mg/kg every 2 weeks; for nonsquamous non-small-cell lung cancer, IV: 15 mg/kg every 3 weeks with carboplatin and paclitaxel for 4-6 cycles; for renal cell cancer, 10 mg/kg every 2 weeks with interferon alfa.

BRENTUXIMAB VEDOTIN, for *adults,* for Hodgkin's lymphoma or systemic anaplastic large-cell lymphoma (sALCL), IV: 1.8 mg/kg up to a maximum of 180 mg every 3 weeks; continue until disease progression is seen, unacceptable toxicities are experienced, or a maximum of 16 cycles is achieved.

CETUXIMAB, for *adults,* for KRAS mutation-negative colorectal cancer or squamous cell head and neck cancer, IV: loading dose is 400 mg/m^2 infused over 120 minutes; maintain at 250 mg/m^2 infused over 60 minutes weekly until disease progression or unacceptable toxicity.

IBRITUMOMAB, for *adults*, for B-cell non-Hodgkin's lymphoma, IV: combined with rituximab, 2 steps are involved: day 1, administer rituximab; on day 7, 8, or 9 of treatment administer rituximab, then Y-90 ibritumomab within 4 hours of the completion of rituximab infusion; if platelet count is 150,000 cells/mm^3 or higher, inject 0.4 mCi/kg (14.8 MBq/kg) over 10 minutes up to a maximum of 32 mCi (1184 MBq); if platelet count is between 100,000-149,000 cells/mm^3, inject 0.3 mCi/kg (11.1 MBq/kg) over 10 minutes up to a maximum of 32 mCi (1184 MBq); if platelet count is less than 100,000 cells/mm^3, do not administer.

IPILIMUMAB, for *adults*, for melanoma, IV: 3 mg/kg every 3 weeks for 4 doses.

OFATUMUMAB, for *adults*, for chronic lymphocytic leukemia (CLL), IV: initiate at 300 mg week 1, followed 1 week later by 2000 mg once weekly for 7 doses, followed 4 weeks later by 2000 mg once every 4 weeks for 4 doses.

PANITUMUMAB, for *adults*, for KRAS mutation-negative colorectal cancer, IV: 6 mg/kg every 14 days as a single agent.

PERTUZUMAB, for *adults*, for HER2+ breast cancer, IV: initiate at 840 mg over 60 minutes followed by a maintenance dose of 420 mg over 30-60 minutes every 3 weeks until disease progression or unacceptable toxicity.

RITUXIMAB, for *adults*, for chronic lymphocytic leukemia (CLL), IV: 375 mg/m^2 on the day prior to fludarabine/cyclophosphamide in cycle 1, then 500 mg/m^2 day 1, every 28 days, of cycles 2-6; for granulomatosis with poly-ngiitis (GPA), aka Wegener's granulomatosis, IV: 375 mg/m^2 once weekly for 4 doses combined with IV methylprednisolone and daily prednisone; for non-Hodgkin's lymphoma (NHL), IV: depending on subtype (various regimens exist) use 375 mg/m^2 per dose with other agents; for rheumatoid arthritis, IV: 1000 mg on days 1 and 15 combined with methotrexate; more courses may be given every 24 weeks but no sooner than every 16 weeks; for microscopic polyangiitis (MPA), IV: 375 mg/m^2 once weekly for 4 doses with IV methylprednisolone and daily prednisone.

TOSITUMOMAB, for *adults*, for non-Hodgkin's lymphoma (NHL), Step 1: tositumomab 450 mg administered over 60 minutes, iodine I^{131} tositumomab (containing I^{131} 5 mCi and tositumomab 35 mg) administered over 20 minutes; Step 2 (7-14 days after step 1): tositumomab 450 mg administered over 60 minutes and iodine I^{131} tositumoma; if platelets are 150,000/mm^3 or higher iodine I^{131} cal-culated to deliver 75 cGy total body irradiation and tositumomab 35 mg over 20 minutes, if platelets are between 100,000/ mm^3 and 150,000/mm^3, iodine I^{131} calculated to deliver 65 cGy total body irradiation and tositumomab 35 mg over 20 minutes.

TRASTUZUMAB, for *adults*, for adjuvant treatment of HER2+ breast cancer, IV: with concurrent paclitaxel or docetaxel, initiate at 4 mg/kg over 90 minutes followed by 2 mg/kg infused over 30 minutes weekly for 12 weeks, followed 1 week later by 6 mg/kg infused over 30-90 minutes every 3 weeks for total duration of 52 weeks; with concurrent docetaxel/carboplatin follow same protocol but initiate for 18 weeks instead of 12; for HER2+ breast cancer, IV: either as a single agent or combined with paclitaxel, initiate at 4 mg/kg infused over 90 minutes followed by 2 mg/kg over 30 minutes weekly until disease regression; for HER2+ gastric cancer, IV: combined with cisplatin and either capecitabine or fluorouracil for 6 cycles followed by trastuzumab monotherapy, initiate at 8 mg/kg over 90 minutes followed by 6 mg/kg over 30-90 minutes every 3 weeks until disease progression.

ADVERSE EFFECTS

Common adverse effects of anticancer agents can occur.

RED FLAGS

Bevacizumab has caused gastrointestinal perforation in .3-2.4% of study patients.

There have been reported cases of progressive multifocal leukoencephalopathy (PML) when using brentuximab vedotin resulting in death.

When using cetuximab, cardiopulmonary arrest and/or sudden death has occurred in 2% of patients receiving concurrent radiation therapy and 3% of patients receiving combination therapy with platinum- and fluoruracil-based agents.

Panitumumab causes skin toxicities in approximately 90% of patients with approximately 12% of patients having severe toxicities.

Trastuzumab can cause cardiomyopathies and pulmonary toxicities.

▨ INTERACTIONS

INTERACTION ISSUES

A:

D:

M: Brentuximab vedotin is a major substrate of CYP3A4.

E:

Pgp:

SECTION 7: TYROSINE KINASE INHIBITORS

AFATINIB (a FA ti nib) PR=D *(Gilotrif)*

AXITINIB (ax I ti nib) PR=D *(Inlyta®)*

BOSUTINIB (boe SOO ti nib) PR-D PR=D *(Bosulif)*

CABOZANTINIB (ka boe ZAN ti nib) PR=D *(Cometriq™)*

CRIZOTINIB (kriz OH ti nib) PR=D *(Xalkori™)*

DASATINIB (da SA ti nib) PR-D *(Sprycel™)*

ERLOTINIB (er LOE tye nib) PR=D *(Tarceva®)*

GEFITINIB (ge FI tye nib) PR=D *(Iressa®)*

IMATINIB (eye MAT eh nib) PR=D *(Gleevec)*

LAPATINIB (la PA ti nib) PR=D *(Tykerb®)*

NILOTINIB (nye LOE ti nib) *(Tasigna)* **PR=D**

PAZOPANIB (paz OH pa nib) *(Votrient™)* **PR=D**

PONATINIB (poe NA ti nib) PR=D *(Iclusig)*

REGORAFENIB PR=D (re goe RAF e nib) *(Stivarga®)*

RUXOLITINIB (rux oh LI ti nib) PR=C *(Jakavi™)*

SORAFENIB (sor AF e nib) PR=D *(Nexavar®)*

SUNITINIB (su NIT e nib) PR=D *(Sutent®)*

VANDETANIB (van DET a nib) PR=D *(Caprelsa)*

This is another relatively recent addition to anti-cancer therapies.

▨ FUNCTION

Afatinib is used to treat very specific types of non-small-cell lung cancer (NSCLC) involving epidermal growth factor receptors (EGFR).

Axitinib is used to treat advanced renal cell cancer (RCC).

Bosutinib is used to treat Philadelphia chromosome-positive chronic myelogenous leukemia in patients intolerant or resistant to prior therapy.

Cabozantinib treats medullary thyroid cancer (MTC).

Crizotinib treats non-small-cell lung cancer (NSCLC) that is anaplastic lymphoma kinase (ALK) positive.

Dasatinib is used in treating chronic myelogenous leukemia (CML) and Philadelphia chromosome-positive CML and ALL. Off label, it can be used to treat gastrointestinal stromal tumors.

Erlotinib is used to treat non-small-cell lung cancer (NSCLC) and pancreatic cancer.

Gefitinib is used to treat non-small-cell lung cancer (NSCLC) after failure of other therapies.

Imatinib is used to treat Philadelphia chromosome-positive CML and ALL, gastrointestinal stromal tumor (GIST), aggressive systemic mastocytosis, dermatofibrosarcoma protuberans, hypereosinophilic syndrome and myelodysplastic/myeloproliferative disease. Off label it treats desmoid tumors and melanoma.

Lapatinib is used to treat advanced or metastatic HER2+ breast cancer.

Nilotinib is used to treat Philadelphia chromosome-positive CML and off label for refractory gastrointestinal stromal tumor (GIST).

Pazopanib treats advanced renal cell cancer

(RCC) and soft-tissue sarcoma as well as, off label, thyroid cancer.

Ponatinib treats chronic myelogenous leukemia (CML) and Philadelphia chromosome-positive (Ph+) acute lymphoblastic leukemia (ALL) that are resistant or intolerant to prior tyrosine kinase inhibitor therapy.

Regorafenib treats colorectal cancer in patients previously treated with several types of chemotherapy and locally advanced or non-resectable gastrointestinal stromal tumor (GIST) in patients previously treated with imatinib and sunitinib.

Ruxolitinib treats intermediate or high-risk myelofibrosis.

Sorafenib treats advanced renal cell cancer (RCC) and non-resectable hepatocellular cancer. Off label, it can treat advanced thyroid cancer, angiosarcomas, or resistant gastrointestinal stromal tumor (GIST).

Sunitinib treats advanced renal cell cancer; gastrointestinal stromal tumor following failure of, or intolerance to, imatinib; and pancreatic neuroendocrine tumors. Off label, it is used to treat advanced thyroid cancer, non-GIST soft tissue sarcomas, and advanced, non-resectable medullary thyroid cancer.

Vandetanib is used to treat locally advanced, non-resectable medullary thyroid cancer.

MECHANISM OF ACTION

Tyrosine kinases are cellular signaling proteins important in several basic functions of a cell including cell proliferation and migration. The agents in this category inhibit several functions that affect cancer, inlcuding angiogenesis of tumors. To grow, tumors require more vasculature to supply nutrients. Stopping angiogenesis is a frequently used strategy to slow or stop tumor growth while minimizing many of the traditional side effects of chemotherapy.

By inhibiting tyrosine kinase and preventing angiogenesis, tumor growth is severely hampered. Axitinib, cabozantinib, sunitinib, sorafenib and pazopanib affect tumors through this mechanism. Regorafenib uses this mechanism as well as inhibiting other kinases involved with starting cancers and creating favorable microenvironments for tumor growth. Vandetanib also inhibits multiple kinases affecting tumor growth

including angiogenesis and cellular proliferation.

Bosutinib, dasatinib, imatinib, nilotinib, and ponatinib target a specific tyrosine kinase created from a mutation of the BCR-ABL gene that results in cell growth. This is involved in chronic myeloid leukemia (CML). By inhibiting this kinase, tumor growth signaling is shut off and the tumor no longer grows. Imatinib can also affect other kinases allowing use in other cancers.

Crizotinib inhibits several tyrosine kinases that support tumor growth including anaplastic lymphoma kinase (ALK), hepatocyte growth factor receptor, and Recepteur d'Origine Nantais.

Since epidermal growth factor receptors (EGFR) are tyrosine kinases, these inhibitors can directly slow or stop the cell-growth effects of this kinase. Afatinib, gefitinib, erlotinib, lapatinib inhibit this subtype of tyrosine kinases.

Ruxolitinib works by targeting Janus associated kinases, which mediate immune function and hematopoiesis. Inhibiting these kinases inhibits the dysregulation present in myelofibrosis.

DOSAGES

AFATINIB, for *adults*, for non-small-cell lung cancer (NSCLC) with specific EGFR specifications, 40 mg once daily until disease progression or unacceptable toxicity.

AXITINIB, for *adults*, for advanced renal cell cancer, initiate with 5 mg bid; if dose is tolerated, for at least 2 consecutive weeks, may increase the dose to 7 mg bid and further to 10 mg bid if tolerance is maintained.

BOSUTINIB, for *adults*, for Philadelphia chromosome-positive chronic myelogenous leukemia, 500 mg once daily.

CABOZANTINIB, for adults, for medullary thyroid cancer, 140 mg once daily, not to exceed 180 mg daily.

CRIZOTINIB, for *adults*, for non-smal-cell lung cancer, 250 mg bid.

DASATINIB, for *adults*, 100 mg once daily.

ERLOTINIB, for adults, for non-small-cell lung cancer (NSCLC), 150 mg once daily; for pancreatic cancer, 100 mg once daily in combination with gemcitabine.

GEFITINIB, for *adults*, for non-small-cell lung cancer (NSCLC), 250 mg once daily.

IMATINIB, for *children* 1 year and older and

adolescents, for Philadelphia chromosome positive ALL or CML, 340 mg/m^2/d to a maximum 600 mg/d. For *adults*, for a variety of cancers including Philadelphia chromosome-positive CML, gastrointestinal stromal tumor (GIST), aggressive systemic mastocytosis, dermatofibrosarcoma protuberans, hypereosinophilic syndrome, and myelodysplastic/myeloproliferative disease, 400 mg once daily, may be increased to 400 mg bid; for Philadelphia chromosome-positive ALL, 600 mg once daily.

LAPATINIB, for *adults*, for HER2+ breast cancer, 1250 mg once daily.

NILOTINIB, for *adults*, for chronic myeloid leukemia (CML), Ph+, 300 mg bid; can be increased to 400 mg bid in resistant or intolerant cases.

PAZOPANIB, for *adults*, for renal cell cancer (RCC), 800 mg once daily; for soft-tissue sarcoma, 800 mg once daily.

PONATINIB, for *adults*, for Philadelphia chromosome-positive (Ph+) acute lymphoblastic leukemia (ALL) or chronic myelogenous leukemia (CML), 45 mg once daily.

REGORAFENIB, for *adults*, for colorectal cancer or gastrointestinal stromal tumor (GIST), 160 mg once daily for the first 21 days of each 28-day cycle.

RUXOLITINIB, for *adults*, for myelofibrosis, initiate using the following platelets counts: if over 200,000/mm^3, 20 mg bid; if between 100,000-200,000/mm$_3$, 15 mg bid; if between 50,000 and 100,000/mm3, 5 mg bid.

SORAFENIB, for *adults*, for advanced renal cell carcinoma (RCC) or hepatocellular cancer, 400 mg bid.

SUNITINIB, for *adults*, for gastrointestinal stromal tumor (GIST) or advanced renal cell cancer (RCC), 50 mg once daily for 4 weeks, then 2 weeks off.

VANDETANIB, for *adults*, for medullary thyroid cancer, 300 mg once daily.

ADVERSE EFFECTS

Common adverse effects of anticancer agents include severe vomiting, stomatitis, anorexia, diarrhea, and hair loss. Many suppress the bone marrow. Treatment-induced neoplasms can occur many years after treatment.

RED FLAGS

Cabozantinib can cause serious and occasionally fatal hemorrhage including hemoptysis and gastrointestinal bleeding according to a boxed warning. Another boxed warning states that GI perforations and fistulas have been reported.

Crizotinib commonly causes ocular toxicities.

Lapatinib, pazopanib, ponatinib, regorafenib, and sunitinib have boxed warnings of hepatotoxicity that may be severe and/or fatal. Ponatinib also has a boxed warning about thromboemboli.

Nilotinib and vandetanib may prolong QT intervals, and sudden deaths have been reported according to a boxed warning.

INTERACTIONS

DRUG

IMATINIB

- *Guan Ye Lian Qiao* (St. John's wort) (C)– Decreases blood concentrations (Izzo & Ernst, 2009) Level 2b evidence.
- *Ren Shen* (Ginseng) (D)–a case study of a chronic myelogenous leukemia showed imatinib-induced hepatitis. The patient was concurrently drinking energy drinks containing *ren shen*. Upon cessation of both the imatinib and the energy drinks, the hepatitis resolved. Reinitiating the imatinib without the energy drinks did not induce hepatitis (Bilgi, Bell & Ananthakrishnan, 2001, May) Level 4 evidence.

INTERACTION ISSUES

A:

D: Afatinib is approximately 95% protein bound; axitinib is over 99% bound; cabozantinib is 99.7% protein bound or higher, dasatinib is 96% bound; erlotinib is 92-95% bound; imatinib is approximately 95% bound; lapatinib is greater than 99% bound; nilotinib is approximately 98% bound; pazopanib and ponatinib are over 99% bound; regorafenib is 99.5% bound; ruxolitinib is approximately 97% bound; sorafenib is 99.5% bound; sunitinib is 95% bound.

M: Axitinib, bosutinib, and cabozantinib are major substrates of CYP3A4; crizotinib is a major substrate of CYP3A4 and a moderate inhibitor of both 2B6 and 3A4; dasatinib and erlotinib are major substrates of CYP3A4; gefitinib is a major substrate of CYP2D6 and 3A4; imatinib is a major substrate of CYP3A4 and a moderate inhibitor of 2D6 and 3A4; lapatinib is a major substrate of CYP3A4 and a moderate inhibitor of 2C8; nilotinib is a major substrate of CYP3A4, a moderate inhibitor of 2C8, 2C9, and 2D6, and a weak or moderate inducer of 2B6, 2C8, and 2C9; pazopanib, regorafenib, and ruxolitinib are major substrates of CYP3A4; sorafenib is a moderate inhibitor of CYP2B6 and 2C9 and a strong inhibitor of 2C8; sunitinib and vandetanib are major substrates of CYP3A4.

E:

Pgp: Afatinib and bosutinib are substrates and inhibitors of Pgp; cabozantinib inhibits Pgp; crizotinib, imatinib, lapatinib, and nilotinib are substrates and inhibitors of Pgp; pazopanib is a substrate of Pgp; ponatinib is a substrate and inhibitor of Pgp; regorafenib, sunitinib, and vandetanib inhibit Pgp.

SECTION 8: OTHER ANTICANCER AGENTS

ALDESLEUKIN (al des LOO kin) PR=C
(Proleukin®)

ALITRETINOIN (a li TRET i noyn) PR=D
(Panretin)

ALTRETAMINE (al TRET a mene) PR=D
(Hexalen®)

ARSENIC TRIOXIDE (AR se nik tri OKS id) PR=C *(Trisenox)*

ASPARAGINASE (*E. COLI*) (a SPEAR a ji nase e KO lye) PR=D *(Elspar)*

ASPARAGINASE (ERWINIA) (a SPEAR a ji nase er WIN i ah) PR=C *(Erwinase®)*

AZACITIDINE (ay za SYE ti dene) PR=D *(Vidaza®)*

BEXAROTENE (beks AIR oh tene) PR=X *(Targretin®)*

DABRAFENIB (da BRAF e nib) PR=D *(Tafinlar)*

DECITABINE (de SYE ta bene) PR=D *(Dacogen)*

DENILEUKIN DIFTITOX PR=D (de ni LOO kin DIF ti toks) *(Ontak)*

ETOPOSIDE (e toe POE side) PR=D *(Toposar®)*

ETOPOSIDE PHOSPHATE *(Etopophos) This is a prodrug of etoposide, and most of its information is similar and not covered.*

IRINOTECAN (eye rye no TEE kan) PR=D *(Camptosar®)*

LENALIDOMIDE (len a LID oh mide) PR=X *(REVLIMID®)*

MITOTANE (MYE toe tane) PR=C *(Lysodren®)*

MITOXANTRONE (mye toe ZAN trone) PR=D

OMACETAXINE (oh ma se TAX ene) PR=D *(Synribo)*

PEGASPARGASE (peg AS par jase) PR=C *(Oncaspar)*

PORFIMER (POR fi mer) PR=C *(Photofrin®)*

ROMIDEPSIN (roe mi DEP sin) PR=D *(Istodax)*

TENIPOSIDE (ten i POE side) PR=D *(Vumon®)*

THALIDOMIDE (tha LI doe mide) PR=X *(Thalomid)*

TOPOTECAN (toe poe TEA kan) PR=D *(Hycamtin)*

TRAMETINIB (tra ME ti nib) PR=D *(Mekinist)*

TRETINOIN (TRET i noyn) PR=D *(Vesanoid®)*

VEMURAFENIB (vem ue RAF e nib) PR=D *(Zelboraf)*

VISMODEGIB (vis moe DEG ib) PR=D *(Erivedge)*

VORINOSTAT (vor IN oh stat) PR=D *(Zolinza®)*

■ FUNCTION

Aldesleukin treats renal cell carcinoma and melanoma on label and AML off label.

Alitretinoin is used to treat AIDS-related Kaposi's sarcoma.

Altretamine treats persistent or recurrent ovarian cancer.

Arsenic trioxide treats relapsed or refractory acute promyelocytic leukemia (APL) on label and is used for initial treatment of APL and myelodysplastic syndrome (MDS) off label.

Asparaginase (*E. coli*) is used treat ALL in combination with other agents on label and lymphoblastic lymphoma off label. Asparaginase (Erwinia) treats ALL in patients with a hypersensitivity to the *E. coli* derived form of asparaginase.

Azacitidine is used to treat myelodysplastic syndrome (MDS) on label and AML off label.

Bexarotene treats cutaneous T-cell lymphoma in patients who are refractory to at least 1 prior systemic therapy.

Dabrafenib and vemurafenib treat nonresectable or metastatic melanoma in patients with a BRAFV600E mutation. Off label, vemur-afenib can also treat melanoma with a BRAF-V600K mutation.

Decitabine treats myelodysplastic syndrome (MDS). Off label, it is used to treat AML and sickle cell anemia.

Denileukin diftitox treats persistent or recurrent cutaneous T-cell lymphoma that expresses the CD25 component of the IL-2 receptor. Off label, it treats relapsed or refractory peripheral T-cell lymphoma.

Etoposide treats refractory testicular tumors and small-cell lung cancer (SCLC). Off label, it treats acute lymphocytic leukemia (ALL); refractory acute myeloid leukemia (AML); breast, merkel cell, non-small-cell lung, refractory ovarian, and prostate cancers; central nervous system tumors; ewing's sarcoma, gestational trophoblastic disease, Hodgkin's and non-Hodgkin's lymphomas; refractory multiple myeloma; neuroblastoma; neuroendocrine tumors; osteosarcoma; retinoblastoma; metastatic soft-tissue sarcoma, thymic malignancies; unknown-primary adenocarcinoma, Wilms's tumor; and is a conditioning regimen for hematopoietic cell transplantation.

Irinotecan treats carcinoma of the colon or rectum. Off label, it also can treat cervical, esophageal, gastric, non-small and small-cell lung, ovarian, and pancreatic cancers, glioblastomas, and Ewing's sarcoma.

Lenalidomide is used to treat relapsed or previously treated mantle cell lymphoma, multiple myelo-ma (with dexamethasone), and myelodysplastic syndromes. Off label it treats relapsed or refractory chronic lymphocytic leukemia (CLL), non-Hodgkin lymphoma, and systemic light chain amyloidosis.

Mitotane treats inoperable adrenocortical carcinoma on label, Cushing's syndrome off label.

Mitoxantrone treats acute non-lymphocytic leukemias, advanced hormone-refractory prostate cancer, and secondary multiple sclerosis (MS). Off label, it can be used to treat Hodgkin's and non-Hodgkin's lymphomas, acute lymphocytic leukemia (ALL), relapsed or pediatric acute myeloid leukemia (AML), breast cancer, and pediatric acute promyelocytic leukemia.

Pegaspargase treats acute lymphocytic leukemia (ALL).

Porfimer is used to treat obstructing esophageal cancer, microinvasive endobronchial or obstructing non-small-cell lung cancer (NSCLC), and high-grade dysplasia in Barrett's esophagus. Off label, it treats actinic keratoses and low-risk basal and squamous cell skin cancers.

Romidepsin treats refractory cutaneous and peripheral T-cell lymphomas.

Teniposide is used in acute lymphoblastic leukemia (ALL) in children in combination with other agents. Off label, it treats ALL in adults.

Thalidomide treats multiple myeloma and cutaneous manifestations of erythema nodosum leprosum (ENL). Off label, it treats refractory Crohn's disease, chronic graft-versus-host disease (GVHD) in hematopoietic stem cell transplantation, AIDS-related aphthous stomatitis, Walden-ström's macroglobulinemia, multiple myeloma (maintenance), and systemic light chain amyloidosis.

Topotecan treats recurrent or resistant cervical cancer in combination with cisplatin, ovarian cancer, and relapsed or refractory small-cell lung cancer (SCLC). Off label it is used to treat AML, CNS lymphoma, Ewing's sarcoma, lung cancer metastases in the CNS, merkel cell cancer, osteosarcoma, and in children, rhabdomyosarcoma and neuroblastoma.

Trametinib treats non-resectable or metastatic melanoma in patients with BRAFV600E or BRAFV600K mutations.

Tretinoin is used to treat acute promyelocytic leukemia (APL).

Vismodegib treats basal cell carcinomas.

Vorinostat treats cutaneous T-cell lymphoma.

MECHANISM OF ACTION

Aldesleukin is a recombinant form of interleukin-2 that promotes the proliferation and activation of T and B cells, natural killer cells, and thymocytes. These then cause interactions with the immune system and the death of cells.

Reinoids act by binding with retinoid receptors, which regulate gene expression, cellular differentiation, and proliferation. Alitretinoin works by activating naturally occurring retinoid receptors, which inhibits growth of Kaposi's sarcoma. Bexarotene is also a retinoid.

Altretamine structurally looks like alkylating agents but has activity in tumors that do not respond to classic alkylating agents. How this agent kills tumor cells is not well understood.

Arsenic Trioxide kills APL cells through morphological changes and fragmentation of DNA. Tretinoin also affects APL cells causing decreased proliferation and increased differentiation.

Asparaginase breaks down asparagine causing a lower amount of this amino acid in lymphoblasts, inhibition of protein synthesis, and cell apoptosis. Pegaspargase is a modified version of asparaginase with a similar mechanism of action.

Azacitidine and decitabine prevent proper methylation of DNA and cause cell death.

Dabrafenib, trametinib, and vemurafenib selectively inhibit the protein kinase B-raf (BRAF), specifically, BRAFV600E mutations resulting in tumor growth inhibition. Trametinib also inhibits other BRAFV600 mutations.

Denileukin diftitox is a drug that combines diphtheria toxin with interleukin-2 creating a targeted delivery system. It interacts with IL-2 receptors and delivers the toxin, which inhibits protein synthesis and causes cell death.

Etoposide and teniposide arrest growth of cells possibly by inhibiting mitochondrial transport of NADH and/or by inhibiting the DNA enzyme topoisomerase II, which causes strands of DNA to break.

Irinotecan and topotecan prevent recleaving of DNA after topoisomerase I cleaves it. This results in accumulation of irreparable DNA breaks and prevention of cell proliferation.

Lenalidomide has several mechanisms of action and can be both anticancer and immunomodulatory. Anticancer effects are due to its effects to increase programmed cell death (apoptosis) and in preventing blood vessel formation. Inhibition of proinflammatory cytokine secretion explains its immunomodulatory effects.

Mitotane affects mitochondria in adrenal cortical cells and decreases cortisol production. It also alters peripheral metabolism of steroids.

Mitoxantrone acts by causing cross-linking and strand breaks in DNA inhibiting DNA and RNA synthesis.

Omacetaxine is a reversible protein synthesis inhibitor that prevents protein synthesis.

Porfimer is retained in neoplastic (cancer) tissues. Exposure to laser light causes production of oxygen free radicals and cytotoxicity.

Romidepsin and vorinostat are histone deacetylases that remove acetyl groups from the protein lysine. This can cause a breakdown in various proteins involving DNA including histones and transcription factors. These then lead to termination of cell growth.

Thalidomide affects both the immune system and angiogenesis of tumors. While the exact mechanisms of action are not known, it is thought that part of its effects can be explained by increasing natural killer cells and increasing interleukin-2 and interferon gamma levels.

Vismodegib is what is known as an inhibitor of the hedgehog pathway. This pathway is normally used in embryo development to regulate cell growth and differentiation. Not normally active in adults, in certain basal cell carcinomas, it can be reactivated causing unregulated proliferation of skin basal cells.

DOSAGES

ALDESLEUKIN, for *adults*, for renal cell carcinoma (RCC) or melanoma, IV: 600,000 units/kg every 8 hours for a maximum of 14 doses; repeat in 9 days.

ALITRETINOIN, for *adults*, for Kaposi's sarcoma, topical: initiate by applying gel bid to skin lesions, may gradually increase application to 3-4 times daily based on lesion tolerance, continue for as long as benefit is observed, usually 2 to over 14 weeks.

ALTRETAMINE, for *adults*, for ovarian cancer, oral: 65 mg/m^2 qid for 14 or 21 days of a 28-day cycle.

ARSENIC TRIOXIDE, for *children* 4 years and older and *adults*, for relapsed or refractory acute promyelocytic leukemia (APL), initiate at 0.15 mg/kg/d administered daily until bone marrow remission up to a maximum of 60 doses; consolidate with 0.15 mg/kg/d starting 3-6 weeks after completion of initiation up to a maximum consolidation of 25 doses over a period of up to 5 weeks.

ASPARAGINASE (*E. COLI*), for *children* and *adults*, for acute lymphoblastic leukemia (ALL), IV, IM: 6000 units/m^2 3 times weekly.

ASPARAGINASE (ERWINIA), for *children* and *adults*, for acute lymphoblastic leukemia (ALL), IV, IM: 25,000 units/m^2 3 times weekly.

AZACITIDINE, for *adults*, for MDS, IV, subcutaneous: 75 mg/m^2/d for 7 days repeated every 4 weeks.

BEXAROTENE, for *adults*, for refractory cutaneous T-cell lymphoma, 300-400 mg/m^2/d taken as a single daily dose; for cutaneous lesions of T-cell lymphoma, topical: apply to lesions once every other day for first week, then increase on a weekly basis to once daily bid, tid, and finally qid as tolerated.

DABRAFENIB, for *adults*, for melanoma with BRAFV600E mutation, 150 mg bid.

DECITABINE, for *adults*, for MDS, IV: 15 mg/m^2 over 3 hours every 8 hours for 3 days every 6 weeks; treatment is recommended for at least 4 cycles or 20 mg/m^2 over 1 hour daily for 5 days every 28 days.

DENILEUKIN DIFTITOX, for *adults*, for persistent or recurrent cutaneous T-cell lymphoma, IV: 9 or 18 mcg/kg once daily on days 1 through 5 every 21 days for 8 cycles.

ETOPOSIDE, for *adults*, for small-cell lung cancer in combination with other agents, 70 mg/m^2/d for 4 days or 100 mg/m^2/d for 5 days every 3-4 weeks.

IRINOTECAN, for *adults*, for colorectal cancer, IV: weekly regimen: 125 mg/m^2 over 90 minutes on days 1, 8, 15, and 22 of a 6-week treatment cycle; may adjust upward to 150 mg/m^2 if tolerated; once-every-3-week regimen: 350 mg/m^2 over 90 minutes once every 3 weeks.

LENALIDOMIDE, for *adults*, 10 mg once/d.

MITOTANE, for *adults*, for adrenocortical carcinoma, initiate at 2-6 g/d in 3-4 divided doses; increase incrementally to 9-10 g/d in 3-4 divided doses up to maximum daily dose of 18 g.

MITOXANTRONE, for *adults*, for acute myeloid leukemia (AML), initiate at 12 mg/m^2 once daily for 3 days with cytarabine; beginning approximately 6 weeks later, 12 mg/m^2 once daily for 2 days with cytarabine; repeat in 4 weeks; for multiple sclerosis, 12 mg/m^2 every 3 months, maximum lifetime cumulative dose is 140 mg/m^2; for advanced, hormone-refractory prostate cancer, 12-14 mg/m^2 every 3 weeks with corticosteroids.

OMACETAXINE, for *adults*, for CML, subcutaneous: induce at 1.25 mg/m^2 bid for 14 days of a 28-day cycle; maintain at same dose for 7 days of a 28-day cycle.

PEGASPARGASE, for children and *adults*, for acute lymphoblastic leukemia (ALL), IM, IV: 2500 units/m^2 as part of a combination chemotherapy regimen.

PORFIMER, for *adults*, for photodynamic therapy in esophageal cancer or endobronchial non-small-cell lung cancer, IV: 2 mg/kg followed by endoscopic exposure to appropriate laser light and debridement; separate repeat courses by at least 30 days up to maximum 3 courses; for photodynamic therapy in Barrett's esophagus dysplasia, IV: 2 mg/kg followed by endoscopic exposure to appropriate laser light; separate repeat courses by at least 90 days to a maximum 3 courses.

ROMIDEPSIN, for *adults*, for cutaneous or peripheral T-cell lymphoma, IV: 14 mg/m^2 days 1, 8, and 15 of a 28-day cycle.

THALIDOMIDE, for *children* 12 years and older and *adults*, for erythema nodosum leprosum (ENL), initiate at 100-300 mg once daily. For adults, for multiple myeloma, 200 mg nocte with dexamethasone 40 mg daily on days 1-4, 9-12, and 17-20 of a 28-day treatment cycle.

TENIPOSIDE, for *children*, for combination therapy of acute lymphoblastic leukemia (ALL), IV: 165 mg/m² twice weekly for 8-9 doses or 250 mg/m² weekly for 4-8 weeks.

TOPOTECAN, for *adults*, for recurrent or resistant cervical cancer, IV: 0.75 mg/m²/d 3 days every 21 days; for ovarian cancer, IV: 1.5 mg/m²/d 5 consecutive days every 21 days; minimum 4 cycles recommended; for relapsed or refractory small-cell lung cancer (SCLC), 2.3 mg/m²/d 5 consecutive days every 21 days; IV: 1.5 mg/m²/d 5 consecutive days every 21 days; minimum 4 cycles recommended.

TRAMETINIB, for *adults*, for melanoma with BRAFV600E or BRAFV600K mutations, 2 mg once daily.

TRETINOIN, for *children* and *adults*, for remission induction, 45 mg/m²/d in 2-3 divided doses for up to 30 days after complete remission; maximum duration of treatment is 90 days; for remission maintenance, 45-200 mg/m²/d in 2-3 divided doses for up to 12 months.

VEMURAFENIB, for *adults*, for melanoma with BRAFV600E mutation, 960 mg bid.

VISMODEGIB, for *adults*, for basal cell carcinoma, 150 mg once daily.

VORINOSTAT, for *adults*, for cutaneous T-cell lymphoma, 400 mg once daily.

ADVERSE EFFECTS

Common adverse effects of anticancer agents include severe vomiting, stomatitis, anorexia, diarrhea, and hair loss. Many suppress the bone marrow. Treatment-induced neoplasms can occur many years after treatment.

High-dose aldesleukin and denileukin diftitox use can lead to capillary leak syndrome according to a boxed warning. Other boxed warnings discuss developing moderate to severe lethargy or sleepiness leading to coma with continuing treatment impaired neutrophil function and increased chance of infection.

Lenalidomide has multiple boxed warnings. One warns against use during pregnancy. Another states neutropenia and thrombocytopenia will occur in 80% of patients with del 5q myelodysplastic syndrome. A third warning states

there is a significant increase in risk for thromboembolic events.

RED FLAGS

Irinotecan has different boxed warnings cautioning about severe myelosuppression and severe and potentially fatal diarrhea.

Mitoxantrone has a boxed warning that may cause myocardial toxicity and potentially fatal heart failure. Another boxed warning describes the risk of developing secondary AML.

Thalidomide and Lenalidomide have a high risk for coagulative events according to a boxed warning. Another one warns of severe birth defects or death of the fetus.

Tretinoin can cause approximately 40% of patients to develop rapidly evolving leukocytosis according to a boxed warning. Another warning describes the high risk of teratogenicity during pregnancy.

INTERACTIONS

DRUG

IRINOTECAN

- *Huang Qin* (Scutellaria) (C) Ameliorates irinotecan-induced gastrointestinal toxicity in cancer patients (Hu, Yang, Ho, Chan *et al.*, 2005) Level 2b evidence; (Izzo & Ernst, 2009) Level 2b evidence.

INTERACTION ISSUES

A:

D: Bexarotene is over 99% protein bound; dabrafenib is 99.7% protein bound; etoposide is 94-98% bound; teniposide is 99.4% bound; trametinib is approximately 97% bound; tretinoin is over 95% bound; vemurafenib and vismodegib are over 99% bound.

M: Bexarotene is a weak or moderate inducer of CYP3A4; dabrafenib is a major substrate of CYP2C8 and 3A4 and a weak or moderate inducer of 2B6, 2C19, 2C8, 2C9, and 3A4; etoposide is a major substrate of CYP3A4; irinotecan is a major substrate of CYP2B6 and 3A4; romidepsin and teniposide are major substrates of CYP3A4; Trametinib is a weak or moderate inducer of CYP3A4; tretinoin is a major substrate of CYP2C8 and a weak or moderate inducer of 2E1; vemurafenib is major substrate and a weak or moderate inducer of CYP3A4 and a moderate inhibitor of 1A2.

E:

Pgp: Dabrafenib, etoposide, irinotecan, omacetaxine, romidepsin, and teniposide are substrates of Pgp; vemurafenib is a substrate and inhibitor of Pgp; vismodegib is a substrate of Pgp.

Anti-Inflammatory Drugs 12

SECTION 1: NON-STEROIDAL ANTI-INFLAMMATORY DRUGS

DICLOFENAC (dye KLOE fen ak) PR=C/D at 30 weeks or greater gestation *(Arthrotec®,[1] Cambia, Cataflam®, Flector, Pennsaid, Solaraze®, Voltaren®, Voltaren®-XR, Zipsor)*

DIFLUNISAL (dye FLOO ni sal) PR=C

ETODOLAC (ee toe DOE lak) PR=C

FENOPROFEN (fen oh PROE fen) PR=C *(Nalfon®)*

FLAVOCOXID (fla vo KOKS id) PR=N *(Limbrel, Limbrel250, Limbrel500)*

FLURBIPROFEN (flure BI proe fen) PR=C *(Ocufen)*

IBUPROFEN (eye byoo PROE fen) PR=C *(Addaprin [O], Advil [O], Advil® Allergy Sinus,[7] Advil Junior Strength [O], Advil Migraine [O], Advil® Multi-Symptom Cold,[7] Advil PM [O],[5] Caldolor; Children's Advil [O], Children's Ibuprofen [O], Children's Motrin [O], Children's Motrin Jr Strength [O], Duexis®,[6] Dyspel [O], EnovaRX-Ibuprofen; Genpril [O], I-Prin [O], Ibudone®,[3] Ibuprofen Children's [O], Ibuprofen Comfort Pac; Ibuprofen Junior Strength [O], Infant's Advil [O], Infant's Ibuprofen [O], KS Ibuprofen [O], Motrin [O], Motrin IB [O], Motrin Infant's Drops [O], Motrin Junior Strength [O], Motrin PM [O],[5] NeoProfen; Provil [O], Reprexain™,[3] Vicoprofen®[3])*

INDOMETHACIN (in doe METH a sin) PR=C/D after 30 weeks gestation *(Indocin®, Indocin® SR)*

KETOPROFEN (kee toe PROE fen) PR=C

KETOROLAC (KEE toe role ak) PR=C *(Acular®, Acular LS™, Acuvail, Sprix)*

MECLOFENAMATE (me kloe fen AM ate) PR=N

MEFENAMIC ACID (me fe NAM ik AS id) PR=C *(Ponstel®)*

MELOXICAM (mel OKS i kam) PR=C/D at 30 weeks or greater gestation *(Meloxicam Comfort Pac, Mobic®)*

NABUMETONE (na BYOO me tone) PR=C

NAPROXEN (na PROKS en) PR=C *(Aleve [O], All Day Pain Relief [O], All Day Relief [O], Anaprox®, Anaprox® DS, EC-Naprosyn®, Flanax Pain Relief [O], Mediproxen [O], Naprelan®, Naprosyn, Naproxen Comfort Pac, Naproxen DR, Treximet®,[9] Vimovo™[8])*

OXAPROZIN (oks a PROE zin) PR=C *(Daypro®)*

PIROXICAM (peer OKS i kam) PR=C *(Feldene®)*

SULINDAC (sul IN dak) PR=C *(Clinoril®)*

TOLMETIN (TOLE met in) PR=C *(Tolectin®)*

COX-2 INHIBITORS:

CELECOXIB (se le KOKS ib) PR=C/D at 30 weeks or greater gestation *(Celebrex®)*

SALICYLATES:

ASPIRIN (ASA) (AS pir in) *(See Chapter 6, Section 9)*

CHOLINE MAGNESIUM TRISALICYLATE (KOE leen mag NEE zhum trye sa LIS i late) PR=C/D at 30 weeks or greater gestation

MAGNESIUM SALICYLATE (mag NEE zhum sa LIS i late) PR=C/D after 30 weeks gestation *(Doans Extra Strength [O], Doans Pills [O], MST 600)*

SALSALATE (SAL sa late) PR=C *(Amigesic®)*

TROLAMINE (TROLE a mene) PR=N *(Analgesic Creme Rub/Aloe [O], Arthricream [O], Arthricream Rub [O], Asper-Flex [O], Mobisyl [O], Myoflex [O], Trumicin [O])*

FUNCTION

Normally, the inflammatory process is part of the body's healthy repair mechanism. It consists of four ancient signs: *calor* (heat), *dolor* (pain), *rubor* (redness), and *tumor* (swelling). However, it can become problematic under various conditions. An autoimmune response can cause inflammation to get out of hand and cause serious harm. Or the inflammatory process can be triggered by an otherwise harmless substance such as in allergies. Sometimes, the inflammatory process doesn't end when the initial insult is repaired. At other times, just the normal inflammatory process causes too much discomfort. Anti-inflammatory agents attempt to stop or reduce the inflammatory process and are useful in treating a large number of conditions. Each agent has **antipyretic**, **analgesic**, and anti-inflammatory effects but differs in how much of each it accomplishes.

In general, non-steroidal anti-inflammatory drugs (NSAIDs) are the drugs of choice for pain involved with inflammation and low to moderate pain especially in the somatic structures. Opioids are better for moderate to severe pain or pain originating in the viscera. And a combination of NSAIDs and opioids is often used to treat pain from cancer, or moderate to severe pain, and to reduce the overall dose of opioids.

Aspirin and the other salicylates are used to treat gout, rheumatic fever, and rheumatoid arthritis. They are also used to prevent adverse cardiac events by inhibiting platelet aggregation. Aspirin may also help reduce the incidence of colorectal cancer.

Acetic acid derivatives, which include indomethacin and sulindac, while having antipyretic properties, are not used to reduce fevers. Indomethacin has relatively high toxicities and is used only in the acute treatment of gouty arthritis, ankylosing spondylitis, and osteoarthritis of the hip. Sulindac is not as potent as indomethacin and is used in treating rheumatoid arthritis, ankylosing spondylitis, acute gout, and osteoarthritis.

Antipyretic: A substance that reduces fever

Analgesic: A drug that relieves pain

Celecoxib is approved for treating rheumatoid arthritis and osteoarthritis. It recently was approved for treating juvenile rheumatoid arthritis in patients 2 years and older. There used to be several other COX-2 inhibiting agents on the market, but all were found to increase the incidence of myocardial infarction and stroke. All but celecoxib were pulled from the market. Their main advantage was a reduction, though not as great as it theoretically should have been, in ulcers, hemorrhages, and perforations in long-term use.

Diclofenac is used in the long-term treatment of rheumatoid arthritis, ankylosing spondylitis, and osteoarthritis.

Nabumetone and tolmetin are used to treat adult or juvenile rheumatoid arthritis and osteoarthritis. They are as potent as aspirin but may have fewer adverse effects.

The oxicam derivatives, meloxicam and piroxicam, are used to treat rheumatoid arthritis, ankylosing spondylitis, and osteoarthritis. Their long half-lives allow for once-a-day dosing.

Propionic acid derivatives, which include ibuprofen, fenoprofen, flurbiprofen, naproxen, and oxaprozin, are often used in the chronic treatment of rheumatoid arthritis and osteoarthritis as their GI effects are generally less than those of aspirin and the salicylates.

A summary of advantages and disadvantages of various NSAIDs is shown in Figure 12.1.

MECHANISM OF ACTION

All non-steroidal anti-inflammatory drugs (NSAIDs) act by inhibiting prostaglandin synthesis. Prostaglandins are cyclic, fatty acid derivatives that act as signals to the local area. What these signals say depend on the specific prostaglandin and the specific tissues it is signaling and varies widely.

The first step in prostaglandin synthesis involves arachidonic acid and can follow two different pathways. The first is the cyclooxygenase pathway. This pathway builds eicosanoids which includes prostaglandins, thromboxanes, and prostacyclins. There are two types of the cyclooxygenase enzyme: COX-1 and COX-2. COX-1 helps

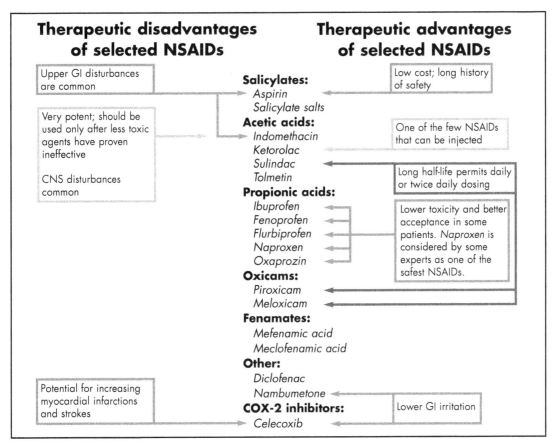

Figure 12.1: A list of non-steroidal anti-inflammatory drugs (NSAIDs) in their subclasses with advantages and disadvantages of individual agents.

build proteins that are used in the normal function of the body and tends to be quite beneficial. Examples of this include protection of the stomach from acid, vascular homeostasis, helping kidney function, and platelet aggregation. COX-2, normally in the brain, kidney, and bone, is increasingly expressed elsewhere during an inflammatory process. In a gross oversimplification, COX-1 is considered to have benefits, while COX-2 is more involved with the inflammatory response. This is summarized in Figure 12.2 on the following page.

The other pathway is the lipoxygenase pathway, which, among other things, builds leukotrienes. Drugs that block leukotrienes are very useful in treating allergic asthma.

NSAIDs act by blocking COX-2. All NSAIDs, except for the COX-2 inhibitors, also inhibit COX-1, which is where many of the adverse effects arise.

Prostaglandin E2 (PGE) is looked at as a mediator of many of the functions of NSAIDs. It is thought to sensitize nerve endings to inflammatory chemicals that increase pain. Therefore its blockage reduces the sensation of pain. PGE, in the hypothalamus, causes fever by resetting the thermoregulatory center. Again, blocking PGE would cause a decrease in fever.

Aspirin is unique among the NSAIDs in that it irreversibly inactivates COX by being converted into salicylate. Most NSAIDs reversibly inhibit COX. Aspirin's antipyretic and anti-inflammatory effects are primarily due to prostaglandin synthesis blockade in the thermoregulatory centers in the hypothalamus and peripheral targets. Salicylates directly reduce the sensitivity of pain receptors. COX also produces a chemical, thromboxane A2 (TXA2), that enhances platelet aggregation. Inhibition of this chemical has an anticoagulant effect. Other salicylates have similar actions.

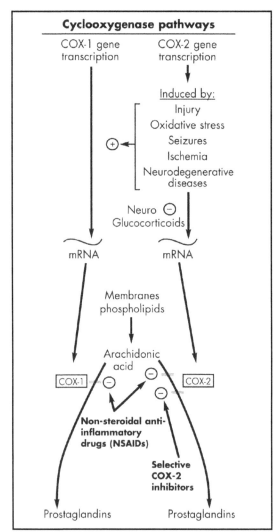

Figure 12.2: Summary of cyclooxygenase pathways and how drugs affect them. The COX-1 pathway is predominantly beneficial; it is interrupted by almost all NSAIDs. The COX-2 pathway is generally used in response to various insults to the body and increases pain and inflammation. This pathway is blocked by both NSAIDs and COX-2 inhibitors. Theoretically, blocking COX-2 with minimal inhibition of COX-1 would create an almost adverse effect free agent for pain and inflammation. This, however, was not the case in reality.

DOSAGES

ASPIRIN, See Chapter 6, Section 9.

CELECOXIB, for *adults*, for acute pain or primary dysmenorrhea, initiate at 400 mg, followed by an additional 200 mg if needed on day 1; maintenance dose is 200 mg bid prn; for ankylosing spondylitis, 200 mg/d as a single dose or in divided doses twice daily; if no effect after 6 weeks, may increase to 400 mg/d; if no response following 6 weeks of treatment with 400 mg/d, consider discontinuation and alternative treatment; for familial adenomatous polyposis, 400 mg bid; for osteoarthritis, 200 mg/d as a single dose or in divided doses twice daily; for rheumatoid arthritis, 100-200 mg bid.

CHOLINE MAGNESIUM TRISALICYLATE, for *children* under 37 kg, 25 mg/kg/d bid; 2250 mg/d for heavier *children*. For *adults*, 500 mg to 1.5 g bid/tid or 3 g nocte; usual maintenance dose is 1-4.5 g/d; for the *elderly*, 750 mg tid.

DICLOFENAC, for *adults*, for analgesia/primary dysmenorrhea, initiate at 50 mg tid; maximum dose 150 mg/d; for rheumatoid arthritis, 150-200 mg/d in 2-4 divided doses (100 mg/d of sustained release product); for osteoarthritis, 100-150 mg/d in 2-3 divided doses (100-200 mg/d of sustained release product); for ankylosing spondylitis, 100-125 mg/d in 4-5 divided doses.

DIFLUNISAL, for *adults*, for mild-to-moderate pain, initiate at 500-1000 mg followed by 250-500 mg every 8-12 hours up to a maximum daily dose of 1.5 g; for arthritis, 250-500 mg bid up to a maximum daily dose of 1.5 g.

ETODOLAC, for *children* 6-16, for juvenile idiopathic arthritis (JIA), extended release, 20-30 kg: 400 mg once daily; 31-45 kg: 600 mg once daily, 46-60 kg: 800 mg once daily; over 60 kg: 1000 mg once daily. For *adults*, for acute pain, immediate release: 200-400 mg every 6-8 hours prn to a maximum 1000 mg/d; for rheumatoid or osteoarthritis, immediate release: 400 mg bid or 300 mg 2-3 times/d or 500 mg bid; extended release: 400-1000 mg once daily.

FENOPROFEN, for *adults*, for rheumatoid arthritis, 300-600 mg 3-4 times/d up to 3.2 g/d; for mild to moderate pain, 200 mg every 4-6 hours prn.

FLAVOCOXID, for *adults*, for osteoarthritis management, 250-500 mg every 12 hours.

FLURBIPROFEN, for rheumatoid arthritis and osteoarthritis, 200-300 mg/d in 2-4 divided doses; do not administer more than 100 mg for any single dose; maximum is 300 mg/d.

IBUPROFEN, for *children*, as an antipyretic, 6

months to 12 years, temperature less than 102.5°F (39°C), 5 mg/kg; over 102.5°F, 10 mg/kg given every 6-8 hours; maximum daily dose is 40 mg/kg/d; for juvenile rheumatoid arthritis, 30-50 mg/kg/d divided every 8 hours; start at lower end of dosing range and increase up to a maximum of 2.4 g/d; as an analgesic, 4-10 mg/kg every 6-8 hours; for *children* 12 years and over, 200 mg every 4-6 hours prn to a maximum 1200 mg/d. For *adults*, for inflammatory disease, 400-800 mg 3-4 times/d; maximum dose 3.2 g/d; for analgesia/pain/fever/dysmenorrhea, 200-400 mg every 4-6 hours; maximum daily dose is 1.2 g unless directed by physician; OTC labeling (analgesic, antipyretic), 200 mg every 4-6 hours prn up to a maximum of 1200 mg/d.

INDOMETHACIN, for *children* over 2, for inflammatory/rheumatoid disorders, 1-2 mg/kg/d in 2-4 divided doses; maximum dose 4 mg/kg/d; not to exceed 150-200 mg/d. For *adults*, for inflammatory/rheumatoid disorders, 25-50 mg 2-3 times/d; maximum dose is 200 mg/d; extended release capsule should be given on a 1-2 times/d schedule; maximum dose for sustained release is 150 mg/d. Patients with arthritis and persistent night pain and/or morning stiffness may take larger portion (up to 100 mg) of the total daily dose at bedtime; for bursitis/tendonitis, initiate at 75-150 mg/d in 3-4 divided doses; usual treatment duration is 7-14 days; for acute gouty arthritis, 50 mg tid until pain is tolerable, then reduce dose; usual treatment less than 3-5 days.

KETOPROFEN, for *adults*, for rheumatoid or osteoarthritis, regular release: 50 mg qid or 75 mg tid up to a maximum 300 mg/d; extended release: 200 mg once daily; for mild-to-moderate dysmenorrhea; regular release: 25-50 mg every 6-8 hours up to a maximum 300 mg/d. For the *elderly*, initiate at 25-50 mg 3-4 times/d; increase up to 150-300 mg/d.

KETOROLAC, for *adults*, the maximum combined duration of treatment is 5 days; for patients under 50 kg and/or 65 years and over, see *elderly* dosing: 20 mg, followed by 10 mg every 4-6

hours; do not exceed 40 mg/d; oral dosing is intended to be a continuation of IM or IV therapy only. For the *elderly* over 65 years, with renal insufficiency or weight under 50 kg, 10 mg every 4-6 hours; do not exceed 40 mg/d; oral dosing is intended to be a continuation of IM or IV therapy only.

MAGNESIUM SALICYLATE, for *children* 12 years and older and *adults*, for relief of mild-to-moderate pain, two caplets every 6 hours prn up to a maximum of 8 caplets/d.

MECLOFENAMATE, for *children* over 14 years and *adults*, for mild-to-moderate pain, 50 mg every 4-6 hours; increases to 100 mg may be required; maximum dose is 400 mg; for rheumatoid arthritis and osteoarthritis, 50 mg every 4-6 hours; increase, over weeks, to 200-400 mg/d in 3-4 divided doses; do not exceed 400 mg/d; maximal benefit for any dose may not be seen for 2-3 weeks.

MEFENAMIC ACID, for *children* over 14 years and *adults*, 500 mg to start, then 250 mg every 4 hours prn; maximum duration is 1 week.

MELOXICAM, for *children* 2 years and over, for JRA, 0.125 mg/kg/d; maximum dose 7.5 mg/d. For *adults*, for osteoarthritis and rheumatoid arthritis, initiate at 7.5 mg once daily, some patients may receive additional benefit from an increased dose of 15 mg once daily; maximum dose is 15 mg/d.

NABUMETONE, for *adults*, 1000 mg/d; an additional 500-1000 mg may be needed in some patients to obtain more symptomatic relief; may be administered once or twice daily up to a maximum dose of 2000 mg/d.

NAPROXEN, for *children* over 2 years, for juvenile arthritis, 5 mg/kg/d bid. For *adults*, for acute gout, initiate at 750 mg, followed by 250 mg every 8 hours until attack subsides; EC-Naprosyn® is not recommended; for pain (mild to moderate), dysmenorrhea, acute tendonitis, bursitis, initiate at 500 mg, then 250 mg every 6-8 hours up to a maximum of 1250 mg/d naproxen base; for rheumatoid arthritis, osteoarthritis, and ankylosing spondylitis, 250-500 mg/d bid; may increase to

1.5 g/d of naproxen base for limited time period.

OXAPROZIN, for *children* 6-16 years, for juvenile rheumatoid arthritis, 22-31 kg: 600 mg once daily; 32-54 kg: 900 mg once daily; 55 kg or over: 1200 mg once daily. For *adults*, for osteoarthritis, 600-1200 mg once daily but decreased to lowest dose possible; patients with low body weight should start with 600 mg daily; for rheumatoid arthritis, 1200 mg once daily, a one-time loading dose of up to 1800 mg/d or 26 mg/kg (whichever is lower) may be given. Maximum doses, patient under 50 kg: 1200 mg/d; patient over 50 kg with normal renal/hepatic function and low risk of peptic ulcer, 1800 mg or 26 mg/kg (whichever is lower) in divided doses.

PIROXICAM, for *adults*, 10-20 mg/d once daily, although associated with increase in GI adverse effects; doses over 20 mg/d have been used (*i.e.*, 30-40 mg/d).

SALSALATE, for *adults*, 3 g/d in 2-3 divided doses.

SULINDAC, for *adults*, maximum daily dose is 400 mg; for osteoarthritis, rheumatoid arthritis, ankylosing spondylitis, 150 mg bid; for bursitis/tendonitis, 200 mg bid; usual treatment duration is 7-14 days; for acute gouty arthritis, 200 mg bid; usual treatment duration is 7 days.

TOLMETIN, for *children* 2 years or over, as an anti-inflammatory, initiate at 20 mg/kg/d in 3 divided doses, then 15-30 mg/kg/d in 3 divided doses; as an analgesic, 5-7 mg/kg every 6-8 hours. For *adults*, 400 mg tid; usual dose is 600 mg to 1.8 g/d; maximum dose is 2 g/d.

TROLAMINE, for *children* 12 years and older and *adults*, for pain: topical: apply to area prn up to 3-4 times/d.

■ ADVERSE EFFECTS

All NSAIDs except for aspirin appear to increase the likelihood of adverse cardiovascular events, including **myocardial infarctions**, cerebrovascular accidents, or initiation or worsening of hypertension. All, including aspirin, increase the risk of

Myocardial infarction: Necrosis of part of the heart muscle; heart attack

Hyperkalemia: Too much potassium in the blood

Anaphylaxis: A severe and occasionally fatal hypersensitivity/allergic reaction to an antigen; symptoms often include respiratory distress, vascular collapse, and severe skin rashes

Hemolytic anemia: An anemia, or loss of hemoglobin, characterized by red blood cell destruction

Tinnitus: Ringing in the ears

gastrointestinal irritation, ulceration, hemorrhage, and perforation. They also may cause kidney toxicity.

When the COX-2 inhibitors came on the market, there was a lot of optimism that the major adverse effects of pain relief were history. Unfortunately, this was not the case, and it appeared that people on COX-2 inhibitors had fewer but more serious adverse effects.

Aspirin and salicylates, at higher doses, may cause respiratory alkalosis and at toxic levels may cause central respiratory paralysis and acidosis and ultimately, coma and death. Various prostaglandins are necessary to increase the stomach's protective mucus lining and reduce acid secretion. Without these protective mechanisms, epigastric distress, ulceration, and hemorrhage are quite common, especially with long-term use. Aspirin can also cause edema and **hyperkalemia** due to sodium and water retention. Aspirin should not be taken for at least one week before surgery. Although **anaphylaxis** is rare, other hypersensitivity reactions may occur in up to 15% of patients.

Celecoxib may still cause GI disorders albeit at a lower incidence than the other NSAIDs. They are contraindicated in patients with allergies to sulfonamides. Celecoxib, and selective COX-2 inhibitors in general, should not be used in patients with chronic renal issues, severe heart disease, volume depletion, or liver failure.

The fenamates, mefenamic acid and meclofenamate, can cause severe diarrhea associated with bowel inflammation. There have been some reports of **hemolytic anemia**.

Propionic acid derivatives may cause headache, dizziness, and **tinnitus**.

■ RED FLAGS

Aspirin given during a viral infection may cause Reye syndrome, a disease with relatively high mortality that involves hepatitis and cerebral edema. This is more common in children, and aspirin should be avoided and acetaminophen (see next section) should be given to children with a fever.

Ibuprofen has been shown to interfere with the

antiplatelet effects of aspirin, and caution should be used when combining these agents in the context of using low-dose aspirin to minimize cardiac risks. Other NSAIDs may have similar effects on aspirin. Occasional use of ibuprofen is probably not problematic. When combining immediate release aspirin with a single dose of ibuprofen of 400 mg, ibuprofen should be taken at least a half hour after the aspirin or 8 hours before.

INTERACTIONS

DRUG

Aspirin and the salicylates interfere with many drugs. They can cause increased plasma concentrations of phenytoin, naproxen, sulfinpyrazone, thiopental, thyroxine, and triodothyronine. Antacids may interfere with the rate of absorption. Anticoagulants with aspirin may lead to hemorrhage. In patients with gout, aspirin should not be combined with probenecid or sulfinpyrazone.

Celecoxib inhibits CYP2D6 and could cause increased levels of some beta-blockers, antidepressants, and antipsychotic drugs. Inhibitors of CYP2C9, such as fluconazole, fluvastatin, and zafirlukast, may increase serum levels of celecoxib.

HERB

ASPIRIN (See Chapter 6, Section 9)
IBUPROFEN
• *Yin Guo Ye* (Ginkgo) (D)—clinical cases indicate interactions of ginkgo with antiepileptics, acetylsalicylic acid, diuretics, ibuprofen, risperidone, rofecoxib, trazodone, and warfarin (Izzo & Ernst, 2009) Level 4 evidence.

INDOMETHACIN
• *Da Suan* (Garlic) (D)—may increase bleeding time due to its decreased platelet aggregation effect and should be used with caution when taking indomethacin and other NSAIDs, expert opinion (Gruenwald, Brendler & Jaenicke, 2004) Level 5 evidence.
• *Da Suan* (Garlic) (D)—potentiates anticoagulant and antiplatelet effects of indomethacin and dypiridamole in bench research (Apitz-Castro, Escalante *et al.*, 1986) Level 5 evidence.
• *Gan Jiang/Sheng Jiang* (D) (Ginger)—extract of

ginger may speculatively enhance anticoagulation of warfarin and other anticoagulants (Mills & Bone, 2000; Gianni & Dreitlein, 1988) [Level 5 evidence] though a 2 g single dose in 8 men did not affect bleeding time, platelet count, or aggregation (Lumb, 1994) [Level 2b evidence]; 10 grams of extract did affect platelet aggregation, while taking 4 grams daily for 3 months did not show significant anticoagulation activity (Bordia, Verma & Srivastava, 1997) Level 3b evidence.

NON-STEROIDAL ANTI-INFLAMMATORY DRUGS (NSAIDs)
• *Da Suan* (Garlic) (D)—may increase bleeding time due to its decreased platelet aggregation effect and should be used with caution when taking indomethacin and other NSAIDs, expert opinion (Gruenwald, Brendler & Jaenicke, 2004) Level 5 evidence.
• *Ma Huang* (Ephedra) (D)—when used with loxoprofen caused an increase in the incidence and severity of gastric lesions in mice (Cho, Hong, Jin, Yoshino, Miura, Aikawa *et al.*, 2002) Level 5 evidence.
• *Yin Guo Ye* (Ginkgo leaf) (D)—may increase bleeding when used with NSAIDs, extrapolation from a study (Gruenwald, Brendler & Jaenicke, 2004) Level 4 evidence.

INTERACTION ISSUES

A:
D: Celecoxib is approximately 97% protein bound; diclofenac, diflunisal, and etodolac are over 99% protein bound; fenoprofen, flurbiprofen, indomethacin, and ketorolac are 99% bound; ibuprofen is 90-99% bound; ketoprofen is over 99% bound; meclofenamate is 99% or greater bound; meloxicam is approximately 99% bound; nabumetone and naproxen are over 99% bound; oxaprozin and piroxicam are 99% bound.
M: Celecoxib is a major substrate of CYP2C9 and a moderate inhibitor of 2C8 and 2D6; piroxicam is a major substrate of 2C9.
E:
Pgp:

SECTION 2: OTHER ANALGESICS

ACETAMINOPHEN (a seet a MIN oh fen) PR=C
(Acephen™ [O], Aceta-Gesic®,[10] Alagesic LQ,[16] Alka-Seltzer Plus® Day Cold [O],[29] All-Nite Multi-Symptom Cold/Flu Relief [O],[28] Anacin® Advanced Headache Formula [O],[22] APAP 500 [O], Aspirin Free Anacin® Extra Strength [O], Benadryl® Allergy and Cold [O],[30] Benadryl® Allergy and Sinus Headache [O],[30] Benadryl® Maximum Strength Severe Allergy and Sinus Headache [O],[30] Bupap,[31] Capital® and Codeine,[18] Cetafen® [O], Cetafen Cold® [O],[12] Cetafen® Extra [O], Cold Control PE [O],[30] Comtrex® Maximum Strength, Non-Drowsy Cold & Cough [O],[29] Contac® Cold + Flu Maximum Strength Non-Drowsy [O],[12] Coricidin HBP® Cold and Flu [O],[32] Cramp Tabs [O],[11] Dolgic Plus,[16] Endocet®,[19] Esgic,[16] Esgic-Plus,[16] Excedrin® Extra Strength [O],[26] Excedrin® Migraine [O],[22] Excedrin PM® [O],[10] Excedrin® Sinus Headache [O],[12] Excedrin® Tension Headache [O], Fem-Prin® [O],[22] Feverall® [O], Fioricet,[16] Fioricet® with Codeine,[20] Goody's® Extra Strength Headache Powder [O],[22] Goody's® Extra Strength Pain Relief [O],[22] Goody's PM® [O],[10] Hycet®,[15] Legatrin PM® [O],[10] Little Fevers™ [O], Lorcet® 10/650,[15] Lorcet® Plus,[15] Lortab®,[15] Magnacet®,[19] Mapap® [O], Mapap® Arthritis Pain [O], Mapap® Children's [O], Mapap® Extra Strength [O], Mapap® Infant's [O], Mapap® Junior Rapid Tabs [O], Mapap® Multi-Symptom Cold [O],[29] Mapap PM [O],[10] Mapap® Sinus PE [O],[12] Margesic,[16] Margesic® H,[15] Maxidone®,[15] Midol® Teen Formula [O],[11] Night Time Multi-Symptom Cold/Flu Relief [O],[28] Non-Aspirin Pain Reliever [O], Norco®,[15] Norel® SR,[27] Nortemp Children's [O], Ofirmev™; One Tab™ Allergy & Sinus [O],[30] One Tab™ Cold & Flu [O],[30] Ornex® [O],[2] Ornex® Maximum Strength [O],[2] Orviban CF,[31] Pain & Fever Children's [O], Pain Eze [O], Pain-Off [O],[22] Percocet®,[19] Percogesic® Extra Strength [O],[10] Phrenilin Forte,[31] Primlev™,[19] Promacet,[31] Q-Pap [O], Q-Pap Children's [O], Q-Pap Extra Strength [O], Q-Pap Infant's [O], RapiMed® Children's [O], RapiMed® Junior [O], Repan,[16] Robitussin® Peak Cold Nasal Relief [O],[12] Robitussin® Peak Cold Nighttime Multi-Symptom Cold [O],[30] Roxicet™,[19] Roxicet™ 5/500,[19] Silapap Children's [O], Silapap Infant's [O], Sinus Pain & Pressure [O],[12] Stagesic™,[15] Sudafed PE® Nighttime Cold [O],[30] Sudafed PE® Pressure + Pain [O],[12] Sudafed PE® Severe Cold [O],[30] Theraflu® Daytime Severe Cold & Cough [O],[29] Theraflu® Nighttime Severe Cold & Cough [O],[30] Theraflu® Sugar-Free Nighttime Severe Cold & Cough [O],[30] Theraflu Warming Relief,® Daytime Multi-Symptom Cold [O],[29] Theraflu Warming Relief® Daytime Severe Cold & Cough [O],[29] Theraflu®Warming Relief™ Flu & Sore Throat [O],[30] Theraflu® Warming Relief™ Nighttime Severe Cold & Cough [O],[30] TopCare® Pain Relief PM [O],[10] Trezix™,[21] Triaminic™ Children's Fever Reducer Pain Reliever [O], Tylenol® [O], Tylenol® 8-Hour [O], Tylenol® Allergy Multi-Symptom Nighttime [O],[30] Tylenol® Arthritis Pain Extended Relief [O], Tylenol® Children's [O], Tylenol® Children's Meltaways [O], Tylenol® Children's Plus Cold and Allergy [O],[30] Tylenol® Cold & Cough Nighttime [O],[28] Tylenol® Cough & Sore Throat Nighttime [O],[28] Tylenol® Cold Head Congestion Daytime [O],[29] Tylenol® Cold Multi-Symptom Daytime [O],[29] Tylenol®Extra Strength [O], Tylenol® Jr. Meltaways [O], Tylenol® PM [O],[10] Tylenol® Severe Allergy [O],[10] Tylenol® Sinus Congestion & Pain Daytime [O],[12] Tylenol® with Codeine No. 3,[18] Tylenol® with Codeine No. 4,[18] Tylenol® Women's Menstrual Relief [O],[11] Ultracet®,[23] Valorin [O], Valorin Extra [O], Vanquish® Extra Strength Pain Reliever [O],[22] Vicks® DayQuil® Cold & Flu Multi-Symptom [O],[29] Vicks® DayQuil® Sinex® Daytime Sinus [O],[12] Vicks® Nature Fusion™ Cold & Flu Multi-Symptom Relief [O],[29] Vicks® Nature Fusion™ Cold & Flu Nighttime Relief [O],[28] Vicks® NyQuil® Cold & Flu Nighttime Relief [O],[28] Vicodin®,[15] Vicodin ES®,[15] Vicodin HP®,[15] Xodol® 10/300,[15] Xodol® 5/300,[15] Xodol® 7.5/300,[15] Zamicet™,[15] Zebutal,[16] Zgesic,[13] Zolvit®,[15] Zydone®[15])

PREGABALIN (pre GAB a lin) *See Chapter 5, Section 8*

FUNCTION

Acetaminophen has antipyretic and analgesic effects but does not have much anti-inflammatory effect. It can be used in many cases where aspirin or an NSAID would be inappropriate: patients with gastric complaints, who cannot have decreased platelet activity, or who do not need anti-inflammatory actions. It is the agent of choice in children with viral infections, as it does not increase the incidence of Reye syndrome. It is also useful for patients who have gout and are taking probenecid. Figure 12.3 shows the differences between acetaminophen and NSAIDs.

Pregabalin is used to treat the pain of diabetic peripheral neuropathy, management of postherpetic neuralgia, and as adjunctive therapy for partial-onset seizure disorder.

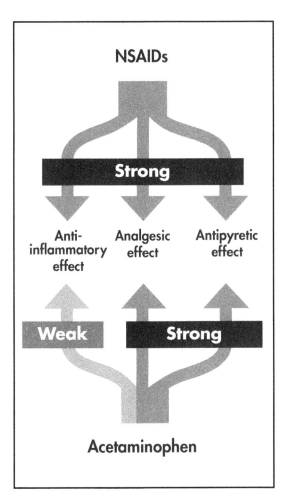

Figure 12.3 The different effects of NSAIDs versus acetaminophen.

MECHANISMS OF ACTION

Just like aspirin and other NSAIDs, acetaminophen inhibits the COX enzyme and the production of prostaglandins. What is different is that it accomplishes this primarily in the CNS with very little peripheral activity. This accounts for its antipyretic effect, which is predominantly controlled in the hypothalamus, and its analgesic effect. In NSAIDs, the anti-inflammatory effect is almost entirely local, and therefore this agent has almost no anti-inflammatory action. It also does not reduce platelet aggregation.

Pregabalin acts by binding to voltage-gated calcium channels in the CNS and inhibits excitatory neurotransmitter release.

DOSAGES

ACETAMINOPHEN, for *children* under 12 years, 10-15 mg/kg every 4-6 hours prn; do not exceed 2.6 g/d. Alternatively, age-based doses may be used: for 0-3 mo, 40 mg; 4-11 mo, 80 mg; 1-2 y, 120 mg; 2-3 y, 160 mg; 4-5 y, 240 mg; 6-8 y, 320 mg; 9-10 y, 400 mg; 11 y, 480 mg. For *adults*, 325-650 mg every 4-6 hours or 1000 mg 3-4 times/d; do not exceed 4 g/d.

PREGABALIN, for *adults*, for diabetes-associated neuropathic pain, initiate at 50 mg 3 times/d; may be increased within 1 week based on tolerability and effect up to a maximum dose of 300 mg/d. For postherpetic neuralgia, initiate at 75 mg 2 times/d or 50 mg 3 times/d; may be increased to 300 mg/d within 1 week based on tolerability and effect, maximum dose is 600 mg/d. For partial-onset seizures as adjunctive therapy, initiate at 75 mg 2 times/d or 50 mg 3 times/d; may be increased based on tolerability and effect to a maximum dose of 600 mg/d. When discontinuing, pregabalin should not be abruptly discontinued; taper dosage over at least 1 week.

ADVERSE EFFECTS

Acetaminophen is very well tolerated by most patients. Infrequently it may cause a skin rash; minor allergic reactions; and minor, transient, lower leukocyte counts. Large doses over time may

Necrosis: Localized tissue death

Ataxia: Incoordination of voluntary muscles resulting in jerky movements that may affect the limbs, head, or trunk

Cystinuria: The abnormal presence of the amino acid cystine in the urine

cause renal tubular **necrosis** or hypoglycemic coma. Overdosage may cause life-threatening hepatic necrosis.

Pregabalin may cause peripheral edema, dizziness, sleepiness, **ataxia**, weight gain, dry mouth, tremor, and vision problems.

▨ RED FLAGS

Large doses of acetaminophen may cause renal tubular necrosis, hypoglycemic coma, or life-threatening hepatic necrosis.

▨ INTERACTIONS

DRUG

Pregabalin may potentiate the sedative effects of other CNS depressants such as ethanol, barbiturates, and narcotics.

INTERACTION ISSUES

The drugs in this category do not greatly affect the ADME scheme or Pgp.

HERB

ACETAMINOPHEN

- *Da Suan* (Garlic) (D)–may prevent hepatotoxicity from acetaminophen. Fresh garlic seems to have this effect, while aged garlic may prophyllactically reduce it (Wang *et al.*, as cited in Brinker, 2001) Level 5 evidence.
- *Dang Gui* (Angelica) (D)–may treat liver damage caused by acetaminophen by promoting hepatocyte generation, expert opinion, (Chen & Chen, 2004) Level 5 evidence.
- *Niu Bang Gen* (Burdock root) (D)–has been shown to have hepatoprotective effects with constituents that are antioxidant and targeted at hepatocytes, alleviating toxicity and treating liver damage due to acetaminophen and carbon tetrachloride in rats (Lin *et al.*) Level 5 evidence.

SECTION 3: DISEASE-MODIFYING ANTIRHEUMATIC DRUGS

Many of the agents in this section are injections and are therefore not covered in this book.

AURANOFIN (ah RANE oh fin) PR=C
(Ridaura®)

HYDROXYCHLOROQUINE *(See Chapter 10, Section 6)*

LEFLUNOMIDE (le FLOO noh mide) PR=X
(Arava®)

METHOTREXATE *(See Chapter 11, Section 9)*

PENICILLAMINE (pen i SIL a mene) PR=D
(Cuprimine®, Depen®)

TOFACITINIB (toe fa SYE tI nIb) PR=C
(Xeljanz)

▨ FUNCTION

Disease-modifying antirheumatic drugs (DMARDs), also called slow-acting antirheumatic drugs (SAARDs), are varied drugs that may reduce or prevent joint damage in patients with rheumatoid arthritis (RA). They are used in treating RA that does not respond to NSAIDs and can slow disease progression and possibly induce remission. There are no drugs of choice in this category, but treatment is often initiated with methotrexate or hydroxychloroquine and supple-

mented with other agents. These agents also can be useful in treating psoriatic arthritis.

Penicillamine has many adverse effects and toxicities, and its use in RA is usually restricted to when gold therapy has failed and before corticosteroids are used. It is also used to treat **cystinuria** and Wilson's disease.

▨ MECHANISMS OF ACTION

Auranofin and other gold compounds are not completely understood, but it is thought the gold is absorbed by macrophages, immune cells that "eat" debris in the interstitial spaces, and it inhibits **phagocytosis**. Various enzymes and chemical complements of the immune and inflammatory responses are also decreased through unknown mechanisms. Ultimately, there is less bone and joint destruction.

Leflunomide acts by inhibiting the enzyme dihydroorotate dehydrogenase (DHODH), which is necessary to synthesize UMP necessary for RNA and ultimately DNA synthesis.

Penicillamine is often used as a chelating agent. Chelators bind with chemicals so that they can be more easily excreted. Chelation with cystine explains its effectiveness in treating cystinuria and the prevention of renal **calculi**. Its action in treating RA is not completely understood, although it does reduce circulating rheumatoid factor and depress T-cell activity.

DOSAGES

AURANOFIN, for *adults*, 6 mg/d in 1-2 divided doses; after 3 months may be increased to 3 mg tid; if still no response after 3 months at 9 mg/d, discontinue drug.

LEFLUNOMIDE, for *adults*, for rheumatoid arthritis, initiate at 100 mg/d for 3 days, followed by 20 mg/d; may be decreased to 10 mg/d.

PENICILLAMINE, for rheumatoid arthritis, in *children*, initiate at 3 mg/kg/d (less than or equal to 250 mg/d) for 3 months, then 6 mg/ kg/d (less than or equal to 500 mg/d) in divided doses twice daily for 3 months to a maximum of 10 mg/kg/d in 3-4 divided doses up to a maximum dose of 750 mg/d; for Wilson's disease, for *children* under 12 years, 20 mg/kg/d in 2-3 divided doses; rounded off to the nearest 250 mg dose up to a maximum dose of 1 g/d. For *adults*, for RA, initiate at 125-250 mg/d; may increase dose at 1-3 month intervals up to 1-1.5 g/d up to a maximum dose in *elderly* of 750 mg/d; for Wilson's disease, 250 mg qid (maximum in *elderly* 750 mg/d).

TOFACITINIB, for *adults*, for rheumatoid arthritis, 5 mg bid.

ADVERSE EFFECTS

Auranofin and other gold compounds require close monitoring so serum levels of gold do not become toxic. Toxicity may manifest as **hematuria**, **proteinuria**, persistent diarrhea, tongue inflammation, and **pruritis** and rash.

Leflunomide can cause headache, diarrhea, nausea, weight loss, and allergic reactions that include symptoms such as a flu-like syndrome, rash, hair loss, and hypokalemia. It has been shown to be **teratogenic** in animals and is therefore contraindicated in pregnant women and women who could become pregnant. It should be used with caution in patients with liver disease.

Prolonged use of penicillamine may cause skin problems, nephritis, and **aplastic anemia**. It has a wide variety of adverse effects, and 20-30% of Wilson's disease patients need to discontinue its use due to them. About one third of patients experience an allergic reaction. Signs of toxicity include fever, sore throat, chills, bruising, or bleeding.

Tofacitinib has a boxed warning regarding increased risk of infections and another one specifically warning about reported incidents of tuberculosis with use. A third one states that there have been reports of lymphomas and other cancers reported in patients taking this agent.

RED FLAGS

No major red flags observed.

INTERACTIONS

No interactions found.

INTERACTION ISSUES

A:

D: Leflunomide is over 99% protein bound.

M: Leflunomide is a moderate inhibitor of CYP2C9; tofacitinib is a major substrate of CYP3A4.

E:

Pgp:

Phagocytosis: A method where certain cells engulf and dispose of cellular debris and microorganisms

Calculus: An abnormal stone formed in body tissues by accumulation of mineral salts; plural: calculi

Hematuria: Abnormal presence of blood in the urine

Proteinuria: The presence of an abnormally large quantity of protein in the urine

Pruritis: Itching

Teratogen: A substance that causes congenital defects in fetuses

Aplastic anemia: A blood disorder characterized by deficiency of all formed elements of the blood; indicates a failure of the bone marrow's ability to generate cells

SECTION 4: DRUGS USED TO TREAT GOUT

ALLOPURINOL (al oh PURE i nole) PR=C
 (Aloprim®, Zyloprim®)

COLCHICINE (KOL chi sene) PR=C *(Colcrys)*

FEBUXOSTAT (feb UX oh stat) PR=C *(Uloric®)*

PROBENECID (proe BEN e sid) PR=B

Gout is a disorder of high levels of uric acid in the blood causing deposition of sodium urate crystals in tissues, especially the kidney and joints. This causes an inflammatory process and **granulocyte** infiltration that **phagocytize** the crystals. As part of the inflammatory process, there is production of lactic acid, which lowers the pH and causes more crystals to form, hence creating a cycle of increasing pathology. Common symptoms of gout include pain, warmth, redness, and swelling. The first area affected is often the first metatarsophalangeal joint. Therapy consists of attempting to lower serum levels of uric acid. Acute attacks are often caused by excessive alcohol intake, a diet rich in purines, or kidney disease. Indomethacin and other NSAIDs (but not aspirin, which is contraindicated) are often used to treat the pain and decrease inflammatory infiltration of granulocytes. Chronic gout is caused by a genetic defect, renal insufficiency, Lesch-Nyhan syndrome, or excessive uric acid production associated with cancer chemotherapy.

> Granulocyte: A form of white blood cell with granules in its cytoplasm; these include basophils, eosinophils, and neutrophils

> Phagocytosis: A method where certain cells engulf and dispose of cellular debris and microorganisms

FUNCTION

Allopurinol treats the primary hyperuricemia of gout and the secondary hyperuricemia of other conditions, such as certain cancers or renal disease.

Colchicine is used to treat acute gouty attacks as it relieves pain and as a prophylactic to reduce the frequency of attacks. Indomethacin has largely supplanted its use in acute attacks.

Probenecid increases the excretion of uric acid.

MECHANISMS OF ACTION

Allopurinol and febuxostat act by competitively inhibiting the last two steps of uric acid production in the body, reducing the amount of uric acid in the blood.

Colchicine binds to tubulin, a protein necessary for many cellular functions including mobility. This prevents granulocyte migration into affected areas and minimizes the inflammatory process by inhibiting synthesis and release of leukotrienes, chemicals that are part of the inflammatory cascade. It also blocks cell division by binding to mitotic spindles, which decreases the number of granulocytes.

The progression of a gouty attack and how allopurinol, colchicine, and febuxostat interfere with this progression are summarized in Figure 12.4.

Probenecid works by inhibiting proximal tubule reabsorption of uric acid in the kidneys.

DOSAGES

ALLOPURINOL, doses over 300 mg should be given in divided doses. For *children* under 6 years, 50 mg tid; 6-10 years, 300 mg/d in 2-3 divided doses. For *children* over 10 years and *adults*, secondary hyperuricemia associated with chemotherapy, 600-800 mg/d in 2-3 divided doses for prevention of acute uric acid nephropathy for 2-3 days starting 1-2 days before chemotherapy; for gout, mild, 200 300 mg/d; severe, 400 600 mg/d; for prophylaxis, initiate dose at 100 mg/d and increase weekly to recommended dosage; for recurrent calcium oxalate stones, 200-300 mg/d in single or divided doses. For the *elderly*, initiate at 100 mg/d and increase until desired uric acid level is obtained.

COLCHICINE, for *adults*, for prophylaxis of acute attacks of gout, 0.6 mg bid, may be decreased in patients at risk of toxicity or in those who are intolerant (including weakness, loose stools, or diarrhea); normal range is 0.6 mg every other day to 0.6 mg tid; for acute attacks of gout, initiate at 0.6-1.2 mg, followed by 0.6 every 1-2 hours; more aggressive approaches have recommended a maximum dose of up to 6 mg. Wait at least 3 days before initiating another course of therapy.

FEBUXOSTAT, for *adults,* for management of hyperuricemia in patients with gout, initiate at 40 mg once daily; may increase to 80 mg once daily in patients who do not achieve a serum uric acid level under 6 mg/dL after 2 weeks.

PROBENECID, for *children* over 50 kg, for gonorrhea, use adult guidelines. For *adults,* for hyperuricemia with gout, 250 mg bid for one week; increase to 250-500 mg/d; may increase by 500 mg/month, if needed, to a maximum of 2-3 g/d (dosages may be increased by 500 mg every 6 months if serum urate concentrations are controlled).

ADVERSE EFFECTS

Allopurinol is generally well tolerated with nausea and diarrhea as the most common side effects. Hypersensitivity reactions occur in about 3% of patients and may occur years into chronic therapy.

Colchicine may cause nausea and vomiting, abdominal pain, and diarrhea. Long-term use can lead to **myopathy, agranulocytosis, aplastic anemia,** and hair loss. It should not be used during pregnancy and should be used with caution in patients with liver, kidney, or cardiovascular disease.

Probenecid has few adverse effects and is generally well tolerated by patients.

RED FLAGS

No major red flags observed.

INTERACTIONS

DRUG

Allopurinol interferes with the metabolism of mercaptopurine, an anticancer agent, and azathioprine, an immunosuppressant. Dosage of these two agents may need to be reduced when used concurrently with allopurinol.

Probenecid is sometimes used to increase serum levels of penicillin as it blocks its excretion in the kidneys. Excretion of naproxen, ketoprofen, and indomethacin is also inhibited.

INTERACTION ISSUES

A:
D: Febuxostat is approximately 99% protein bound.
M: Colchicine is a major substrate of CYP3A4 and a weak or moderate inducer of 2C9, 2E1, and 3A4.
E:
Pgp: Colchicine is a substrate of Pgp.

Myopathy: An abnormal condition of the skeletal muscles that includes wasting and weakness

Agranulocytosis: The extreme reduction in the number of leukocytes, or white blood cells, in the blood

Aplastic anemia: A blood disorder characterized by deficiency of all formed elements of the blood; indicates a failure of bone marrow's ability to generate cells

Figure 12.4: The cascade of chemicals that create gout and how agents interfere. DNA and RNA metabolism ultimately form uric acid. This formation can be blocked by allopurinol. Uric acid can form crystals that are phagocytized by neutrophils. Lysosomes, where uric acid is stored intracellularly, can rupture, killing the neutrophil and setting up an inflammatory reaction. Colchicine can limit inflammatory reactions.

SECTION 5: DRUGS USED TO TREAT MIGRAINES

ALMOTRIPTAN (al moh TRIP tan) PR=C
(Axert™)

ELETRIPTAN (el e TRIP tan) PR=C (Relpax®)

ERGOTAMINE (er GOT a meen) PR=X
(Cafergot®, Ergomar®, Migergot[24])

FROVATRIPTAN (froe va TRIP tan) PR=C
(Frova®)

NARATRIPTAN (NAR a trip tan) PR=C
(Amerge®)

RIZATRIPTAN (rye za TRIP tan) PR=C (Maxalt®,
Maxalt-MLT®)

SUMATRIPTAN (soo ma TRIP tan) PR=C
(Alsuma, Imitrex®, Imitrex STATdose Refill,
Imitrex STATdose System, Sumavel DosePro,
Treximet[®9])

ZOLMITRIPTAN (zohl mi TRIP tan) PR=C
(Zomig®, Zomig-ZMT™)

Migraines affect 18% of women and 6% of men during their lifetime. It often manifests as unilateral, throbbing pain worse with exertion and accompanied by autonomous symptoms such as nausea, **photophobia**, and/or sensitivity to sound or odors. Symptoms can last from a few hours to 3 days. About 15% of sufferers may have auras, neurological symptoms such as visual, sensory, speech, and/or motor disturbances, prior to an episode. Patients with severe migraines can have up to 5 attacks per month. They are quite disabling. Diagnosis is clinical, based on presentation, signs, and symptoms. Treatment is based in using serotonin[1D] receptor agonists (most of the "triptans"), **antiemetics**, and analgesics. Changes of lifestyle, such as sleeping patterns and diet, β-blockers, amitryptilline, valproate, and topiramate are prophylactic. Migraines are caused by arterial dilation both inside and outside the head that causes stretching and release of the pain increasing neurochemical substance P. Auras are caused by a transient decrease of neural activity and blood flow in the cortex and other areas of the brain.

Photophobia: Abnormal sensitivity to light, especially by the eyes

---

Antiemetic: An agent that suppresses nausea and vomiting

FUNCTION

There are two types of migraine specific agents: the triptans and ergot derivatives. Both are agonists of serotonin[1D] receptors. The triptans, which all end with the suffix triptan, are effective in about 70% of patients in stopping a migraine once it has begun. They differ in their effectiveness and side effect profiles, and patients may need to try several

before determining which works best. The ergot derivatives all have ergot somewhere in their name. While they are about as strong as the triptans, their adverse effects may be more severe.

As mentioned above, β-blockers, tricyclic antidepressants, antiseizure medications, and calcium channel blockers may be given to prevent or minimize the occurrence of a migraine. Anti-inflammatory agents and, in severe cases, opioids may be helpful in treating the pain during an attack. Treatment, both prophylactic and symptomatic, is summarized on the timeline in Figure 12.5 on the facing page.

MECHANISM OF ACTION

These agents act by activating serotonin[1D] receptors, which cause vasoconstriction especially in the head. This vasoconstriction counteracts the vasodilation that is the basis for migraines. The [1D] receptors are primarily located on intracranial peripheral nerves innervating the vasculature. They may also reduce the amount of pain potentiating and proinflammatory neurochemicals.

DOSAGES

ALMOTRIPTAN, for *adults*, for migraine, initiate at 6.25-12.5 mg in a single dose; if the headache returns, repeat the dose after 2 hours up to a maximum of 2 doses in a 24-hour period.

ELETRIPTAN, for *adults*, for acute migraine, 20-40 mg; if the headache improves but returns, dose may be repeated after 2 hours up to a maximum of 80 mg/d.

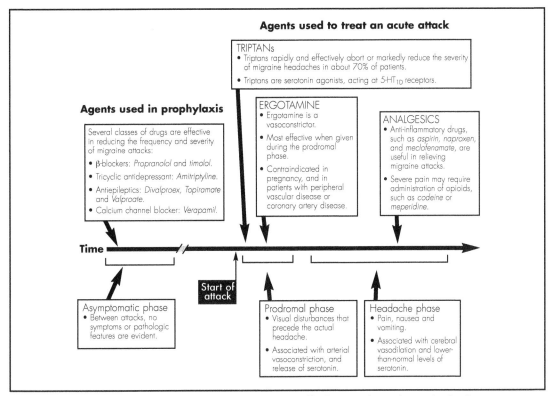

Figure 12.5: A timeline for a migraine attack and what agents are effective at a given point on the timeline.

ERGOTAMINE, 1 tablet under tongue at first sign, then 1 tablet every 30 minutes if needed up to a maximum of 3 tablets/d and 5 tablets/wk.

FROVATRIPTAN, for *adults*, for migraine, 2.5 mg; if headache recurs, a second dose may be given if first dose provided some relief and at least 2 hours have elapsed up to a maximum daily dose of 7.5 mg.

NARATRIPTAN, for *adults*, 1-2.5 mg at the onset of headache; if headache returns or does not fully resolve, the dose may be repeated after 4 hours up to maximum of 5 mg/d. Not recommended for use in the *elderly*.

RIZATRIPTAN, 5-10 mg, repeat after 2 hours if relief not attained up to a maximum 30 mg/d.

SUMATRIPTAN, for *adults*, a single dose of 25 mg, 50 mg, or 100 mg; if a satisfactory response has not been obtained at 2 hours, a second dose may be taken; the total daily dose should not exceed 200 mg.

ZOLMITRIPTAN, for *adults*, for migraine, initiate at 2.5 mg or under at the onset of headache.

ADVERSE EFFECTS

The triptans commonly cause a headache 24-48 hours after administration that usually can be aborted with another dose. While they may cause nausea and vomiting, these symptoms are much worse with the ergot derivatives. Neither class of agents should be used in patients with peripheral vascular disease or coronary artery disease.

The ergot derivatives are contraindicated during pregnancy.

RED FLAGS

No major red flags observed.

INTERACTIONS

DRUG

Ergot derivatives inhibit CYP3A4 and may interact with many drugs. Azole-derived antifungals, clarithromycin, diclofenac, doxycycline, protease inhibitors (antivirals), erythromycin, imatinib, isoniazid, nefazodone, nicardipine, propofol, quinidine, telithromycin, and verapamil should not be combined with the ergots as they may increase serum levels. Serotonin syndrome, a life-threatening condition of too much serotonin activation, can be caused when combined with other agents that activate receptors of or increase levels of serotonin such as MAO inhibitors, buspirone, SSRIs, TCAs, nefazodone, sibutramine, sumatriptan, and trazodone.

HERB

ERGOT ALKALOIDS

- *Ma Huang* (Ephedra) (D)–may cause hypertension when combined with ergot alkaloids or oxytocin, expert opinion (Blumenthal, 1998) Level 5 evidence.

ELETRIPTAN

- *Guan Ye Lian Qiao* (St. John's wort) (C) decreases blood concentrations (Izzo & Ernst, 2009) Level 4 evidence.

INTERACTION ISSUES

A:

D:

M: Eletriptan and ergotamine are major substrates of CYP3A4.

E:

Pgp:

SECTION 6: DRUGS USED TO TREAT ULCERATIVE COLITIS

BALSALAZIDE (bal SAL a zide) PR=B
(Colazal®, Giazo®)

MESALAMINE (me SAL a mene) PR=B *(Apriso, Asacol HD, Canasa™, Delzicol, Lialda™, Pentasa®, Rowasa®, SfRowasa)*

OLSALAZINE (ole SAL a zene) PR=C
(Dipentum®)

SULFASALAZINE (sul fa SAL a zene) PR=B *(Azulfidine®, Azulfidine® EN-tabs®, Sulfazine, Sulfazine EC)*

Ulcerative colitis (UC) is a chronic inflammatory disease, related to Crohn's disease, that involves ulcerations of the large intestine. Its most common sign is bloody diarrhea with mucus along with urgency and cramping. Systemic signs and symptoms can include arthritis, malaise, fever, anemia, anorexia, and weight loss. Diagnosis is based upon signs and symptoms and confirmed by sigmoidoscopy or colonoscopy and ruling out of various infectious agents. It is a disease of exacerbations and remissions. It increases the risk of colon cancer. Diet changes may minimize symptoms; however, various pharmaceutical agents are used to treat the disease. These include corticosteroids, immunomodulators, anticytokines, antibiotics, and 5-ASA derivatives, the subject of this section. Rarely, surgery may be necessary.

FUNCTION

The agents in this class all treat ulcerative colitis. Mesalamine can be used rectally to treat proctosigmoiditis or proctitis.

Sulfasalazine, as enteric coated tablets, is used to treat rheumatoid arthritis (including juvenile) when analgesics and NSAIDs are not effective.

MECHANISMS OF ACTION

5-Aminosalicylic acid derivatives (5-ASAs) act by topical action in the colon mucosa to decrease inflammation through blocking production of arachidonic acid metabolites necessary for inflammation.

Sulfasalazine acts systemically by inhibiting prostaglandin synthesis. Prostaglandins are chemicals involved with the inflammatory process.

DOSAGES

BALSALAZIDE, for *children* 5-17 years, 750 mg tid for up to 8 weeks or 2.25 g tid for 8 weeks. For *adults*, 2.25 g tid for 8-12 weeks.

MESALAMINE, for *adults*, for treatment of UC, capsule: 1 g qid or initiate tablets at 2.4-4.8 g/d for up to 8 weeks.

OLSALAZINE, for *adults*, 0.5 g bid.

SULFASALAZINE, for *children* 2 years or older, for UC, initiate at 40-60 mg/kg/d in 3-6 divided doses; maintain at 20-30 mg/kg/d in 4 divided doses. For *children* 6 years or older, for juvenile rheumatoid arthritis, use enteric coated tablet, 15-25 mg/kg/d bid,;initiate at 1/4 to 1/3 of this dose; increase weekly up to a maximum of 2 g/d typically. For *adults*, for UC, initiate at 1 g 3-4 times/d; maintain at 2 g/d in divided doses; may initiate therapy with 0.5-1 g/d; for rheumatoid arthritis, use enteric coated tablet, initiate at 0.5-1 g/d, increase weekly to maintenance dose of 1 g bid up to a maximum 3 g/d.

ADVERSE EFFECTS

These agents commonly cause headache and abdominal pain. Less common adverse effects include insomnia, fatigue, fever, and GI disturbances. Rarely, they may cause bronchospasm, erythema nodosum, hemorrhage, hypertension, palpitations, pericarditis, pancreatitis, and liver problems.

RED FLAGS

Patients with sulfonamide allergies should avoid these agents.

INTERACTIONS

DRUG

These agents may decrease absorption of cardiac glycosides. They may decrease metabolism and therefore increase levels of thiopurine analogs such as azathioprine, mercaptopurine, and thioguanine.

INTERACTION ISSUES

A:

D: Balsalazide is 99% or over protein bound, olsalazine and sulfasalazine are over 99% bound.

M:.

E:

Pgp:

ENDNOTES

[1] Combination of Diclofenac and Misoprostol.

[2] Combination of Acetaminophen and Pseudoephedrine.

[3] Combination of Ibuprofen and Hydrocodone.

[4] Combination of Naproxen and Lansoprazole.

[5] Combination of Ibuprofen and Diphenhydramine.

[6] Combination of Ibuprofen and Famotidine.

[7] Combination of Ibuprofen, Pseudoephedrine, and Chlorpheniramine.

[8] Combination of Naproxen and Esomeprazole.

[9] Combination of Naproxen and Sumatriptan.

[10] Combination of Acetaminophen and Diphenhydramine.

[11] Combination of Acetaminophen and Pamabrom.

[12] Combination of Acetaminophen and Phenylephrine.

[13] Combination of Acetaminophen and Phenyltoloxamine.

[14] Combination of Acetaminophen, Dichloralphenazone, and Isometheptene.

[15] Combination of Acetaminophen and Hydrocodone.

[16] Combination of Acetaminophen, Butalbital, and Caffeine.

[17] Combination of Acetaminophen and Propoxyphene.

[18] Combination of Acetaminophen and Codeine.

[19] Combination of Acetaminophen and Oxycodone.

[20] Combination of Acetaminophen, Butalbital, Caffeine, and Codeine.

[20] Combination of Acetaminophen, Caffeine, Hydrocodone, Chlorpheniramine, and Phenylephrine.

[21] Combination of Acetaminophen, Caffeine, and Dihydrocodeine.

[22] Combination of Acetaminophen, Aspirin, and Caffeine.

[23] Combination of Acetaminophen and Tramadol.

[24] Combination of Ergotamine and Caffeine.

[27] Combination of Acetaminophen, Chlorpheniramine, Phenylephrine, and Phenyltoloxamine.

[28] Combination of Acetaminophen, Dextromethorphan, and Doxylamine.

[29] Combination of Acetaminophen, Dextromethorphan, and Phenylephrine.

[30] Combination of Acetaminophen, Diphenhydramine, and Phenylephrine.

[31] Combination of Acetaminophen and Butalbital.

[32] Combination of Acetaminophen and Chlorpheniramine.

CHINESE MEDICAL DESCRIPTION

The Chinese medical explanation of the drug categories in this chapter may be found in Chapter 15 on pages 385–417.

Miscellaneous Drugs 13

SECTION 1: AGENTS USED IN ERECTILE DYSFUNCTION

SILDENAFIL (sil DEN a fil) PR=B *(Revatio®, Viagra®)*

TADALAFIL (tah DA la fil) PR=B *(Adcirca®, Cialis®)*

VARDENAFIL (var DEN a fil) PR=B *(Levitra®, Staxyn™)*

Erectile dysfunction affects up to 30 million men in the United States. Normal erection is caused by sexual stimulation initiating a cascade of chemical release and enzymatic reactions. First, there is release of nitric oxide (NO), which causes increased activity of the enzyme guanylyl cyclase, which transforms guanosine triphosphate (GTP) into cyclic guanosine monophosphate (cGMP). cGMP causes relaxation of the smooth muscle of the corpus cavernosum of the penis by reducing the intracellular calcium. This allows more blood flow and creates an erection. This cascade is summarized in Figure 13.1 on the next page.

▓ FUNCTION

These agents are used to treat erectile dysfunction in cases of organic or psychogenic causes. They differ in their time of onset and duration of action. Tadalafil is often called the "weekender" as it is advertised to have effects for up to 36 hours. The other drugs do not have as long a duration.

Sildenafil is also used to treat pulmonary arterial hypertension.

▓ MECHANISM OF ACTION

These agents are phosphodiesterase inhibitors. There are many different subtypes of phosphodiesterase; these agents act on the fifth subtype and are known as PDE-5 inhibitors. The PDE-5 enzyme normally helps the breakdown of cGMP to its inactive form of GMP. Blocking this means

that it is easier to initiate and maintain an erection. One of the interesting aspects of PDE-5 inhibitors is that they cannot work without sexual stimulation. These effects are summarized in Figure 13.2 on the following page.

▓ DOSAGES

SILDENAFIL, for erectile dysfunction (Viagra®), recommended dose is 50 mg prn approximately 1 hour before sexual activity. Based on effectiveness and tolerance, may be increased to maximum recommended dose of 100 mg or decreased to 25 mg. The maximum recommended dosing frequency is once daily. For pulmonary arterial hypertension (Revatio®), 20 mg tid taken 4-6 hours apart.

TADALAFIL, for erectile dysfunction, 10 mg prior to anticipated sexual activity; dosing range 5-20 mg; do not take more than once daily.

VARDENAFIL, for *adults*, for erectile dysfunction, take 10 mg 60 minutes prior to sexual activity with a dose range of 5-20 mg; to be given as one single dose no more than once daily. For the *elderly* 65 years or over, initiate at 5 mg 60 minutes prior to sexual activity.

▓ ADVERSE EFFECTS

While common, the most frequent adverse effects rarely cause discontinuation of these agents. These effects include headache, flushing, GI upset, and nasal congestion.

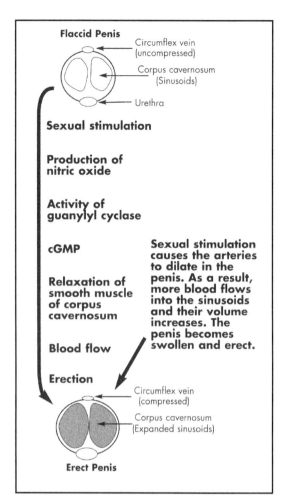

Figure 13.1: How sexual stimulation causes an erection of the penis in a normal male

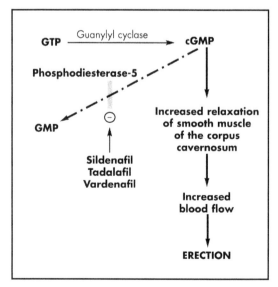

Figure 13.2: Phosphodiesterase 5 (PDE-5) inhibitors act by blocking the inactivation of cGMP which allows for more smooth muscle relaxation and blood flow.

Sildenafil may cause disturbances in color vision due to some PDE-6 inhibition. PDE-6 is a subtype of PDE that is located in the retina and is important in color vision.

RED FLAGS

Rare cases of sudden vision loss attributed to nonarteritic ischemic optic neuropathy (NAION) have been reported from postmarketing surveillance of these agents. NAION is where blood flow is blocked to the optic nerve. Risk factors for this condition include patients with heart disease, diabetes, hypertension along with those who smoke, are over 50, or have certain eye problems.

INTERACTIONS

DRUG

Because these agents potentiate the activity of NO, organic nitrates, as used to treat angina, are absolutely contraindicated. The use of α-adrenergic antagonists, used to treat BPH, are also contraindicated. There is one exception to this last contraindication: tamsulosin can be used with tadalafil.

HERB

SILDENAFIL

• *Yin Yang Huo* (Epimedi) (D)–*Yin Yang Huo* decreases the pharmacokinetics of sildenafil in rats (Hsueh, Wu, Lin, Chiu *et al.*, 2013) Level 5 evidence.

INTERACTION ISSUES

A:

D: Sildenafil is approximately 96% protein bound; vardenafil approximately 95% bound.

M: Sildenafil, tadalafil, and vardenafil are major substrates of CYP3A4.

E:

Pgp:

SECTION 2: AGENTS USED TO TREAT OSTEOPOROSIS

ALENDRONATE (a LEN droe nate) PR=C
(Binosto, Fosamax®, Fosamax Plus D®1)

CLODRONATE (KLOE droh nate) PR=N
(Bonefos®, Clasteon®)

ETIDRONATE (e ti DROE nate) PR=C
(Didronel®)

IBANDRONATE (eye BAN droh nate) PR=C
(Boniva®)

RISEDRONATE (ris ED roe nate) PR=C
(Actonel®, Atelvia®)

TILUDRONATE (tye LOO droe nate) PR=C
(Skelid®)

FUNCTION

These agents are primarily used for treating osteoporosis. Many are also used to treat Paget's disease, a disease of unknown etiology where there is excessive bone destruction and disorganized bone remodeling. In both osteoporotic patients and patients with Paget's disease, there is an increased rate of bone fractures.

These agents have also been shown to reduce the chances of bone and organ metastases in breast cancer patients.

MECHANISMS OF ACTION

These agents fall under the chemical category of bisphosphonates. They inhibit the action of **osteoclasts**, cells that have the normal function of breaking down bone. This inhibition has three forms. The first mechanism is to inhibit the proton pump, which is crucial for breaking down **hydroxyapatite**. The second mechanism is a decrease in the formation and activation of osteoclasts. The third mechanism is to increase osteoclast **apoptosis**. Each agent may weigh these functions differently, and the exact mechanisms of these functions are not completely understood. The end result of these activities is to have a small but significant gain in bone mass.

DOSAGES

ALENDRONATE, for *adults*, for osteoporosis in postmenopausal females, for prophylaxis, 5 mg once daily or 35 mg once weekly; for treatment, 10 mg once daily or 70 mg once weekly; for osteoporosis in males, 10 mg once daily or 70 mg once weekly; for osteoporosis secondary to glucocorticoids in males and females,

treatment; 5 mg once daily, a dose of 10 mg once daily should be used in postmenopausal females who are not receiving estrogen; for Paget's disease of bone in males and females, 40 mg once daily for 6 months.

CLODRONATE, recommended daily maintenance dose following IV therapy is 1600 mg (4 capsules) to 2400 mg (6 capsules) in single or 2 divided doses; maximum recommended daily dose is 3200 mg (8 capsules); should be taken at least 1 hour before or after food, as food may decrease absorption.

ETIDRONATE, for Paget's disease, initiate at 5-10 mg/kg/d (not to exceed 6 months) or 11-20 mg/kg/d (not to exceed 3 months); doses over 20 mg/kg/d are not recommended; for retreatment, initiate only after etidronate-free period of at least 90 days; monitor patients every 3-6 months; retreatment regimens the same as initial treatment; for heterotopic ossification caused by spinal cord injury, 20 mg/kg/d for 2 weeks, then 10 mg/kg/d for 10 weeks; total treatment period 12 weeks; complicating total hip replacement, 20 mg/kg/d for 1 month preoperatively, then 20 mg/kg/d for 3 months postoperatively; total treatment period is 4 months.

IBANDRONATE, for treatment of postmenopausal osteoporosis, 2.5 mg/d or 150 mg once a month; for prevention of postmenopausal osteoporosis, 2.5 mg/d, 150 mg once a month may be considered.

RISEDRONATE, for Paget's disease of bone, 30 mg once daily for 2 months; retreatment may be

> **Osteoclast:** A cell located in the bone that functions to break down bone during remodeling

> **Hydroxyapatite:** A chemical made of calcium, phosphate, and hydroxide that forms a lattice-like structure that helps bones and teeth become rigid

> **Apoptosis:** Programmed cell death

considered following post-treatment observation of at least 2 months if relapse occurs or if treatment fails to normalize serum alkaline phosphatase; dose and duration of therapy same as initial treatment; for osteoporosis (postmenopausal) prevention and treatment, 5 mg once daily or 35 mg once weekly; for osteoporosis (glucocorticoidinduced) prevention and treatment, 5 mg once daily.

TILUDRONATE, should be taken with 6-8 oz of plain water and not taken within 2 hours of food. For *adults*, 400 mg (2 tablets of tiludronic acid) daily for a period of 3 months; allow an interval of 3 months to assess response.

Osteomalacia: Abnormal condition of the bone characterized by loss of calcification resulting in softening of the bone and weakness

Sympathomimetic: Either mimicking or stimulating the sympathetic nervous system

ADVERSE EFFECTS

Adverse effects of bisphosphonates include diarrhea, nausea, and abdominal pain. Esophageal ulcers are also a possibility especially with alendronate, etidronate, and risedronate. Long-term use of etidronate may cause **osteomalacia.**

Because of the potential for esophageal ulcers, it is recommended that the patient remain upright for at least 30-60 minutes after taking agent.

RED FLAGS

No major red flags observed.

INTERACTIONS

No interactions reported.

INTERACTION ISSUES

A:
D: Ibandronate is 85.7-99.5% protein bound.
M:
E:
Pgp:

SECTION 3: AGENTS USED TO TREAT OBESITY

BENZPHETAMINE (benz FET a mene) PR=X *(Didrex®, Regimex)*

DIETHYLPROPION (dye eth il PROE pee on) PR=B

LORCASERIN (lor KA ser in) PR=X *(Belviq)*

ORLISTAT (OR li stat) PR=X *(Xenical®)*

PHENDIMETRAZINE (fen dye ME tra zene) PR=X *(Bontril PDM®, Bontril® Slow-Release, Melfiat®)*

PHENTERMINE (FEN ter mene) PR=X *(Adipex-P®, Qsymia™,[2] Suprenza)*

FUNCTION

These drugs are used to treat obesity. Except for orlistat, every agent above is an anorexiant or an appetite suppressor. Orlistat is in a different class known as a lipase inhibitor and has a completely different method of treating obesity.

MECHANISM OF ACTION

The anorexiants are, in general, **sympathomimetic** and act by inhibiting reuptake of serotonin and norepinephrine into the presynaptic neuron. This increases the levels that remain in the synaptic cleft, and they exert greater activity. Phentermine also increases release of dopamine, while sibutramine slightly inhibits the reuptake of dopamine. Diethylpropion exerts its effects primarily through norepinephrine and dopamine. Since all of these are sympathomimetic, they may also treat obesity by increasing the metabolic rate.

Orlistat is a lipase inhibitor. These agents work in the intestine by binding and inhibiting gastric and pancreatic lipases, enzymes that break down fats. This causes an approximate decrease in fat absorption of 30%. This reduction in calories is thought to cause weight loss, though other GI effects may also contribute to a decreased food intake. Orlistat also lowers total and LDL cholesterol.

Lorcaserin is a serotonin 2C receptor agonist that activates receptors in the hypothalamus and results in a feeling of satiety and reduced food intake.

DOSAGES

BENZPHETAMINE, for *children* 12 years and over and *adults*, initiate at 25-50 mg once daily; increase to 25-50 mg 1-3 times/d; once-daily dosing should be administered midmorning or midafternoon; maximum dose is 50 mg tid.

DIETHYLPROPION, for *adults*, tablet, 25 mg tid before meals or food; for controlled release tablet, 75 mg at midmorning.

LORCASERIN, for *adults*, for weight management, 10 mg bid; evaluate response by week 12; if patient has not lost 5% or more of baseline body weight, discontinue.

ORLISTAT, for *children* 12 years and over and *adults*, 120 mg tid with each fat-containing meal either during or up to 1 hour after the meal; omit dose if meal is occasionally missed or contains no fat.

PHENDIMETRAZINE, for *adults*, for tablet, 35 mg 2 or 3 times daily 1 hour before meals; for timed release capsule, 105 mg once daily in the morning before breakfast.

PHENTERMINE, for *adults*, 8 mg tid 30 minutes before meals or food or 15-37.5 mg/d before breakfast or 10-14 hours before retiring.

ADVERSE EFFECTS

Most anorexiants are Schedule IV drugs and are tightly controlled by the government due to their potential for dependency and abuse. Common side effects with these agents include an increase in heart rate and blood pressure, headache, insomnia, constipation, and a dry mouth.

Orlistat can cause oily spotting, flatulence with discharge, fecal urgency, and increased defecation.

RED FLAGS

No major red flags observed.

INTERACTIONS

DRUG

Benzphetamine, diethylpropion, and sibutramine should not be used with MAO inhibitors. Benzphetamine and sibutramine are both sub-strates of CYP3A4 and may interfere with various drugs including ketoconazole, erythromycin, and cimetidine. They also shouldn't be used with SSRIs, serotonin agonists, lithium, dextromethorphan, or pentazocine.

HERB

BENZPHETAMINE

- *Hei Hu Jiao* (Black pepper) (D)–an active ingredient was shown to reduce metabolism of benzphetamine in rats (Dalvi & Dalvi, 1991) Level 5 evidence.

SYMPATHOMIMETIC

- *Chen Pi* (Tangerine peel) (Indeterminate)–contains constituents that stimulate the sympathetic nervous system. Use with caution in those taking antihypertensives, antidiabetic, antihyperthyroid, and/or antiseizure medications (Chinese language article cited in Chen & Chen, 2004) Indeterminate level of evidence.
- *Ma Huang* (Ephedra) (D)–based on ephedrine content, may increase activity of sympathomimetic drugs such as furazolidone and procarbazine, expert opinion (Gruenwald, Brendler & Jaenicke, 2004) Level 5 evidence. (D)–may potentiate sympathomimetic drugs and induce hypertension, expert opinon (Mills & Bone, 2000) Level 5 evidence.
- *Qing Pi* (Citrus Viride) (Indeterminate)–contains constituents that stimulate sympathetic nervous system. Use with caution in those taking antihypertensives, antidiabetic, antihyperthyroid, and antiseizure medications (Chinese language article cited in Chen & Chen, 2004) Indeterminate level of evidence.
- *Rou Cong Rong* (Cistanche) (Indeterminate)–may interact with sympathomimetics, MAOIs, SSRIs, and TCAs by increasing activities of neurotransmitters such as norepinephrine, dopamine, and serotonin (Chinese language article cited in Chen & Chen, 2004) Indeterminate level of evidence.
- *Zhi Ke* (Aurantium fruit, bitter orange), *Zhi Shi* (Aurantium Immaturus) (Indeterminate)–both contain constituents that stimulate the sympathetic nervous system. Use with caution in those taking antihypertensives, antidiabetic,

antihyperthyroid, and antiseizure medications (Chinese language article cited in Chen & Chen, 2004) Indeterminate level of evidence.

VITAMIN

Orlistat may interfere with the absorption of fat-soluble vitamins A, D, E, and K as well as beta-carotene and carotenoids.

INTERACTION ISSUES

A:

D:

M: Benzphetamine is a major substrate of CYP3A4; lorcaserin is a moderate inhibitor of CYP2D6.

E:

Pgp:

SECTION 4: AIDS FOR SMOKING CESSATION

BUPROPION *(See Chapter 5, Section 4, Class 5)*

NICOTINE (nik oh TENE) PR=D *(Commit [O], Nicoderm CQ [O], Nicorelief [O], Nicorette [O], Nicorette Mini [O], Nicorette Refill [O],*

Nicorette Starter Kit [O], Nicotrol; Nicotrol NS; Thrive [O])

VARENICLINE (var e NI klene) *(Chantix, Chantix Continuing Month Pak, Chantix Starting Month Pak)*

▓ FUNCTION

These agents are used to treat smoking and to aid in its cessation.

▓ MECHANISM OF ACTION

Varenicline acts as a partial nicotinic receptor agonist and prevents nicotine stimulation of the mesolimbic dopamine system. This system is thought to be the center of the addiction apparatus of the brain. Basically, it stimulates dopamine, the addiction neurochemical, activity but to a much smaller degree than nicotine. This results in decreased craving and withdrawal symptoms.

▓ DOSAGES

NICOTINE, for *adults,* for tobacco cessation, patients should be advised to completely stop smoking upon initiation of therapy; gum: chew 1 piece of gum when having an urge to smoke, up to 24 pieces/d; patients who smoke under 25 cigarettes/d should start with 2 mg strength; those smoking 25 cigarettes/d or more should start with the 4 mg strength; oral inhaler: usually 6-16 cartridges per day; recommended duration of treatment is 3 months, then wean by gradual reduction of dose over 6-12 weeks; lozenge: patients who smoke their first cigarette within 30 minutes of waking

should use the 4 mg strength; otherwise the 2 mg strength; weeks 1-6, one lozenge every 1-2 hours; weeks 7-9, one lozenge every 2-4 hours; weeks 10-12, one lozenge every 4-8 hours; nasal spray: 1-2 sprays/hr, not to exceed more than 10 sprays/hr up to a maximum of 80 sprays/d; transdermal patch: apply new patch every 24 hours to nonhairy, clean, dry skin on the upper body or upper outer arm; each patch should be applied to a different site.

VARENICLINE, for *adults,* initiate as follows: days 1-3, 0.5 mg once daily; days 4-7, 0.5 mg bid; maintain (weeks 2-12) at 1 mg bid.

▓ ADVERSE EFFECTS

Varenicline commonly causes insomnia, headache, abnormal dreams, and nausea. Less common adverse effects include a rash and GI disturbances. Use in caution with renal dysfunction. There are increased adverse effects when combined with nicotine therapy.

▓ RED FLAGS

No major red flags observed.

▓ INTERACTIONS

No interactions reported.

SECTION 5: SKELETAL MUSCLE RELAXANTS

BACLOFEN (BAK loe fen) PR=C *(Ed Baclofen, Gablofen, Lioresal®)*

CARISOPRODOL (kar eye soe PROE dole) PR=C *(Soma®, Soma® Compound⁴)*

CHLORZOXAZONE (klor ZOKS a zone) PR=B *(Lorzone, Parafon Forte® DSC)*

CYCLOBENZAPRINE (sye kloe BEN za prene) PR=C *(Amrix, Fexmid)*

DANTROLENE (DAN troe lene) PR=C *(Dantrium®, Revonto)*

METAXALONE (me TAKS a lone) PR=N *(Skelaxin®)*

METHOCARBAMOL (meth oh KAR ba mole) PR=C *(Robaxin®)*

ORPHENADRINE (or FEN a drene) PR=C *(Norflex™)*

▓ FUNCTION

These agents are used to relax muscles and relieve discomfort.

Baclofen treats reversible spasticity associated with multiple sclerosis or spinal cord lesions. Off-label uses of this agent include intractable hiccups, intractable pain relief, bladder spasticity, trigeminal neuralgia, cerebral palsy, and Huntington's chorea.

Many of these agents are used to treat muscle spasms and pain associated with acute temporomandibular joint (TMJ) syndrome.

Dantrolene is used to treat spinal cord injury spasticity, stroke, cerebral palsy, multiple sclerosis, and malignant hyperthermia. An off-label use is to treat neuroleptic malignant syndrome.

Methocarbamol is also used as supportive treatment for tetanus.

▓ MECHANISMS OF ACTION

Baclofen acts by inhibiting transmission of reflexes at the spinal cord level, possibly through hyperpolarization of the primary afferent fiber in a reflex arc. This causes muscle spasticity reduction. Chlorzoxazone works similarly.

Carisoprodate and metaxalone have an unknown mechanism of action but are thought to be from their central depressant effects.

Cyclobenzaprine is a centrally acting skeletal muscle relaxant related to tricyclic antidepressants. It reduces tonic somatic motor activity influencing both alpha and gamma motor neurons.

Dantrolene acts directly on skeletal muscle by interfering with release of calcium ions from the sarcoplasmic reticulum. This prevents or reduces the increase in myoplasmic calcium ion concentration and reduces the contraction or counteracts malignant hyperthermia.

Methocarbamol causes skeletal muscle relaxation through CNS depressant effects.

Orphenadrine is an indirect skeletal muscle relaxant thought to work by central atropine-like effects. It has some euphoric and analgesic properties.

▓ DOSAGES

BACLOFEN, for *children* 2-7 years, initiate at 10-5 mg tid; increase dose every 3 days in increments of 5-15 mg/d to maximum 40 mg/d; for 8 years or over, maximum dose 20 mg/d tid. For *adults*, 5 mg tid; may increase 5 mg every 3 days up to a maximum of 80 mg/d.

CARISOPRODOL, for *children* 16 years or over and *adults*, 350 mg 3-4 times/d; take last dose at bedtime.

CHLORZOXAZONE, for *adults*, 250-500 mg 3-4 times/d to a maximum 750 mg 3-4 times/d.

CYCLOBENZAPRINE, do not use longer than 2-3 weeks. For *children* 15 years or older and *adults*, initiate at 5 mg tid; may increase to 7.5-10 mg tid if needed. For the *elderly*, 5 mg tid.

DANTROLENE, for *children* for spasticity, initiate at 0.5 mg/kg bid; increase to 3-4 times/d in 4-7 day intervals, then increase by 0.5 mg/kg to a maximum 3 mg/kg 2-4 times/d up to 400 mg/d; for *children* and *adults* for malignant hyperthermia preoperative prophylaxis, 1-2 mg/kg qid, begin 1-2 days prior to surgery; last dose 3-4 hours prior to surgery; for postcrisis follow-up,

1-2 mg/kg qid 1-3 days. For *adults* for spasticity, initiate at 25 mg/d; increase to 2-4 times/d, then increase dose by 25 mg every 4-7 days to a maximum of 100 mg 2-4 times/d or 400 mg/d.

METAXALONE, for *children* over 12 years and *adults*, 800 mg 3-4 times/d.

METHOCARBAMOL, for *children* 16 or older and *adults*, 1.5 g qid for 2-3 days (up to 8 g/d may be given in severe conditions), then decrease to 4-4.5 g/d in 3-6 divided doses.

ORPHENADRINE, for *adults*, 100 mg bid.

▧ ADVERSE EFFECTS

These agents commonly cause drowsiness, vertigo, psychiatric disturbances, insomnia, slurred speech, ataxia, and hypotonia. Less common adverse effects include hypotension, rash, nausea, and constipation. Rarely palpitations, syncope, depression, hallucinations, xerostomia, anorexia, impotence, paresthesias, and dyspnea may occur. Withdrawal reactions can occur with abrupt cessation of many of these agents.

▧ RED FLAGS

These agents may cause CNS depression. Patients should not perform tasks that require mental alertness such as driving or operating heavy machinery.

An FDA black box warns against rapid withdrawal of these agents as serious withdrawal effects can occur.

Carisoprodate may, rarely, cause seizures.

Cyclobenzaprine may cause QT prolongation, arrhythmias, and tachycardia.

Dantrolene has a box warning that it may cause hepatotoxicity.

▧ INTERACTIONS

DRUG

These agents should not be combined with CNS depressants.

Carisoprodate is a major substrate of CYP2C19 and should be used with caution with delavirdine, fluconazole, fluvoxamine, gemfibrozil, isoniazid, omeprazole, and ticlopidine.

Chlorzoxazone is a major substrate of CYP2E1 as well as a minor substrate for many other CYP isozymes. Caution should be used when combined with disulfiram, isoniazid, and miconazole.

Cyclobenzaprine should not be combined with MAO inhibitors and only with caution with tricyclic antidepressants. It is also a major substrate of CYP1A2 and should be used with caution with amiodarone, ciprofloxacin, fluvoxamine, ketoconazole, norfloxacin, ofloxacin, and rofecoxib. Because of its propensity for QT prolongation, cyclobenzaprine should not be combined with droperidol and fluoxetine.

Dantrolene is a major substrate of CYP3A4. Therefore caution should be used when combined with the following agents: aminoglutethimide, carbamazepine, nafcillin, nevirapine, phenobarbital, phenytoin, rifamycins, azole antifungals, clarithromycin, diclofenac, doxycycline, erythromycin, imatinib, isoniazid, nefazodone, nicardipine, propofol, protease inhibitors, quinidine, telithromycin, and verapamil. Toxicity may occur when combined with estrogens, MAO inhibitors, phenothiazines, clindamycin, warfarin, clofibrate, and tolbutamide.

HERB

CHLORZOXAZONE

- *Da Suan* (Garlic) (B-)—may induce increased metabolism of chlorzoxazone by inducing cyto-chrome P450 2E1 (Gurley, Gardner *et al.*, 2002) Level 3b evidence (Izzo & Ernst, 2009) Level 2b evidence.
- *Guan Ye Lian Qiao* (St. John's wort) (C)—decreases blood concentrations (Izzo & Ernst, 2009) Level 2b evidence.

INTERACTION ISSUES

A:

D:

M: Carisoprodol is a major substrate of CYP2C19; cyclobenzaprine is a major substrate of CYP1A2; dantrolene is a major substrate of CYP3A4.

E:

Pgp:

SECTION 6: ACNE DRUGS

ADAPALENE (a DAP a lene) PR=C *(Differin®, Epiduo®5)*

BENZOYL PEROXIDE (BEN zoe il peer OKS ide) PR=C *(Acanya®,7 Acne-Clear [O], Acne Medication [O], Acne Medication 10, Acne Medication 5 [O], Benzac AC Wash, Benzac W Wash, BenzaClin®,7 Benzamycin®,8 Benza-mycin® Pak,8 BenzEFoam, BenzEFoam Ultra, BenzePrO, BenzePrO Short Contact, Benziq, Benziq LS, Benziq Wash, Benzoyl Peroxide Cleanser [O], Benzoyl Peroxide Wash [O], BP Cleansing [O], BP Gel [O], BP Wash [O], BPO, BPO Creamy Wash, BPO Creamy Wash [O], BPO Foaming Cloths, BPO-10 Wash [O], BPO-5 Wash [O], Clearplex V [O], Clearplex X, Clearskin [O], Desquam-X Wash [O], Duac®,7 Epiduo®,5 Inova, Lavoclen-4 Acne Wash, Lavoclen-4 Creamy Wash, Lavoclen-8 Acne Wash, Lavoclen-8 Creamy Wash, Neutrogena Clear Pore [O], OC8 [O], Oscion Cleanser, PanOxyl [O], PanOxyl Wash [O], PanOxyl-4 Creamy Wash [O], PanOxyl-8 Creamy Wash [O], PR Benzoyl Peroxide Wash, SE BPO Wash, Vanoxide-HC®,6 Zaclir Cleansing)*

ERYTHROMYCIN *(see Chapter 10, Section 2)*

ISOTRETINOIN (eye soe TRET i noyn) PR=X *(Absorica, Amnesteem, Claravis, Myorisan, Zenatane)*

SALICYLIC ACID (sal i SIL ik AS id) PR=C *(Ala seb [O],10 Aliclen, Betasal [O], Calicylic [O], Clear Away 1-Step Wart Remover [O], Corn Remover One Step [O], Corn Remover Ultra Thin [O], DHS Sal [O], Exuviance Blemish Treatment [O], Gordofilm, Hydrisalic [O], Ionil [O], Keralyt, Keralyt [O], Keralyt Scalp, Medi-plast [O], Neutrogena Oil-Free Acne Wash [O], One Step Callus Remover [O], P & S [O], Pernox® Lemon [O],10 Pernox® Regular [O],10 Psoriasin [O], Sal-Plant [O], SalAc [O], Salactic Film [O], Salacyn, Salex, Salicylic Acid Wart Remover, Salkera, Salvax, Scalpicin 2-in-1 [O], Scholl's Callus Removers [O], Scholl's Corn Removers [O], Scholl's Corn Removers Extra [O], Scholl's Corn Removers Small [O], Seba-sorb [O], Sebex [O],10 Sebulex® [O],10 Stri-Dex Maximum Strength [O], Stri-Dex Sensitive Skin [O], Stridex Essential [O], Tarsum® [O],9 Tinamed Corn/Callus Remover [O], Tinamed Wart Remover [O], Trans-Ver-Sal AdultPatch [O], Trans-Ver-Sal PediaPatch [O], Trans-Ver-Sal PlantarPatch [O], Virasal, X-Seb T® Pearl [O],9 X-Seb T® Plus [O]9)*

SULFACETAMIDE *(see Chapter 10, Section 3)*

TAZAROTENE (taz AR oh tene) PR=X *(Avage™, Fabior, Tazorac®)*

TRETINOIN (TRET i noyn) PR=X *(Atralin, Avita, Refissa, Renova, Renova Pump, Retin-A, Retin-A Micro, Retin-A Micro Pump, Tretin-X)*

■ FUNCTION

These agents, through various means, treat acne.

Salicylic acid is also used to treat seborrheic dermatitis or psoriasis of body and scalp, dandruff, and other scaling dermatoses, warts, corns, and calluses.

Tazarotene also treats stable plaque psoriasis, facial skin wrinkling, facial mottled hyper- or hypopigmentation, and benign facial lentigines. Tretinoin treats similar conditions except for psoriasis. It has also been used off label to treat some skin cancers.

■ MECHANISMS OF ACTION

Adapalene is retinoid-like and modulates cell differentiation, kerantization, and inflammation, all of which contribute to acne vulgaris. Adapalene and tazarotene are retinoid-like in addition to the drugs that have a suffix of -retinoin.

Benzoyl peroxide releases free-radical oxygen killing bacteria in sebaceous follicles by oxidizing bacterial proteins.

Salicylic acid, depending on its concentration, either breaks down keratin or, at higher concentrations, destroys tissue. It accomplishes this by dissolving the intercellular cement causing tissue to swell, soften, and shed squamous cells.

■ DOSAGES

ADAPALENE, for *children* 12 years and older and *adults*, for acne, topical: apply nocte.

BENZOYL PEROXIDE, for *children* 12 years and

older and *adults*, for acne, topical: apply sparingly once daily; gradually increase to 2-3 times/d prn; topical cleansers: wash once or twice daily.

ISOTRETINOIN, for *children* 12-17 years, for severe recalcitrant nodular acne, 0.25-.5 mg/kg bid for 15-20 weeks; may stop if the total cyst count decreases by 70%; a second course may be initiated after at least 2 months off of therapy. For *adults*, for severe recalcitrant nodular acne, 0.25-.5 mg/kg bid for 15-20 weeks; may stop if the total cyst count decreases by 70%; patients with very severe disease or scarring or acne that primarily involves the trunk may require up to 2 mg/kg/d; a second course may be initiated after at least 2 months off of therapy.

SALICYLIC ACID, for *children* and *adults*, for acne, topical: cream, cloth, foam, or liquid cleansers (2%): use to cleanse skin once or twice daily by gently massaging into the skin, working into a lather and rinsing thoroughly; gel (0.5% or 2%): apply small amount to face in the morning or evening; pads (0.5% or 2%): use pad to cover area with a thin layer 1-3 times/d; patch (2%): at bedtime, wash face, dry at least 5 minutes, and apply directly over pimple, then remove in the morning; shower/bath gels or soap (2%): use once daily by massaging into acne-prone skin and rinse well. For calluses, corns, or warts, topical: before applying product on warts, soak area in warm water for 5 minutes; remove loosened wart tissue with a brush, wash cloth, or emery board and dry area thoroughly before applying medication; foam: apply bid by rubbing into skin until absorbed; gel or liquid (17%): apply to each wart and allow to dry; may repeat once or twice daily for up to 12 weeks; gel (6%): apply once daily; generally used at night and rinsed off in the morning; liquid (27.5%): apply to each wart, allow to dry, then apply a second application; may repeat this process once or twice daily for up to 6 weeks; transdermal patch (15%): apply over affected area nocte and remove in the morning; may continue for up to 12 weeks; transdermal patch (40%): apply and leave in place for 48 hours; may continue for up to 12 weeks. For dandruff, psoriasis, or seborrheic dermatitis, topical: cream (2.5%): apply 3-4 times daily; may be left in place overnight; foam: apply bid by rubbing into skin until absorbed; ointment (3%): apply to scales or plaques up to 4 times per day, not for scalp or face; shampoo (1.8% to 3%): 2-3 times a week massage into wet hair or affected area; leave in place for several minutes, then rinse thoroughly.

TAZAROTENE, for *children* 12 and older and adults, for psoriasis, topical: Tazorac® gel: initiate at 0.05% by applying once daily to lesions to cover only the lesion with a thin film; may increase strength to 0.1%. For acne, for *children* 12 years and older and *adults*, topical: Tazorac® cream/gel 0.1%: apply a thin film once daily. For *children* 17 and older and *adults*, for helping fine facial wrinkles, facial mottled hyper- or hypo-pigmentation or benign facial lentigines: topical: Avage™: apply a pea-sized amount once daily.

TRETINOIN, for *children* 12 years and older and *adults*, for acne vulgaris, topical: begin with a weaker formulation of tretinoin (0.025% cream, 0.04% microsphere gel, or 0.01% gel) and increase the concentration as tolerated; apply once daily to lesions before bed or on alternate days; if stinging or irritation develop, decrease frequency of application. For *adults*, for fine wrinkles, mottled hyperpigmentation, and tactile roughness of facial skin, topical: pea-sized amount of the 0.02% or 0.05% cream applied to entire face nocte.

ADVERSE EFFECTS

Retinoid-like agents can cause photosensitivity and susceptibility to sunburns. Caution should also be used when applying heat and infrared lamps. A boxed warning on retinoids notes severe birth defects when a fetus is exposed to them.

INTERACTION ISSUES

A:

D: Isotretinoin is 99-100% protein bound; tazarotene is over 99% bound.

M:

E:

Pgp:

SECTION 7: IMMUNOSUPPRESSIVE DRUGS

AZATHIOPRINE (ay za THYE oh prene) PR=D *(Azasan®, Imuran®)*

CYCLOPHOSPHAMIDE *(See Chapter 11)*

CYCLOSPORINE (CsA) (SYE kloe spor ene) PR=C *(Gengraf®, Neoral®, Restasis®, Sandimmune®)*

EVEROLIMUS *(See Chapter 11)*

INFLIXIMAB *(See Chapter 12, Section 3)*

MERCAPTOPURINE *(See Chapter 11)*

METHOTREXATE *(See Chapter 11)*

MYCOPHENOLATE (mye koe FEN oh late)

PR=C *(CellCept®, CellCept® Intravenous, Myfortic®)*

PIMECROLIMUS (pim e KROE li mus) PR=C *(Elidel®)*

RITUXIMAB *(See Chapter 11)*

SIROLIMUS (SRL) (sir OH li mus) PR=C *(Rapamune®)*

TACROLIMUS (FK506 or TAC) (ta KROE li mus) PR=C *(Hecoria, Prograf®, Protopic®)*

Many of the adrenocorticoid drugs are also used as immunosuppressive agents. Please see Chapter 7, Section 4.

These agents primarily are used to treat patients who have undergone organ or tissue transplants. An allograft is a graft from one patient to another that is not genetically identical. When this occurs, rejection of the transplant is nearly universal if immunosuppressant therapy is not undertaken to prevent this rejection. Most often, these agents are used in combination with each other in order to minimize the doses of individual agents and maximize their effectiveness.

Many of these agents are also used in various autoimmune disorders where the body's immune system is attacking itself.

FUNCTION

While azathioprine has been the mainstay of immunosuppressive therapy for decades, mycophenolate is beginning to replace it because of its safety and efficacy. It is used in renal, hepatic, and cardiac transplants.

Cyclosporine is used to treat many transplants including kidney, liver, and heart transplants. It is often used in combination with corticosteroids for this purpose. It is also used to treat rheumatoid arthritis and recalcitrant psoriasis.

Sirolimus is approved for use in kidney transplants with cyclosporine and glucocorticoids, reducing the doses and adverse effects of each of these agents. It is also used in vascular **stents** to prevent **restenosis**. It is also effective in preventing graft vascular disease.

Tacrolimus, used in liver and kidney transplants, is more often used than cyclosporine due to its potency and lower doses of concomitant corticosteroids.

Stent: A device that is designed to anchor skin grafts or support body openings or cavities

Stenosis: Narrowing

MECHANISM OF ACTION

Azathioprine is converted in the body to mercaptopurine, an anticancer drug. Ultimately, this prevents cell reproduction, and since the immune response is predicated on rapid proliferation, this agent primarily prevents lymphocyte generation.

Mycophenolate is converted to mycophenolic acid (MPA), which inhibits formation of guanosine phosphate, necessary for RNA, DNA, and protein synthesis. Ultimately it works like mercaptopurine and azathioprine in preventing B- and T-cell proliferation.

Cytokines are signaling proteins used by the immune system to activate and recruit various other immune cells. Common cytokines are interleukins (IL), interferons (IFN), tumor necrosis factors (TNF), growth factors, and colony-stimulating factors (CSF). IL-2 is a particularly important cytokine that activates helper T cells that release more IL-2 along with IFN and TNF. These activate other cells of the immune system including natural killer (NK) cells, macrophages, and cytotoxic T cells. In other

words, blocking IL-2 will prevent or slow down a full-blown immune response.

Cyclosporine and tacrolimus act by blocking IL-2 synthesis and subsequent T-cell proliferation. They do this by blocking an enzyme, calcineurin, that causes the inactive form of another protein (NFATc) to become active and ultimately promote cytokine synthesis. Cyclosporine inhibits calcineurin by forming a complex with cyclophilin. In contrast, tacrolimus accomplishes the same outcome but binds with a protein known as FK-binding protein (FKBP) that inhibits calcineurin. This cascade is shown in Figure 13.3.

While sirolimus, like tacrolimus, binds with FKBP, it doesn't block activation of NFATc. Instead it forms a complex with mammalian tar-

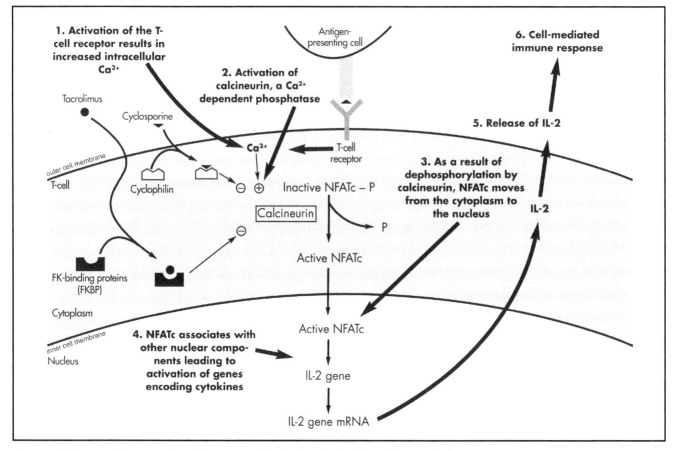

Figure 13.3: Summary of the normal cascade resulting in interleukin 2 (IL-2) and how drugs can block it. 1: Activating a T-cell receptor allows calcium ions intracellularly. 2: This activates calcineurin. Calcineurin is the point that both cyclosporine and tacrolimus act. Cyclosporine prevents activation of calcineurin by activating cyclophillin. Tacrolimus prevents activation by binding FK-binding proteins. 3: Activated calcineurin allows NFATc to enter the nucleus. 4: NFATc activates genes encoding cytokines. 5: This causes greater translation and ultimately the release of IL-2. 6: IL-2 increases the cell-mediated immune response.

get of rapamycin (mTOR). Rapamycin is the original name of sirolimus. This inhibits the normal action of mTOR and prevents proliferation of T cells. Unlike cyclosporine and tacrolimus, sirolimus does not interfere with IL-2 production, but rather inhibits the cell's response to it. This is summarized in Figure 13.4.

DOSAGES

AZATHIOPRINE, for *adults*, for reduction of steroid use in CD or UC, maintenance of remission in CD or fistulizing disease (unlabeled uses), initiate at 50 mg daily; may increase by 25 mg/d every 1-2 weeks as tolerated to a target dose of 2-3 mg/kg/d.

CYCLOSPORINE, Neoral®/Genraf® and Sandimmune® are not bioequivalent and cannot be used interchangeably. For *children*, for transplant, refer to adult dosing; children may require, and are able to tolerate, larger doses than adults. For *adults*, for newly transplanted patients, adjunct therapy with corticosteroids is recommended; initial dose should be given 4-12 hours prior to transplant or may be given postoperatively; adjust initial dose to achieve desired plasma concentration, dose is dependent upon type of transplant and formulation: cyclosporine (modified), renal: 9 ± 3 mg/kg/d divided twice daily; liver: 8 ± 4 mg/kg/d divided twice daily; heart: 7 ± 3 mg/kg/d divided twice daily; cyclosporine (non-modified): initial dose is 15 mg/kg/d as a single dose (range 14-18 mg/kg); lower doses of 10-14 mg/kg/d have been used for renal transplants\; continue initial dose daily for 1-2 weeks; decrease by 5% per week to a maintenance dose of 5-10 mg/kg/d; some renal transplant patients may be dosed as low as 3 mg/kg/d; for rheumatoid arthritis, cyclosporine (modified): initiate at 1.25 mg/kg/d bid; dose may be increased by 0.5-0.75 mg/kg/d if insufficient response is seen after 8 weeks of treatment; additional dosage increases may be made again at 12 weeks up to a maximum dose of 4 mg/kg/d; discontinue if no benefit is seen by 16 weeks of therapy; for psoriasis, cyclosporine (modified):

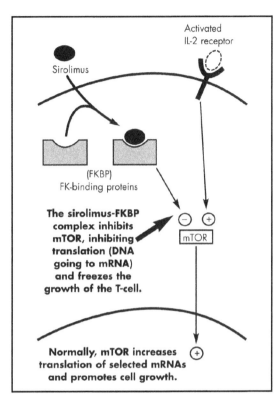

Figure 13.4: How sirolimus decreases an immune response. Sirolimus binds FK-binding proteins in a T cell, which inhibits mTOR and ultimately prevents the cell from proliferating.

initiate at 1.25 mg/kg/d bid; may be increased by 0.5 mg/kg/d if insufficient response is seen after 4 weeks of treatment; additional dosage increases may be made every 2 weeks if needed up to a maximum dose of 4 mg/kg/d; discontinue if no benefit is seen by 6 weeks of therapy; once patients are adequately controlled, the dose should be decreased to the lowest effective dose; doses lower than 2.5 mg/kg/d may be effective; treatment longer than 1 year is not recommended.

MYCOPHENOLATE, for *children*, for renal transplant, CellCept® suspension: 600 mg/m^2/ dose bid; maximum dose is 1 g bid; Myfortic®: 400 mg/m^2/dose bid; maximum dose is 720 mg bid. For *adults*, for renal transplant, CellCept®: 1 g bid; doses over 2 g/d are not recommended; Myfortic®: 720 mg bid (1440 mg/d); for cardiac transplantation, Cell-Cept®: 1.5 g bid.

PIMECROLIMUS, for *children* 2 years and older and *adults*, for mild to moderate atopic dermatitis, topical: apply thin layer to affected area bid and rub in gently and completely.

SIROLIMUS, combination therapy with cyclosporine, doses should be taken 4 hours after cyclosporine and should be taken consistently either with or without food. For *children* 13 and older and *adults*, dose by body weight: under 40 kg, loading dose is 3 mg/m^2 on day 1 followed by maintenance dosing of 1 mg/m^2 once daily; 40 kg or over, loading dose is 6 mg on day 1; maintenanc,: 2 mg once daily.

TACROLIMUS, for *children*, it is recommended that therapy be initiated at high end of the recommended *adult* dosing ranges; dosage adjustments may be required; for liver transplant, initiate at 0.15-0.20 mg/kg/d in 2 divided doses every 12 hours; begin oral dose no sooner than 6 hours post-transplant. For *adults*, for heart transplant, initiate at 0.075 mg/kg/d in 2 divided doses every 12 hours; begin oral dose no sooner than 6 hours post-transplant; for kidney transplant, initiate at 0.1 mg/kg/d bid every 12 hours; initial dose may be given within 24 hours of transplant but should be delayed until renal function has recovered; *African American* patients may require larger doses to maintain an active concentration; for liver transplant, initiate at 0.1-0.15 mg/kg/d in 2 divided doses every 12 hours; begin oral dose no sooner than 6 hours post-transplant.

ADVERSE EFFECTS

Azathioprine can cause suppression of the bone marrow as well as nausea and vomiting.

Cyclosporine commonly causes kidney and liver toxicity, and serum enzymes from these organs should be closely monitored. It may cause lymphoma formation, hypertension, hyperkalemia, tremor, hirsutism, glucose intolerance, and gum hyperplasia.

Mycophenolate can cause pain, diarrhea, **leukopenia**, **sepsis**, and lymphoma.

Sirolimus frequently causes hyperlipidemia. It is nephrotoxic: more so

Leukopenia: A decreased number of white blood cells in the blood; defined as fewer than 5,000 cells per cubic millimeter

Sepsis: The presence of pathogenic organisms or their toxins in the blood or tissues

when combined with cyclosporine, less so when used with tacrolimus. It can also cause headache, nausea, diarrhea, hypertension, leukopenia, and thrombocytopenia.

Tacrolimus has similar adverse effects as cyclosporine but does not cause hirsutism or gum hyperplasia. It can also cause tremor, seizures, hallucinations, and insulin-dependent diabetes mellitus especially in black and Hispanic patients.

RED FLAGS

Agents in this class can make a patient prone to infections that can be life threatening.

INTERACTIONS

DRUG

Combining azathioprine with ACE inhibitors or co-trimoxazole can exaggerate the luekopenic response in renal transplant patients.

Cyclosporine and tacrolimus should be used with caution with other agents that can cause kidney dysfunction such as aminoglycoside antibiotics, diclofenac, naproxen, sulindac, cimetidine, and ranitidine. Also, potassium-sparing diuretics should not be used as they may increase the chances of hyperkalemia.

Absorption of mycophenolate can be reduced when administered with magnesium- or aluminum-containing antacids or cholestyramine.

HERB

CYCLOSPORINE
- *Dong Chong Xia Cao* (Cordyceps, Chinese caterpillar fungus) (D)–improved clinical outcomes in humans from the use of cyclosporine A (Xu, Huang, Jiang, Xu & Mi, 1995) Indeterminate level of evidence; ameliorated kidney damage in rats (Zhao & Li, 1993) Level 5 evidence.
- *Dong Chong Xia Cao* (Cordyceps, Chinese caterpillar fungus) (D)–was shown to interfere with absorption of oral cyclosporine but not intravenous injection in rats. Recommendation from the study was to avoid concurrent use (Chiang, Hou, Tsai, Yang, Chao, Hsiu *et al.*, 2005) Level 5 evidence.

- *Guan Ye Lian Qiao* (St. John's wort, hypericum) (C)–cases have been reported where decreased cyclosporin concentrations led to organ rejection (Hu, Yang, Ho, Chan *et al.*, 2005) Level 3b evidence; (Zhou, Chan, Pan, Huang & Lee, 2004) Level 2b evidence.
- *Huang Qi* (Astragulus) (D)–may stimulate T-cell activity and may decrease the immunosuppressant effects of cyclosporine and corticosteroids, expert opinion (Miller, 1998) Level 5 evidence.

TACROLIMUS

- *Guan Ye Lian Qiao* (St. John's wort) (C)–decreases blood concentrations (Zhou, Chan, Pan, Huang & Lee, 2004) Level 2b evidence, (Izzo & Ernst, 2009) Level 4 evidence.
- *Wu Wei Zi* (Nan) (S. Chinese magnolia vine) (D)–a rat study showed significant changes to pharmacokinetics of tacrolimus when schisandra sphenanthera was administered a half hour before. There were no significant interactions when it was administered 1.5 hours after tacrolimus dose (Wei, Tao, Di, Yang *et al.*, 2103) Level 5 evidence.
- *Zhi Shi* (Aurantium Immaturus) (D)–A rat study showed that administering *Zhi Shi* lowered the C(max) and AUC of tacrolimus significantly (Lin, Wu, Hou, Tsai *et al.*, 2011) Level 5 evidence.

INTERACTION ISSUES

A:

D: Cyclosporine is 90-98% protein bound; mycophenolate is over 97% bound; tacrolimus is approximately 99% bound.

M: Cyclosporine is a major substrate and moderate inhibitor of CYP3A4; sirolimus and tacrolimus are major substrates of CYP3A4.

E:

Pgp: Cyclosporine is a substrate and inhibitor of Pgp; sirolimus is a substrate of Pgp; Tacrolimus is a substrate and an inhibitor of Pgp.

ENDNOTES

[1] Combination of Alendonate, Cholecalciferol, and vitamin D.

[2] Combination of Phentermine and Topiramate.

[3] Combination of Aspirin and Carisoprodate.

[4] Combination of Aspirin, Codeine, and Carisoprodate.

[5] Combination of Adapalene and Benzoyl Peroxide.

[6] Combination of Benzoyl Peroxide and Hydrocortisone.

[7] Combination of Benzoyl Peroxide and Clindamycin.

[8] Combination of Benzoyl Peroxide and Erythromycin.

[9] Combination of Salicylic Acid and Coal Tar.

[10] Combination of Salicylic Acid and Sulfur.

CHINESE MEDICAL DESCRIPTIONS

The Chinese medical explanation of the drug categories in this chapter may be found in Chapter 15 on pages 415–417.

Drugs of Abuse

Drugs of abuse are included here for several reasons. They are obviously relevant to clinical practice. In addition, they are required knowledge for the National Certification Commission of Acupuncture and Oriental Medicine biomedical exam (as of February 1, 2014). It also seems relevant since many drugs of abuse are pharmaceuticals and are already explained in this book. Those that have not been still follow the basic principles of other drugs in regard to pharmacokinetics and pharmacodynamics.

Addiction is defined by the Drug Enforcement Administration (DEA) as "compulsive drug-seeking behavior where acquiring and using a drug becomes the most important activity in the user's life." The basis of drug abuse comes down to positive primary or secondary effect(s) of an agent in combination of that agent causing dependence and tolerance. Withdrawal syndromes can also play a role in maintaining an addiction.

Primary effects generally refer to the "feel-good" aspects of various agents. Secondary effects can mean anything from social interactions to "life avoidance" aspects of drug use. Primary effects generally seem straight-forward, while secondary effects can be quite convoluted.

Dependence is defined as the necessity of continuing a substance in order to avoid negative effects such as withdrawal symptoms. It can be physical and/or psychological in nature. Physical dependence is where a drug, after continued use, will cause withdrawal symptoms if ceased. Therefore, a patient needs to continue using the drug or negative physical effects will occur. Psychological dependence generally refers to the perceived need or craving for a drug rather than having a physical reaction to not taking the drug.

Generally, physical dependence will diminish and disappear rather quickly (days to weeks); psychological dependence can remain for a lifetime and is the primary cause for a relapse into addiction.

Tolerance refers to the body's ability to form a "resistance" to a particular agent. It means that an individual must take more and more of a substance in order to have the same effect. In other words, the effective dose of the agent must increase over time to have the desired effect. While tolerance may not be technically necessary in an addiction, every drug of abuse does create tolerance.

Withdrawal refers to the physical symptoms that occur from stopping an agent after repeated use. They can be relatively mild to life threatening, though they usually last a relatively short time. Many addiction treatments attempt to eliminate or minimize withdrawal symptoms as they are seen as a substantial barrier to breaking the addiction cycle. Generally, programs based on this tactic have limited success when looking at the research literature.

Having said that, treatment in general is very difficult in addiction. By its very nature, addiction is a disease of recurrence. This is where the saying "Once an addict, always an addict" originates. There are no highly effective means of "breaking" an addiction. Even the most successful treatments have a 5-10% success rate. The best of current treatments tend to be peer-led groups such as the anonymous movements. Some people are put off by their perceived religious bent, and similar, less religious alternatives are also available. Intensive counseling and rehabilitation programs can also be effective, though remittance is common once out of the drug-free and controlled confines of the program. Buprenorphine and methadone clinics have mixed-to-poor results according to the scientific literature, though individuals may swear by them.

The DEA uses a "schedule" to rank controlled substances and the amount of control the federal government imposes on their use. This schedule goes from Schedule I drugs with very high poten-tial for misuse and addiction to Schedule V drugs with low potential for abuse. These are summa-rized below.

There are several hypotheses of addiction. Two leading models include the dopamine hypothesis and the self-medication hypothesis.

SCHEDULE	POTENTIAL FOR ABUSE	MEDICAL USE	SAFETY	EXAMPLES
I	High	None	No accepted safe usage	Heroin, gamma hydroxybutyric acid (GHB), lysergic acid diethylamide (LSD), marijuana,[1] and methaqualone
II	High	Yes, with severe restrictions	Use may lead to severe physical or psychological dependence	Morphine, phencyclidine (PCP), cocaine, methadone, hydrocodone, fentanyl, and methamphetamine
III	Less than Schedule I and II drugs	Yes	Use may lead to low to moderate physical or high psychological dependence	Anabolic steroids, codeine and hydrocodone products with aspirin or acetaminophen, and some barbiturates
IV	Low compared with Schedule III drugs	Yes	Use may lead to limited physical or psychological dependence	Alprazolam, clonazepam, and diazepam
V	Low compared with Schedule IV drugs	Yes	Use may lead to limited physical or psychological dependence relative to schedule IV drugs	Cough medicines with codeine

Figure 14.1: Schedule of drugs. This is a summary of the Drug Enforcement Administration's (DEA) schedule of drugs, which helps guide enforcement strategies. Note: 1. While many states are currently legalizing use of marijuana, the DEA, at this time, does not recognize it as safe or appropriate for medical use.

Many others as well as different interpretations of these models exist and are hotly debated among experts.

The dopamine hypothesis is very biologically based and states that all addictions stem from a release of dopamine, the feel-good neurotrans-mitter, in certain areas of the brain. So what addicts are actually addicted to is dopamine, not the agent, or activity, causing the dopamine release. Eventually addiction is caused by the changes in neuro cells in the brain involved in dopamine release and reception.

The self-medication theory states that addicts are using drugs to medicate for a psychological deficit or condition of some sort. So one takes marijuana in order to reduce stress. This is much more psychologically oriented and has the appeal of "if we can only figure out what the problem is, we can solve it."

Again these are only theories, and neither is complete in and of itself. There is a lot more research to be done in discovering the nature of addiction and how to treat it.

Illicit drugs break down into several different types as explored in the sections of this chapter. Many of these agents do have therapeutic benefit and have already been discussed in this book but are listed here as a reminder of their addictive potential. In addition, since tolerance is such an integral part of addiction, dosages will not be discussed unless specifically relevant to a particular agent. Likewise, most of the other headings will not be discussed unless relevant. The names in parentheses in this section refer to the drugs, street names, not their brand names. Of course a list of street names is usually incomplete due to ever-evolving slang. This is followed by a roman numeral referring to its DEA schedule number. There are also sections on administration methods, effects on the body, and overdose symptoms.

SECTION 1: NARCOTICS

HEROIN (HER oh in) *(Acetomorphine, Big H, Black Tar, Brown Sugar, Chasing the Dragon, Chiva, Diacetylmorphine, Diamorphine Hydrochloride, Dope, Hell Dust, Heroin Hydrochloride, Horse, Junk, Negra, Nose Drops, Smack, Thunder) I*

HYDROMORPHONE (hye droe MOR fone) *(D, Dillies, Dust, Footballs, Juice, Smack) II (see Chapter 5, Section 8)*

METHADONE (METH a done) *(Amidone, Chocolate Chip Cookies, Fizzies, Maria, Pastora, Salvia, Street Methadone, Wafer) II (see Chapter 5, Section 8)*

MORPHINE (MOR fene) *(Dreamer, Emsel, First Line, God's Drug, Hows, M.S., Mister Blue, Morf, Morpho, Unkie) II, (see Chapter 5, Section 8)*

OPIUM (OH pee um) *(Ah-pen-yen, Aunti, Aunti Emma, Big O, Black Pill, Chandoo, Chandu, Chinese Molasses, Chinese Tobacco, Dopium, Dover's Powder, Dream Gun, Dream Stick, Dreams, Easing Powder, Fi-do-nie, Gee, God's Medicine, Gondola, Goric, Great Tobacco, Guma, Hop/hops, Joy Plant, Midnight Oil, Mira, O, O.P., Ope, Pen Yan, Pin Gon, Pox, Skee, Toxy, Toys, When-shee, Ze, Zero) II (see Chapter 5, Section 8)*

OXYCODONE (oks i KOE done) *(Hillbilly Heroin, Kicker, OC, Ox, Perc, Roxy, Oxy) II (see Chapter 5, Section 8)*

The term narcotics is derived from the Greek word for stupor. Originally, they referred to any drug that dulled the senses and relieved pain; currently they only refer to opioids. They tend to impart feelings of euphoria and relaxation, and they relieve pain.

ADMINISTRATION

HEROIN: Injected (usually lower quality), smoked, sniffed, or snorted.

HYDROMORPHONE: Tablets, injection.

METHADONE: Swallowed, injection.

MORPHINE: Oral solutions, immediate and sustained release tablets and capsules, suppositories, injection.

OPIUM: Smoked, injection, or pills. Used in combination with other drugs.

OXYCODONE: Oral, inhaled, injection.

EFFECTS

HEROIN: Drowsiness, respiratory depression, constricted pupils, nausea, a warm flushing of the skin, dry mouth, and heavy extremities.

HYDROMORPHONE: Constipation, pupillary constriction, urinary retention, nausea, vomiting, respiratory depression, dizziness, impaired coordination, loss of appetite, rash.

METHADONE: Anxiety, muscle tremors, nausea, diarrhea, vomiting, and abdominal cramps.

MORPHINE: Decreased hunger, cough reflex inhibition, euphoria, and pain relief.

OPIUM: Euphoria, constipation, dry mouth and nose, pain relief.

OXYCODONE: Euphoria, pain relief, sedation, respiratory depression, constipation, pupillary constriction, cough suppression.

OVERDOSAGE

HEROIN: Slow and shallow breathing, blue lips and fingernails, clammy skin, convulsions, coma, possibly death.

HYDROMORPHONE: Severe respiratory depression, drowsiness progressing to stupor or coma, lack of skeletal muscle tone, cold and clammy skin, constricted pupils, and reduction in blood pressure and heart rate.

METHADONE: Slow and shallow breathing, blue fingernails and lips, stomach spasms, clammy skin, convulsions, weak pulse, coma, and possibly death.

MORPHINE: Cold, clammy skin, lowered blood pressure, sleepiness, slowed breathing, slow pulse rate, coma, and possibly death.

OPIUM: Slow breathing, seizures, dizziness, weakness, loss of consciousness, coma, and possibly death.

OXYCODONE: Extreme drowsiness, muscle weakness, confusion, cold and clammy skin, pinpoint pupils, shallow breathing, slow heart rate, fainting, coma, and possibly death.

SECTION 2: STIMULANTS

AMPHETAMINE (am FET a mene) *(Bennies, Black Beauties, Crank, Ice, Speed, Uppers) I (see Chapter 5, Section 3)*

COCAINE (koh CANE) *(Coca, Coke, Crack, Flake, Snow, Soda Cot) II*

KHAT (CAT) *(Abyssinian Tea, African Salad, Catha, Chat, Kat, Oat); one of its main constituents is Schedule I, while another is*

Schedule IV. To be clear, it is an illegal agent in the United States.

METHAMPHETAMINE (meth am FET a mene) *(Batu, Biker's Coffee, Black Beauties, Chalk, Chicken Feed, Crank, Crystal, Glass, Go-Fast, Hiropon, Ice, Meth, Methlies Quick, Poor Man's Cocaine, Shabu, Shards, Speed, Stove Top, Tina, Trash, Tweak, Uppers, Ventana, Vidrio, Yaba, Yellow Bam) II*

Stimulants activate the sympathetic nervous system and speed up metabolism and the body's systems. Khat is a plant with stimulant properties native to East Africa and the Arabian Peninsula.

ADMINISTRATION

AMPHETAMINE: Oral, injection, smoked.

COCAINE: Snorted, injection, smoked.

KHAT: Usually chewed and retained (like chewing tobacco) but can be smoked, eaten, or made into a tea.

METHAMPHETAMINE: Swallowed, snorted, injected, smoked.

EFFECTS

AMPHETAMINE: Increased blood pressure and pulse rate, insomnia, loss of appetite, and physical exhaustion. Chronic abuse produces a psychosis that resembles schizophrenia, characterized by paranoia, picking at the skin, preoccupation with one's own thoughts, and auditory and visual hallucinations.

COCAINE: Euphoria, increased blood pressure and heart rate, dilated pupils, insomnia, and loss of appetite.

KHAT: Increase in blood pressure and heart rate,

insomnia, gastric disorders, and possible manic behavior. Chronic use can result in violence, suicidal depression, and physical exhaustion.

METHAMPHETAMINE: Euphoria, increased wakefulness and physical activity, decreased appetite, rapid breathing and heart rate, irregular heartbeat, increased blood pressure, and hyperthermia. Chronic users can exhibit violent behavior, anxiety, confusion, insomnia, and psychotic features such as paranoia, aggression, visual and auditory hallucinations, mood disturbances, and delusions.

OVERDOSAGE

AMPHETAMINE: Agitation, increased body temperature, hallucinations, convulsions, and possibly death.

COCAINE: Cardiac arrhythmias, ischemic heart conditions, sudden cardiac arrest, convulsions, strokes, and death.

KHAT: Delusions, loss of appetite, difficulty with breathing, and increases in both blood pressure and heart rate.

METHAMPHETAMINE: Death from stroke, heart attack, or multiple organ problems caused by overheating.

SECTION 3: DEPRESSANTS

BARBITURATES (bar BICH yoor ates) *(Barbs, Block Busters, Christmas Trees, Goof Balls, Pinks, Red Devils, Reds & Blues, Yellow Jackets) II, III, IV depending on individual agent (see Chapter 5, Section 2)*

BENZODIAZEPINES (ben zo die AZ uh pene) *(Benzos, Downers) IV, (see Chapter 5, Section 2)*

FLUNITRAZEPAM *(Circles, Forget Pill, Forget-Me-Pill, La Rocha, Lunch Money drug, Mexican Valium, Pingus, R2, Reynolds, Roach, Roach 2, Roaches, Roachies, Roapies, Robutal, Rochas Dos, Rohypnol, Roofies, Rophies, Ropies, Roples, Row-Shay, Ruffies, Wolfies) IV*

GHB/SODIUM OXYBATE (SOW dee um ox i BATE) *(Easy Lay, G, Georgia Home Boy, GHB, Goop, Grievous Bodily Harm, Liquid Ecstasy, Liquid X, Scoop) I*

These agents therapeutically help individuals sleep, relieve anxiety and muscle spasms, and can be antiseizure. Illicitly they can induce euphoria, and are sometimes used in conjuction with stimulants and other drugs to minimize side effects. GHB and Nitrazepam (Rohypnol®), a benzodiazepine, can be used in sexual assault. Agents in this section can also cause amnesia.

⬛ ADMINISTRATION

BARBITURATES: Oral, injection.
BENZODIAZEPINES: Oral, snorting crushed pills.
FLUNITRAZEPAM: Tablets can be swallowed, crushed and snorted, or dissolved in liquid.
GHB/SODIUM OXYBATE: Usually a liquid or powder mixed into a liquid such as water, juice, or alcohol.

⬛ EFFECTS

BARBITURATES: Can slow down the central nervous system and cause sleepiness. Higher doses can cause impairment of memory, judgment, and coordination; irritability; and paranoid and suicidal ideation.
BENZODIAZEPINES: Sleepiness, amnesia, hostility, irritability, and vivid or disturbing dreams.
FLUNITRAZEPAM: Sedation, decreased anxiety, increased or decreased reaction time, impaired mental functioning and judgment, confusion, aggression, excitability, amnesia, slurred speech, loss of motor coordination, weakness, headache, and respiratory depression.
GHB/SODIUM OXYBATE: Euphoric and calming effects, drowsiness, decreased anxiety, confusion and memory impairment, increased libido, suggestibility, passivity.

⬛ OVERDOSAGE

BARBITURATES: Shallow respiration, clammy skin, dilated pupils, weak and rapid pulse, coma, and possibly death.
BENZODIAZEPINES: Shallow respiration, clammy skin, dilated pupils, weak and rapid pulse, coma, and possibly death.
FLUNITRAZEPAM: Can cause severe sedation, unconsciousness, slow heart rate, and suppression of respiration that may be sufficient to result in death especially when combined with other drugs such as alcohol or heroin.
GHB/SODIUM OXYBATE: Unconsciousness, seizures, slowed heart rate, greatly slowed breathing, lower body temperature, vomiting, nausea, coma, and death.

Hallucinogens alter human perception and/or

SECTION 4: HALLUCINOGENS

ECSTASY/MDMA (3,4-methylenedioxy-N-methylamphetamine) *(Adam, Beans, Clarity, Disco Biscuit, E, Ecstasy, Eve, Go, Hug drug, Lover's Speed, MdMA, Peace, StP, X, XtC) I*

K2/SPICE *(Bliss, Black Mamba, Bombay Blue, Fake Weed, Genie, Spice, Zohai) I*

KETAMINE (KEY tuh mene) *(Cat Tranquilizer, Cat Valium, Jet K, Kit Kat, Purple, Special K, Spe-cial La Coke, Super Acid, Super K, Vitamin K) III*

LSD (LYSERGIC ACID DIETHYLAMIDE) *(Acid, Blotter Acid, Dots, Mellow Yellow, Window Pane) I*

PEYOTE (pay OH tee) MESCALINE (MES kuh lene) *(Buttons, Cactus, Mesc, Peyoto) I*

PSILOCYBIN (sie low SIE bin) *(Magic Mushrooms, Mushrooms, Shrooms) I*

mood. Several are naturally occurring and others completely synthetic. K2/Spice can be one of several synthetic compounds similar to psychoactive chemicals in marijuana. Mescaline is the active ingredient in peyote and is produced synthetically.

ADMINISTRATION

ECSTASY/MDMA: Tablets that can be crushed, snorted, or occasionally smoked.

K2/SPICE: Smoked and occasionally made into tea.

KETAMINE: Powder is snorted or smoked, while the liquid is injected or mixed into drinks.

LSD: Oral.

PEYOTE: Chewed or soaked in water and imbibed, or ground into a powder and swallowed or smoked with tobacco or marijuana.

PSILOCYBIN: Oral.

EFFECTS

ECSTASY/MDMA: As a form of amphetamines, these agents increase the release and activity of serotonin, dopamine, and norepinephrine causing changes in perception, including euphoria, increased sensitivity to touch, energy, sensual/sexual arousal, need to be touched, need for stimulation, and increased motor activity, alertness, heart rate, and blood pressure. Unwanted effects include confusion, anxiety, depression, paranoia, sleep problems, drug craving, muscle tension, tremors, involuntary teeth clenching, muscle cramps, nausea, faintness, chills, sweating, and blurred vision.

K2/SPICE: Similar to those of marijuana, para-noia, panic attacks, and giddiness and increased heart rate and blood pressure.

KETAMINE: Distorts perception of sight and sound; makes user feel disconnected and not in control. May cause agitation, depression, cognitive difficulties, unconsciousness, amnesia, increased heart rate and blood pressure, involuntarily rapid eye movement, dilated pupils, salivation, tear secretions, nausea, and stiffening of the muscles.

LSD: Visual changes, extreme changes in mood, dilated pupils, higher body temperature, increased heart rate and blood pressure, sweating, loss of appetite, sleeplessness, dry mouth, and tremors. After use, anxiety and depression can occur.

PEYOTE: Euphoria, anxiety, hallucinations, altered perception of space, time, and body image, intense nausea, vomiting, dilation of the pupils, increased heart rate and blood pressure, a rise in body temperature causing heavy perspiration, headaches, muscle weakness, and impaired motor coordination.

PSILOCYBIN: Hallucinations and an inability to discern fantasy from reality, nausea, vomiting, muscle weakness, and lack of coordination. Panic reactions and psychosis also may occur.

OVERDOSAGE

ECSTASY/MDMA: Can interfere with the ability to regulate temperature, which can lead to hyperthermia resulting in liver, kidney, and cardiovascular system failure and death.

K2/SPICE: No reported deaths due to use.

KETAMINE: Can cause unconsciousness and dangerous bradypnea.

LSD: Psychosis and possibly death.

PEYOTE: No strong overdosage effects are noted.

PSILOCYBIN: Longer, more intense "trip" episodes, psychosis, and possible death.

SECTION 5: MARIJUANA, OR CANNABIS

CANNABIS (CAN uh bis) *(Aunt Mary, BC Bud, Blunts, Boom, Chronic, Dope, Gangster, Ganja, Grass, Hash, Herb, Hydro, Indo, Joint, Kif, Mary Jane, Mota, Pot, Reefer, Sinsemilla, Skunk, Smoke, Weed, Yerba) I*

Cannabis, or marijuana, is a psychoactive drug that is grown in many parts of the world including the United States, Canada, Mexico, South America, and Asia. Currently in the U.S., several states have legalized its use to varying degrees. However, it remains illegal at the federal level.

ADMINISTRATION

Usually smoked but can be mixed with foods and eaten or brewed as a tea.

EFFECTS

Known cannaboid receptors on neurons influence brain activity areas involved in pleasure, memory, thought, concentration, sensory and time perception, and coordinated movement. This can result in problems with memory and learning, distorted perception, difficulty in thinking and problem-solving, loss of coordination, dizziness, nausea, tachycardia, facial flushing, dry mouth merriment, happiness, and even exhilaration at high doses, disinhibition, relaxation, increased sociability and talkativeness, enhanced sensory perception, impaired judgment, reduced coordination and ataxia, emotional lability, incongruity of affect, dysphoria, disorganized thinking, inability to converse logically, agitation, paranoia, confusion, restlessness, anxiety, drowsiness, and panic attacks. Increased appetite and short-term memory impairment are common. Heightened imagination, illusions, delusions, and hallucinations are rare except at high doses.

OVERDOSAGE

No death from overdose of marijuana has been reported.

SECTION 6: STEROIDS

STEROID (STER oid) *(Arnolds, Juice, Pumpers, Roids, Stackers, Weight Gainers) III*

(see Chapter 7, Section 3)

Steroids or anabolic steroids, also known as androgens, are synthetic variants of testosterone. As these are anabolic, they build muscle mass and are taken to improve athletic and physical performance and improve physical appearance. Commonly abused steroids include testosterone, nandrolone, stanozolol, methandienone, and boldenone.

ADMINISTRATION

These drugs are used orally, through intramuscular injection, or absorbed through the skin.

EFFECTS

High doses can cause mood and behavioral changes including dramatic mood swings, increased feelings of hostility, impaired judgment, and increased levels of aggression ("roid rage").

In adolescents, anabolic steroid use can stunt the ultimate height that an individual achieves. In boys, steroid use can cause early sexual development, acne, and stunted growth.

In adolescent girls and women, anabolic

steroid use can induce permanent physical changes, such as deepening of the voice, increased facial and body hair growth, menstrual irregularities, male pattern baldness, and lengthening of the clitoris.

In men, anabolic steroid use can cause shrinkage of the testicles, reduced sperm count, enlargement of the male breast tissue, sterility, and an increased risk of prostate cancer.

In both men and women, anabolic steroid use can cause high cholesterol levels, which may increase the risk of coronary artery disease, strokes, and heart attacks. Anabolic steroid use can also cause acne and fluid retention. Oral preparations of anabolic steroids, in particular, can damage the liver.

OVERDOSAGE

Overdosage does not have known consequences, and the adverse effects come from long-term usage.

SECTION 7: INHALANTS

INHALANTS (in HEY lints) *(Gluey, Huff, Rush, Whippets)*

Inhalants are volatile chemicals found in common household products that are inhaled to induce psychoactive effects.

ADMINISTRATION

Inhalation is the only method of administration, though there are several methods to accomplish this: sniffing or snorting; "bagging", which is sniffing or snorting from fumes sprayed or placed in a paper or plastic bag; and "huffing", where a rag soaked with an inhalant is placed over the mouth or from inhalant-filled balloons.

EFFECTS

Abuse can cause damage to the parts of the brain that control thinking, moving, seeing, and hearing resulting in feeling less inhibited; loss of consciousness; slurred speech; an inability to coordinate movements; euphoria; dizziness; spots or sores around the mouth; red or runny eyes or nose; chemical breath; drunk, dazed, or dizzy appearance; nausea; loss of appetite; anxiety; excitability; and irritability. After heavy use of inhalants, abusers may feel drowsy for several hours and experience a lingering headache. Long-term inhalant abuse can cause weight loss, muscle weakness, disorientation, inattention, depression, damage to the nervous system and other organs, and cognitive abnormalities that can range from mild impairment to severe dementia.

OVERDOSAGE

Prolonged sniffing can induce irregular and rapid heart rhythms and lead to heart failure and death within minutes. Death by asphyxiation from displacing oxygen is an ever-present risk.

SECTION 8: DRUGS OF CONCERN

BATH SALTS OR DESIGNER CATHINONES *(Bliss, Blue Silk, Cloud Nine, Drone, Energy-1, Ivory Wave, Lunar Wave, Meow Meow, Ocean Burst, Pure Ivory, Purple Wave, Red Dove, Snow Leopard, Stardust, Vanilla Sky, White Dove, White Knight, White Lightning)*

DXM (DEXTROMETHORPHAN) *(CCC, Dex, Poor Man's PCP, Robo, Rojo, Skittles, Triple C, Velvet) (see Chapter 5, Section 7)*

SALVIA DIVINORUM (SAL vee uh dih veh NOR uhm) *(Maria Pastora, Sally-d, Salvia)*

Drugs of concern are not currently illegally (though they may be in individual states). They do pose risks to abusers and are being watched by many state and federal authorities.

Bath salts are synthetic stimulants found in a number of retail products. Derivatives of cathinone, a central nervous system stimulant, they are active chemicals found naturally in the khat plant. Mephedrone and MDPV (3-4-methylenedioxypyrovalerone) are two of the designer cathinones most commonly found in these products.

Dextromethorphan is an over-the-counter opioid used as a cough suppressant and is available in numerous retail medications.

Salvia divinorum is an herb native to Oaxaca, Mexico, and is abused for its hallucinogenic effects.

ADMINISTRATION

BATH SALTS: Most commonly sniffed or snorted but can be taken orally, smoked, or injected after being placed in a solution.

DXM: Oral liquid or tablets.

SALVIA DIVINORUM: Chewed, smoked, or vaporized.

EFFECTS

BATH SALTS: Agitation, insomnia, irritability, dizziness, depression, paranoia, delusions, suicidal thoughts, seizures, panic attacks, impaired perception of reality, reduced motor control, rapid heart rate, chest pains, nosebleeds, sweating, nausea and vomiting, and decreased ability to think clearly.

DXM: Euphoria and visual and auditory hallucinations, confusion, inappropriate laughter, agitation, paranoia, overexcitability, lethargy, loss of coordination, slurred speech, sweating, hypertension, and involuntary spasmodic movement of the eyeballs.

SALVIA DIVINORUM: Perceptions of bright lights, vivid colors, shapes, and body movement as well as body or object distortions, fear and panic, uncontrollable laughter, a sense of overlapping realities, hallucinations, loss of coordination, dizziness, and slurred speech.

OVERDOSAGE

BATH SALTS: Unknown.

DXM: Can be treated in an emergency room and generally does not result in severe medical consequences or death.

SALVIA DIVINORUM: No major overdosage effects noted.

Provisional Chinese Medical Descriptions of Western Drugs by Category

Trying to work out at least provisional Chinese medical descriptions of Western drugs is no easy task. It requires a great deal of knowledge about Chinese medicine and a great deal of thought. It also requires the ability to discriminate between what information about a drug should be taken into account and what information should be set aside.

By and large, this means setting aside biochemical information and cellular and molecular pharmacodynamics. Instead, the focus should be on the signs and symptoms that would otherwise be knowable to the Chinese doctor via the four examinations.

In most cases, trying to determine flavor (味 *wei*), nature (性 *xing*, i.e., temperature), and channel gatherings (归 经 *gui jing*) or channel enterings (入 经 *ru jing*) is not particularly profitable or even possible; although, in some cases, we may posit nature.

Instead, the emphasis should be on the general Chinese medical classification of the drug and its seeming Chinese medical functions (功 用 *gong yong*). The drug's indications (主 治 *zhu zhi*) and contraindications (宣 忌 *xuan ji*) are already specified in the Western pharmacologic literature as are its dosages (用 量 *zhong liang*).

In general, one begins this process by listing the drug's intended therapeutic effects and its possible side effects in terms of Chinese medical symptoms. Next one lists the disease mechanisms (病 机 *bing ji*) that might account for each of these "symptoms." Then one looks for the single Chinese medical mechanism that would account for both its intended therapeutic effects and its possible side effects.

In doing this kind of problem-solving, an important principle is to start from what is most assuredly known and then identifying are the mostly likely mechanisms accounting for the remaining unknown.

This is very much like doing a Chinese medical pattern discrimination (辨 证 *bian zheng*) and requires a sophisticated understanding of disease mechanisms. Often it feels like an impossible task because of many seeming contradictions. However, by thinking deeply, one should be able to reconcile the apparent contradictions and come to a provisional Chinese medical description of the drug under discussion. I say *provisional* because it has taken Chinese doctors a thousand years to reach consensus on the current standard Chinese medical descriptions of our most important Chinese medicinals (中 药 *zhong yao*).

Therefore, it should not be expected that a single person or two will be able to correctly describe scores of Western medicinals (西药 *xi yao*). It will take a number of great minds to eventually arrive at what may become these drugs' standard Chinese medical descriptions.

CHAPTER 4: DRUGS AFFECTING THE AUTONOMIC NERVOUS SYSTEM

SECTION 1: CHOLINERGIC AGONISTS

Cholinergic agonists are used to:

1. Stimulate an atonic bladder with urinary retention postpartum or postoperatively

2. Treat the muscular weakness of myasthenia gravis and Eaton-Lambert syndrome

3. Stimulate salivation in cases of xerostomia due to radiation and Sjögren's syndrome

In Chinese medicine, urinary retention is called non-exiting of urination (小 便 不 出 *xiao bian bu chu*), muscular weakness is referred to as loss or lack of strength (失 力 *shi li*), and xerostomia corresponds to dry mouth (口 干 *kou gan*).

Cholinergic agonists may cause the side effects listed below.

Those side effects that are recognized Chinese medical disease categories in their own right or Chinese medical signs and symptoms are indicated by their Chinese names in parentheses. Chinese correspondences are only given the first time such a disease or symptom is listed.

- Diaphoresis (汗 *han*)
- Headache (头 痛 *tou tong*)
- Urinary urgency (尿 急 *niao ji*)
- Nausea (恶 心 *e xin*)
- Diarrhea (泄 泻 *xie xie*)
- Hypotension
- Salivation (流 涎 *liu xian*)
- Flushing (赤 面 *chi mian*, literally, red face)
- Abdominal pain and cramps (肤 痛 *fu tong*)
- Bronchospasm, *i.e.*, panting (喘 *chuan*)
- Heart palpitations (心 悸 *xin ji*)
- Tremors (震 颤 *zhen chan*)
- Tachycardia, *i.e.*, a rapid pulse (数 脉 *shu mai*)

The main symptom of hypotension is orthostatic dizziness, which, in Chinese medicine, is simply dizziness (眩 晕 *xuan yun*).

In this case, the thing that is absolutely known about the above intended therapeutic effects is that the muscular weakness of both myasthenia gravis and Eaton-Lambert syndrome is due to spleen qi vacuity/deficiency, which may also be called central qi falling downward. Secondly, atonic bladder with urinary retention postpartum and postoperatively is mostly due again to qi vacuity/deficiency, in which case there is not enough qi to move the urine out of the body. This may also be seen as a manifestation of central qi falling downward. As for the xerostomia, this may be due to either of two mechanisms. Either there simply are insufficient yin fluids to moisten the mouth or yin fluids are not being transported upward to the mouth.

What do we know for sure about the side effects? We know that there is only one basic Chinese medical mechanism for hypotension, and that is also spleen vacuity. So here there appears to be a contradiction. Nausea is always a symptom of upwardly counterflowing stomach qi. Flushing is also a symptom of upwardly counterflowing yang qi or heat, and a rapid pulse is also always a symptom of heat.

Urinary urgency can be a symptom of damp heat or of qi vacuity. Diarrhea is most commonly also due to either damp heat or qi vacuity. Tremors are a symptom of qi flowing chaotically in the body, *i.e.*, wind.

Heart palpitations may be due to a large number of mechanisms. However, the most common are qi, blood, and/or yin vacuity, heat, or phlegm.

Salivation, meaning hypersalivation, may be due to either damp rheum spilling over or qi vacuity failing to contain water fluids.

Panting may be due to some evil qi blocking the diffusion of the lungs or a lung qi vacuity failing to diffuse, and sweating is due either to the upbearing and out-thrusting of the righteous qi or failure of the defensive qi to secure the exterior. And finally, abdominal pain and cramps indicate that there is a failure of free flow. However, there are a number of reasons the abdominal qi may not be freely flowing.

If we know that cholinergic agonists treat central qi falling downward because they treat the muscular weakness of myasthenia gravis and Eaton-Lambert syndrome and postpartum and postoperative urinary retention, then we must think about the different classes of Chinese medicinals that are used to remedy this disease mechanism, and these are divided into two: qi supplements and qi rectifiers. Now, can qi supplements cause the side effects listed above? And the answer to that is, except for abdominal pain and cramps, no. Therefore, it does not appear that cholinergic agonists are qi-supplementing medicinals. That then leaves qi rectifiers, similar to *Chai Hu* (Radix Bupleuri), which actually is an exterior resolver that upbears clear yang. *Chai Hu* administered to the wrong person could certainly cause sweating and headache.

Because such acrid, windy-natured medicinals tend to plunder or consume yin, they could also cause flushing, heart palpitations, tremors, and a rapid pulse. Because they upbear and outthrust the righteous qi, in a person who was qi vacuous, they could also cause symptoms of qi vacuit, such as hypotension, urinary urgency, panting, and diarrhea, and because they are upbearing, they could cause upward counterflow of the stomach qi resulting in nausea.

If there is xerostomia because of insufficient qi to move water fluids upward to the mouth, upbearing, qi-moving medicinals might reasonably remedy xerostomia. However, if they over-disperse the qi, they might also result in hypersalivation because the qi is no longer able to contain water fluids within the body. As for the abdominal pain and cramping, if this is insidious pain, it could be due to spleen qi vacuity. How-ever, unfortunately, we do not know the actual type of stomach pain caused by cholinergic agonists. So this side effect must be set aside until more about its exact quality can be learned.

Given what we do know, we would say that the closest fit in terms of the Chinese medical categorization of cholinergic agonists is as acrid, windy-natured, upbearing, and exterior-resolving medicinals (解 表 药 *jie biao yao*). If this categorization is correct, then they might be expected to cause problems in patients who tend to be yin vacuous. In addition, dose might be the deciding factor between upbearing clear yang in a good way, thus remedying signs and symptoms of central qi falling downward, and simply over-dispersing the righteous qi in a bad way, causing even more symptoms of qi vacuity.

This hypothetical Chinese medical categorization of cholinergic agonists is further supported by the fact that *Gan Cao* (Radix Glycyrrhizae) may treat overdoses of pilocarpine. *Gan Cao* is a qi supplement that also helps engender fluids. Therefore, it reasonably could offset overdispersing of the qi and plundering of yin fluids.

SECTION 2: ANTICHOLINESTERASES (REVERSIBLE)

Anticholinesterases are used to treat:

1. The muscular weakness of myasthenia gravis
2. The cognitive weakness (神 志 昏 乱 *shen zhi hun luan* or 恍 惚 善 忘 *huang hu shan wang*) of Alzheimer's disease
3. Attention deficit–hyperactivity disorder (ADHD) in children

Attention deficit–hyperactivity disorder is composed of two elements: impaired memory (健 忘 *jian wang*) and excessive stirring (多 动 *duo dong*) or agitation (躁 *zao*).

The side effects of anticholinesterases include:

- Diaphoresis
- Headache
- Hypotension
- Urinary urgency
- Salivation
- Flushing
- Abdominal pain and cramps
- Bronchospasm, *i.e.*, panting
- Diarrhea

We have discussed the Chinese medical disease mechanisms of myasthenia gravis above. The cognitive weakness of Alzheimer's is due to either one or a combination of two reasons: (1) qi vacuity and (2) phlegm and/or stasis. Similarly, the attention deficit part of ADHD is mostly due to qi vacuity, remembering that children's spleens are inherently vacuous and weak, and the spleen is the root of the engenderment and transformation of qi. Since the side effects are all the same as cholinergic agonists, it would similarly appear that anticholinesterases are acrid, windy-natured upbearing qi rectifiers. This is further supported by the fact that medicinals that move and rectify the qi would also help treat the phlegm and blood stasis of Alzheimer's as well as the depressive heat, which is commonly the cause of the hyperactivity of ADHD.

As long as such medicinals did not overdisperse the qi, they would have a salutary effect on the central qi falling downward of the myasthenia gravis as well as the qi vacuity causing the cognitive weakness of Alzheimer's and the attention deficit of ADHD.

SECTON 3: ANTIMUSCARINIC AGENTS

Antimuscarinic agents treat:

1. Spasms of the gastrointestinal tract, including irritable bowel syndrome (IBS), *i.e.*, abdominal pain (肤 痛 *fu tong*)
2. Tremors (震 颤 *zhen chan*) due to Parkinson's and the extrapyramidal side effect of other drugs
3. Coughing (咳 嗽 *ke sou*)
4. Nausea and vomiting (呕 恶 *ou e*)

The side effects of antimuscarinic agents include:

- Blurred vision (花 眼 *hua yan*)
- Confusion (神 志 昏 乱 *shen zhi hun luan*)
- Drowsiness (嗜 卧 *shi wo*)
- Constipation (便 必 *bian bi*)
- Dry mouth (口 干 *kou gan*)
- Restlessness, *i.e.*, agitation
- Headache
- Urinary retention
- Tachycardia, *i.e.*, a rapid pulse

Spasms of the gastrointestinal tract mostly have to do with qi stagnation, while IBS always includes an element of liver depression qi stagnation. Liver depression qi stagnation may also cause strangury, thus resulting in a feeling of spasming of the bladder. Tremors are due to internal stirring of wind. However, internally stirring wind is nothing other than frenetically and chaotically flowing qi.

Coughing is due to upward counterflow of the lung qi, while nausea and vomiting are due to upward counterflow of the stomach qi. The lung qi may counterflow upward if a replete, hot liver rebels against the lungs' normal control, and the stomach qi may counterflow upward if liver depression horizontally counterflows to attack the stomach. Therefore, qi-rectifying medicinals would have a beneficial effect on any of these four types of conditions. However, because qi rectifiers are also acrid and windy-natured and tend to disperse the qi and plunder yin fluids, they could also cause all of the listed side effects. For

instance, the most common mechanism of blurred vision is blood vacuity.

Constipation may be due to fluid dryness of the large intestine, and dry mouth may be due to stomach yin vacuity. Similarly, urinary retention may be due to kidney yin vacuity. A rapid pulse and agitation are due to heat, in this case most likely yin vacuity heat. Headache could be due to yin vacuity with ascendant yang hyperactivity.

Drowsiness, meaning fatigue, is a definite qi vacuity symptom. If too much qi is dispersed, then there might be qi vacuity. In the same way, confusion is commonly due to qi vacuity and/or yin-blood vacuity. All this is supported by the facts that *Fu Ling* (Poria), *Ren Shen* (Radix Ginseng), *Yuan Zhi* (Radix Polygalae), plus *Shi Chang Pu* (Rhizoma Acori Tatarinowii) have been shown to alleviate impaired memory due to scopolamine. All these medicinals supplement the heart spirit, and the heart spirit is nothing other than an accumulation of heart qi.

In addition, *Dang Gui* (Radix Angelicae Sinensis), a blood supplement, has been found to relieve amnesia in rats caused by scopolamine and cycloheximide.

SECTION 4: DIRECT-ACTING ADRENERGIC AGONISTS

Direct-acting adrenergic agonists treat:

1. Asthma, *i.e.*, panting and wheezing (喘 哮 *chuan xiao*)
2. Hypotension, *i.e.*, dizziness
3. Hypertension
4. Muscle spasm (肌 急 *ji ji*)

The side effects of direct-acting adrenergic agents include:

- Cardiac arrhythmias, *i.e.*, heart palpitations
- Hyperactivity, *i.e.*, agitation
- Headache
- Insomnia (不 眠 *bu mian*)
- Nausea
- Dry mouth
- Sedation, *i.e.*, fatigue (疲 倦 *pi juan*) or somnolence (嗜 卧 *shi wo*)
- Tachycardia, *i.e.*, a rapid pulse
- Bradycardia, *i.e.*, a slow pulse (迟 脉 *chi mai*)

In Chinese medicine, asthma is treated by exterior-resolving medicinals that diffuse the lung qi. As we have seen above, hypotension is always a symptom of spleen qi vacuity in Chinese medicine, and spleen qi vacuity is commonly treated with a combination of qi-supplements and qi rectifiers. Both exterior resolvers and qi rectifiers tend be to acrid, windy-natured medicinals that upbear and out-thrust.

Hypertension is commonly associated with ascendant liver yang hyperactivity, liver fire flaming upward, phlegm heat, or internal stirring of liver wind. The root mechanism of all four of these patterns is depressive heat. Depressive heat means there is liver depression that has transformed heat. If one resolves this depression and clears this heat, the blood pressure often goes down. Interestingly, a qi-rectifying exterior resolver such as *Chai Hu* (Radix Bupleuri) can raise blood pressure in those who are hypotensive and lower blood pressure in those who are hypertensive.

Muscle spasm, especially low back muscle spasm, may be a symptom of qi stagnation, which might be treated with acrid, windy-natured medicinals in Chinese medicine.

In terms of side effects, hyperactivity and a rapid pulse are both symptoms of heat. Activity is a function of yang qi. The more yang qi, the more activity. However, the more yang qi, the more heat. Heat is yang qi. If an acrid, windy-natured drug damaged yin fluids, there could be dry mouth and insomnia. If an upbearing medicinal upbore too much, there could be headache and nausea. If a qi-moving, scattering, and dispersing medicinal drained too much qi, there could be fatigue and a slow pulse.

As for heart palpitations, if associated with a rapid pulse, they are due to heat and yin-blood malnourishment, while if they are associated with a slow pulse, they would be due in this case to qi vacuity.

Thus the Chinese medicinal description of direct-acting adrenergic agonists once again appears to be that of acrid, windy-natured, exterior-resolving (解 表 *jie biao*), qi-rectifying medicinals (理 气 药 *li qi yao*). If you ask why so

many Western medicinals are described this way in Chinese medicine, we would remind you of Zhu Dan-xi's famous saying, "Hundreds of diseases are due to depression" as well as the *Nei Jing's (Inner Classic)* advice, "For depression, out-thrust."

SECTION 5: MIXED ACTION ADRENERGIC AGONISTS

Mixed action adrenergic agonists treat:
1. Asthma, *i.e.*, panting and wheezing
2. Complete heart block
3. Narcolepsy
4. Nasal congestion (鼻 塞 *bi sai*)

The side effects of mixed action adrenergic agonists include:
- Insomnia
- Hypertension
- Nausea
- Dry mouth

We have discussed asthma and narcolepsy above as we have all of the side effects of these drugs. Nasal congestion is due to the non-diffusion of the lung qi and the accumulation of phlegm in the nose, the orifice of the lungs. Thus nasal congestion in Chinese medicine is treated by exterior-resolving medicinals. The symptoms of complete heart block in Chinese medicine correspond to heart palpitations and a bound or regularly intermittent pulse. A bound pulse is a slow, irregularly intermittent pulse, while a regularly intermittent pulse is also defined as a slow pulse. In this case, there is usually phlegm plus qi stagnation at the least.

Once again, we believe this all adds up to a Chinese medical description of acrid, windy-natured, upbearing and out-thrusting, exterior-resolving (解 表 *jie biao*), qi-rectifying medicinals (理 气 药 *li qi yao*).

SECTION 6: ALPHA-ADRENERGIC BLOCKING AGENTS

The main condition these drugs are used to treat is benign prostatic hypertrophy (BPH), although they are sometimes also used to treat intractable hypertension.

The side effects of these drugs include:

- Orthostatic hypotension (眩晕 *xuan yun, i.e.,* dizziness)
- Nausea and vomiting
- Nasal congestion and runny nose (清涕 *bi sai liu qing ti*)
- Inhibition of ejaculation (精不射出 *jing bu she chu*)
- Tachycardia, *i.e.*, a rapid pulse

In Chinese medicine, BPH is due to qi vacuity, blood stasis, and phlegm. However, since we know that orthostatic hypotension is a qi vacuity symptom, we also know that this group of drugs does not supplement the qi. In fact, the nasal congestion and runny nose caused by these drugs indicates a lung qi vacuity failing to secure and astringe water fluids.

Nausea and vomiting definitely involve upward counterflow of the stomach qi, but this may in turn be due to spleen qi vacuity. If the spleen qi does not upbear, the stomach qi cannot downbear.

The tachycardia definitely indicates heat, and the most likely type of heat caused as a drug reaction is vacuity heat due to the plundering of yin. Since we have ruled out qi supplementation as these drugs' way of treating BPH, that leaves some method of dispelling stasis and eliminating phlegm, and the one method that is common to both is qi rectification (理气 *li qi*). By moving the qi, we move the blood. By moving the qi, we move water fluids and, therefore, phlegm, dampness, and turbidity.

Qi rectifiers can damage yin fluids and lead to a rapid pulse. They can also damage the qi and lead to orthostatic hypotension. But how might they lead to failure to ejaculate? Ejaculation is a species of transformation whereby pent-up qi is discharged and, along with it, essence and fluids. Normally, failure to ejaculate or orgasm is impugned in Chinese medicine to liver depression. However, it might be possible for over-attacking and over dispersing to prevent a build-up of qi to be discharged. This is only a guess.

SECTION 7. BETA-ADRENERGIC BLOCKING AGENTS (a.k.a. BETA-BLOCKERS)

When taken internally, beta-blockers treat:

1. Hypertension
2. Migraines (偏头痛 *pian tou tong*)
3. Hyperthyroidism
4. Angina pectoris and myocardial infarction (MI), *i.e.*, chest impediment (胸痹 *xiong bi*)

The side effects of these drugs include:

- Decreased libido
- Failure to ejaculate
- Cold extremities (肢冷 *zhi leng*)
- Fatigue
- Insomnia
- Nightmares
- Depression
- Bradycardia, *i.e.*, a slow pulse

We have seen above that the overwhelming majority of hypertension is rooted in liver depression, which then gives rise to yang hyperactivity, liver fire, liver wind, and phlegm heat. Migraines in Chinese medicine can either be due to vacuity or repletion. When due to repletion, we are mostly talking about liver repletion, which counterflows upward into the boney box of the head from which it has no outlet. Hyperthyroidism in Chinese medicine is mostly due to depressive heat that transforms into fire and eventually damages yin. Once it has damaged yin, the replete heat transforms into vacuity heat. The symptoms of angina pectoris and MI correspond to chest impediment, and the main repletions in chest impediment are qi stagnation, blood stasis, and phlegm. However, these are often associated with heat and hyperactivity even though heat and hyperactivity themselves may not be causing chest impediment. Therefore, the conditions that beta-blockers are meant to treat are all associated with liver depression and the heat that transforms from liver depression.

In Chinese medicine, the liver and kidneys share a common source. In addition, the libido is a function of the life-gate ministerial fire or kidney yang, and the life-gate ministerial fire has a very close relationship with the liver. Flaming and hyperactivity of the one causes flaming and hyperactivity of the other. If we put together the intended therapeutic effects of beta-blockers with their side effect of decreased libido, this suggests excessive heat clearing. Excessive heat-clearing would also explain the chilled extremities and slow pulse. Since heat is nothing other than qi, excessive heat clearing could lead to fatigue. Interestingly, one of the symptoms of most people's depression is also fatigue. A decrease in righteous qi can lead to a decline in the engenderment and transformation of blood. If the blood then fails to nourish the heart spirit, there can be insomnia and nightmares. Therefore, it appears that beta-blockers are heat-clearing medicinals (清 热 药 *qing re yao*) that clear heat from the liver and heart, remembering that most heat in

the heart arises from depressive liver heat, and, in the process, also affects kidney yang.

Interestingly, beta-blockers can also exacerbate angina pectoris and induce congestive heart failure as well as asthma. If one adversely drains kidney yang, this will cause a decrease in heart yang. If heart yang becomes vacuous and insufficient, then blood stasis and phlegm obstruction will be engendered or worsened. Thus the worsening of angina and the causation of congestive heart failure. Since the heart and lung qi together form the ancestral or combined qi of the chest, anything that causes damage to the heart may likewise cause damage to the lungs and vice versa. In this case, it would appear that blood stasis and phlegm also inhibit the diffusion and downbearing of the lung qi and thus the asthma.

CHAPTER 5: DRUGS AFFECTING THE CENTRAL NERVOUS SYSTEM

SECTION 1: DRUGS FOR PARKINSON'S DISEASE

Drugs for Parkinson's disease are mainly used to treat Parkinson's and extrapyramidal symptoms caused by other drugs, that is tremors.

The side effects of drugs for Parkinson's disease include:

- Visual and auditory hallucinations
- Agitation
- Dizziness
- Confusion
- Orthostatic hypotension
- Urinary retention
- Peripheral edema (肢 肿 *zhi zhong*)
- Dry mouth
- Toxic psychosis, *i.e.*, mania (狂 *kuang*)
- Anorexia
- Nausea and vomiting
- Fatigue
- Somnolence
- Anxiety (焦 急 *jiao ji*)
- Depression
- Insomnia

Since tremors in Chinese medicine are a symptom of internal stirring of liver wind, these drugs should likely be classified as wind-extinguishing, tremor-stopping medicinals (息 风 止 震 药 *xi feng zhi zhen yao*). The Chinese medicinals in this category are definitely attacking and draining medicinals that typically should not be used in those with qi and blood vacuities.

Judging from such side effects as dizziness, confusion, orthostatic hypotension, urinary retention, peripheral edema, anorexia, nausea and vomiting, fatigue, somnolence, anxiety, depression, and insomnia, these drugs can damage the spleen (and possibly the kidneys) and lead to or aggravate qi and blood vacuities.

Since blood and essence (meaning yin) share a common source, it appears that, in susceptible individuals, they can also damage yin leading to internal engenderment of heat. This is supported by such heat symptoms as visual and auditory hallucinations, agitation, dry mouth, and mania. It is interesting to note that some of the Chinese medicinals in this category can cause many of the same side effects.

SECTION 2: DRUGS FOR OTHER NEURODEGENERATIVE DISEASES

See Chapter 4, Section 3 for information on some of these drugs. Corticosteroids used for these diseases are discussed under Chapter 7, Section 4. No other information on these drugs is available.

SECTION 3: NEUROLEPTIC OR ANTIPSYCHOTIC DRUGS

A. TYPICAL NEUROLEPTICS

Typical neuroleptics treat:

1. Schizophrenia and psychoses, *i.e.*, mania and withdrawal
2. Nausea and vomiting
3. Intractable hiccup (呃 逆 不 止 *e nib u zhi*)
4. The spasms and contractures (痉 挛 *jing luan*) of Tourette's syndrome

The side effects of these drugs include:

- Tremors
- Tardive dyskinesia, *i.e.*, involuntary movements or excessive stirring
- Blurred vision
- Dry mouth
- Fatigue
- Somnolence
- Orthostatic hypotension
- Confusion
- Constipation
- Urinary retention
- Amenorrhea (闭 经 *bi jing*)
- Galactorrhea (乳 汁 自 出 *ru zhi zi chu*)
- Infertility (不 孕 症 *bu yun zheng*)
- Impotence (阳 痿 *yang wei*)

Schizophrenia and psychoses are categorized as mania in Chinese medicine and are a type of hyperactivity. Nausea, vomiting, and intractable hiccup are all species of upward counterflow of the stomach qi, and the spasms and contractures of Tourette's syndrome are usually seen as internally stirring liver wind and/or ascendant hyperactivity of liver yang. As stated above, if there is mania, there is heat. However, mania is also treated by subduing yang and downbearing counterflow, and Chinese medicinals that downbear counterflow are also used to treat nausea, vomiting, and hiccup (*i.e.*, *Dai Zhe Shi*, Haemititum).

Again, it is the heavy, settling spirit-quieting medicinals that subdue yang, and these medicinals can definitely damage the spleen qi and lead to fatigue, somnolence, orthostatic hypotension, and

confusion. Qi vacuity can also cause both galatorrhea and urinary retention. In the first case, there is insufficient qi to contain fluids within the body. In the second, there is insufficient qi to move urine out of the body. Similarly, impotence may also be due to qi vacuity.

Amenorrhea, blurred vision, dry mouth, constipation, and infertility may all be due to blood vacuity due to spleen vacuity. Tremors and tardive dyskinesia may be due to blood vacuity failing to control yang qi and giving rise to internally stirring wind. Thus antipsychotic drugs also look like heavy, settling, spirit-quieting medicinals (重 镇 安 神 药 *zhong zhen an shen yao*). The phenothiazines are known to cause the tongue fur to develop white plaques resembling milk curds. This indicates the internal engenderment of dampness due to spleen qi vacuity.

SECTION 4: ANXIOLYTIC AND HYPNOTIC DRUGS

Anxiolytic and hypnotic drugs are used mainly to treat anxiety and insomnia.

The side effects of these drugs include:

- Fatigue
- Confusion
- Impaired memory
- Weakness
- Headache
- Blurred vision
- Vertigo (眩 *xuan*)
- Nausea and vomiting
- Diarrhea
- Joint pain (骨 结 疼 痛 *gu jie teng tong*)
- Chest pain
- Urinary incontinence (尿 失 禁 *niao shi jin*)
- Rebound insomnia (in Chinese medicine, this would simply be insomnia)

It is tempting to simply categorize these Western drugs as spirit-quieting medicinals based on their intended therapeutic effects. However, of the two subcategories of spirit-quieting medicinals in Chinese medicine, the spirit-nourishing medicinals would not cause the kind of side effects that these drugs do. That then leaves the heavy, settling spirit-quieting medicinals, and these can cause the kinds of side effects that these medicines do.

Because of the combination of fatigue, confusion, impaired memory, blurred vision, vertigo, nausea and vomiting, diarrhea, urinary incontinence, and rebound insomnia, it is clear that these medications are attacking and draining and can damage the spleen, thus resulting in or aggravating qi and blood vacuities. If the joint pain is due to malnourishment of the sinews and bones rather than impediment by some sort of evil qi, then this would make sense. Similarly, the chest pain could be due to a heart qi and blood vacuity. Unfortunately, we would need more information on the exact nature of the joint and chest pain to conclude this for sure. In any case, it appears that these drugs function similarly to heavy, settling spirit-quieting medicinals (重 镇 安 神 药 *zhong zhen an shen yao*). Alprazolam is known to cause dry mouth and tongue, suggesting its ability to damage blood and yin.

SECTION 5: CNS STIMULANTS

CNS stimulants are used to treat:

1. Obesity
2. Narcolepsy
3. Asthma

The side effects of these drugs include:

- Headache
- Chilliness
- Palpitations
- Fatigue
- Depression
- Angina
- Hyper- or hypotension
- Sweating
- Dry mouth
- Nausea and vomiting
- Anorexia
- Diarrhea
- Agitation
- Insomnia
- Dizziness
- Talkativeness
- Lack of strength
- Anxiety
- Confusion
- Deranged speech (言 语 错 乱 *yan yu cuo luan*)
- Decreased libido
- Mania

All three conditions of obesity, narcolepsy, and asthma involve phlegm, dampness, and turbidity, while these drugs' side effects mostly appear to be due to qi vacuity and yin-blood-fluid vacuity engendering vacuity heat. Therefore, this class of drugs is very similar to *Ma Huang* (Herba Ephedrae) in both its intended therapeutic effects and potential side effects. Therefore, it appears that these drugs are very powerful exterior-resolving medicinals (解 表 药 *jie biao yao*).

Another category of CNS stimulants is the indirect-acting adrenergic agonists.

Indirect-acting adrenergic agonists treat:

1. Obesity (肥 胖 *fei pang*)
2. Narcolepsy, *i.e.*, somnolence (嗜 卧 *shi wo*)
3. ADHD
4. Obstructive sleep apnea (OSA)
5. The fatigue of MS

The side effects of indirect-acting adrenergic agonists include:

- Headache
- Chilliness (恶 寒 *e han*, aversion to cold)
- Heart palpitations
- Fatigue
- Depression (郁 症 *yu zheng*)
- Hyper- or hypotension
- Sweating
- Dry mouth
- Nausea and vomiting
- Anorexia, *i.e.*, torpid intake or lack of appetite (纳 呆 *na dai*)
- Diarrhea
- Abdominal cramping

Overdosages of indirect-acting adrenergic agonists may result in:

- Restlessness, *i.e.*, agitation
- Irritability (易 怒 *yi nu*)
- Insomnia
- Dizziness (眩 晕 *xuan yun*)
- Tremor
- Talkativeness (多 说 *duo shuo*)

In Chinese medicine, obesity is seen as a pathologic accumulation of phlegm, dampness, and turbidity. People who are obese typically suffer from a combination of spleen vacuity and liver depression. Because the spleen qi moves and transforms water fluids, spleen qi vacuity leads to dampness, which then leads to phlegm. However, because the qi moves water fluids, liver depression qi stagnation may also lead to dampness, which leads to phlegm. Therefore, there are two main ways of dealing with being overweight: supplementing the spleen and moving the qi.

Narcolepsy is considered a strange disease in Chinese medicine. Although it would be easy to equate narcolepsy with fatigue and, therefore, spleen qi vacuity, in fact it is typically associated with phlegm confounding the clear orifices. As we have just seen, liver depression qi stagnation can lead to phlegm, and moving the qi can help eliminate phlegm.

Attention deficit–hyperactivity disorder is likewise usually a combination of spleen vacuity and liver depression. However, in this case, liver depression has transformed depressive heat and thus the hyperactivity. By resolving the depression, one clears the heat causing the hyperactivity.

As for the fatigue associated with MS, it would also be easy to simply say that these medicines fortify the spleen and supplement the qi. However, as we'll see, the side effects suggest this is not so. According to Yan De-xin, all sufferers of chronic disease must also present liver depression. In that case, if the liver is depressed, this will cause or aggravate any tendency to spleen vacuity. Therefore, by coursing the liver and resolving depression, one can indirectly benefit the spleen and relieve fatigue.

The side effects and results of overdoses of these drugs clearly indicate that they damage yin and cause yang hyperactivity. These include agitation, talkativeness, insomnia, tremors, heart palpitations, and dry mouth. However, they also seem to damage and consume the qi as evidenced by fatigue, dizziness, chilling, lack of appetite, and sweating and possibly by diarrhea.

In addition, they seem to upbear the qi. This is indicated by nausea, vomiting, and headache. And emotional depression always includes an element of liver depression. All of this again suggests acrid, windy-natured, exterior-resolving (解表 *jie biao*), qi-rectifying medicinals (理气药 *li qi yao*).

This is further supported by these drugs causing hypertension in some and hypotension in others. However, the irritability does appear a bit of a paradox. Irritability is a symptom of liver depression. It has no other root cause.

Therefore, if these drugs act similarly to exterior resolvers and qi rectifiers, should they not alleviate irritability rather than cause it? I believe the answer to that conundrum lies in the fact that these medicinals can clearly damage yin fluids. Yin and blood are both necessary in order to nourish and enrich the liver. Without sufficient nourishment by blood and enrichment by yin, the liver cannot perform its function of governing, coursing, and discharge. So the liver becomes depressed in spite of the acrid, moving medicinals, and there is irritability.

SECTION 6: ANTIDEPRESSANTS

A. TRICYCLIC ANTIDEPRESSANTS

This class of drugs mainly treats depression.

The side effects of these drugs include:

- Blurred vision
- Dry, scratchy eyes (干涩目 *gan se mu*)
- Urinary retention
- Constipation
- Epilepsy (癫痫 *dian xian*)
- Fatigue
- Somnolence
- Orthostatic hypotension
- Palpitations
- Tachycardia, *i.e.*, a rapid pulse
- Weight gain, *i.e*, fatness or obesity
- Lack of strength

There is no emotional depression without liver depression qi stagnation. However, in the overwhelming majority of patients with depression, there is also an element of spleen vacuity. If we posit that these drugs are acrid, windy, qi-rectifying medicinals (理气药 *li qi yao*), then all their side effects make sense.

All these side effects can be explained as due

to either qi vacuity or yin-blood-fluid vacuity. For instance, fatigue, somnolence, orthostatic hypotension, and lack of strength are all qi vacuity signs and symptoms. Since the spleen is the root of the engenderment and transformation of the qi and blood, damage to the qi may also damage the spleen and explain the weight gain.

Blurred vision, dry and scratchy eyes, constipation, and heart palpitations are all yin-blood-fluid insufficiency conditions. If yin vacuity fails to control yang, this can give rise to vacuity heat and a rapid pulse or internal stirring of liver wind and epilepsy. At least one tricyclic antidepressant, imipramine, is known to cause the tongue fur to develop white plaques resembling milk curds. This indicates the internal engenderment of dampness due to spleen qi vacuity. The amitriptylines are known to cause dry mouth and tongue, suggesting their ability to damage blood and yin.

B. SELECTIVE SEROTONIN REUPTAKE INHIBITORS (SSRIs)

This class of drugs treats:
1. Depression
2. Generalized anxiety disorder (GAD), social anxiety disorder, and panic disorder
3. Premenstrual dysphoric disorder (PMDD)
4. Post-traumatic stress disorder (PTSD)
5. Obsessive-compulsive disorder (OCD)

In Chinese medicine, GAD, PTSD, and OCD can all be described as types of anxiety or fear and fright (恐 惊 kong jing). The Chinese medical diagnosis of PMDD would depend on the exact symptoms experienced. However, as a generalization, it could be seen as a species of mania and withdrawal (狂 癫 kuang dian).

The side effects of these medications include:
- Nausea and vomiting
- Headache
- Decreased libido
- Delayed or inability to ejaculate and anorgasmia

All of the intended therapeutic uses of this class of antidepressants typically include a combination of liver depression with spleen vacuity complicated on a case-by-case basis with phlegm

and depressive heat. We now know that all depression includes some anxiety. Anxiety is a form of fear and is commonly due to non-construction and malnourishment of the heart spirit because of a liver-spleen disorder.

All premenstrual syndrome (PMS) or PMDDs (an especially severe form of PMS) involve a liver-spleen disharmony, while PTSD and OCD both also involve a lot of fear and fright. Given their side effects, it appears that these drugs are attacking and draining and, therefore, can damage and consume the qi. Therefore, they appear to be qi-rectifying medicinals (理 气 药 li qi yao), which particularly affect the spleen's relationship with the kidneys. We posit this latter point because of the decreased libido, delayed or inability to ejaculate, and anorgasmia.

C. MONOAMINE OXIDASE INHIBITORS (MAOIs)

Monoamine oxidase inhibitors are mainly used to treat depression.

The side effects of these drugs include:
- Fatigue
- Orthostatic hypotension
- Blurred vision
- Dry mouth
- Constipation
- Dysuria, i.e., urinary strangury (淋 症 lin zheng)

Based on these facts, it appears that MAOIs should be classified as acrid, windy-natured qi-rectifying medicinals (理 气 药 li qi yao), which can consume the qi and damage yin, blood, and fluids.

D. ALPHA-2 ANTAGONISTS

This class of drugs is also used to treat depression.

The side effects of these drugs include:
- Fatigue
- Lack of strength
- Dry, scratchy eyes
- Dizziness
- Increased appetite (善 饥 shan ji)
- Weight gain
- Mania

Like the other antidepressants, this class of

drugs seems to be windy-natured qi-rectifying medicinals (理 气 药 *li qi yao*), which can consume the qi and damage yin. If it damages yin, this can lead to vacuity heat or fire effulgence and cause mania. Increased appetite is also always a symptom of stomach heat. In this case, damage to stomach yin may aggravate stomach heat and lead to increased appetite. However, because of damage to the spleen qi, increased appetite coupled with spleen vacuity may lead to weight gain.

E. DOPAMINE REUPTAKE INHIBITORS

Once again, this class of medications is mainly used to treat depression.

The side effects of these drugs include:
- Dizziness
- Headache
- Insomnia
- Nausea
- Dry, scratchy eyes
- Agitation
- Mania
- Heart palpitations
- Hyper- or hypotension
- Tachycardia, *i.e.*, a rapid pulse
- Seizures, *i.e.*, epilepsy in Chinese medicine

The side effects of these drugs yet again fall into two main groups:

(1) qi vacuity and

(2) yin vacuity with or without yang hyperactivity, flaming fire, or liver wind. Therefore, these drugs should probably be classified as acrid, windy, qi-rectifying medicinals (理 气 药 *li qi yao*).

SECTION 7: DRUGS FOR MANIA

Drugs for mania treat mania.

The side effects of this type of drug are minimal but can include:
- Nausea and vomiting
- Diarrhea
- Fatigue
- Hypotension
- Polyuria (多 尿 *duo niao*)
- Polydipsia (多 饮 *duo yin*)
- Heart palpitations
- Tremors, *i.e.*, tetany (痉 *jing*)

- Acne (粉 刺 *fen ci*)

In Chinese medicine, mania is called *kuang* (狂) and always involves heat or fire. Therefore, it would be tempting to say that this class of medication clears heat. However, acne is always a heat sign, and polydipsia also suggests stomach heat. So if this class of medication causes heat, such drugs are not likely to be heat-clearing medicinals. However, in the Chinese medical treatment of mania, we may also use heavy, settling, spirit-quieting medicinals that also subdue yang (潜 阳 *qian yang*) and downbear counterflow (降 逆 *jiang ni*), and these medicinals may cause the side effects of this class of medication.

Heavy, settling, spirit-quieting medicinals may damage the spleen qi and also may aggravate depressive heat. If they downbear yang without also clearing heat, this may cause even more depressive heat. So now, looking at the rest of the side effects of this type of medication, tetany always involves wind, and wind may be internally engendered from heat or from yin vacuity, while heart palpitations may be due to qi, blood, yin, or yang vacuity with or without heat.

When taken together, the rest of the side effects suggest damage to the spleen qi. Therefore, we suggest that this class of medication be thought of as types of heavy, settling, spirit-quieting medicinals (重 镇 安 神 药 *zhong zhen an shen yao*).

B. ATYPICAL NEUROLEPTICS

Atypical neuroleptics treat schizophrenia and psychoses and have the same side effects as typical neuroleptics. Therefore, we believe that their Chinese medical categorization should also be the same.

SECTION 8: OPIOID ANALGESICS AND ANTAGONISTS

Opioid analgesics are primarily used to treat pain (痛 *tong*).

The side effects of these drugs include:
- Respiratory depression (少 气 *shao qi*)
- Constipation

- Nausea and vomiting
- Urinary retention

Opium has been known in China for hundreds of years, and Chinese medical descriptions of it exist. It is classified as a securing and astringing medicinal (固 涩 药 *gu se yao*). It represses and constrains the lung qi and stops cough, astringes the intestines, and stops pain. Thus the side effects of respiratory depression, constipation, and urinary retention are due to opioids' overastringing and oversecuring. The nausea and vomiting are most likely due to the inherent "toxins" (毒 *du*) in these substances.

SECTION 9: DRUGS USED TO TREAT EPILEPSY

Drugs used to treat epilepsy are meant to treat seizures.

The side effects of these drugs include:
- Nausea and vomiting
- Headache
- Dizziness
- Confusion
- Ataxia
- Hallucinations
- Fatigue
- Somnolence
- Blurred vision
- Alopecia (脱 发 *tuo fa*)
- Urticaria (风 癮 疹 *feng yin zhen*)
- Tremors
- Agitation

Epilepsy in Chinese medicine is referred to as *dian xian* (癫 痫). This includes all types of seizures. In general, epilepsy is due to some combination of phlegm, internally engendered wind, and kidney vacuity along with the ramifications of these. Obviously from the side effects of this class of drug, they can cause qi and blood vacuity. Fatigue, somnolence, confusion, ataxia, and dizziness all suggest qi vacuity, while blurred vision, alopecia, and tremors suggest blood vacuity and, in the case of the last symptom, wind. Urticaria is commonly associated with qi and blood vacuities mixed with externally contracted wind. Agitation suggests heat, perhaps due to a yin-blood vacuity. Headache is too various in terms of Chinese medicine to say anything definite about it. However, most of these side effects could be due to the attacking and draining nature of wind-extinguishing, tremor-stopping medicinals (息 风 止 震 药 *xi feng zhi zhen yao*). Therefore, we suggest that is how this class of medications should be provisionally classified.

CHAPTER 6: DRUGS AFFECTING THE CARDIOVASCULAR SYSTEM

SECTION 1: INHIBITORS OF THE RENNIN-ANGIOTENSIN SYSTEM

Inhibitors of the rennin-angiotensin system treat:
1. Hypertension
2. Heart failure
3. Arrhythmia
4. Myocardial infarction

The side effects of this group of medications include:
- Hypotension
- Cough
- Maculopapular rash
- Sore throat (咽 痛 *yan tong*)
- Fever (发 热 *fa re*)

Based on published Chinese reports on the Chinese medical treatment of ACEI-induced cough, we know that such coughs are due to drug-induced yin vacuity. Therefore, it would seem reasonable to assume that so are the sore throat and fever. In that case, the maculopapular rash would be due to vacuity heat in the blood aspect.

Arrhythmia equals heart palpitations and/or a bound or regularly intermittent pulse, and heart failure also typically manifests these two pulse images. These two pulse images indicate obstruction of the flow of the heart qi and blood due to phlegm and/or blood stasis.

Myocardial infarction corresponds to chest

impediment also typically associated with phlegm and/or blood stasis. However, as we have seen above, phlegm and blood stasis as well as the disease mechanisms of hypertension are all related to liver depression. Therefore, it would appear that these medications are attacking and draining qi-rectifying medicinals (理气药 *li qi yao*). If they overattack and overdrain, then they would not only damage yin but also consume the qi, thus resulting in hypotension.

SECTION 2: BETA-ADRENERGIC BLOCKING AGENTS

These drugs are covered in Chapter 4, Section 8.

SECTION 3: DIURETICS

Diuretics by definition induce urination.

The side effects of diuretics are mostly the symptoms of dehydration:

- Fatigue
- Lack of strength
- Orthostatic hypotension
- Muscle cramps
- Headache
- Arrhythmias, *i.e.*, heart palpitations

It seems obvious that diuretics should be classified as medicinals that seep dampness and free the flow of urination (渗湿痛尿药 *shen shi tong niao yao*). When we urinate, we move fluids out of the body. Since it is the qi that moves these fluids out of the body, we lose qi every time we urinate. This would explain the symptoms of qi vacuity, such as fatigue, weakness, and orthostatic hypotension.

Because blood and fluids share a common source, fluid desertion may lead to blood vacuity with such symptoms as headache and muscle cramps.

SECTION 4: VASODILATORS

Vasodilators are mainly used to treat:

1. Hypertension
2. Angina pectoris
3. Congestive heart failure
4. MI

The side effects of these drugs include:

- Orthostatic hypotension
- Headache
- Facial flushing
- Tachycardia, *i.e.*, a rapid pulse
- Nausea and vomiting
- Sweating
- Skin rash

Above, we have discussed the disease mechanisms of hypertension, angina pectoris, heart failure, and MI and that these conditions are treated with attacking and draining medicinals that move the qi and, therefore, promote the movement of blood and phlegm. These kinds of medicinals can also consume the qi and damage yin in susceptible individuals or at high enough doses.

Orthostatic hypotension, sweating, and nausea and vomiting are due to spleen vacuity, while facial flushing, tachycardia, and skin rashes most probably are due to yin vacuity engendering internal heat. Thus these medicines appear to be acrid, windy-natured qi-rectifying medicinals (理气药 *li qi yao*) that resolve depression.

SECTION 5: ANTIARRHYTHMIC AGENTS

Antiarrhythmic agents are subdivided into four types:

(1) sodium channel blockers,
(2) beta-blockers,
(3) potassium channel blockers, and
(4) calcium channel blockers.

We have already discussed beta-blockers in Chapter 4, Section 8, and calcium channel blockers will be discussed in the following section of this chapter. Therefore, **here we will only discuss sodium channel blockers and potassium channel blockers.**

In terms of what these two antiarrhythmic agents treat from the Chinese medical point of view, they both treat palpitations. Within Chinese medicine, heart palpitations may be due to qi, blood, yin, and/or yang vacuities, blood stasis, phlegm obstruction, and/or replete or vacuity heat. In addition, heart palpitations are also treated by Chinese medicinals that nourish the heart and quiet the spirit as well as heavy, settling, spirit-quieters. Therefore, there is no single ategory of Chinese medicinals that treats palpitations.

That being said, looking at **the side effects of types 1 and 3 antiarrhythmic agents,** we can rule out the four types of supplements and heart-nourishing spirit-quieters. These would not cause:

- Dry mouth
- Urinary retention
- Blurred vision
- Constipation
- Lack of strength
- Photosensitivity
- Neuropathy, *i.e.*, tingling and numbness (麻木 *ma mu*) if we are talking about peripheral neuropathy
- Tremor
- Ataxia

We can also rule out heat-clearing medicinals. If this were the case, we would expect to see nausea and vomiting, anorexia, and diarrhea besides the general qi vacuity symptoms.

Nor do we think these medicines should be categorized as phlegm transformers or blood quickeners. If so, their scope of application would be too narrow since not all patients with arrhythmias present with blood stasis and/or phlegm.

That leaves the heavy, settling, spirit-quieting medicinals (重镇安神药 *zhong zhen an shen yao*), and we have already seen that these medicinals can damage the qi and blood. Most of the above side effects of type 1 and 3 antiarrhythmic agents are manifestations of blood vacuity: blurred vision, constipation, photosensitivity, tingling and numbness, and tremor, while the remaining side effects are manifestations of qi and fluid vacuities, remembering that blood and fluids share a common source.

Inotropic agents, included in this section, are used to treat:

1. Congestive heart failure
2. Peripheral vascular disease

The side effects of these drugs include:

- Anorexia
- Nausea and vomiting
- Diarrhea
- Headache
- Fatigue
- Lack of strength
- Dizziness
- Confusion
- Blurred vision
- Skin rashes
- Palpitations
- Tachycardia, *i.e.*, a rapid pulse

In Chinese medicine, peripheral vascular disease is primarily associated with blood stasis, and blood stasis is also usually a part of congestive heart failure. Since quickening the blood is an attacking and draining treatment, it can consume the qi and damage yin and, therefore, could cause all of the side effects listed above. Thus, it appears that inotropic agents are blood-quickening medicinals (活血药 *huo xue yao*).

SECTION 6: CALCIUM CHANNEL BLOCKERS

Calcium channel blockers are used to treat:

1. Hypertension
2. Arrhythmias
3. Raynaud's disease, *i.e.*, chilled extremities
4. Angina pectoris
5. Migraines

The side effects of these drugs include:

- Hypotension
- Fatigue
- Vertigo
- Constipation
- Headache
- Peripheral edema
- Coughing and wheezing (咳哮 *ke xiao*)

Based on the principle of starting with what we are sure of, it appears that these medications are attacking and draining as opposed to supplementing and supporting. We say this because of the obvious qi vacuity side effects of hypotension and fatigue.

Given that these drugs appear to be able to damage the qi, and blood is the mother of qi, it is likely that the constipation is due to blood vacuity as may be the headache.

Vertigo coupled with coughing and wheezing suggest the presence of phlegm, and the spleen is the root of phlegm engenderment. If the spleen were vacuous, this would also explain the side effect of peripheral edema.

If we look at hypertension, arrhythmias, and migraines, a common class of Chinese medicinals used in all three of these conditions is heavy, settling, spirit-quieting medicinals (重镇安神药 *zhong zhen an shen yao*). In the case of hypertension and migraines, these medicinals are not used to quiet the spirit but to subdue yang and downbear counterflow. As we have seen above, these can damage the spleen and cause both qi and blood vacuities.

If spleen qi vacuity gets bad enough, it will become yang vacuity, in which case it might cause Raynaud's, especially if it were combined with liver depression. These drugs would not cause or directly aggravate the liver depression, but an element of liver depression certainly tends to complicate conditions such as hypertension, arrhythmias, and migraines. As for the angina pectoris, our guess is that, by reducing blood pressure and quieting the spirit, this might also help indirectly relieve chest impediment pain.

SECTION 7: OTHER ANTIHYPERTENSIVES
No discussion.

SECTION 8: PLATELET INHIBITORS

Platelet inhibitors are used to prevent the formation of thromboses. It seems reasonable to think that they should be categorized as blood-quickening medicinals (活血药 *huo xue yao*). Like over- or wrong use of Chinese blood-quickening medicinals, these can cause unwanted bleeding.

SECTION 9: ANTICOAGULANTS

Like the platelet inhibitors above, anticoagulants should probably also be categorized as blood-quickening medicinals (活血药 *huo xue yao*).

SECTION 10: DRUGS USED TO STOP BLEEDING

In Chinese medicine, we also have a category of bleeding-stopping medicinals (止血药 *zhi xue yao*). Since these Western drugs may also cause unwanted thrombosis as can Chinese bleeding-stopping medicinals, we propose that these drugs also be classified as bleeding-stopping medicinals from the Chinese medical point of view.

SECTION 11: DRUGS USED TO TREAT ANEMIA

The clinical symptoms of anemia, fatigue, lack of strength, and orthostatic hypotension are qi vacuity symptoms. Therefore, we propose to classify these drugs as qi-supplementing medicinals (补气药 *bu qi yao*). This would be consistent with their harmlessness and lack of adverse effects.

SECTION 12: DRUGS USED TO TREAT SICKLE CELL DISEASE

These drugs are used to treat:
1. Sickle cell anemia
2. Cancers such as melanoma, chronic myelocytic leukemia, ovarian cancer, and squamous cell cancer
3. HIV
4. Psoriasis
5. Polycythemia vera
6. Essential thrombocytopenia

The side effects of these drugs include:
- Edema (水肿 *shui zhong*)
- Dizziness
- Fever
- Hallucinations
- Headache
- Nausea and vomiting

• Diarrhea

• Constipation

The signs and symptoms of sickle cell anemia during acute crises include pain in the extremities, severe abdominal pain, and chest pain. These symptoms all suggest blood stasis, and certainly cancers are typically complicated by blood stasis as is HIV disease (*e.g.,* Kaposi's sarcoma). Similarly, psoriasis, polycythemia vera, and thrombocytopenia almost always include an element of blood stasis.

Additionally, Chinese blood-quickening medicinals can consume the qi and damage yin-blood. Thus, the wrong or excessive use of blood-quickening medicinals are capable of causing all of the side effects of drugs used to treat sickle cell anemia. Therefore, we propose that these drugs be classified provisionally as blood-quickening medicinals (活 血 药 *huo xue yao*).

SECTION 13: HMG-COA REDUCTASE INHIBITORS (*I.E.*, STATINS)

HMG-COA reductase inhibitors are used to treat high serum cholesterol.

The side effects of these drugs include:

• Muscle cramps

• Liver failure

• Acute kidney failure

In Chinese medicine, the clinical symptoms of high cholesterol are all associated with blood stasis, such as chest impediment and angina pectoris, while muscle cramps are mainly due to blood vacuity.

We have seen that excessive or inappropriate use of blood-quickening medicinals can damage the blood. The signs and symptoms of acute renal failure include peripheral edema, weight gain, anorexia, lack of strength, nausea and vomiting, and other such symptoms of qi vacuity. The signs and symptoms of liver failure also indicate spleen qi vacuity, such as jaundice, fatigue, somnolence, lack of strength, and orthostatic hypotension.

Therefore, we believe that these drugs should also be classified as blood-quickening medicinals (活 血 药 *huo xue yao*).

SECTION 14: OTHER AGENTS TO TREAT HYPERLIPIDEMIA

This group of Western drugs is actually made up of four subclasses:

(1) bile sequestrants,

(2) fibrates,

(3) cholesterol absorption inhibitors, and

(4) niacin.

All are meant to help treat high cholesterol, which might otherwise lead to coronary heart disease (CHD).

The side effects of bile sequestrants include:

• Nausea

• Constipation

• Flatulence (下 气 *xia qi*)

The side effects of fibrate include:

• Nausea

• Muscle pain and weakness

• Increased risk of cholelithiasis

The side effects of cholesterol absorption inhibitors include:

• Fatigue

• Abdominal pain

• Muscle pain and weakness

The side effects of niacin are:

• Skin flushing and itching (瘙 痒 *sao yang*)

• Peptic ulcers

• Liver damage

Our assumption is that these drugs should be classified as windy-natured, qi-rectifying medicinals (理 气 药 *li qi yao*) or blood-quickening medicinals (活 血 药 *huo xue yao*), which move the qi within the blood. When used in excess or in the wrong patients, they appear to consume the qi and damage yin-blood.

CHAPTER 7: DRUGS AFFECTING THE ENDOCRINE SYSTEM

SECTION 1: HORMONES OF THE PITUITARY AND THYROID GLANDS

A. HORMONES OF THE POSTERIOR PITUITARY

Hormones of the posterior pituitary primarily are used to treat:

1. Diabetes insipidus, *i.e.*, polyuria
2. Nocturnal enuresis (夜 多 尿 *ye duo niao*)

The side effects of these drugs include:

- Thrombosis
- MI

In Chinese medicine, both diabetes insipidus and nocturnal enuresis are treated by securing and astringing medicinals (固 涩 药 *gu se yao*), and the side effects of clot formation and myocardial infarction might logically be caused by oversecuring and overastringing. The word "astringe" (涩 *se*) is the same word translated as "choppy" or "rough" when discussing pulse images, and the choppy pulse indicates blood stasis. Thus we suggest that this class of drug be considered a type of securing and astringing medicinals (固 涩 药 *gu se yao*).

B. DRUGS AFFECTING THE THYROID

i. Thyroid supplements

Thyroid supplements are used to treat thyroid insufficiency as characterized by:

1. Fatigue
2. Lack of strength
3. Weight gain
4. Hair loss
5. Poor healing
6. Aversion to cold
7. Cold hands and feet

The side effects of these drugs include:

- Arrhythmia
- Hypertension
- Insomnia
- Anxiety
- Fatigue
- Headache
- Irritability
- Nervousness
- Sweating
- Heat intolerance, *i.e.*, aversion to heat (恶 热 *e re*)

The clinical symptoms of thyroid deficiency are a combination of qi, blood, and yang vacuities. However, it should be remembered that yang vacuity includes qi vacuity within it, since yang is nothing other than enough qi in one place to experience the qi's inherent warmth. When taken as a whole, the side effects of thyroid supplements appear to be yang repletion and yin vacuity symptoms. Therefore, we suggest that this class of Western drugs should be considered yang-supplementing medicinals (补 阳 药 *bu yang yao*).

ii. Antithyroid medications

Antithyroid medications treat hyperthyroidism.

The side effects of these drugs include:

- Susceptibility to infection
- Fever
- Rash
- Lymphadenopathy

Obviously, in hyperthyroidism, there is a hyperactivity of yang. Therefore, these drugs must be attacking and draining. Of the various types of attacking and draining medicinals, we propose that this group of drugs be classified as heat-clearing medicinals (清 热 药 *qing re yao*).

If one overclears heat and drains fire, then one causes a qi vacuity. If the central qi falls downward and causes depression in the lower burner with depressive heat, this may inflame life-gate ministerial fire and give rise to what Li Dong-yuan called yin fire. This yin fire can then float upward causing qi vacuity fever and rash. Certainly a susceptibility to infection suggests a defensive qi vacuity.

As for the lymphadenopathy, the swollen lymph nodes are phlegm binding or nodulation in Chinese medicine. If the spleen qi is too vacuous and weak to move and transform water fluids, these collect and transform into dampness. If dampness is stewed and boiled by heat, including vacuity heat, this may congeal dampness into phlegm and thus the lymphadenopathy.

SECTION 2: ANTIDIABETIC DRUGS

Antidiabetic drugs do one of two things:
(1) They increase secretion of insulin, or
(2) They decrease insulin resistance.

The side effect of the first subcategory is drug-induced hypoglycemia, that is:
- Fatigue
- General discomfort, uneasiness, or ill feeling (malaise)
- Nervousness
- Irritability
- Tremors
- Headache
- Hunger
- Cold sweats
- A rapid pulse
- Blurred vision
- Confusion
- Convulsions
- Coma

In Chinese medicine, diabetes mellitus is typically treated by some combination of qi and yin supplements, heatclearers, dampness-eliminators, and bloodquickeners. Fatigue is, ipso facto, a symptom of qi vacuity. We also know that the rapid pulse indicates heat, the blurred vision indicates blood vacuity, and the tremors and convulsions indicate internally stirring wind due to blood and yin vacuity.

Similarly, irritability indicates liver depression, which, in this case, is due to blood vacuity failing to nourish the liver. Nervousness then would also be a symptom of yin failing to control yang, which stirs frenetically. Malaise is too vague to be processed by the logic of Chinese medicine, and headache also can be due to too many disease mechanisms.

Coma tells us that there has been desertion of at least the qi and maybe, because of the cold sweats, even yang. So of the various classes of Chinese medicinals which are used to treat diabetes, that could cause these symptoms? The answer, we think, are heat-clearing, dampness-

eliminating medicinals (清 热 除 湿 药 *qing re chu shi yao*). Heat-clearing medicinals can damage qi and eventually yang, while dampness-eliminating medicinals can damage yin-blood. In this case, the hunger is a symptom of qi vacuity, not stomach heat. It is an indication of the spleen needing more raw materials from which to engender and transform qi and blood.

SECTION 3: SEX HORMONES

This category of drugs is subdivided into androgens, antiandrogens, antiprogestin, progestins, and estrogens.

ANDROGENS are used to treat:
1. Hypogonadism
2. Osteoporosis
3. Speed recovery from burns and wounds

The side effects of androgens include:
- Acne
- Facial hair, *i.e.*, hirsutism
- Baldness

In Chinese medicine, recovery from wounds is dependent upon the qi, specifically the defensive qi, which is a part of the yang qi. Osteoporosis is typically treated with a combination of spleen qi supplements and kidney yang supplements. Acne is a symptom of hyperactive ministerial fire.

According to the *Nei Jing (Inner Classic)*, the reason men have hair on their faces is because, having more yang qi then women, their blood travels upward to the face; whereas, in females, their blood moves downward to become the menses and to nourish the fetus. So increased hair on the face also indicates hyperactivity of ministerial fire.

Ironically, this type of baldness in Chinese medicine is also due to hyperactivity of ministerial fire. In this case, too much yang ascends to the vertex where it damages the blood and dries out the scalp. Therefore, we would suggest that androgens be seen as a species of yang-supplementing medicinals (补 阳 药 *bu yang yao*).

ANTIANDROGENS are used primarily to treat prostate cancer.

Their side effects include impotence in men. This suggests that they are attacking and draining medicinals that damage the yang qi. Since prostate cancer usually involves significant damp heat, we would suggest that these medicinals are heat clearing and perhaps also dampness eliminating. However, they do not cause enough or varied enough side effects to determine their Chinese medical classification for sure other than that they may damage yang qi.

ANTIPROGESTINS are used as an abortifacient and their main side effect is incomplete abortion. Miscarriage may be due to any combination of qi vacuity, heat, and/or blood stasis. In this case, our assumption is that antiprogestins are heat-clearing medicinals (清 热 药 *qing re yao*), which may damage the yang qi.

PROGESTINS are commonly used in contraception and to treat progesterone insufficiency. In Chinese medicine, conditions associated with progesterone insufficiency, such as luteal phase defect and habitual miscarriage, are routinely and very successfully treated with a combination of spleen qi supplements and kidney yang supplements.

Since qi supplements alone do not successfully treat progesterone insufficiency but yang-supplementation includes a certain amount of qi supplementation, our assumption is that progestins should be classified as yang-supplement medicinals (补 阳 药 *bu yang yao*). This would also be consistent with their potentially causing hirsutism and acne.

ESTROGENS are used in contraception and to treat estrogen insufficiency.

The symptoms of estrogen deficiency include:
1. A rapid pulse
2. Fatigue
3. Poor memory
4. Hot flashes
5. Joint pain, swelling, and stiffness, *i.e.*, impediment condition (痹 证 *bi zheng*)
6. Decreased libido
7. Depression
8. Headache
9. Osteoarthritis, *i.e.*, impediment condition
10. Low back pain (腰 痛 *yao tong*)
11. Dry skin (皮 枯 *pi ku*)
12. Vaginal dryness

The side effects of these drugs include:
• Headache
• Depression
• Hypertension
• Nausea and vomiting
• Thrombosis
• Weight gain
• Hirsutism
• Increased risk of breast and uterine cancer

When taken together, dry skin, vaginal dryness, joint swelling and stiffness, and poor memory indicate a yin-blood vacuity. In that case, a rapid pulse and hot flashes suggest internally engendered heat due to yin vacuity failing to control yang. Because the kidneys are the root of true yin in the body, and the low back is their mansion, there is low back pain. Because the kidneys govern the bones, there is osteoarthritis. Because yin vacuity always includes an element of qi vacuity, there is fatigue.

The irritability is due to blood and yin failing to nourish and enrich the liver. Thus liver depression qi stagnation is caused or aggravated. The headaches may be due to qi and blood vacuity alone or yin vacuity with ascendant liver yang hyperactivity.

The decreased libido is specifically a yang vacuity symptom. However, yin and yang are mutually rooted. So if there is kidney yin vacuity, there typically is also some element of yang vacuity, at least below. This is even so if yang is hyperactive above. All of this suggests that estrogens are yin-supplementing medicinals (补阴 药 *bu yin yao*).

As for the side effects, nausea and vomiting may be due to dampness. Because yin includes blood and water fluids, supplementation of yin may cause excessive dampness, which damages the spleen and stomach. This would also explain the weight gain. One of the patterns of hypertension is phlegm turbidity obstructing the center, and headache may also be due to phlegm turbidity that has counterflowed up to the head. Because fluids and blood move together, excessive fluids may give rise to dampness and phlegm, which then obstruct the free flow of the blood. This may then lead to blood stasis manifesting as thromboses. In addition, breast and uterine cancer typically involve blood stasis and phlegm binding or nodulation. Hirsutism in this case is due to a superabundance of yin-blood, the surplus of which sprouts as excess hair. Therefore, it appears that estrogens are definitely a species of yin supplements.

SECTION 4: ADRENOCORTICOSTEROID HORMONES

Corticosteroids are used to treat:
1. Addison's disease
2. Adrenocorticotropic hormone (ACTH) insufficiency
3. Corticotropin-releasing hormone (CRH) deficiency
4. Inflammation
5. Asthma

The side effects of corticosteroids include:
- Moon facies
- Buffalo hump
- Hirsutism
- Acne
- Insomnia
- Increased appetite
- Osteoporosis
- Decreased immunity
- Reduced wound healing
- Whole body edema
- Hypertension

The signs and symptoms of Addison's disease and CRH deficiency are weakness; fatigue; orthostatic hypotension; anorexia; nausea and vomiting; diarrhea; decreased cold tolerance; and brown, black, and bluish black discolorations and/or vitiligo. The first of these up through decreased cold tolerance are all qi vacuity signs and symptoms, specifically spleen qi vacuity. The skin discolorations would then most likely be explained as

lack of qi to stir the blood leading to blood stasis.

The signs and symptoms of CRH insufficiency are also similar to those of Addison's disease. Therefore, these medicinals would, at first glance, appear to be qi supplements. However, if this is the case, then how do they also clear heat?

In Chinese medicine, there are several ways to clear heat. The first is to clear heat by counteracting it with cold-natured medicinals. The second way is to out-thrust it with windy-natured, upbearing, and out-thrusting medicinals. The third way is to drain heat downwards via urination or to precipitate it via defecation.

Upbearing and out-thrusting, exterior-releasing medicinals (解表药 jie biao yao) are commonly used along with qi supplements in order to benefit the spleen. The spleen governs upbearing of the clear. Therefore, by upbearing the clear, we promote spleen function. In addition, these medicinals can clear heat, relieve pain, and move fluids via out-thrusting. The fact that corticosteroids are used to treat asthma substantiates this hypothesis. However, because these drugs out-thrust the defensive qi, they may also result in decreased immunity and slow wound healing. Because their windy, moving nature can damage yin, they may lead to insomnia and hypertension.

In addition, if they damage stomach yin, they may increase stomach heat, thus leading to increased appetite and acne. Because they push the qi upward and outward, and the qi moves the blood, they may cause hirsutism. Because they consume qi and ultimately yang, they may lead to failure to move and transform water fluids, leading to moon facies, buffalo hump, and generalized edema. Finally, damage of both yin and yang may lead to osteoporosis.

In fact, Chinese doctors in China are well experienced in the treatment of long-term or excessive use of corticosteroids, and it is well documented that corticosteroids first cause qi and yin vacuity followed by yin and yang vacuity.

SECTION 5: AIDS FOR REPRODUCTION
Information not available.

CHAPTER 8: DRUGS AFFECTING THE RESPIRATORY SYSTEM

SECTION 1: AGENTS USED TO TREAT ASTHMA INCLUDE:

1. Corticosteroids
2. Anticholinergic agents
3. Theophylline derivatives
4. Mast cell stabilizers
5. Leukotriene receptor antagonists
6. 5-Lipoxygenase inhibitors
7. In Chinese medicine, there is a category of Chinese medicinals called the medicinals that stop coughing and stabilize panting (止 咳 定 喘 药 *zhi ke ding chuan yao*), and panting and coughing (喘 咳 *chuan ke*) is one of the terms for asthma in Chinese medicine.

Therefore, it is tempting to simply say that all the Western drugs in this section correspond to coughing-stopping, panting-stabilizing medicinals. However, the different subcategories of medicines in this category act in different ways, and asthma itself is a complex phenomenon. Therefore, we believe each of these subcategories should be handled separately. Since we have dealt with **CORTICOSTEROIDS** in the preceding chapter, they will not be discussed here. In addition, **ANTICHOLINERGICS** have been dealt with in Chapter 4, Section 4.

Asthma in Chinese medicine is typically due to a defensive qi insecurity stemming from a spleen vacuity and deep-lying phlegm rheum. If wind evils take advantage of this vacuity and attack, they disrupt the lungs' diffusion and downbearing. Fluids accumulate and add to the deep-lying phlegm rheum. Depending on the patient's constitution, they then either manifest phlegm heat or simply phlegm dampness.

The side effects of theophylline derivatives include:

- Skin rash and hives
- Headache
- Dizziness
- Tremors
- Fatigue
- Lack of strength
- Loss of appetite, nausea and vomiting, diarrhea
- Anxiety
- Confusion
- Muscle twitching, seizures
- Hypotension
- Worsening of ulcers

As we have seen before, these side effects and adverse reactions are all due to qi and yin vacuity. Therefore, we would suggest that theophylline derivatives be categorized as acrid, windy-natured exterior-resolving medicinals (解 表 药 *jie biao yao*) similar to *Ma Huang* (Herba Ephedrae).

MAST CELL STABILIZERS are used to prevent asthma attacks, not for their acute treatment. This immediately suggests that they supplement and secure the defensive qi. Chinese medicinals that supplement the defensive qi are of two varieties:
1) qi supplements such as *Huang Qi* (Radix Astragali), and
2) securing and astringing medicinals such as *Wu Wei Zi* (Fructus Schisandrae).

The side effects of these Western drugs include:

- Skin rash, hives, itching
- Headache, dizziness, drowsiness
- Nausea and vomiting
- Urinary urgency and pain

These adverse reactions do not appear to be the work of qi supplements. However, they might be due to oversecuring and astringing. For instance, if there were deep-lying wind evils in the exterior, closing the pores (气 门 *qi men*) would trap the wind evils in the exterior and might lead to their stirring.

Wu Wei Zi is known to have sedative properties. Therefore, we know that at least one securing and astringing Chinese medicinal might cause drowsiness. Interestingly, overdoses of *Wu Wei Zi* are known to cause allergic papular rashes and abdominal discomfort.

While urinary urgency is hard to explain, urinary pain might be due to oversecuring and astringing. Thus we propose that these medicinals be classified as securing and astringing medicinals (固 涩 药 *gu se yao*).

LEUKOTRIENE RECEPTOR ANTAGONISTS and **5-LIPOXYGENASE INHIBITORS** are the two remaining categories of asthma drugs.

The side effects of these drugs include:
- Headache
- Fatigue
- Lack of strength
- Nausea or abdominal pain

These two classes of drugs are used preventively and not in the case of acute asthma. Therefore, they must either supplement the qi, secure the exterior, or transform phlegm. The transformation of phlegm is an attacking and draining treatment method, and the symptoms of fatigue and lack of strength are definitely qi vacuity symptoms. Therefore, we would suggest that these medicinals be seen as phlegm-transforming medicinals (化 痰 药 *hua tan yao*).

SECTION 2: AGENTS USED TO TREAT ALLERGIC RHINITIS

Agents used to treat allergic rhinitis include:
1. Alpha-adrenergic agonists
2. Corticosteroids
3. Mast cell stabilizers
4. Antihistamines

ALPHA-ADRENERGIC AGONISTS have been dealt with in Chapter 4, Section 4. **CORTICO-STEROIDS** have been dealt with in Chapter 7, Section 4, and **MAST CELL STABILIZERS** have been dealt with in the preceding section of this chapter. Clinically speaking, these medicines relieve nasal congestion, runny nose (流 涕 *liu ti*), sneezing (喷 嚏 *pen ti*), and itching.

The side effects of antihistamines include:
- Fatigue
- Drowsiness
- Hypotension
- Dry mouth and eyes
- Urinary retention
- Tachycardia, *i.e.*, a rapid pulse
- Increased appetite

When taken together, fatigue, drowsiness, hypotension, and urinary retention suggest qi vacuity. Dry eyes and mouth suggest damage to yin fluids. In that case, tachycardia suggests yin vacuity failing to control yang and, therefore, the engenderment of internal heat and hyperactivity. In that case, the increased appetite would be due to damage of stomach yin with heat. Thus we propose that these drugs be classified as exterior-resolving medicinals (解 表 药 *jie biao yao*).

SECTION 3: AGENTS USED TO TREAT CHRONIC OBSTRUCTIVE PULMONARY DISEASE (COPD)

BETA-ADRENERGIC AGONISTS have been discussed in Chapter 4, Section 4. **CORTICO-STEROIDS** have been discussed in Chapter 7, Section 4, and **ANTICHOLINERGIC AGENTS** have been discussed in Chapter 4, Section 3.

SECTION 4: AGENTS USED TO TREAT COUGH

Agents used to treat cough are subdivided into antitussives and expectorants. It would appear that the antitussives should be categorized as stop-coughing medicinals (止 咳 药 *zhi ke yao*), while the expectorants should be classified as phlegm-transforming medicinals (化 痰 药 *hua tan yao*). The side effects of at least one expectorant (guaifenesin) is the possible causation of kidney stones. Phlegm-transforming medicinals may damage yin, and damage to yin fluids may lead to the formation of kidney stones.

CHAPTER 9: DRUGS AFFECTING THE GASTROINTESTINAL SYSTEM

SECTION 1: AGENTS USED TO TREAT PEPTIC ULCER DISEASE

Agents used to treat peptic ulcer disease include the following subcategories:

1. Antimuscarinic agents
2. Antimicrobial agents
3. H₂-histamine antagonists
4. Prostaglandins
5. Proton-pump inhibitors

6. The clinical symptoms of peptic ulcer disease are abdominal pain that may wake you at night, may be relieved by antacids or milk, may occur 2-3 hours after a meal, or may be worse if you do not eat; nausea; abdominal pain; indigestion; vomiting, especially vomiting blood; blood in stools or black, tarry stools; unintentional weight loss; and fatigue. In Chinese medicine, the most common pattern presentation is a liver-spleen-stomach disharmony commonly complicated by heat and/or dampness. The hematemesis is usually due to heat. The hemafecia may be due to heat or qi vacuity. Therefore, the main categories of Chinese medicinals used to treat this disorder are qi supplements, qirectifiers, heat-clearers, and dampnesseliminators.

ANTIMUSCARINIC AGENTS have been dealt with in Chapter 4, Section 3, while **ANTIMICROBIAL AGENTS** will be dealt with in Chapter 10.

The side effects of H₂-histamine agonists include:

- Headache
- Diarrhea
- Dizziness
- Muscle pain

Therefore, given the main categories of Chinese medicinals used to treat peptic ulcer disease, we believe these medicinals are qi-rectifying medicinals (理 气 药 *li qi yao*), which course the liver and harmonize the stomach. Since such medicinals are typically acrid, windy, upbearing, moving, and draining medicinals, this would explain the headache, dizziness, and diarrhea. In

that case, the muscle pain would be due to malnourishment by damaged blood.

While the side effects of prostaglandins are uncommon, they include:

- Skin rash
- Headache
- Dizziness
- Nausea and vomiting
- Diarrhea
- Flatulence
- Constipation
- Dysmenorrhea (痛 经 *tong jing*)
- Menorrhagia (月 经 过 多 *yue jing guo duo*)
- Midcycle spotting
- Postmenopausal bleeding
- Unwanted uterine contractions

In Chinese medicine, both midcycle spotting and postmenopausal bleeding fall under the category of flooding and leaking (崩 漏 *beng lou*).

Dysmenorrhea and unwanted uterine contractions are both species of pain and, where there is pain, there is no free flow. Either there is some evil qi obstructing the free flow or there is a vacuity failing to nourish the vessels or move the blood. Menorrhagia, midcycle spotting, and postmenopausal bleeding are all species of bleeding, and the three causes of bleeding (other than traumatic injury) are qi vacuity, heat, and blood stasis.

Given that these medicinals either supplement the qi, rectify the qi, clear heat, or eliminate dampness, our choice is again the qi-rectifying medicinals (理 气 药 *li qi yao*). As stated previously, qi-rectifying medicinals are acrid, windy, upbearing, and out-thrusting and have the potential for damaging both the qi and yin, blood, and fluids. Dizziness, nausea, vomiting, and diarrhea all point towards a qi vacuity. Skin rash suggests either blood vacuity or heat. If yin vacuity fails to control yang, there can be vacuity heat, and constipation is often due to intestinal fluid insufficiency. Postmenopausal women are prone both to spleen qi vacuity and to vacuity heat, and vacuity heat can definitely cause midcycle and postmenopausal bleeding, while the combination of vacuity heat and spleen qi vacuity can cause menorrhagia. Then why the dysmenorrhea and uterine contractions? If these drugs damaged yin-blood so that it no longer nourished the vessels properly, then there would be lack of free flow. In addition, miscarriage or premature delivery would be all the more likely if there were vacuity heat and spleen qi vacuity.

The side effects of proton-pump inhibitors include:

- Skin rash
- Headache
- Dizziness
- Fatigue
- Nausea
- Diarrhea

Thus they appear to function from a Chinese medical point of view similarly to the above two groups of medicinals, *i.e.*, as qi-rectifying medicinals (理 气 药 *li qi yao*).

SECTION 2: ANTIEMETIC AGENTS

Antiemetic agents treat nausea and vomiting.

They are subdivided into:

1. Anticholinergic agents
2. Antihistamines
3. Antipsychotics
4. Corticosteroids
5. Cannabinoids
6. Selective 5-HT3-receptor antagonists
7. Substance P/neurokinin 1 receptor antagonists

ANTICHOLINERGIC AGENTS have been discussed in Chapter 4, Section 3. **ANTIHISTAMINES** have been discussed in Chapter 8, Section 2. **ANTIPSYCHOTICS** have been discussed in Chapter 5, Section 6, Class 1, and **CORTICOSTEROIDS** have been discussed in Chapter 7, Section 4.

We believe that the remaining three subdivisions can all be dealt with at the same time. In Chinese medicine, the two classes of Chinese medicinals that treat nausea and vomiting per se are the qi-rectifying medicinals and the heavy, settling, spirit-quieting medicinals. Of these two,

we believe that these drugs are all qi-rectifying medicinals (理 气 药 *li qi yao*).

CANNABINOIDS cause sedation and vertigo. This suggests that they upbear the qi at the same time as they out-thrust the qi.

SELECTIVE 5-HT3-RECEPTOR ANTAGONISTS commonly cause headaches. Such headaches could be due to a combination of upbearing as well as lack of yin-blood.

SUBSTANCE P/NEUROKININ 1 RECEPTOR ANTAGONISTS can cause fatigue (qi vacuity) and constipation (yin, blood, fluid vacuity).

SECTION 3: ANTIDIARRHEALS

There are three main types of antidiarrheals:

(1) antimotility agents,
(2) adsorbents, and
(3) agents they modify fluid and electrolyte transport.

ANTIMOTILITY AGENTS decrease peristalsis and slow the action of the intestines by activating opioid receptors in the enteric nervous system. As we have seen in Chapter 5, Section 7, drugs that function this way should probably be categorized as securing and astringing medicinals (固 涩 药 *gu se yao*) in Chinese medicine.

ADSORBENTS can cause constipation and dry out the stools. This can be due either to excessively clearing heat or excessively seeping dampness. Since the main adsorbent is psyllium husks, psyllium is a member of the Plantagin aceae family, and it is a known diuretic, we propose that it should be seen as a dampness-seeping medicinal (渗 湿 药 *shen shi yao*).

AGENTS THAT MODIFY FLUID AND ELECTROLYTE TRANSPORT include aspirin and indomethacin. Both of these two drugs will be dealt with in Chapter 11, Section 1.

SECTION 4: LAXATIVES

Laxatives in Western medicine fall under three subcategories:

() irritants and stimulants,
(2) bulking agents, and
(3) stool softeners.

Of those discussed in this book, lactulose and

polyethelene glycol are osmotic agents that cause water to stay in the intestines causing similar effects as bulking agents. In Chinese medicine, medicinals that promote defecation are subdivided into harsh, attacking, precipitating medicinals and moistening, precipitating medicinals. We believe that the above two drugs should be classified as moistening, precipitating medicinals (润下药 *run xia yao*).

Psyllium husks, the third medicine discussed in this section, has already been described as a dampness-seeping medicinal (渗湿药 *shen shi yao*). Interestingly, in many Chinese formulas for constipation, *Ze Xie* (Rhizoma Alismatis), a similar diuretic, dampness-seeping medicinal, is added to move water fluids downward to the lower burner.

SECTION 5: MISCELLANEOUS DRUGS OF THE GASTROINTESTINAL SYSTEM

No information available.

CHAPTER 10: ANTIMICROBIAL AGENTS

SECTION 1: INHIBITORS OF CELL WALL SYNTHESIS

These agents are used to treat bacterial infections.

The side effects of these antibiotics include:
- Gastrointestinal disturbances
- Diarrhea
- Nephritis
- Eosinophilia

Long and extensive use of these agents in China have determined that they function similarly to bitter, cold heat-clearing medicinals (清热药 *qing re yao*), which have the potential for damaging the spleen. Some of the drugs in this category, such as the penicillins, are known to cause the tongue fur to turn black, and black tongue fur may be an indication of internal cold (内寒 *nei han*).

SECTION 2: PROTEIN SYNTHESIS INHIBITORS

Protein inhibitors are also used to treat bacterial infections.

The side effects of these drugs include:
- Nausea and vomiting
- Headache
- Dizziness
- Blurred vision
- Hypoplasia of the teeth
- Stunted growth in children
- Nephrotoxicity
- Neuromuscular paralysis

These side effects are due to excessive heat-clearing damaging the spleen and kidneys, remembering that the former and latter heavens are mutually rooted and that spleen disease may eventually reach or affect the kidneys.

Because of spleen vacuity, there is also liver blood vacuity. Chinese experience with these drugs suggests that they are cold heat-clearing medicinals (清热药 *qing re yao*). Some drugs in this category, such as the tetracyclines, are known to cause the tongue fur to turn black, and black tongue fur may be an indication of internal cold (内寒 *nei han*). Tetracyclines are also known to cause the tongue fur to develop thick, white plaques resembling milk curds. This indicates the accumulation of dampness due to spleen vacuity.

SECTION 3: DNA AND RNA SYNTHESIS INHIBITORS AND URINARY TRACT ANTISEPTICS

These antibiotics are mostly used to treat bacterial urinary tract infections (UTIs).

The side effects of these drugs include:
- Nausea and vomiting
- Diarrhea
- Headache
- Dizziness
- Anemia
- Albuminuria
- Hematuria

These side effects all are due to excessive cold heat-clearing. For instance, because of spleen qi vacuity, clear and turbid are not separated, and the clear pours downwards to cause albuminuria. Because of qi vacuity not containing the blood, there is hematuria. Thus, Chinese experience suggests that these drugs should be classified as cold heat-clearing medicinals (清热药 *qing re yao*).

SECTION 4: ANTIMYCOBACTERIAL DRUGS

Antimycobacterial drugs treat rod-shaped bacteria as in tuberculosis (TB).

The side effects of these drugs include:
- Nausea and vomiting
- Anemia, neutropenia, and/or leukopenia
- Peripheral neuropathy
- Decreased visual acuity
- Paresthesias, *i.e.*, numbness and tingling
- Hepatitis
- Jaundice (黄疸 *huang dan*)

Like the previous three groups of medications, these should also probably be classified as cold heat-clearing medicinals (清热药 *qing re yao*). Remember that paresthesias are mostly due to qi and blood vacuity, that fatigue and anorexia with pale or white stools are symptoms of hepatitis, and that jaundice may be a symptom of spleen vacuity dampness. Therefore, these medicinals have the potential to damage the spleen and, therefore, the qi and blood.

SECTION 5: ANTIFUNGAL DRUGS

Antifungal drugs are used to treat fungal infections, such as candidiasis. In Chinese medicine, most fungal infections present as damp heat patterns. However, there is typically or at least often an underlying spleen vacuity that is responsible for the dampness in the damp heat.

These agents' side effects include:
- Gastrointestinal disturbances, such as nausea and vomiting
- Neutropenia, thrombocytopenia, and bone marrow depression
- Edema
- Headache
- Decreased libido
- Impotence
- Hepatitis

Based on these adverse reactions, we believe these drugs should be classified as cold heat-clearing medicinals (清热药 *qing re yao*). In this case, the decreased libido and impotence are examples of spleen disease eventually affecting the kidneys, thus causing a dual spleen-kidney vacuity.

SECTION 6: ANTIPROTOZOAL DRUGS

Antiprotozoal drugs are used to treat protozoal infections.

The side effects of these drugs include:
- Gastrointestinal upset
- Diarrhea
- Blurred vision
- Dizziness
- Headache
- Anemia
- Pruritis
- Peripheral neuropathy
- Heart palpitations
- Cinchonism or quininism

By now, most readers should see that the side effects of these drugs mostly are due to damage to the spleen and qi and, therefore, also the blood. The symptoms of mild cases of cinchonism include fatigue, somnolence, tinnitus, dysphonia, and occasionally loss of hearing, blurred vision, and gastrointestinal upset.

More severe cases show headache, photophobia, altered color perception, and possibly confusion, delirium, and psychosis. Other symptoms observed include palpitations, convulsions, faintness and flushing, localized edema, vertigo, tremor, light-headedness, excitement, apprehension, coma, and even death. Again, more symptoms of spleen qi vacuity leading to concomitant blood vacuity.

Therefore, we suggest that these drugs also be classified as cold heat-clearing medicinals (清热药 *qing re yao*). Some of the drugs in this category, such as metronidazole, are known to cause the tongue fur to turn black, which may be an indication of internal cold (内寒 *nei han*).

SECTION 7: ANTHELMINTHIC DRUGS

Antihelminthic drugs are used to treat various types of parasitic worms. In Chinese medicine, parasitic worms are categorized as *chong* (虫, worms). Since at least the time of Zhu Dan-xi, they have been associated with great spleen vacuity and damp heat with concomitant qi stagnation.

The side effects of these drugs include:

- Fever
- Headache
- Dizziness
- Nausea and vomiting
- Abdominal pain
- Diarrhea
- Fatigue, somnolence
- Anorexia

Yet again it appears that we are dealing with cold heat-clearing medicinals (清 热 药 *qing re yao*), which can damage the spleen and cause qi and blood vacuity. In this case, it would also appear that the fever is a qi vacuity fever as described by Li Dong-yuan in his discussion on yin fire.

SECTION 8: ANTIVIRAL AGENTS

Antiviral agents are used to treat viral infections.

The side effects of these drugs include:

- Nausea and vomiting
- Diarrhea
- Headache
- Dizziness
- Fatigue
- Lack of strength
- Paresthesias
- Anemia, leukopenia, and/or bone marrow suppression
- Jaundice
- Hepatitis
- Peripheral neuropathy
- Buffalo hump and/or enlarged breasts

In Chinese medicine, most viral infections are pattern discriminated as wind heat, heat toxins, or damp heat. Therefore, use of heat-clearing medicinals is the main method of treating them. Similarly, it appears that we are dealing here with cold heat-clearing medicinals (清 热 药 *qing re yao*).

CHAPTER 11: ANTICANCER DRUGS

Anticancer drugs are of various different sorts because cancers are also various. No one anticancer agent works for all types of cancers. In Chinese medicine, anticancer drugs are described as using toxins to treat toxins.

Common adverse effects of anticancer drugs include:

- Severe vomiting
- Stomatitis
- Anorexia
- Diarrhea
- Hair loss
- Somnolence
- Lack of strength
- Dizziness
- Peripheral neuropathy
- Erythema, rash, or urticaria
- Fever

Within integrated Chinese-Western medicine (中 西 医 结合 *zhong xi yi jie he*) in China, there is a relatively huge amount of experience in the treatment of cancer with anticancer drugs. This experience suggests that these medicinals as a whole are cold, toxic, heat-clearing medicinals (清 热 药 *qing re yao*), which easily damage the spleen and result in such severe blood vacuity that it evolves into yin vacuity with vacuity heat. It is also possible that some of these chemotherapeutic drugs are hot and toxic.

Another, easier way of classifying these drugs in Chinese medical terms would be to simply call them anticancer medicinals (抗 癌 药 *kang ai yao*) and leave it at that.

SECTION 1: ALKALYTING AGENTS

A major side effect of these agents is pulmonary fibrosis, symptoms of which may include:

- Shortness of breath (dyspnea)

- A dry cough
- Fatigue
- Unexplained weight loss
- Aching muscles and joints

These symptoms suggest spleen and lung qi dual vacuity. Also, spleen vacuity over time leads to liver blood vacuity, which can lead to muscle and joint pain due to lack of nourishment.

SECTION 2: ANTIMETABOLITES

SECTION 3: ANTIBIOTICS

SECTION 4: MICROTUBULE INHIBITORS

SECTION 5: STEROID HORMONES AND THEIR ANTAGONISTS

Drugs in all these categories cause the typical adverse reactions common to many chemotherapeutic agents, such as vomiting, diarrhea, stomatitis, erythema and rash, loss of appetite, and hair loss.

SECTION 6: MONOCLONAL ANTIBODIES

No information about these drugs.

SECTION 7: TYROSINE KINASE INHIBITORS

Drugs in this category cause typical adverse reactions common to many chemotherapeutic agents, such as vomiting, diarrhea, stomatitis, erythema and rash, loss of appetite, and hair loss.

Hemorrhaging caused by cabozantinib is most likely due to severe toxic heat causing the blood to move forcefully outside its channels.

SECTION 8: OTHER ANTICANCER AGENTS

Most drugs in this category can cause typical adverse reactions common to many chemotherapeutic agents, such as vomiting, diarrhea, stomatitis, erythema and rash, loss of appetite, and hair loss.

Other toxic responses discussed in this section reflect the general discussion of cancer drugs on the previous page.

CHAPTER 12: ANTI-INFLAMMATORY DRUGS

SECTION 1: NON-STEROIDAL ANTI-INFLAMMATORY DRUGS (NSAIDs)

Non-steroidal anti-inflammatory drugs are mainly used to treat pain associated with inflammation, and the basic Chinese medical statement about pain is that if there is pain, there is no free flow. Because these agents stop pain, they must move the qi and/or quicken the blood. However, because they are all also antipyretic, they must also clear heat.

That being said, their side effects include:
- Epigastric upset
- Ulceration and hemorrhage
- Edema
- Hyperkalemia, *i.e.*, nausea, irregular heart beat, and slow, weak, or absent pulse
- Anemia, *i.e.*, fatigue, orthostatic hypotension, lack of strength
- Headache

- Dizziness
- Tinnitus

Our hypothesis is that these medicinals are cold-natured, blood-quickening medicinals (活血药 *huo xue yao*). As such, they are attacking and draining and may damage the qi, blood, and yin. Because they are cold, they may damage the spleen. With prolonged use, it also appears that long-term spleen disease eventually reaches or affects the kidneys.

Aspirin is known to cause burning, soreness, tenderness, and inflammation of the tongue. This suggests severe damage not just to blood but to yin with the engenderment of vacuity heat.

SECTION 2: OTHER ANALGESICS

Acetominophen is the main drug in this class, and it is antipyretic and analgesic.

Its side effects:
- Skin rash

Pregabalin's side effects include:
- Peripheral edema
- Dizziness
- Fatigue
- Somnolence
- Ataxia
- Weight gain
- Dry mouth
- Tremors
- Vision problems

While acetaminophen has few side effects, based on those of pregabalin, we would say that these medicines clear heat and stop pain. Therefore, they free the flow of the qi and blood. Pregabalin also appears to damage the spleen, causing qi and blood vacuity symptoms, internally engendered dampness (*i.e.*, edema), and vacuity wind (*i.e.*, tremors). Thus we would say that these drugs are cold-natured, blood-quickening medicinals (活 血 药 *huo xue yao*).

Acetominophen is known to cause burning, soreness, tenderness, and inflammation of the tongue. This suggests severe damage not just to blood but to yin with the engenderment of vacuity heat.

SECTION 3: DISEASE-MODIFYING ANTIRHEUMATIC DRUGS (DMARDs)

Disease-modifying antirheumatic drugs are a varied group of drugs that may reduce or prevent joint damage in patients with rheumatoid arthritis (RA). In Chinese medicine, the boney deformations associated with advanced RA are seen as mainly due to blood stasis resulting in loss of nourishment of the sinews and bones. Therefore, it would seem reasonable to think that these drugs might also be blood-quickening medicinals (活 血 药 *huo xue yao*).

The side effects of these drugs include:
- Hematuria (尿 血 *niao xue*)
- Persistent diarrhea
- Tongue inflammation, *i.e.*, red tongue
- Pruritis and rash
- Hair loss
- Hypokalemia, *i.e.*, irregular heartbeat, muscle weakness, cramping, or flaccid paralysis (limpness), leg discomfort, extreme thirst, frequent urination, and confusion
- Anemia

When taken together, anemia, hematuria, and persistent diarrhea indicate qi vacuity, while hair loss, pruritis, tongue inflammation, and the symptoms of hypokalemia suggest a liver-blood-kidney yin vacuity with vacuity heat. Therefore, at the very least, we know these drugs are attacking and draining.

SECTION 4: DRUGS USED TO TREAT GOUT

These drugs are all used to treat gouty arthritis. Gouty arthritis in Chinese medicine is mostly seen as damp heat impediment complicated by blood stasis. Therefore, these medications are probably either heat-clearing or blood-quickening medicinals (or both).

The side effects of these drugs include:
- Nausea and vomiting
- Diarrhea
- Anemia
- Hair loss

Once again, we have the signs and symptoms of qi and blood vacuity. Of the two classes of Chinese medicinals mentioned above, heat-clearing medicinals (清 热 药 *qing re yao*) are the most likely to damage the spleen, thus resulting in qi and blood vacuity.

SECTION 5: DRUGS USED TO TREAT MIGRAINES

There are two types of migraine-specific agents:
(1) triptans, and
(2) ergot derivatives.

However, both are receptor agonists of serotonin$_{1D}$ inhibitors. Therefore, we feel comfortable classifying both these two subcategories in the same way.

Because these medications stop pain, it would seem that they are moving or quickening medicinals. However, because they should not be used in patients with peripheral vascular disease or coronary artery disease, such an easy assumption does not appear to be correct.

Both peripheral vascular disease and coronary artery disease are strongly associated with blood stasis. So why would medicinals that move the qi and/or quicken the blood aggravate those two conditions?

The side effects of these agents may help us solve this conundrum:
• Nausea and vomiting
• A rebound headache 24-48 hours later

If these medicinals were, in fact, securing and astringing medicinals that also quieted the spirit, they might have a pain-stopping effect, and they might also aggravate any condition associated with marked blood stasis. However, this does not explain the nausea and vomiting, which are the most common side effects of these drugs.

On the other hand, if these medicinals were heavy, settling, spirit-quieting medicinals (重镇

安神药 *zhong zhen an shen yao*), they would subdue upwardly counterflowing yang but might also easily damage the spleen and stomach, thus causing nausea and vomiting. When their administration was withdrawn or their effect had worn off, then the yang counterflow upward again, hence the rebound headache.

SECTION 6: DRUGS USED TO TREAT ULCERATIVE COLITIS)

The side effects of these drugs include:
• Headache
• Abdominal pain
• Insomnia
• Fatigue
• GI disturbances

Ulcerative colitis is most often treated with a combination of NSAIDs, discussed on page 413, and corticosteroids, discussed on page 405.

CHAPTER 13: MISCELLANEOUS DRUGS

SECTION 1: AGENTS USED TO TREAT ERECTILE DYSFUNCTION (ED)

These agents are used to treat ED due to either organic or psychogenic causes.

The side effects of these drugs include:
• Headache
• Flushing
• Gastrointestinal upset
• Nasal congestion

In Chinese medicine, ED is treated by one or a combination of several methods: yang- supplementation, qi supplementation, blood quickening, and dampness eliminating. In the first two methods, the issue is insufficient yang qi. In the second two methods, the issue is some evil qi preventing the qi and blood flow to the penis. Since three out of the four side effects of these drugs suggest ascendant yang (with counterflowing qi upbearing phlegm in the case of nasal congestion), it is likely that these drugs are yang-supplementing medicinals (补阳药 *bu yang*

yao) in terms of Chinese medicine. In that case, the GI upset may be due to stomach heat and yin vacuity due to damage by excessive yang. This is further supported by the fact that at least one of the Chinese yang-supplementing medicinals that are most commonly used to treat ED, *Xian Ling Pi* (Herba Epimedii), does contain icariin, a phosphodiesterase inhibitor.

SECTION 2: AGENTS USED TO TREAT OSTEOPOROSIS

These drugs are mainly used to treat osteoporosis. They all inhibit the action of the osteoclasts. Therefore, it seems reasonable that they all can be classified as a single category of Chinese medicinals.

Their side effects include:
• Nausea
• Abdominal pain
• Diarrhea
• Esophageal ulcers

In Chinese medicine, osteoporosis is typically

treated with a combination of yang supplements (which also do nourish liver blood), qi supplements, and blood quickeners. It is not likely that qi supplements would cause nausea and diarrhea. Nor would they be likely to cause esophageal ulcers, which are mostly associated with stomach heat. If they were yang supplements, they might increase stomach heat, leading to all four of the listed adverse reactions. Therefore, we propose that these drugs also be seen as yang-supplementing medicinals (补 阳 药 *bu yang yao*) in terms of Chinese medicine.

SECTION 3: AGENTS USED TO TREAT OBESITY

Most of the drugs in this class are appetite suppressors, and all are sympathomimetic. Thus they all may increase the metabolic rate.

Their side effects mostly include:
- Increased heart rate, *i.e.*, a rapid pulse
- Headache
- Insomnia
- Constipation
- A dry mouth

In Chinese medicine, obesity is seen as a pathological accumulation of phlegm, dampness, and turbidity. This accumulation may be due to or complicated by qi stagnation and/or blood stasis. However, in most cases, there are yang vacuity and yin repletion. One method of increasing yang in relation to yin is to use acrid, windy-natured, yang-upbearing and out-thrusting exterior resolvers, such as *Ma Huang* (Herba Ephedrae). However, this may result in damaging yin. Thus we can see that such an approach could result in all of the side effects listed above. Therefore, we propose that this class of medicinals be considered (acrid, warm) exterior-resolving medicinals (解 表 药 *jie biao yao*).

SECTION 4: AIDS FOR SMOKING CESSATION

These drugs commonly cause side effects including:
- Insomnia
- Headache

- Abnormal dreams
- Nausea

Therefore, it seems reasonable to state that they cause or exacerbate liver blood (and possibly heart blood) vacuity, which accounts for the insomnia and/or dream-disturbed sleep and may cause headache as well. Liver stomach disharmony with counterflow qi leads to nausea and possibly adds to the tendency to have a headache.

SECTION 5: SKELETAL MUSCLE RELAXANTS

No information available.

SECTION 6 ACNE DRUGS

No information available.

SECTION 7: IMMUNOSUPPRESSIVE DRUGS

These drugs are mainly used to treat patients who have undergone organ transplant. However, they may also be used in autoimmune disorders.

The side effects of these drugs include:
- Nausea and vomiting
- Diarrhea
- Fatigue
- Peripheral edema
- Blurred vision
- Dizziness
- Tremors
- Headache
- Pruritis
- Rash
- Hirsutism (多 发 *duo fa*)
- Bone marrow suppression
- Thrombocytopenia and/or leukopenia
- Lymphoma

From this list, we know we are dealing with attacking and draining medicinals, not supplements. In Chinese medicine, the overwhelming majority of patients with autoimmune disorders (except myasthenia gravis) present with combinations of liver-spleen disharmony and some sort of heat, be it depressive, damp, or vacuity heat. Since the above signs and symptoms rule out supplements and clearly point to qi and blood vacuity with eventual vacuity heat, our guess is that these medicinals are cold heat-clearing medicinals (清 热 药 *qing re yao*).

If there is tremor, there is wind due to blood vacuity. Signs and symptoms of lymphoma include lymph node enlargement but also fatigue, lack of strength, weight loss, night sweats, chills, and pruritis. Taken together, these are qi and yin vacuity symptoms plus phlegm binding, and the spleen is the source of phlegm engenderment.

Hirsutism in this context is anomalous and difficult to rationalize. It may indicate blood moving upward and outward due to vacuity heat.

CHAPTER 14: DRUGS OF ABUSE

This chapter on Drugs of Abuse was added only in the second edition of this text. Since the author who wrote this final chapter on hypothetical Chinese medical descriptions of Western drugs, Bob Flaws, is now retired and unavailable to update it, there is no information available about some of the agents discussed in Chapter 14.

That said, many of these drugs are described already in this chapter because their medical uses are listed in other chapters in this book. These include (locations here designate a location in this chapter, not the actual chapters stated:

- morphine, heroin, hydrocodone, and oxycodone, which are covered in depth in Chapter 5, Section 8

.

- Barbiturates and other depressants are covered in Chapter 5, Section 2
- Stimulants are discussed under Chapter 5, Section 3
- Steroids are covered under Chapter 7, Section 3
- Cannabis is mentioned briefly in Chapter 9, Section 2

For the other agents in Chapter 14 not covered in this chapter, perhaps using Dr. Flaws's methodology for working out Chinese medical descriptions of Western drugs as set forth in the beginning of this chapter, readers may take it upon themselves to puzzle out a working hypothesis for one or more of the other drugs of abuse discussed in Chapter 14.

Appendix A: Drug-Herb Interaction Tables

TABLE A-1: HERBS THAT MAY INTERACT WITH CYTOCHROME P450

A discussion of the Cytochrome P450 system may be found on pages 9-11 in Chapter 2.

HERBS	CYP1A2	CYP2B6	CYP2C9	CYP2C19	CYP2D6	CYP2E1	CYP3A4
Bai Guo Ye				*induces*			*induces*
Bai Hua She She Cao							*induces*
Da Huang						*induces*	*inhibits*
Da Suan							*induces*
Dan Shen	*inhibits*						*inhibits*
Dang Gui	*inhibits*						*inhibits*
Fu Zi							*induces*
Gan Cao							*induces*
Gan Jiang/Sheng Jiang				*induces*			
Guan Ye Lian Qiao	*induces*		*induces*	*induces*		*induces at low doses, inhibits at higher*	*strong inducer*
Hei Hu Jiao			*strong inhibitor*				*strong inhibitor*
Hu Zhang							*inhibits*
Huang Lian					*inhibits*		
Huang Qi							*strong inhibitor*
Huang Qin			*inhibits*			*inhibits*	*~strong inhibitor*
Lu Cha							*inhibits*
Mu Dan Pi							*strong inhibitor*
Mu Zei	*induces*						
Ren Shen			*inhibits*		*inhibits*		*strong inhibitor*
Rou Gui			*strong inhibitor*				*strong inhibitor*
Sheng Di Huang							*induces*
Sheng Jiang/Gan Jiang			*strong inhibitor*	*inhibits*			*strong inhibitor*
Sheng Ma		*induces*					*induces*
Shu Di Huang							*induces*
Tian Ma			*inhibits*				*inhibits*
Xiao Hui Xiang							*inhibits*
Xin Yi Hua							*~moderate inhibitor*
Yin Guo Ye							
Yin Yang Huo						*inhibits*	*inhibits*
Yu Jin			*strong inhibitor*				*strong inhibitor*

TABLE A-2: DRUGS THAT ARE HIGHLY PROTEIN BOUND

Implications of protein binding are discussed in Chapter 3, Section 2: Distribution

Drug	% Protein Binding				
Abiraterone acetate	>99%	Dexlansoprazole	96-99%	Isotretinoin	99-100%
Afatinib	>99%	Diazepam	98.0%	Isradipine	95.0%
Ambrisentan	~95%	Diclofenac	>99%	Itraconazole	99.8%
Amiodarone	99.0%	Dicloxacillin	96.0%	Ketoconazole	93-96%
Amlodipine	93-98%	Diflunisal	>99%	Ketoprofen	>99%
Aprepitant	>95%	Diphenhydramine	98.5%	Ketorolac	99.0%
Aripiprazole	>=99%	Dipyridamole	91-99%	Lansoprazole	97.0%
Artemether	95.0%	Docetaxel	~94-97%	Lapatinib	>99%
Asenapine	95.0%	Donepezil	96.0%	Leflunomide	>99%
Atomoxetine	98.0%	Doxazosin	~98%	Levothyroxine	>99%
Atorvastatin	>=98%	Dronabinol	97-99%	Liotrix[1]	>99%
Atovaquone	>99%	Dronedarone	>98%	Lopinavir	98-99%
Axitinib	>99%	Dutasteride	99.0%	Losartan	99.7%
Azilsartan	>99%	Efavirenz	>99%	Lovastatin	>95%
Balsalazide	>=99%	Entacapone	98.0%	Lumefantrine	99.7%
Beclomethasone	94-96%	Eprosartan	98.0%	Lurasidone	~99%
Bedaquiline	~100%	Enzalutamide	97-98%	Mebendazole	90-95%
Benazepril	~97%	Erlotinib	92-95%	Meclofenamate	>=99%
Bendamustine	94-96%	Esomeprazole	97.0%	Mefloquine	~98%
Bexarotene	>99%	Etodolac	>=99%	Meloxicam	~99%
Bicalutamide	96.0%	Etoposide	94-98%	Metolazone	95.0%
Bosentan	>98%	Etravirine	99.9%	Midazolam	~97%
Bumetanide	94-96%	Febuxostat	~99%	Mifepristone	98.0%
Buprenorphine	~96%	Felodipine	>99%	Mometasone	98-99%
Buspirone	86-95%	Fenofibrate	>99%	Montelukast	>99%
Cabozantinib	>=99.7%	Fenofibric acid	~99%	Mycophenolate	>97%
Canagliflozin	99.0%	Fenoprofen	99.0%	Nabumetone	>99%
Candesartan	>99%	Fingolimod	>99.7%	Naproxen	>99%
Carvedilol	>98%	Fluoxetine	95.0%	Nateglinide	98.0%
Celecoxib	~97%	Fluoxymesterone	98.0%	Nebivolol	~98%
Chlorambucil	~99%	Flurazepam	~97%	Nefazodone	>99%
Chlordiazepoxide	90-98%	Flurbiprofen	99.0%	Nelfinavir	>98%
Chlorpromazine	92-97%	Flutamide	94-96%	Nicardipine	>95%
Ciclesonide	>=99%	Fluticasone	99.0%	Nifedipine	92-98%
Ciclopirox	94-98%	Fluvastatin	>98%	Nilotinib	~98%
Cilostazol	95-98%	Fosinopril	95.0%	Nimodipine	>95%
Cisapride	97.5-98.0%	Fosphenytoin	95-99%	Nisoldipine	>99%
Clomipramine	97.0%	Furosemide	91-99%	Nitazoxanide	>99%
Clopidogrel	98.0%	Gemfibrozil	99.0%	Olmesartan	99.0%
Clorazepate	metabolite is 97-98%	Glimepiride	>99.5%	Olsalazine	>99%
Clozapine	97.0%	Glipizide	98-99%	Omeprazole	~95%
Cyclosporine	90-98%	Glyburide	>99%	Ospemifene	>99%
Dabrafenib	99.7%	Ibandronate	85.7-99.5%	Oxaprozin	99.0%
Darunavir	~95%	Ibuprofen	90-99%	Oxazepam	86-99%
Darifenacin	98.0%	Idarubicin	94-97%	Paclitaxel	89-98%
Dasatinib	96.0%	Iloperidone	~95%	Pantoprazole	98.0%
Deferasirox	~99%	Imatinib	~95%	Paroxetine	93-95%
Delavirdine	~98%	Indacaterol	~95%	Pazopanib	>99%
		Indomethacin	99.0%	Penbutolol	80-98%

Perampanel	95-96%	Ruxolitinib	~97%	Ticagrelor	>99%
Phenytoin	90-95%	Salmeterol	96.0%	Ticlopidine	98.0%
Pimozide	99.0%	Saquinavir	~98%	Tipranavir	>99%
Pioglitazone	>99%	Sertraline	98.0%	Tolbutamide	~95%
Piroxicam	99.0%	Sildenafil	~96%	Tolcapone	>99%
Pitavastatin	>99%	Silodosin	~97%	Tolterodine	>96%
Ponatinib	>99%	Simvastatin	~95%	Toremifene	>99.5%
Posaconazole	>98%	Sorafenib	99.5%	Torsemide	>99%
Prasugrel	~98%	Spironolactone	91-98%	Trametinib	~97%
Prazosin	92-97%	Sulfasalazine	>99%	Trazodone	85-95%
Propafenone	95.0%	Sunitinib	95.0%	Tretinoin	>95%
Quazepam	>95%	Tacrolimus	~99%	Trimipramine	95.0%
Quinapril	97.0%	Tamoxifen	99.0%	Valsartan	95.0%
Rabeprazole	~96%	Tamsulosin	94-99%	Vardenafil	~95%
Raloxifene	>95%	Tazarotene	>99%	Vemurafenib	>99%
Regorafenib	99.5%	Telmisartan	>99.5%	Vilazodone	~96-99%
Repaglinide	>98%	Temazepam	96.0%	Vinblastine	99.0%
Reserpine	96.0%	Teniposide	99.4%	Vismodegib	>99%
Rifapentine	~98%	Terazosin	90-95%	Warfarin	99.0%
Rilpivirine	99.7%	Terbinafine	>99%	Zafirlukast	>99%
Riluzole	96.0%	Testosterone	98.0%	Ziprasidone	>99%
Ritonavir	98-99%	Thyroid[2]	>99%		
Rosiglitazone	98.8%	Tiagabine	96.0%		

Notes:

1   Only the T4 component of liotrix is >99% bound.

2   Only the T4 component of desiccated thyroid is >99% bound.

TABLE A-3: DRUGS THAT AFFECT P-GLYCOPROTEIN

A discussion of P-Glycoprotein may be found in Chapter 3, Section 6, page 24.

Drug	Effect	Drug	Effect
Abiraterone acetate	inhibits	Darunavir	inhibits
Afatinib	substrate, inhibits	Desloratadine	substrate
Ambrisentan	substrate	Dexamethasone	substrate, inhibits, induces
Amiodarone	substrate, inhibits	Diltiazem	substrate
Atorvastatin	substrate, inhibits	Dipyridamole	inhibits
Azithromycin	inhibits	Docetaxel	substrate
Bendamustine	substrate	Dronedarone	inhibits
Boceprevir	substrate, inhibits	Enzalutamide	inhibits
Bosutinib	substrate, inhibits	Erythromycin	substrate, inhibits
Cabozantinib	substrate	Estradiol	substrate
Carbamazepine	substrate	Etoposide	substrate
Carvedilol	inhibits	Fexofenadine	substrate
Cetirizine	substrate	Fosamprenavir	substrate
Cimetidine	substrate	Hydrocortisone	substrate
Ciprofloxacin	substrate	Idarubicin	substrate
Clarithromycin	inhibits	Imatinib	substrate, inhibits
Clobazam	substrate	Indinavir	substrate
Colchicine	substrate	Irinotecan	substrate
Crizotinib	substrate, inhibits	Itraconazole	inhibits
Cyclosporine	substrate, inhibits	Ivermectin	substrate
Dabrafenib	substrate		

continued on the following page...

continued from previous page...

Drug	Effect
Ketoconazole	inhibits
Lapatinib	substrate inhibits
Linagliptin	substrate
Loperamide	substrate
Loratadine	substrate
Lovastatin	substrate
Maraviroc	substrate
Mefloquine	inhibits
Methotrexate	substrate
Mifepristone	inhibits
Mitomycin	substrate
Nadolol	substrate
Nefazodone	induces
Nelfinavir	substrate, inhibits
Nicardipine	substrate
Nilotinib	substrate, inhibits
Omacetaxine	substrate
Ondansetron	substrate
Paclitaxel	substrate
Paliperidone	substrate
Pazopanib	substrate
Ponatinib	substrate, inhibits
Pravastatin	substrate
Prazosin	induces
Progesterone	induces
Propranolol	inhibits
Quinidine	substrate, inhibits
Quinine	substrate, inhibits
Ranitidine	substrate
Ranolazine	substrate, inhibits
Regorafenib	inhibits
Reserpine	inhibits
Rifampin	substrate, induces
Risperidone	substrate
Ritonavir	substrate, inhibits
Romidepsin	substrate
Saquinavir	substrate, inhibits
Saxagliptin	substrate
Silodosin	substrate
Sirolimus	substrate
Sitagliptin	substrate
Sunitinib	inhibits
Tacrolimus	substrate, inhibits
Tamoxifen	inhibits
Telaprevir	substrate, inhibits
Teniposide	substrate
Tenofovir	induces
Tipranavir	induces
Trazodone	induces
Ulipristal	inhibits
Vandetanib	inhibits
Vemurafenib	substrate, inhibits
Verapamil	substrate, inhibits
Vinblastine	substrate, induces
Vincristine	substrate
Vincristine (Liposomal)	substrate
Vismodegib	substrate

TABLE A-4: HERBS THAT MAY AFFECT P-GLYCOPROTEIN

Da Suan	induces
Dang Gui	inhibits
Guan Ye Lian Qiao	induces
Wu Wei Zi	inhibits
Yin Guo Ye	inhibits

TABLE A-5: DRUGS WITH NARROW THERAPEUTIC INDICES (NTI)

A discussion of therapeutic index may be found in Chapter 3, Section 5, page 24.

Drug	Notes		
Aminophylline		Levothyroxin	2
Amitriptyline	1	Lithium	2
Amoxapine	1	Methadone	
Carbamazepine	2	Mycophenolate	3
Clomipramine	1	Nortriptyline	1
Cyclosporine	2	Phenytoin	2
Desipramine	1	Procainamide	2
Digoxin	2	Protriptyline	1
Doxepin	1	Sirolimus	
Ethosuximide	2	Tacrolimus	2
Fosphenytoin	4	Theophylline	2
Imipramine	1	Trimipramine	1
		Warfarin	2

Notes:

1   Tricyclic antidepressants are considered to have a narrow therapeutic index by some experts but are not included on major lists of NTI drugs.

2   On the North Carolina list of NTI drugs.

3   Debated among experts, not on any approved NTI lists

4   Fosphenytoin is not on most lists of narrow therapeutic index drugs. However, it is a prodrug of phenytoin and therefore should be considered as potentially having a narrow index.

Appendix B: Bibliography

Abascal, K. & Yarnell, E. (2002, Oct). Herbs and drug resistance: part 2—clinical implications of research on microbial resistance to antibiotics. Alternative & Complementary Therapies. 8(5):284-90.

n.d.) Abbreviations. Retrieved January 13, 2013, from http://www.medicalterm.com.au/Free%20Pdf%20note s/Medical%20Terminology%20Abbreviations.pdf.

American Psychiatric Association. (2000). Diagnostic and statistical manual of mental disorders (4th ed., text revision). Arlington, VA: American Psychiatric Assoc.

American Psychological Association. (2001). Publication manual of the American Psychological Association (5th ed.). Washington, DC: American Psychological Assoc.

Anderson, K. N. & Anderson, L. E. (1994). Mosby's pocket dictionary of medicine, nursing, & allied health. St. Louis: Mosby.

Apitz-Castro, R., Escalante, J., Vargas, R. & Jain, M. K. (1986, May). Ajoene, the antiplatelet principle of garlic, synergistically potentiates the antiaggregatory action of prostacyclin, forskolin, indomethacin, and dypiridamole on human platelets. Thromb Res. 42(3):303-11.

Arora, A. & Scholar, E. M. (2005, Dec.). Role of tyrosine kinase inhibitors in cancer therapy. JPET. (315) 3: 971-979. Retrieved 8/6/13 from http://jpet.aspetjournals.org/content/315/3/971.full.

Astrup, A., Breum, L., Toubro, S., Hein, P. & Quaade, F. (1992). The effect and safety of an ephedrine/caffeine compound compared to ephedrine, caffeine, and placebo in obese subjects on an energy restricted diet. A double-blind trial. Int. J. Obesity. 16(4):269-277.

Astrup, A. & Toubro, S. (1993). Thermogenic, metabolic, and cardiovascular responses to ephedrine and caffeine in man. Int. J. Obes. Relat. Metab. Disord. 17(Suppl 1):S41-3.

Astrup, A., Toubro, S., Cannon, S., Hein, P. & Madsen, J. (1991, Mar). Thermogenic synergism between ephedrine and caffeine in healthy volunteers: A double-blind, placebo-controlled study. Metabolism. 40(3):323-9.

Awang, D. V. C. (1996). Siberian ginseng toxicity may be case of mistaken identity. Can. Med. Assoc. J. 155(9):1237.

Bano, G., Amla, V., Raina, R. K., Zutshi, U. & Chopra, C. L. (1987). The effect of piperine on pharmacokinetics of phenytoin in healthy volunteers. Planta Med. 53(6):568-9.

Bano, G., Raina, R. K., Zutshi, U., Bedi, K. L., Johri, R. K. &

Sharma, S.C. (1991, Dec). Effect of piperine on bioavailability and pharmacokinetics of propranolol and theophylline in healthy volunteers. Eur. J. Clin. Pharmacol. 41(6):615-7.

Bao, Z. D., Wu, Z. G. & Zheng, F. (1991). Amelioration of aminoglycoside nephrotoxicity by Cordyceps sinensis in old patients. Chinese J. Integrated Traditional Western Med. 14(5):271-3.

Beckman, C. R. B., Ling, F. W., Laube, D. W., Smith, R. P., Barzansky, B. M. & Herbert, W. N. P. (2002). Obstetrics and Gynecology (4th ed.). Baltimore

Beers, M. H. (Ed.). (2006). The Merck manual of diagnosis and therapy (18th ed.). Whitehouse Station, NJ: Merck Research Laboratories.

Beers, M. H. & Berkow, R. (Eds.). (1999). The Merck manual of diagnosis and therapy (17th ed.). Whitehouse Station, NJ: Merck Research Laboratories.

Bernardi, M., D'Intino, P. E., Trevisani, F., Cantelli-Forti, G., Raggi, M. A., Turchetto, E. & Gasbarrini, G. (1994). Effects of prolonged ingestion of graded doses of licorice by healthy volunteers. Life Sci. 55(11):863-72.

Bilgi, N., Bell, K., Ananthakrishnan, A. N. Atallah, E. (2101, May). Imatinib and Panax ginseng: a potential interaction resulting in liver toxicity. Ann. Pharmacother. 44(5):926-8.

Blumenthal, M. (Ed.). (1998). The complete German commission E monographs. Boston, MA: Integrative Medicine Communications.

Bone, K. (1996). Clinical applications of ayurvedic and Chinese herbs. Warwick, Queensland, Australia: Phytotherapy Press.

Boozer, C. N., Daly, P. A., Homel, P., Solomon, J. L., Blanchard, D., Nasser, J. A., Strauss, R, & Meredith, T. (2002). Herbal ephedra/caffeine for weight loss: A 6-month randomized safety and efficacy trial. International Journal of Obesity. 26:593–604.

Bordia, A., Verma, S. K. & Srivastava, K. C. (1997). Effect of ginger (Zingibera Officinale rose.) and fenugreek (Trigonella foenumgraecum l.) on blood lipids, blood sugar, and platelet aggregation in patients with coronary artery disease. Prostaglandins Leukot. Essent. Fatty Acids. 56(5):379-84.

Brater, D. C., Kaojarern, S., Benet, L. Z., Lin, E. T., Lockwood, T., Morris, R. C., McSherry, E. J. & Melmon, K. L. (1980, Nov). Renal excretion of pseudoephedrine. Clin. Pharmacol. Ther. 28(5):690-4.

Brinker, F. (1995). Eclectic dispensary of botanical therapeutics (Vol. 2). Sandy, OR: Eclectic Medical.

Brinker, F. (2001). Herb contraindications & drug interactions (3rd ed.). Sandy, OR: Eclectic Medical Publications.

Bristol-Myers Squibb Company. (2003, Nov) Buspar. Retrieved September 1, 2005 from http://www.bms.com/cgi-bin/anybin.pl?sql=select%20PPI%0A%09%09%09%09%20%20%20from%20TB_PRODUCT_PPI%20%0A%09%09%09%09%20%20%20where%20PPI_SEQ%20=%2035&key=PPI.

Brooks, S. M., Sholiton, L. J., Werk Jr., E. E. & Altenau, P. (1977). The effects of ephedrine and theophylline on dexamethasone metabolism in bronchial asthma. Clinical Pharmacology. 17:308-18.

Brunton, L. L. (Ed.). (2006). Goodman and Gilman's the pharmacological basis of therapeutics (11th ed.). New York: McGraw-Hill.

Champe, P. C. & Harvey, R. A. (1994). Lippincott's illustrated reviews: Biochemistry (2nd ed.). Philadelphia: Lippincott, Williams & Wilkins.

Chandra, R. H. Rajkumar, M. & Veeresham, C. (2009). Pharmacokinetic interaction of ginkgo biloba with carbamazepine. Planta Medica. (4):454.

Chang, L. (2006). Herbal inhibitory interactions with the CYP3A4 isozyme of the cytochrome P450 system. Unpublished raw data.

Chen, J. (1998/1999). Recognition and prevention of herb-drug interactions. Medical Acupuncture. 10 (2):9-13.

Chen, J. C. & Chen, T. T. (2004). Chinese medical herbology and pharmacology. City of Industry, CA: Art of Medicine Press.

Chi, Y. C., Lin, S. P. Hou, Y. C. (2012, Sep 15). A new herb-drug interaction of Polygonum cuspidatum, a resveratrol-rich nutraceutical, with carbamazepine in rats. Toxicol. Appl. Pharmacol. 263(3):315-22.

Chiang, H. M., Hou, Y. C., Tsai, S. Y., Yang, S. Y., Chao, P. D. L., Hsiu, S. L. & Wen, K. C. (2005). Marked decrease of cyclosporin absorption caused by coadministration of Cordyceps sinensis in rats. Journal of Food and Drug Analysis. 13(3):239-43.

Chien, C. F., Wu, Y. T., Lee, W. C., Lin, L. C. & Tsai, T. H. (2010, Mar 30). Chem. Biol. Interact. 184(3):458-65.

Cho, S., Hong, T., Jin, G. B., Yoshino, G., Miura, M., Aikawa, Y., Yasuno, F. & Cyong, J. C. (2002). The combination therapy of ephedra herb and loxoprofen caused gastric lesions in mice. American Journal of Chinese Medicine. 30(4):571-7.

Chu, D., Sun, Y., Lin, J., Wong, W. & Mavligit, G. (1990, Jan). F3, a fractionated extract of Astragalus membranaceus, potentiates lymphokine-activated killer cell cytotoxici-

ty generated by low-dose recombinant interleukin-2 [Article in Chinese]. Zhong Xi Yi Jie He Za Zhi. 10(1):34-6, 35.

Circosta, C., De Pasquale, R., Palumbo, D. R., Samperi, S. & Occhiuto, F. (2006). Estrogenic activity of standardized extract of Angelica sinensis. Phytotherapy Research. 20(8):665-9.

Cotran, R. S., Vinay, V. & Collins, T. (1999). Robbin's pathologic basis of disease (6th ed.). Philadelphia: W. B. Saunders.

Crossman, A. R. & Neary, D. (1998). Neuroanatomy, an illustrated colour text. London: Harcourt, Brace.

Dalvi, R. R. & Dalvi, P. S. (1991). Differences in the effects of piperine and piperonyl butoxide on hepatic drug-metabolizing enzyme system in rats. Drug Chemical Toxicology. 14(1-2):219-29.

Dasgupta, A., Kidd, L., Poindexter, B. J. & Bick, R. J. (2010, Aug). Interference of hawthorn on serum digoxin measurements by immunoassays and pharmacodynamic interaction with digoxin. Arch. Pathol. Lab. Med. 134(8):1188-92. Retrieved January 3, 2014, from http://www.archivesofpathology.org/doi/full/10.1043/2009-0404-OA.1.

Dawson, J. K., Earnshaw, S. M. & Graham, C. S. (1995). Dangerous monoamine oxidase inhibitor interactions are still occurring in the 1990s. Journal of Accident and Emergency Medicine. 12(1):49-51.

de Klerk, G. J., Nieuwenhuis, M. G. & Beutler J. J. (1997). Hypokalemia and hypertension associated with use of liquorice flavoured chewing gum. BMJ. 314:731.

de Lima Toccafondo Vieira, M. & Huang, S. M. (2012, Sep). Botanical-drug interactions: A scientific perspective. Planta Med. 78(13):1400-15.

Deahl, M. (1989). Betel nut–induced extrapyramidal syndrome: An unusual drug interaction. Movement Disorders. 4(4):330-2.

Dingemanse, J. (1993, Jan). An update of recent moclobemide interaction data. Internal. Clin. Psychopharm. 7(3-4):167-80.

Duda, R. B., Zhong, Y., Navas, V., Li, M. Z. C., Toy, B. R. & Alavarez, J. G. (1999). American ginseng and breast cancer therapeutic agents synergistically inhibit MCF-7 breast cancer cell growth. J. Surg. Oncol. 72:230.

Dulloo, A. G. & Miller, D. S. (1986a). The thermogenic properties of ephedrine/methylxanthine mixtures: Animal studies. Am. J. Clin. Nutr. 43:388-94.

Dulloo, A. G. & Miller, D. S. (1986b). The thermogenic properties of ephedrine/methylxanthine mixtures: Human Studies. Int. J. Obes. 10(6):467-81.

Durr, D., Stieger, B., Kullak-Ublick, G. A., Rentsch, K. M., Steinert, H. C., Meier, P. J. & Fattinger, K. (2000). St.

John's wort induces intestinal P-glycoprotein/MDR1 and intestinal and hepatic CYP3A4. Clin. Pharmacol. Ther. 68:598-604.

Engelsen, J., Nielsen, J. D. & Hansen, K. F. (2003, April 28). Effect of coenzyme Q10 and ginkgo biloba on warfarin dosage in patients on long-term warfarin treatment. A randomized, double-blind, placebo-controlled crossover trial [Article in Danish]. Ugeskr Laeger. 165(18): 1868-71.

Etheridge, A. S. Kroll, D. J. & Mathews, J. M. (2009). Inhibition of paclitaxel metabolism *in vitro* in human hepatocytes by Ginkgo biloba preparations. J. Diet. Suppl. 6(2):104-10.

Fan, L., Mao, X. Q., Tao, G. Y., Wang, G., Jiang, F., Chen, Y., Li, Q., Zhang, W., Lei, H. P., Hu, D. L., Huang, Y. F., Wang, D. & Zhou, H. H. (2009). Effect of Schisandra chinensis extract and Ginkgo biloba extract on the pharmacokinetics of talinolol in healthy volunteers. Xenobiotica. 39:249-254.

Fan, L., Tao, G. Y., Wang, G., Chen, Y., Zhang, W., He, Y. J., Li, Q., Lei, H. P., Jiang, F., Hu, D. L., Huang, Y. F. & Zhou, H. H. (2009, May). Effects of Ginkgo biloba extract ingestion on the pharmacokinetics of talinolol in healthy Chinese volunteers. Ann. Pharmacother. 43(5):944-9. Retrieved December 18, 2013, from http://www.ncbi.nlm.nih.gov/pubmed/19401473?ordinalpos=2&itool=Email.EmailReport.Pubmed_ReportSelector.Pubmed_RVDocSum.

Fasinu, P. S., Bouic, P. J. & Rosenkranz, B. (2012). An overview of the evidence and mechanisms of herb-drug interactions. Front. Pharmacol. 3:69.

Folkersen, L., Knudsen, N. A. & Teglbjaerg, P. S. (1996, Dec 16). Licorice: A basis for precautions one more time! [Article in Danish]. Ugeskr Laeger. 158(51):7420-1.

Fowler, J. S., Wang, G. J., Volkow, N. D., Logan, J., Franceschi, D., Franceschi, M., MacGregor, R., Shea, C., Garza, V., Liu, N. & Ding, Y. S. (2000, Jan 21). Evidence that gingko biloba extract does not inhibit MAO A and B in living human brain. Life Sci. 66(9):PL141-6.

Francischetti, I. M., Monteiro, R. Q. & Guimaraes, J. A. (1997, Jun 9). Identification of glycyrrhizin as a thrombin inhibitor. Biochem. Biophys. Res. Commun. 235(1):259-63.

Fugh-Berman, A. (2000). Herb-drug interactions. Lancet. 355(9198):134.

Gianni, L. & Dreitlein, W. B. (1988, May). Some popular OTC herbals can interact with anticoagulant therapy. Pharmacist: 80,83,84,86.

GlaxoSmithKline. (2006). Dexedrine (dextroamphetamine sulfate). Food and Drug Administration. Retrieved August 27, 2006, from http://www.fda.gov/ medwatch/safety/2006/safety06.htm#Dexedrine.

Goso, Y., Ogata, Y., Ishihara, K. & Hotta, K. (1996). Effects of traditional herbal medicine on gastric mucin against ethanol-induced gastric injury in rats. Comp. Biochem. Physiol. 113C(1):7-21.

Gotink, K. J. & Verheuf, H. M. W. (2010, Mar). Anti-angiogenic tyrosine kinase inhibitors: What is their mechanism of action? Angiogenesis. 13(1):1–14. Retrieved August 6, 2013, from http://www.ncbi.nlm.nih.gov/pmc/articles/PMC2845892/.

Grace, J. M., Skanchy, D. J. & Aguilar, A. J. (1999, July). Metabolism of artelinic acid to dihydroqinghaosu by human liver cytochrome P4503A. Xenobiotica. 29(4):703-17.

Greenway, F. L., de Jonge, L., Blanchard, D., Frisard, M. & Smith, S. R. (2004, Jul). Effect of a dietary herbal supplement containing caffeine and ephedra on weight, metabolic rate, and body composition. Obesity Research. 12(7):1152-7.

Gruenwald, J., Brendler, T. & Jaenicke, C. (Eds.) (2004). PDR for herbal medicines (3rd ed.). Montvale, NJ: Thomson PDR.

Gurley, B. J., Gardner, S. F., Hubbard, M. A., Williams, D. K., Gentry, W. B., Cui, Y. & Ang, C. Y. (2002, Sep). Cytochrome P450 phenotypic ratios for predicting herb-drug interactions in humans. Clin. Pharmacol. Ther. 72(3):276-87.

Han, Y. L., Yu, H. L., Li, D., Meng, X. L., Zhou, Z. Y., Yu, Q., Zhang, X. Y., Wang, F. J. & Guo, C. (2011, Nov). In vitro inhibition of Huanglian (Rhizoma coptidis [L.]) and its six active alkaloids on six cytochrome P450 isoforms in human liver microsomes. Phytother. Res. 25(11):1660-5.

Harada, T., Ohtaki, E., Misu, K., Sumiyoshi, T. & Hosoda, S. (2002). Congestive heart failure caused by digitalis toxicity in an elderly man taking a licorice-containing Chinese herbal laxative. Cardiology. 98:218-20.

Hardman, J. G. & Limbird, L. E. (Eds.). (2001). Goodman & Gilman's the pharmacological basis of therapeutics (10th ed.). New York: McGraw-Hill.

Hatano, T., Fukuda, T., Miyase, T. Noro, T. & Okuda, T. (1991, May). Phenolic constituents of licorice. III. Structures of glicoricone and licofuranone and inhibitory effects of licorice constituents on monoamine oxidase. Chem. Pharm. Bull. (Tokyo). 39(5):1238-43.

Heck, A. M., Dewitt, B. A. & Lukes, A. L. (2000). Potential interactions between alternative therapies and warfarin. Am. J. Health-Syst. Pharm. 57(13):122.

Hellum, B. H., Hu, Z. & Nilsen, O. G. (2009, Jul). Trade herbal products and induction of CYP2C19 and CYP2E1 in cultured human hepatocytes. Basic Clin. Pharmacol. Toxicol. 105(1):58-63. Retrieved December 18, 2013, from http://www.ncbi.nlm.nih.gov/pubmed/19371257?ordinalpos=1&itool=Email.EmailReport.Pubmed_ReportSelector.Pubmed_RVDocSum.

Hikino, H., Takahashi, M., Otake, K. & Konno, C. (1986, March-April). Isolation and hypoglycemic activity of eleutherans A, B, C, D, E, F, and G: Glycans of eleutherococcus sentlcosus roots. Journal of Natural Products. 49(2):293-7.

Hirata, J. D., Small, R., Swiersz, L. M., Ettinger, B. & Zell, B. (1997, Dec). Does *Dong Quai* have estrogenic effects in postmenopausal women? A double-blind, placebo-controlled trial. Fert. Steril. 68(6):981-6.

Howland, R. D. & Mycek, M. J. (2006). Lippincott's illustrated reviews: Pharmacology (3rd ed.). Baltimore: Lippincott, Williams & Wilkins.

Hsieh, M. T., Lin, Y. T., Lin, Y. H. & Wu, C. R. (2000). Radix Angelica sinensis extracts ameliorate scopolamine- and cycloheximide-induced amnesia, but not p-chloroamphetamine-induced amnesia in rats. Am. J. Chin. Med. 28(2):263-72.

Hsieh, M. T., Wu, C. R., Wang, W. H. & Lin, L. W. (2001, Jan). The ameliorating effect of the water layer of Fructus schisandrae on cycloheximide-induced amnesia in rats: Interaction with drugs acting at neurotransmitter receptors. Pharmacological Research. 43(1):17-22.

Hsueh, T. Y., Wu, Y. T., Lin, L. C., Chiu, A. W., Lin, C. H. & Tsai, T. H.(2013, Jun 21). Herb-drug interaction of Epimedium sagittatum (Sieb. et Zucc.) maxim extract on the pharmacokinetics of sildenafil in rats. Molecules. 18(6):7323-35.

Hu, Z., Yang, X., Ho, P. C., Chan, S. Y., Heng, P. W., Chan, E., Duan, W., Koh, H. L. & Zhou, S. (2005). Herb-drug interactions: A literature review. Drugs 65(9):1239-82.

Huang, Y., Zheng, S. L., Xu, Z. S. & Hou, Y. (2013, Nov 27). Effects of unprocessed vs. cooked-processed Gastrodia elata on cytochrome P450 enzymes in rats. Drug Res. Retrieved December 2, 2013, from http://www.ncbi.nlm.nih.gov/pubmed/24285404.

Hulley, S. B., Cummings, S. R., Browner, W. S., Grady, D., Hearst, N. & Newman, T. B. (2001). Designing clinical research (2nd ed.). Philadelphia: Lippincott, Williams & Wilkins.

Hussain, R. M. (2003). The sweet cake that reaches parts other cakes can't! Postgrad. Med. J. 79:115-11.

Ishihara, K., Kushida, H., Yuzurihara, M., Wakui, Y., Yanagisawa, T., Kamei, H., Ohmori, S. & Kitada, M. (2000, Aug). Interaction of drugs and Chinese herbs: Pharmacokinetic changes of tolbutamide and diazepam caused by extract of Angelica dahurica. Journal of Pharmacy and Pharmacology. 52(8):1023-9.

Izzat, M. B., Yim, A. P. C. & El-Zufari, M. H. (1998). A taste of Chinese medicine. Ann. Thorac. Surg. 66:941-42.

Izzo, A. A. & Ernst, E. (2009). Interactions between herbal medicines and prescribed drugs: An updated systematic review. Drugs 69(13):1777-98.

Johne, A., Brockmöller, J., Bauer, S., Maurer, A., Langheinrich, M. & Roots, I. (1999, Oct). Pharma-cokinetic interaction of digoxin with an herbal extract from St. John's wort (Hypericum perforatum). Clin. Pharmacol. Ther. 66(4):338-45.

Jung, H., Sok, D. E., Kim, Y., Min et al. (2000, Feb). Potentiating effect of obacunone from Dictamnus dasycarpus on cytotoxicity of microtuble inhibitors, vincristine, vinblastine, and taxol. Plant Med. 66(1):74-6.

Kim, I. S., Kim, S. Y. & Yoo, H. H. (2012, Dec). Effects of an aqueous-ethanolic extract of ginger on cytochrome P450 enzyme-mediated drug metabolism. Pharmazie. 67(12):1007-9.

Kimura, Y., Ito, H. & Hatano, T. (2010). Effects of mace and nutmeg on human cytochrome P450 3A4 and 2C9 activity. Biol. Pharm. Bull. 33(12):1977-82. Retrieved January 7, 2014, from https://www.jstage.jst.go.jp/article/bpb/33/12/33_12_1977/_pdf.

King, D. E., Malone, R. & Lilley, S. H. (2000, May 1). New classification and update on the quinolone antibiotics. American Family Physician. 61(9):2741-8.

Koo, M. W. L. (1999). Effects of ginseng on ethanol induced sedation in mice. Life Sci. 64(2):153-60.

Kowalak, J. F. & Mills, E. J. (Eds.). (2001). Professional guide to complementary & alternative therapies. Bethlehem Pike, PA: Springhouse.

Kwan, C. Y. (1995, Dec). Vascular effects of selected antihypertensive drugs derived from traditional medicinal herbs. Clin. Exp. Pharmacol. Physio. Suppl., 22(1):S297-9.

Laird, J. (2011, Dec). Interactions between supplements and drugs: Deciphering the evidence. JAAPA. 24:12:44-6, 48-9.

Langhammer, A. J. & Nilsen, O. G. (2013, Jul 10). In vitro inhibition of human CYP1A2, CYP2D6, and CYP3A4 by six herbs commonly used in pregnancy. Phytother. Res. [Epub ahead of print]

Lau, C., Mooiman, K. D., Maas-Bakker, R. F., Beijnen, J. H., Schellens, J. H. & Meijerman, I. (2013, Sep 16). Effect of Chinese herbs on CYP3A4 activity and expression in vitro. J. Ethnopharmacol. 149(2):543-9.

Laughren, T. (2007). NDAs 18-936/S-078, 21-235/S-008 & 20-101/S-036. Retrieved December 31, 2012, from http://www.accessdata.fda.gov/drugsatfda_docs/applet ter/2007/018936s078,021235s008,020101s036ltr.pdf.

Lee, C. M., Wong, H. N., Chui, K. Y., Choang, T. F., Hon, P.

M. & Chang, H. M. (1991, Jun 24). Miltirone, a central benzodiazepine receptor partial agonist from a Chinese medicinal herb Salvia miltiorrhiza. Neurosci. Lett. 127(2):237-47.

Levinson, W. & Jawetz, E. (2000). Medical microbiology & immunology: Examination & board review (6th ed.). New York: McGraw-Hill.

Lewis, S. J., Oakey, R. E. & Heaton, K. W. (1998, Jan). Intestinal absorption of oestrogen: The effect of altering transit-time. Eur. J. Gastroenterol. Hepatol. 10(1):33-9.

Lexi-Comp Online. [Database on Internet]. (1978-2006). Hudson, OH: Lexi-Comp, Inc. Available from http://www.lexi.com/web/index.jsp.

Lexi-Comp, Inc. (2005). Lexi-drugs (comp + specialties) [PDA software]. Retrieved September 3, 2005, from http://connect.lexi.com/dbupdate/lexi_connect_windows.jsp.

Lilly, L. S. (1998). Pathophysiology of heart disease (2nd ed.). Baltimore: Lippincott, Williams & Wilkins.

Lin, S. C., Chung, T. C., Lin, C. C., Ueng, T. H., Lin, Y. H., Lin, S. Y. & Wang, L. Y. (2000). Hepatoprotective effects of Arctium lappa on carbon tetrachloride- and acetaminophen-induced liver damage. Am. J. Chin. Med. 28(2):163-73.

Lin, S. H., Yang, S. S., Chau, T. & Halperin, M. L. (2003, Mar, 3). An unusual cause of hypokalemic paralysis: chronic licorice ingestion. Am J Med Sci. 25(3):153-6.

Lin, S. P., Wu, P. P., Hou, Y. C., Tsai, S. Y., Wang, M. J., Fang, S. H. & Chao, P. D. (2011). Different influences on tacrolimus pharmacokinetics by coadministrations of zhi ke and zhi shi in rats. Evid. Based Complement. Alternat. Med. 2011. Retrieved January 3, 2014, from http:// www.ncbi.nlm.nih.gov/pmc/articles/PMC3035000/.

Liu, I. X., Durham, D. G. & Richards, R. M. E. (2000, Mar). Baicalin synergy with β-lactam antibiotics against methicillin-resistant Staphylococcus aureus and other β-lactam-resistant strains of S. aureus. Journal of Pharmacy and Pharmacology. 52(3):361-6.

Lo, A. C., Chan, K., Yeung, J. H. & Woo, K. S. (1995, Jan-Mar). *Dang Gui* (Angelica sinensis) affects the pharmacodynamics but not the pharmacokinetics of warfarin in rabbits. Eur. J. Drug. Metab. Pharmacokinet. 20(1):55-60.

Lumb, A. B. (1994). Effect of dried ginger on human platelet function. Thromb. Haemostasis. 71(10):110-1.

Malchow-Moller, A., Larsen, S., Hey, H., Stokholm, K. H., Juhl, E. & Quaade, F. (1981). Ephedrine as an anorectic: The story of the 'Elsinore pill'. Internat. J. Obesity. 5:183-7.

Marco, D. (2011). The dopamine hypothesis of drug addiction and its potential therapeutic value. Front.

Psychiatry. 2:64. Retrieved 02/18/2014 from http://www.ncbi.nlm.nih.gov/pmc/articles/PMC3225760/.

Marieb, E. N. (2004). Human anatomy & physiology (6th ed.). San Francisco: Pearson Benjamin Cummings.

Mateo-Carrasco, H., Gálvez-Contreras, M. C., Fernández-Ginés, F. D. & Nguyen, T. V. (2012). Elevated liver enzymes resulting from an interaction between raltegravir and Panax ginseng: a case report and brief review. Drug Metabol. Drug. Interact. 27(3):171-5.

Matheny, C. J., Lamb, M. W., Brouwer, K. L. R. & Pollack, G. M. (2001). Pharmacokinetic and pharmacodynamic implications of P-glycoprotein modulation. Pharmacotherapy. 21(7). Retrieved August 4, 2011, from http://www.medscape.com/viewarticle/409741_4.

McKinley, M. & O'Loughlin, V. D. (2006). Human anatomy. New York: McGraw-Hill.

McRae, S. (1996). Elevated serum digoxin levels in a patient taking digoxin and Siberian ginseng. Canadian Medical Association Journal. 155(3):293-5.

Miller, L. G. (1998). Herbal medicinals: selected clinical considerations focusing on known or potential drug-herb interactions. Arch. Intern. Med. 158(20):2200-11.

Mills, S. & Bone, K. (2000). Principles and practice of phytotherapy. Edinburgh: Churchill Livingstone.

Mycek, M. J., Harvey, R. A. & Champe, P. C. (2000). Lippincott's illustrated reviews: Pharmacology (2nd ed.). Philadelphia: Lippincott, Williams & Wilkins.

Nagababu, E. & Lakshmaiah, N. (1994, Apr). Inhibition of microsomal lipid peroxidation and monooxygenase activities by eugenol. Free Radic. Res. 20(4):253-66.

National Institute of Health. (2002, May). Seventh report of the Joint National Committee on Prevention, Detection, Evaluation, and Treatment of High Blood Pressure (JNC 7). Retrieved October 15, 2013, from http://www.nhlbi.nih.gov/guidelines/hypertension/phycard.pdf.

National Institute of Neurological Disorders and Stroke. (2006). NINDS Lennox-Gastaut syndrome information page. Retrieved May 27, 2006, from http://www.ninds.nih.gov/disorders/lennoxgastautsyndrome/lennoxgastautsyndrome.htm

Nieminen, T. H., Hagelberg, N. M., Saari, T. I., Neuvonen, M., Laine, K., Neuvonen, P. J. & Olkkola, K. T. (2010, Sep). St. John's wort greatly reduces the concentrations of oral oxycodone. Eur. J. Pain. 14(8):854-9. Retrieved January 3, 2014, from http://onlinelibrary.wiley.com/doi/10.1016/j.ejpain.2009.12.007/abstract.

Nishikawa, T., Kimura, T., Taguchi, N. & Dohi, S. (1991, Apr). Oral clonidine preanesthetic medication augments the pressor responses to intravenous ephedrine in awake or anesthetized patients. Anesthesiology. 74(4):705-10.

Nishimura, N., Naora, K., Hirano, H. & Iwamoto, K. (1999). A Chinese traditional formula, *Sho-Saiko-To (Xiao-Chai-Hu-Tang)*, reduces bioavailability of tol-butamide after oral administration in rats. Am. J. Chin. Med. 27(3-4):355-63.

Nishiyama, N., Zhou, Y., Takashina, K. & Saito, H. (1994, Nov). Effects of DX-9386, a traditional Chinese preparation, on passive and active avoidance performances in mice. Biol. Pharm. Bull. (11):1472-6.

Norred, C. L. & Brinker, F. (2001, Nov-Dec). Potential coagulation effects of preoperative complementary and alternative medicines. Altern. Ther. Health Med. 7(6):58-67.

North Carolina Board of Pharmacy (n.d.). Pharmacist FAQs. Retrieved December 31, 2012, from http://www.ncbop.org/faqs/Pharmacist/faq_NTIDrugs.htm.

Oesterheld, J. (n.d.). P-gp (ABCB1) Introduction. Retrieved August 4, 2011, from http://www.genemedrx.com/PGP_Introduction.php.

Page, R. L. & Lawrence, J. D. (1999, Jul). Potentiation of warfarin by *Dong Quai*. Pharmacotherapy. 19(7):870-6.

Pao, L. H., Hu, O. Y., Fan, H. Y., Lin, C. C., Liu, L. C. & Huang, P. W. (2012). Herb-drug interaction of 50 Chinese herbal medicines on CYP3A4 activity in vitro and in vivo. Am. J. Chin. Med. 40(1):57-73.

Pavithra, B. H., Prakash, N. & Jayakumar, K. (2009, Dec). Modification of pharmacokinetics of norfloxacin following oral administration of curcumin in rabbits. J. Vet. Sci. 10(4):293-7. Retrieved January 3, 2014, from http://www.ncbi.nlm.nih.gov/pmc/articles/PMC2807264/

PBM Pharmaceuticals, Inc. (2004, Aug). Donnatal Elixir prescribing information. Retrieved August 31, 2005, from http://www.donnatal.com/donnatal/pi_elixir.asp.

PBM Pharmaceuticals, Inc. (2004, Jun). Donnatal Extentabs prescribing information. Retrieved August 31, 2005, from http://www.donnatal.com/donnatal/pi_extentabs.asp.

PDRhealth. (n.d.). Atarax. Retrieved September 1, 2005, from http://www.pdrhealth.com/drug_info/rxdrug profiles/drugs/ata1035.shtml.

Phillips, B., Ball, C., Sackett, D., Badenoch, D., Straus, S., Haynes, B. & Dawes, M. (2001). Levels of evidence and grades of recommendation. Centre for Evidence-Based Medicine. Retrieved May 10, 2006, from http://www.cebm.net/levels_of_evidence.asp.

Physicians Desk Reference (59th ed.). (2005). Montvale, NJ: Thomson PDR.

Piscitelli, S. C., Burstein, A. H., Chaitt, D., Alfaro, R. M. & Falloon, J. (2000, Feb 12). Indinavir concentrations and St.John's wort. Lancet. 355 (9203):547-8.

Piscitelli, S. C., Burstein, A. H., Welden, N., Gallicano, K. D. & Falloon, J. (2002, Jan 15). The effect of garlic supplements on the pharmacokinetics of saquinavir. Clinical Infectious Diseases. 34:234-8.

Qi, L. W., Wang, C. Z., Du, G. J., Zhang, Z. Y., Calway, T. & Yuan, C. S. (2011, Nov 1). Metabolism of ginseng and its interactions with drugs. Curr. Drug Metab. 12(9):818–22.

Richter, P. (2006). Pharmacology lecture notes. Unpublished manuscript. Pacific College of Oriental Medicine at San Diego.

Rivera, C. A., Ferro, C. L., Bursua, A. J. & Gerber, B. S. (2012, Jan 31). Probable interaction between lycium barbarum (Goji) and warfarin. Pharmacotherapy.

Robertson, S. M., Davey, R. T., Voell, J., Formentini, E., Alfaro, R. M. & Penzak, S. R. (2008). Effect of Ginkgo biloba extract on lopinavir, midazolam, and fexofenadine pharmacokinetics in healthy subjects. Curr. Med Res Opin. 24: 591-599.

Rodrigues, M., Alves, G. & Falcão, A. (2013, Jul 22). Investigating herb-drug interactions: The effect of Citrus aurantium fruit extract on the pharmacokinetics of amiodarone in rats. Food Chem. Toxicol. [Epub ahead of print].

Satoh, K., Nagaia F. & Kano, I. (2000, April). Inhibition of H+,K+-ATPase by hinesol, a major component of *Sojutsu*, by interaction with enzyme in the E1 state. Biochemical Pharmacology. 59(7):881-6.

Saw, D., Leon, C., Kolev, S. & Murray, V. (1997, Nov). Traditional remedies and food supplements, 5-year toxicological study (1991-1995). Drug Saf. 17(5):342-56.

Seidel, H. M., Ball, J. W., Dains, J. E. & Benedict, G. W. (2003). Mosby's guide to physical examination (5th ed.). St. Louis: Mosby.

Sepracor, Inc. (2005, Feb). Lunesta. Retrieved September 2, 2005, from http://www.lunesta.com/PostedApproved LabelingText.pdf.

Shen, P., Chen, D. & Zhang, G. (1998, May). Study on efficacy of Chinese kidney-tonifying recipe in male rats with osteoporosis induced by dexamethasone and its mechanism [Article in Chinese]. *Zhong Guo Zhong Xi Yi Jie He Za Zhi*. 18(5):290-2.

Shinozuka, K., Umegaki, K., Kubota, Y., Tanaka, N., Mizuno, H., Yamaguchi, J., Nakamura, K. & Kunitomo, M. (2002, Apr 26). Feeding of Ginkgo biloba extract (GBE) enhances gene expression of hepatic cytochrome P-450 and attenuates the hypotensive effect of nicardipine in rats. Life Sci. 70(23):2783-92.

Shintani, S., Murase, H., Tsukagoshi, H. & Shiigai, T. (1992). Glycyrrhizin (licorice)-induced hypokalemic myopathy: Report of 2 cases and review of the literature. Eur. Neurol. 32(1):44-51.

Silagy, C. & Neil, A. (1994). Garlic as a lipid-lowering agent: a metaanalysis. J. Royal Coll. Phys. 28(l):2-8.

Sloley, B. D., Urichuk, L. J., Morley, P., Durkin, J., Shan, J. J., Pang, P. K. T. & Coutts, R. T. (2000, Apr). Identification of kaempferol as a monoamine oxidase inhibitor and potential neuroprotectant in extracts of Ginkgo biloba leaves. Journal of Pharmacy and Pharmacology. 52(4):451-9.

Sperber, G. & Andersen-Hefner, T. (2011). Playing the game A step-by-step approach to accepting insurance as an acupuncturist. Boulder, CO: Blue Poppy Press.

Spinella, M. & Eaton, L. A. (2002, Ap). Hypomania induced by herbal and pharmaceutical psychotropic medicines following mild traumatic brain injury. Brain Injury. 16(4):359-67.

Srivastava, R., Puri, V., Srimal, R. C. & Dhawan, B. N. (1986, Apr). Effect of curcumin on platelet aggregation and vascular prostacyclin synthesis. Arzneimittelforschung. 36(4):715-7.

Steadman's Medical Dictionary [PDA software]. (2004). Philadelphia: Lippincott, Williams & Wilkins.

Stockley, I. H. (1996). Drug interactions (4th ed.). London: Pharmaceutical Press.

Tam, L. S., Chan, T. Y. K., Leung, W. K. & Critchley, J. A. J. H. (1995). Warfarin interactions with Chinese traditional medicines: *Dan Shen* and methyl salicylate medicated oil. Aust. NZ J. Med. 225:258.

Tanaka, S., Yoon, Y. H., Fukui, H., Tabata, M., Akira, T., Okano, K., Iwai, M., Iga, Y. & Yokoyama, K. (1989, Jun). Antiulcerogenic compounds isolated from Chinese cinnamon. Planta Med. 55(3):245-8.

Tankanow, R., Tamer, H. R., Streetman, D. S., Smith, S. G., Welton, J. L., Annesley, T., Aaronson, K. D. & Bleske, B. E. (2003). Interaction study between digoxin and a preparation of hawthorn (Crataegus oxyacantha). J. Clin. Pharmacol. 43:637-42.

Tatro, D. S. (Ed.). (2002). A2zDrugs (version5.1.101/2002.5.23) [Computer software]. Facts and Comparisons.

Todar, K. (2006). Todar's online textbook of bacteriology. Retrieved August 5, 2006, from http://www.textbookof bacteriology.net/.

Toubro, S., Astrup, A. V., Breum, L. & Quaade, F. (1993, Feb). Safety and efficacy of long-term treatment with ephedrine, caffeine, and an ephedrine/caffeine mixture. Int. J. Obes. Relat. Metab. Disord. 17(Suppl 1):S69-72.

Ueng, Y. F., Tsai, C. C., Lo, W. S. & Yun, C. H. (2010). Induction of hepatic cytochrome P450 by the herbal medicine Sophora flavescens extract in rats: Impact on the elimination of theophylline. Drug Metab. Pharmacokinet. 25(6):560-7. Retrieved January 7, 2014, from https://www.jstage.jst.go.jp/article/dmpk/25/6/25_DMPK-10-RG-055/_pdf.

Upton, R. (Ed.). (1999). Astragalus root. Santa Cruz: American Herbal Pharmacopoeia.

U.S. Department of Justice Drug Enforcement Administration. (2011). Drugs of Abuse 2011 Edition A DEA Resource Guide. Retrieved 01/28/2014 from http://www.justice.gov/dea/docs/drugs_of_abuse_2011.pdf.

Van Strater, A. C. & Bogers, J. P. (2012, Mar). Interaction of St. John's wort (Hypericum perforatum) with clozapine. Int. Clin. Psychopharmacol. 27(2):121-4.

Vereshchagin, I. A., Geskina, O. D. & Bukhteeva, R. R. (1982). Increasing antibiotic therapy efficacy with adaptogens in children suffering from dysentery. Antibiotiki. 27(l):65-9.

Vohora, S. B., Shah, S. A. & Dandiya, P. C. (1990, Feb). Central nervous system studies on an ethanol extract of Acorus calamus rhizomes. J. Ethnopharmacol. 28(1):53-62.

Vuksan, V., Sievenpiper, J. L., Wong, J., Xu, Z., Beljan-Zdravkovic, U., Arnason, J. T., Assinewe, V., Stavro, M. P., Jenkins, A. L., Leiter, L. A. & Francis, T. (2001, Apr). American ginseng (Panax quinquefolius l.) attenuates postprandial glycemia in a time-dependent but not dose-dependent manner in healthy individuals. American Journal of Clinical Nutrition. 73(4):753-758.

Vuksan, V., Stavro, M. P., Sievenpiper, J. L., Beljan-Zdravkovic, U., Leiter, L. A., Josse, R. G. & Xu, Z. (2000). Similar postprandial glycemic reductions with escalation of dose and administration time of American ginseng in type 2 diabetes. Care, Diabetes. 23(9:1221-1226.

Wahed, A. & Dasgupta, A. (2001, Sep). Positive and negative *in vitro* interference of Chinese medicine *Dan Shen* in serum digoxin measurement: Elimination of interference by monitoring free digoxin concentration. American Journal of Clinical Pathology. 116(3):403-8.

Wang, E. J., Li, Y., Lin, M., Chen, L., Stein, A. P., Reuhl, K. R. & Yang, C. S. (1996). Protective effects of garlic and related organosulfur compounds on acetaminophen-induced hepatotoxicity in mice. Toxicol. Appl. Pharmacol. 136:146-54.

Wanwimolruk, S., Wong, K. & Wanwimolruk, P. (2009). Variable inhibitory effect of different brands of commercial herbal supplements on human cytochrome P-450 CYP3A4. Drug Metabol. Drug Interact. 24(1):17-35.

White, H. L., Scates, P. W. & Cooper, B. R. (1996, Mar 15). Extracts of Ginkgo biloba leaves inhibit monoamine oxidase. Life Sci. 58(16):1315-21.

White, L. M., Gardner, S. F., Gurley, B. J., Marx, M. A., Wang, P. L. & Estes, M. (1997, Feb). Pharmacokinetics and cardiovascular effects of *Ma Huang* (Ephedra sinica) in normotensive adults. J. Clin. Pharmacol. 37(2):116-22.

Wichtl, M (Ed.). (1994). Herbal drugs and phytopharmaceuticals. Boca Raton, FL: CRC Press.

Wilkinson, G. R. & Beckett, A. H. (1968). Absorption, metabolism, and excretion of the ephedrines in man. I: The influence of urinary pH and urine volume output. Journal of Pharmacology and Experimental Therapeutics 162:139-147.

Xu, F., Huang, J. B., Jiang, L., Xu, J. & Mi, J. (1995). Amelioration of cyclosporin nephrotoxicity by Cordyceps sinensis in kidney-transplanted recipients. Nephrol. Dial. Transplant. 10(1):142-3.

Xu, X. & Malavé, A. (2001, May). Protective effect of berberine on cyclophosphamide-induced hemorrhagic cystitis in rats. Basic & Clinical Pharmacology & Toxicology. 88(5):232-7.

Yamahara, J., Rong, H. Q., Naitohh, Y., Kitani, T. & Fujimura, H. (1989). Inhibition of cytotoxic drug-induced vomiting in suncus by a ginger constituent. J. Ethnopharmacol. 27(3):353-5.

Yao, M., Gao, J., Li, G. Q. & Xie, Z. (2012, Nov). Quantifying four-probe metabolites in a single UPLC-MS/MS run to explore the effects of cooked rhubarb on cytochrome P450 isozymes. Bioanalysis. 4(22):2693-703.

Yi, S., Cho, J. Y., Lim, K. S., Kim, K. P., Kim, J., Kim, B. H., Hong, J. H., Jang, I. J., Shin, S. G. & Yu, K. S. (2009, Oct). Effects of Angelicae tenuissima radix, Angelicae dahuricae radix, and Scutellariae radix extracts on cytochrome P450 activities in healthy volunteers. Basic Clin. Pharmacol. Toxicol. 105(4):249-56. Retrieved December 18, 2013 from http://www.ncbi.nlm.nih.gov/pubmed/19422358?ordinalpos=1&itool=Email.EmailReport.Pubmed_ReportSelector.Pubmed_RVDocSum.

Yokooji, T., Kida, M., Mori, M., Akashi, H., Mori, N., Yoshihara, S. & Murakami, T. (2010, May). Interaction of Rhei rhizoma extract with cytochrome P450 3A and efflux transporters in rats. Pharmazie. 65(5):367-74.

Yokotani, K., Chiba, T., Sato, Y., Nakanishi, T., Murata, M. & Umegaki, K. (2013). Effect of three herbal extracts on cytochrome P450 and possibility of interaction with drugs. Shokuhin Eiseigaku Zasshi. 54(1):56-64.

Yu, C. M., Chan, J. C. N. & Sanderson, J. E. (1997). Chinese herbs and warfarin potentiation by 'Dan Shen'. J. Int. Med. 241:337-9.

Yu, C. P., Tsai, S. Y., Kao, L. J., Chao, P. D. & Hou, Y. C. (2013, May 15). A Chinese herb formula decreases the monocarboxylate transporter–mediated absorption of valproic acid in rats. Phytomedicine. 20(7):648-53.

Yuan, C. S., Wei, G., Dey, L., Karrison, T., Nahlik, L., Maleckar, S., Kasza, K., Ang-Lee, M. & Moss, J. (2004). American ginseng reduces warfarin's effect in healthy patients. Annals of Internal Medicine. 141(1):23-27.

Yuan, Y., Zhang, H., Ma, W., Sun, S., Wang, B., Zhao, L., Zhang, G. & Chai, Y. (2013, May 30). Influence of compound *Danshen* tablet on the pharmacokinetics of losartan and its metabolite EXP3174 by liquid chromatography coupled with mass spectrometry. Biomed. Chromatogr. 27(9):1219-24. Retrieved 12/2/2013 from http://www.ncbi.nlm.nih.gov/pubmed/23722257.

Yun-Choi, H. S., Kim, J. H. & Lee, J. R. (1987, Nov-Dec). Potential inhibitors of platelet aggregation from plant sources, III. J. Nat. Prod. 50(6):1059-64.

Zava, D. T., Dollbaum, C. M. & Blen, M. (1998, Mar). Estrogen and progestin bioactivity of foods, herbs, and spices. Proc. Soc. Exp. Biol. Med. 217(3):369-78.

Zhang, G., Zhu, L., Zhou, J., Tang, L., Liu, Z. & Ye, Z. (2012, Aug). Effect of Aconiti laterlis radix compatibility of Glycyrrhizae radix on CYP3A4 in vivo. *Zhongguo Zhong Yao Za Zhi*. 37(15):2206-9. Chinese.

Zhang, Z. J., Tan, Q. R., Tong, Y., Wang, X. Y., Wang, H. H., Ho, L. M., Wong, H. K., Feng, Y. B., Wang, D., Ng, R., McAlonan, G. M., Wang, C. Y. & Wong, V. T. (2011, Feb 16). An epidemiological study of concomitant use of Chinese medicine and antipsychotics in schizophrenic patients: Implication for herb-drug interaction. PLoS One. 6(2). Retrieved 12/7/2014 from http://www.ncbi.nlm.nih.gov/pmc/articles/PMC3040227/.

Zhao, X. & Li, L. (1993, Jul). Cordyceps sinensis in protection of the kidney from cyclosporine A nephrotoxicity. *Zhong Hua Yi Xue Za Zhi*. 73(7):410-2, 447.

Zhao, K. S., Mancini, C. & Doria, G. (1990, Nov-Dec). Enhancement of the immune response in mice by Astragalus membranaceus extracts. Immunopharmacol. 20(3):225-33.

Zhou, S., Chan, E., Pan, S. Q., Huang, M. & Lee, E. J. (2004, Jun). Pharmacokinetic interactions of drugs with St. John's wort. J. Psychopharmacol. 18(2):262-76.

Zhu, J. S., Halpern, G. M, & Jones, K. (1998). The scientific rediscovery of a precious ancient Chinese herbal regimen: Cordyceps sinensis—part II. J. Alt. Compl. Med. 4(4):429-57.

Zhu, M., Wong, P. Y. & Li, R. C. (1999a). Effects of Taraxacum mongolicum on the bioavailability and disposition of ciprofloxacin in rats. J. Pharm. Sci. 88(6):632-4.

Zhu, M., Wong, P. Y. K. & Li, R. C. (1999b). Influence of Sanguisorba officinalis, a mineral-rich plant drug, on the pharmacokinetics of ciprofloxacin in the rat. Journal of Antimicrobial Chemotherapy. 44(1):125-8.

Appendix C: Abbreviations

3TC: 2'-deoxy-3'-thiacytidine, lamivudine

5-FC: Flucytosine, an antifungal

5-FdUMP: 5-flurodeoxyuridine 5'-monophosphate, an active metabolite of 5-FC

5HT: 5-hydoxytriptamine, the chemical name of the neurotransmitter serotonin

6-MP: Mercaptopurine, an anticancer agent

6-TG: Thioguanine, an anticancer agent

α: Alpha

A: In DNA, adenine; in RNA, adenosine

aa: Amino acids

ABE: Acute bacterial endocarditis

ABG: Arterial blood gas

ac: *Ante cibum* (Latin), before meals

ACE: Angiotensin converting enzyme

ACEI: Angiotensin converting enzyme inhibitor

ACh: Acetylcholine, a common neurotransmitter

AChE: Acetylcholinesterase, an enzyme that breaks down acetylcholine in the synaptic cleft

ACTH: Adrenocorticotropic hormone, also known as corticotrophin

AD: Latin abbreviation for right ear, an error prone abbreviation

ADE: Adverse drug event

ADH: Antidiuretic hormone, also called vasopressin

ADHD: Attention deficit–hyperactivity disorder

ADLs: Activities of daily living

ADP: Adenosine diphosphate

ADR: Adverse drug reaction

AED: Anti-epileptic drug

AF: Atrial fibrillation

AIDS: Acquired immunodeficiency syndrome

ALK: Anaplastic lymphoma kinase

ALL: Acute lymphocytic leukemia

ALS: Amyotrophic lateral sclerosis

AMD: Age-related macular degeneration

AMI: Acute myocardial infarction

AML: Acute myelocytic leukemia

ANS: Autonomic nervous system

APL: Acute promyelocytic leukemia

ARB: Angiotensin-receptor blockers

ART: Assisted reproductive techniques/technologies

AS: Latin abbreviation for left ear, an error prone abbreviation

ASA: Acetylsalicylic acid, aspirin

ASD: Atrial septal defect

ATP: Adenosine triphosphate

AU: Latin abbreviation for both ears, an error prone abbreviation

AUC: Area under the curve

AV: Atrioventricular, refers to the AV node in the heart

AZT: 3'-azido-3'-deoxythymidine, zidovudine

β: Beta

BBB: Blood-brain barrier

BBT: Basal body temperature

BCC: Basal cell carcinoma

Bid: *Bis in die* (Latin), twice daily

BM: Bowel movement

BMR: Basal metabolic rate

BMT: Bone marrow transplant

BP: Blood pressure

BPH: Benign prostatic hypertrophy

BPM: Beats per minute

BS: Bowel sounds or breath sounds, depending on context

BUN: Blood urea nitrogen

C: Plasma concentration of a drug

C: In DNA, cytosine; in RNA, cytidine

Ca: Carcinoma/cancer

Ca2+: Calcium ions

CABG: Coronary artery bypass graft surgery

CAD: Coronary artery disease

CAM: Complementary and alternative medicine

cAMP: Cyclic AMP, or adenosine monophosphate

CAT: Computerized axial tomography

CBC: Complete blood count

CC: Chief complaint

cc: Cubic centimeters, an error prone abbreviation

CCU: Cardiac care unit

CD: Crohn's disease

cGMP: Cyclic GMP, or guanosine monophosphate

CHC: Chronic hepatitis C

CHD: Coronary heart disease

CHF: Congestive heart failure

CIC: Chronic idiopathic constipation

CIE: Chemotherapy-induced emesis

CIV: Continous intravenous (infusion)

CL: Clearance, the removal of a drug from the body

Cl-: Chlorine ions

CLL: Chronic lymphocytic leukemia

cm: centimeter

C_{max}:   Maximum plasma concentration of a drug

CML: Chronic myelocytic leukemia

CMS: Center for Medicare/Medicaid Services

CMV: Cytomegalovirus

CNS: Central nervous system

CO: Cardiac output

CoA: Coenzyme A, a cofactor in many physiological reactions

COAD: Chronic obstructive airways disease

COMT: Catechol-O-methyltransferase

COPD: Chronic obstructive pulmonary disease

COX-1:   Cyclooxygenase subtype 1

COX-2:   Cyclooxygenase subtype 2

CPAP: Continuous positive airway pressure

CPR: Cardiopulmonary resuscitation

CPT: Current procedural terminology

CR: Controlled release, a drug preparation that allows a drug to release a uniform stream to the absorption site over a relatively long period of time

CRH: Corticotropin releasing hormone

CsA: Cyclosporine

CSF: Cerebrospinal fluid

CSF: Colony-stimulating factors

Css: Steady state concentration of a drug

CT: Computerized tomography

CTCL: Cutaneous T-cell lymphoma

CVA: Cerebral vascular accident

CXR: Chest X-ray

CYP: Cytochrome P450

CYP3A4:   The most relevant cytochrome P450 subtype for drug-drug and drug-herb interactions

D: Total amount of drug in the body (not in the blood)

d4T: Stavudine

D & C: Dilation and curettage (of the uterus)

DA: Dopamine, a neurotransmitter

DAG: Diacylglycerol

DCIS: Ductal carcinoma in situ, a form of breast cancer

ddC: Dideoxycytidine, zalcitabine

ddI: Dideoxyinosine, didanosine

DEA: Drug Enforcement Administration

DHFR: Dihydrofolate reductase, the enzyme responsible for converting folic acid to the active form, tetrahydrofolate

DHODH: Dihydroorotate dehydrogenase, an enzyme necessary for production of UMP

DHT: 5-dihydrotestosterone

DI: Diabetes insipidus

DIC: Disseminated intravascular coagulation

DIP: Distal interphalangeal

DMARD: Disease-modifying antirheumatic drug

DNA: Deoxyribonucleic acid, the basic building block of our genes

DOB: Date of birth

DOT: Directly observed therapy

DVT: Deep-vein thrombosis

Dx: Diagnosis

EBV: Epstein-Barr virus

EC: Enteric coated, a coating on a drug that allows it to pass through the stomach without breaking down, only releasing the medicine in the intestines

EC50:   The concentration of the drug when it has achieved 50% of the maximum effect of the drug; the potency of the drug

ECG: Electrocardiogram

ED: Erectile dysfunction

ED50:   The drug dose that produces a therapeutic effect in 50% of the population

EE: Erosive esophagitis

EEG: Electroencephalogram

EGFR: Epidermal growth factor receptor

EHR: Electronic health-care records

EKG: Electrocardiogram

E_{max}:   The maximal effect of a drug

EMG: Electromyogram

EMR: Electronic medical records

ENL: Erythema nodosum leprosum

EPS: Extrapyramidal symptoms

EPSP: Excitatory postsynaptic potential, an event that increases the likelihood of an action potential in the neuron after a synapse

ER: Extended release, a drug formulation that allows release of the drug over time

ESR: Erythrocyte sedimentation rate

FAP: Familial adenomatous polyposis

FDA: Food and Drug Administration

FH: Family history

FH2:   Dihydrofolate

FH4:   Tetrahydrofolate, the active form of the vitamin folic acid

FK506:   Tacrolimus, an immunosuppressive agent

FKBP: FK binding protein

FOM: Floor of mouth

FSH: Follicle stimulating hormone

FT4:   Free thyroxine

FUO: Fever of unknown origin

γ: Gamma

g: Gram

G: In DNA, guanine; in RNA, guanosine

GABA: Gamma-aminobutyric acid, a neurotransmitter

GAD: Generalized anxiety disorder

GDP: Guanosine diphosphate

GERD: Gastroesophageal reflux disease

GFR: Glomerular filtration rate

GH: Growth hormone

GI: Gastrointestinal

GIFT: Gamete intrafallopian tube transfer

GMP: Guanosine monophosphate

GnRH: Gonadotropin-releasing hormone, a pituitary hormone that stimulates release of gonadotropins

GP: Glycoprotein

GTP: Guanosine triphosphate, an energy molecule similar to ATP, also used in forming DNA and RNA

GTT: Glucose tolerance test

GU: Genitourinary

GVHD: graft-versus-host disease

Gyn: Gynecology

HAART: Highly active antiretroviral therapy

HbS: Sickle cell hemoglobin variant

HBV: Hepatitis B virus

HCTZ: Hydrochlorothiazide, error prone abbreviation, should not be used

HCV: Hepatitis C virus

HDL: High-density lipoprotein, the "good" cholesterol

HER2: human epidermal growth factor receptor 2 protein

Hg: Mercury

HIV: Human immunodeficiency virus

HMG: 3-hydroxy-3-methylglutarate, a precursor of cholesterol

HMO: Health maintenance organization

HPV: Human papilloma virus

HR: Heart rate

HRT: Hormone replacement therapy

HS: Half-strength, an error prone abbreviation

HSV: Herpes simplex virus

HSV-1: Herpes simplex virus type 1

HSV-2: Herpes simplex virus type 2

HUS: Hemolytic uremic syndrome

Hx: History

IBD: Inflammatory bowel disease, includes Crohn's disease and ulcerative colitis

IBS: Irritable bowel syndrome

ICD: International classification of disease

IDDM: Insulin-dependent diabetes mellitus (no longer used)

IFN: Interferon, a immune system cytokine

IL: Interleukin, a immune system cytokine

IM: Intramuscular, an injection given into a muscle

IMP: Inosine monophosphate

INH: Isoniazid, also known as isonicotinic acid hydrazide

INR: International normalized ratio

IOP: Intraocular pressure

IP3: Inositol-1, 4, 5-triphosphate system, a second messenger system used to amplify intracellular actions

IPSP: Inhibitory postsynaptic potential, an event that reduces the likelihood of an action potential in the neuron after a synapse

ISMP: Institute for Safe Medication Practices

IT: Intrathecal, within the cerebrospinal space of the spinal cord

ITP: Idiopathic thrombocytopenia purpura

IU: International unit, an error prone abbreviation, can be interpreted as IV

IUCD: Intrauterine contraceptive device

IUD: Intrauterine device

IV: Intravenous

IVC: Inferior vena cava

IVF: In vitro fertilization

IVPB: Intravenous piggyback

JIA: Juvenile idiopathic arthritis

JRA: Juvenile rheumatoid arthritis

K+: Potassium ions

K_d: Describes the affinity of a drug for its receptor

Ke: A rate constant for drug elimination from the total body

kg: Kilogram, 1,000 grams, or approximately 2.2 pounds

KS: Kaposi's sarcoma

L: Left

L: Liter

LABA: Long-acting beta$_2$-agonist

lb: *Libra pondo* (Latin), abbreviation for a pound in weight

LDL: Low density lipoprotein, the "bad" cholesterol

LFT: Liver function tests

LH: Luteinizing hormone

Li+: Lithium ions

LLQ: Left lower quadrant (of the abdomen)

LOC: Loss of consciousness

LPS: Lipopolysaccharide, present in Gram-negative bacteria

LRTI: Lower respiratory tract infection

LSD: Lysergic acid diethylamide, a hallucinogen

LTBI: Latent tuberculosis infection

LUQ: Left upper quadrant (of the abdomen)

LVD: Left ventricular dysfunction

LVF: Left ventricular failure

Mane: (Latin) in the morning

MBC: Minimum bactericidal concentration,;in other words, at what concentration a drug kills an organism

Mg+: Magnesium ions

MAO: Monoamine oxidase

MAOI: Monoamine oxidase inhibitor

mcg: Microgram, 1/1,000,000 of a gram; for safety reasons, this abbreviation should not be used

MD: Medical doctor

MDR: Multidrug resistance

MDS: Myelodysplastic syndrome

mg: Milligram, 1/1,000 of a gram

MG: Myasthenia gravis

MI: Myocardial infarction, a heart attack

MIC: Minimum inhibitory concentration; in other words, at what concentration a drug stops growth of an organism

MPA: Mycophenolic acid

MPA: microscopic polyangitis

MRI: Magnetic resonance imaging

mRNA: Messenger RNA, the basic template used to create proteins

MRSA: Methicillin-resistant Staphylococcus aureus, a serious bacterial infection that is highly resistant to antibiotic therapy

MRSE: Methicillin-resistant Staphylococcus epidermidis, a serious bacterial infection that is highly resistant to antibiotic therapy

MS: Multiple sclerosis

MSU: Midstream urine

MTC: Medullary thyroid cancer

mTOR: Mammalian target of rapamycin

MTX: Methotrexate

MVA: Motor vehicle accident

Na+: Sodium ions

NAD: No abnormality detected

NAION: Non-arteritic ischemic optic neuropathy

NE: Norepinephrine

NFATc: Cytosolic nuclear factor of activated T-cells

NIDDM: Non-insulin-dependent diabetes mellitus (no longer used)

NK: Natural killer cells, part of the immune system

NMDA: N-methyl-D-aspartate

NMS: Neuroleptic malignant syndrome

NO: Niric oxide

Nocte: (Latin), at night/bedtime

NNRTI: Non-nucleoside reverse transcriptase inhibitor, a class of antivirals

NOF: Neck of femur

NPO: Nil (none) by oral

NRTI: Nucleoside reverse transcriptase inhibitor, a class of antivirals

NSAID: Non-steroidal anti-inflammatory drug, *e.g.,* aspirin

NTG: Normal tension glaucoma

NV: Nausea and vomiting

OA: Osteoarthritis

Obs: Obstetrics

OCD: Obsessive-compulsive disorder

OCP: Oral contraceptive pills

OD: Latin abbreviation for right eye

OHSS: Ovarian hyperstimulation syndrome

OS: Latin abbreviation for left eye

OSA: Obstructive sleep apnea

OSAHS: Obstructive sleep apnea/hypopnea syndrome

OTC: Over the counter

OU: Latin abbreviation for both eyes

PABA: p-Aminobenzoic acid, important in folic acid synthesis in bacteria

PAH: Pulmonary arterial hypertension

PAP: Papanicolaou smear

PAT: Paroxysmal atrial tachycardia

PBP: Penicillin-binding proteins

pc: *Post cibum* (Latin), after meals

PCP: Phencyclidine, illicit drug commonly known as "angel dust"

PCP: Pneumocystis carinii pneumonia

PCP: Primary care physician

PDE: Phosphodiesterase enzyme

PE: Phenytoin sodium equivalents

PE: Pulmonary embolism

PGE: Prostaglandin E_2

pH: Inverse log of the concentration of hydrogen ions

PH: Past history

PHN: Postherpetic neuralgia

PHS: Public Health Service

PI: Protease inhibitor, a class of antivirals

PID: Pelvic inflammatory disease

PIP: Proximal interphalangeal

pKa: The inverse log of the acid constant

PMDD: Premenstrual dysphoric disorder

PML: Progressive multifocal leukoencephalopathy

PMS: Practice management software

PMS: Premenstrual syndrome

PNS: Peripheral nervous system

PO: *Per os* (Latin), by mouth

POAG: Primary open-angle glaucoma

PONV: Postoperative nausea and vomiting

PP: Postprandial (after meals)

PPAR: Peroxisome proliferator-activated receptor

PPO: Preferred provider organization

PR:	Rectally
PRN:	*Pro re nata* (Latin), as needed
PSCC:	Polysystemic chronic candidiasis
PSE:	Portal systemic encephalopathy
Pt:	Patient
PT:	Prothrombin time
PTCA:	Percutaneous transluminal coronary angioplasty
PTCL:	Peripheral T-cell lymphoma
PTP:	Primary treating physician
PTSD:	Post-traumatic stress disorder
PV:	Per vagina
PVC:	Premature ventricular contraction
PVD:	Peripheral vascular disease
q:	*Quaque* (Latin), every; for safety reasons, this abbreviation should not be used
q6h:	Every 6 hours
q8h:	Every 8 hours
Qd	*Quaque die* (Latin), every day; for safety reasons, this abbreviation should not be used
Qid:	*Quater in die* (Latin), four times per day
QME:	Qualified medical examiner
Qod:	Every other day; for safety reasons, this abbreviation should not be used
R:	Right
RA:	Rheumatoid arthritis
RBC:	Red blood cell
RCC:	Renal cell cancer
RF:	Rheumatoid factor
RHF:	Right heart failure
RLQ:	Right lower quadrant (of abdomen)
RLS:	Restless legs syndrome
RNA:	Ribonucleic acid, used in translating DNA to proteins
rRNA:	Ribosomal RNA, a specific type of RNA that is part of the structure of ribosomes, which produce proteins in the cell
ROM:	Range of motion
RSV:	Respiratory syncytial virus
RTI:	Reverse transcriptase inhibitor, a class of antivirals
RUQ:	Right upper quadrant (of abdomen)
Rx:	Prescription
SA:	Sinoatrial, refers to the SA node in the heart
SAARD:	Slow-acting antirheumatic drug
SAD:	Seasonal affective disorder
sALCL:	Systemic anaplastic large-cell lymphoma
SC:	Subcutaneous, an error prone abbreviation
SCC:	Squamous cell carcinoma
SERM:	Selective estrogen receptor modulators
SIADH:	Syndrome of inappropriate antidiuretic hormone secretion
SL:	Sublingually
SLE:	Systemic lupus erythematosus
SNRI:	Serotonin and norepinephrine reuptake inhibitor
SOAP:	Subjective, objective, assessment, and plan
SOAPE:	Subjective, objective, assessment, plan, and education
SOB:	Shortness of breath
SOC:	Standards of care
SQ:	Subcutaneous; for safety reasons, this abbreviation should not be used
SR:	Sustained release
SRL:	Sirolimus, an immunosuppressant drug
s/s:	Signs and symptoms
SSRI:	Selective serotonin reuptake inhibitor
STD:	Sexually transmitted disease
STI:	Sexually transmitted infection
SubQ:	Subcutaneous injection
SV:	Cardiac stroke volume
SVC:	Superior vena cava
SVF:	Supraventricular fibrillation
SVT:	Supraventricular tachycardia
SWSD:	Shift work sleep disorder
Sx:	Symptom
T:	In DNA, thymine; in RNA, thymidine
$t_{1/2}$:	Half-life
T3:	Triiodothyronine, one of the endogenous thyroid hormones
T4:	Thyroxine, one of the endogenous thyroid hormones
TAC:	Tacrolimus, an immunosuppressive agent
TB:	Tuberculosis, caused by Mycobacterium tuberculosis
TCA:	Tricyclic antidepressant
TD50:	The drug dose that produces toxic effects in 50% of the population
TFT:	Thyroid function tests
TGMP:	Thioguanosine monophosphate
TH:	Thyroid hormone refers to a class of hormones that are the major effectors of thyroid function
THC:	Tetrahydrocannabinol, the active ingredient in marijuana
TI:	Therapeutic index
TIA:	Transient ischemic attack
Tid:	*Ter in die* (Latin), three times a day
TIMP:	6-thioinosinic acid or 6-mercaptopurine-ribose-phosphate, the active form of anticancer agent mercaptopurine
TIW:	Three times a week, an error prone abbreviation
TLC:	Total lung capacity
TMP:	Thymine monophosphate

TNF:	Tumor necrosis factor, an immune system cytokine	Ung:	*Unguentum* (Latin), ointment
TOP:	Topically	URTI:	Upper respiratory tract infection
TPR:	Total peripheral resistance	UTI:	Urinary tract infection
TRH:	Thyroid releasing hormone	VAS:	Visual acuity scale
tRNA:	Transfer RNA, used to bring individual amino acids to the ribosome to produce proteins	Vd:	Volume of distribution
		VF:	Ventricular fibrillation
		VLDL:	Very low-density lipoprotein, the "very bad" cholesterol
TSH:	Thyroid stimulating hormone		
TSS:	Toxic shock syndrome	VP-16:	Etoposide, an anticancer agent
TTP:	Thrombotic thrombocytopenia purpura	VPB:	Ventricular premature beats
TURP:	Transurethral resection of the prostate	VRE:	Vancomycin-resistant enterococci
Tx:	Treatment	VZV:	Varicella-zoster virus
TXA2:	Thromboxane A2	WBC:	White blood cells
U:	In DNA, uracil; in RNA, uridine	WC:	Workers' compensation
UA:	Urinalysis	WNL:	Within normal limits
UC:	Ulcerative colitis, an inflammatory bowel disease	WPW:	Wolff-Parkinson-White syndrome
UMP:	Uridine 5'-monophosphate		

Appendix D: Glossary

Abortifactant: A substance that can induce the termination of a pregnancy.

Acetylcholine: A common, usually excitatory, neurotransmitter especially present in the autonomic nervous system.

Acetylsalicylic acid (ASA): Aspirin.

Acidosis: Abnormal increase in the amount of hydrogen ions in the body.

Active transport: The transport of a drug across a cell membrane by using a transport protein that takes energy, usually in the form of adenosine triphosphate (ATP). P-glycoprotein is a common example of this.

Adenocarcinoma: A cancer stemming from the epithelium of a gland.

Adenosine triphosphate (ATP): The main energy storage chemical in the body.

Adipose tissue: Connective tissue consisting of fat cells.

Adrenergic: Pertaining to nerve fibers in the SNS that react to epinephrine, norepinephrine, or dopamine neurotransmitters.

Adrenoceptors: Membrane receptors that are sensitive to adrenergic neurotransmitters such as epinephrine or norepinephrine.

Adrenocorticotropic hormone (ACTH): Stimulates release of most gluco- and mineralocorticoids from the adrenal glands. Release of this pituitary hormone is stimulated by corticotropin releasing hormone (CRH) released from the hypothalamus. Also known as corticotropin.

Agglutination: The aggregation or clumping of cells due to interaction with antibodies called agglutinins.

Agonist: Substance that mimics the effects of endogenous compounds.

Agranulocytosis: The extreme reduction in the number of leukocytes, or white blood cells, in the blood.

Akathisia: The inability to remain seated; includes motor restlessness and a feeling of muscle twitching; may be a side effect of antipsychotic medication.

Akinesia: Difficulty in initiating movement, a common symptom of Parkinson's disease.

Albuminuria: Abnormal presence of albumin and possibly other proteins in the urine.

Alkylation: To add a chemical group to another molecule.

Allosteric: Agents that act at sites on the receptor that are different from and do not interfere with active sites for endogenous molecules. See non-competitive binding.

Alopecia: Partial or complete hair loss.

Amines: Any molecule that includes the element nitrogen.

Amyotrophic lateral sclerosis: Also known as Lou Gehrig's disease, it is a progressive degeneration of motor neurons that eventually causes paralysis and death.

Anabolism: Biological processes that primarily build up large compounds from smaller chemicals.

Anaerobic: Able to grow and function without oxygen.

Analgesic: A drug that relieves pain.

Analog: A drug or other chemical that is similar in structure or constituents to another but differs in effects.

Anaphylaxis: A severe and occasionally fatal hypersensitivity/allergic reaction to an antigen; symptoms often include respiratory distress, vascular collapse, and severe skin rashes.

Anaplasia: A condition where a cell changes its structure into a less differentiated, more primitive form; generally seen in malignancies.

Anesthetic: A drug that reversibly decreases nerve function and causes loss of ability to perceive pain and/or other sensations.

Angioedema: Large circumscribed area of subcutaneous edema of sudden onset frequently caused by an allergic reaction.

Angiotensin converting enzyme: An enzyme in the renin-angiotensin-aldosterone hormone cascade that converts angiotensin I to angiotensin II. Inhibitors of this enzyme are prime drugs in treating hypertension.

Anhedonia: Inability to feel pleasure or happiness from activities that would normally provide such feelings.

Anorexia: Lack or loss of appetite.

Anorexiant: An appetite suppressor.

Anorgasmia: Inability to have an orgasm.

Antagonist: Interference of one chemical with the action of another.

Anterograde amnesia: Loss of memory of events after the trauma, disease, or agent is consumed.

Antiarrhythmic: An agent that counteracts an arrhythmia or abnormal heartbeat rhythm.

Antidiuretic hormone (ADH): A hormone produced by the hypothalamus, stored in the posterior lobe of the pituitary gland and released in response to decreased blood volume or increased sodium concentration or other blood constituents; causes increased reabsorption of water in the renal tubules; also called vaso-pressin.

Antiemetic: An agent that suppresses nausea and vomiting.

Antihelminthics: Agents used to treat worm infections.

Antimuscarinic agents: A class of anticholinergics that act on acetylcholine receptors that are responsive to muscarine.

Antineoplastic agents: Drugs used to treat cancer.

Antipyretic: A substance that reduces fever.

Antitussive: A cough suppressant.

Anxiolytic: Means "splitting anxiety"; agents used to treat anxiety and similar disorders.

Aplastic anemia: A blood disorder characterized by deficiency of all formed elements of the blood; indicates a failure of the bone marrow's ability to generate cells.

Apnea: Absence of breathing.

Apoptosis: Programmed cell death.

Area under the curve (AUC): A measurement of bioavailability; indicates plasma drug concentration over time.

Arrhythmias An irregular heartbeat.

Asphyxia: Severe hypoxia leading to loss of consciousness and death.

Asthenia: The lack or loss of strength or energy; weakness; debility.

Asystole: Non-contraction of the heart.

Ataxia: Incoordination of voluntary muscles resulting in jerky movements. May affect limbs, head, or trunk.

Atonic: Without tone.

Atrial fibrillation: A rapid, irregular atrial rhythm. It causes considerable symptoms including palpitations and occasional weakness and presyncope. Thrombi can form and embolize to the brain causing a CVA.

Atrial flutter: A rapid regular atrial rhythm due to an atrial reentrant circuit. The main symptom is palpitations. Thrombi may form and embolize.

Atrioventricular node: Part of the electrical conducting system of the heart, considered the "gateway" between the conducting system of the atria and the ventricular conducting system.

Atrophy: A wasting, loss of size, or reduction in physiological activity of a body part.

Autocoid: Chemical substance produced by one type of cell that affects different cells in the same region; a local hormone or messenger.

Autolysis: Destruction of a cell as a result of enzymes or proteins produced by the same organism.

Autoreceptors: A receptor located on a neuron, that binds a neurotransmitter from the same neuron which then regulates that neuron.

AV block: Where there is a partial or incomplete transmission of the impulse from the atria to the ventricles.

Axial: Pertaining to the central part of the body; not including the limbs.

Bactericidal agents: Drugs that kill existing bacteria.

Bacteriostatic agents: Drugs that do not decrease colony count of bacteria but prevent it from getting larger.

Barbiturates: A class of anxiolytic agents.

Basal nuclei (basal ganglia): Area of the brain that primarily aids in motor movements especially starting, stopping, and monitoring intensity of movements, especially slow or stereotyped.

Benzodiazepines: A class of anxiolytic agents.

Bioavailability: The amount of a drug that is available to act on its target site.

Blood dyscrasia: Abnormal condition of the blood.

Bolus: A dose.

Bradyarrhythmia: An arrhythmia that has an overall rate slower than 60 beats per minute (bpm).

Bradycardia: A heart rate that is too slow, defined as less than 60 bpm.

Bradykinesia: Slow movement, a common symptom of Parkinson's disease.

Bradykinin: A chain of 9 amino acids that causes histamine-like effects such as vasodilation, contraction of non-vascular smooth muscle, and an increase in capillary permeability.

Bronchoconstriction: A decrease in the diameter of the lungs' bronchi causing less airflow.

Bronchodilation: Relaxation and an increase in the diameter of the lung's bronchi allowing for more airflow.

Bronchospasm: A muscle spasm causing narrowing of the airways of the lung, usually accompanied by a cough and wheezing.

Buffalo hump: An accumulation of fat on the back of the neck caused by high doses of glucocorticoids or Cushing's syndrome.

C: Plasma concentration of a drug.

Cachexia: Severe weight loss and weakness due to serious disease.

Calculus: An abnormal stone formed in body tissues by accumulation of mineral salts; plural: calculi.

Capsid: The layer of protein encapsulating a virus.

Cardiac output: The volume of blood ejected by contraction of the ventricles of the heart.

Cardiogenic shock: A condition where the heart cannot pump adequate blood to the body due to damaged ventricles often associated with a myocardial infarction.

Cardiomegaly: An enlarged heart.

Catabolism: Biological processes that primarily break down large storage and other chemicals, often releasing energy in the process.

Catechol-o-methyltransferase (COMT): An enzyme that breaks down catecholamines such as norepinephrine and epinephrine especially in the synaptic cleft.

Catecholamines: Sympathomimetic neurotransmitter family that includes epinephrine, norepinephrine, and dopamine.

Cestodes: "True tapeworms" that are flat, have a segmented body, and generally attach to the host's intestines.

Chelator: A substance that binds with chemicals so that they can be more easily excreted.

Chemoattractant: A chemical that influences the migration of cells.

Cholelithiasis: The presence of gallstones.

Cholestatis: An interruption in the flow of bile at any point in the biliary system from liver to duodenum.

Chorea: An abnormal involuntary movement disorder usually like quick movements of the hand and feet that resemble dancing.

Cinchonism: A condition characterized by deafness, headache, tinnitus, and cerebral congestion.

Circumoral: Around the mouth.

CL: Clearance describes the removal of a drug from the body.

Class I drugs: Drugs where the dose is less than albumin's capacity to bind.

Class II drugs: Drugs given in doses that are much greater than the ability of albumin to bind them.

Clonic convulsion: A convulsion characterized by rhythmic alternating contractions and relaxations of muscle groups.

C_{max}: Maximum plasma concentration of a drug.

Cogwheel rigidity: Muscle rigidity that appears to stop and start, a common symptom of Parkinson's disease.

Colitis: An inflammatory condition of the large intestine.

Competitive binding: Where an agent competes with an endogenous substance for the active binding site of the receptor and the ability to exert an action.

Coomb's test: A test for antibodies damaging red blood cells,;may indicate many blood diseases.

Cor pulmonale: Damage to the heart and lungs due to a pathology in the pulmonary circulation.

Corpus striatum: See striatum.

Corticotropin: See adrenocorticotropic hormone.

Corticotropin releasing hormone (CRH): A hormone released from the hypothalamus that causes secretion of adrenocorticotropic hormone (ACTH), also known as corticotropin, which in turn stimulates the release of most gluco- and mineralocorticoids from the adrenal glands.

Crystalluria: The presence of crystals in the urine.

Css: Steady state concentration of a drug. In other words, the plasma concentration where the amount of drug entering the blood equals the amount of drug removed from the blood by elimination mechanisms.

Cyclothymic disorder: Involves numerous alternating episodes of hypomaniac and depressive symptoms.

Cyst: In the context of protozoa, a dormant phase wherein the organism is non-motile and is highly resistant to environmental extremes and treatment.

Cystinuria: The abnormal presence of the amino acid cystine in the urine.

Cystitis: Inflammation and/or infection of the urinary bladder and ureters.

Cytochrome P450 system: System involved in metabolizing endogenous compounds and exogenous toxins.

Cytosol: A synonym for cytoplasm, what is inside the cell.

D: Total amount of drug in the body (not in the blood).

Defibrillation: Reversal of ventricular fibrillation by applying an electric shock to the heart.

Delusion: A false belief or wrong judgment held with conviction despite overwhelming evidence to the contrary.

Dependence: The psychological and physical need for a substance.

Depolarization: The state where a neuron's membrane is more electrically positive than normal and therefore closer to initiating an action potential.

Dermatitis: Inflammation of the skin.

Detrussor: Pertaining to the detrussor urinae muscle, which forms the external muscle layer of the bladder.

Diabetes insipidus: A disease defined by excretion of large amounts of dilute urine due to the kidney's inability to concentrate it. While there are several types, the most common by far is a problem with the posterior pituitary and deficiency of antidiuretic hormone; also known as vasopressin.

Diaphoresis: The act of perspiring or sweating.

Dynorphins: A member of a group of endogenous neurochemicals which includes endorphins and enkephalins that have morphine-like effects on the body .

Dyskinesia: Impairment or inability to execute voluntary movements.

Dopamine: A neurotransmitter that is primarily sympathomimetic. The main pathology of Parkinson's disease is a lack of this neurotransmitter.

Dopamine-receptor agonists: A class of drugs generally used in the treatment of Parkinson's disease.

Down-regulation: Less synthesis of a protein because the DNA is not being transcribed as frequently, or, more generally, the inhibition of a particular biological function.

Drug fever: A fever associated with the use of a drug. This can be caused by an immune reaction, the inherent effects of the drug, or a complication.

Dysarthria: A disturbance of speech and language caused by a brain injury or inability of the speech muscles to perform.

Dysgeusia: An alteration or loss of taste.

Dysphonia: Any disorder affecting voice quality or the ability to produce voice.

Dysphoria: A disorder of mood characterized by depression and anguish.

Dyspnea: Shortness of breath or difficulty breathing.

Dysuria: Painful urination.

Eaton-Lambert syndrome: A form of muscle weakness that tends to be associated with lung cancer.

EC_{50}: The concentration of the drug when it has achieved 50% of its maximum effect; the potency of the drug.

Ectopic supraventricular rhythms: Where cells in the atria become pacemaker-like cells causing a discharge similar to the SA node that triggers an extra heartbeat. Many are asymptomatic and require no intervention.

ED_{50}: The drug dose that produces a therapeutic effect in 50% of the population.

Efficacy: The maximal effect of a drug. See E_{max}.

E_{max}: The maximal effect of a drug.

Emesis: Vomiting.

Emetogenic: Causes nausea and vomiting.

Emulsify: To disperse a liquid into another liquid.

Encephalopathy: Pathology of the structure or tissues of the brain.

Endocytosis: A method of transporting a large molecule to the cell interior where the cell engulfs the substance and transports it into the cell by pinching off the cell membrane and creating a vesicle.

Endogenous: Originating from within the body.

Endorphins: Morphine-like pain-relieving chemicals produced naturally within the body.

Enkephalins: A neurochemical that activates opiate receptors and increases the threshold of pain.

Enteral: Of the intestines, drugs that are oral or rectal in administration.

Enteric nervous system: A semiautonomous system of nerves located within the digestive system; while a separate system from the CNS and ANS, it can still receive modifying input from these systems. Two plexuses primarily constitute this system: the submucosal nerve plexus and the myenteric nerve plexus.

Enterocolitis: An inflammatory condition of both the small and large intestines.

Eosinophils: A type of leukocyte that stains yellow-red or orange with Wright stain; they are motile phagocytes with antiparasitic function; they also may play a role in allergies.

Epinephrine: A neurotransmitter and hormone that stimulates the sympathetic nervous system.

Erythema: Redness or inflammation of the skin.

Erythema multiforme: A hypersensitivity reaction characterized by skin and mucous membrane eruptions.

Erythema nodosum leprosum (ENL): A systemic inflammatory complication of leprosy that manifests as painful papules or nodules that may pustulate and ulcer and may produce, among many manifestations, fever and arthritis.

Erythrocytes: Red blood cells.

Esophagitis: Inflammation of the esophagus.

Ethanol: Scientific name for drinking alcohol.

Euthyroid: A thyroid gland that is functioning within normal limits; not hypo- or hyperthyroid.

Excipients: Additives to a drug formulation that affect the bulk, delivery, or availability of a drug. They are biologically inert.

Excitatory postsynaptic potential: An increase of voltage that increases the likelihood of an action potential and a nerve impulse.

Exocytosis: A method of transporting a large molecule or numerous molecules from the interior of a cell to the exterior by allowing a vesicle to merge with the cell membrane and spilling its contents.

Expectorants: An agent that acts by loosening mucous in the lungs for easier expulsion.

Extrapyramidal symptoms: Exhibiting movement disorders, especially postural and locomotor, resembling Parkinson's disease.

Facilitated diffusion: A method of transporting a substance into a cell by using a carrier protein in the cell membrane. It does not require energy in order to produce this effect.

Fasciculations: Involuntary twitchings of muscle fibers.

Feedback inhibition: Where an intermediate or final product of a biological pathway stops or slows down one of the initiating steps and eventually reduces the end results of that pathway.

Festination: Tendency to fall when the center of gravity is displaced, a common symptom of Parkinson's disease.

Fetal hydantoin syndrome: A rare disorder caused by fetal exposure to phenytoin. Symptoms include skull and facial abnormalities, underdevelopment of the nails and overall growth, mild developmental delays, and possibly a cleft lip and palate.

Fibrillation: Recurrent, abnormal muscle contraction that is not physiologically useful.

Fibrosis: An abnormal proliferation of fibrous connective tissue.

Flight of ideas: Streams of ideas and unrelated words that

occur at a rate faster than the patient's ability to speak them.

Functional antagonist: The appearance that an agent has antagonistic effects on one receptor while it actually agonizes a different receptor.

Galactorrhea: Abnormal production and secretion of milk from the beasts or any white discharge from the nipple.

Gamma-aminobutyric acid (GABA): A common inhibitory neurotransmitter.

Ganglion: A collection of nerve cells outside of the CNS.

Gastrins: Hormones secreted in the mucosa of the stomach that stimulate hydrochloric acid secretion.

Genotype: The complete genetic makeup of an organism.

Glaucoma: A condition of the eye where the intraocular pressure (pressure within the eye) rises and threatens blindness.

Glossitis: Inflammation of the tongue.

Glucagon: A pancreatic hormone that causes the break down of glycogen and elevates serum glucose levels.

Glutamate: An amino acid and neurotransmitter.

Glycine: A common inhibitory neurotransmitter.

Glycogenolysis: Splitting of glycogen to release glucose.

Glycosuria: An abnormal increase of glucose in the urine.

Glucocorticoids: Hormones produced in the zona fasciculata of the adrenal gland that are used in regular body metabolism and stress reactions; cortisol is the prime example.

Gluconeogenesis: The formation of glycogen, a glucose-storing compound, from fatty acids and proteins rather than carbohydrates.

Goiter: An enlarged thyroid gland. The gland may be hypo-, hyper-, or euthyroid.

Gram stain: This is a histological stain that shows if there are lipopolysaccharides surrounding the cell wall of a bacteria; generally, Gram-negative bacteria are more difficult to treat than Gram-positive bacteria.

Granulocyte: A form of white blood cells with granules in their cytoplasm; these include basophils, eosinophils, and neutrophils.

Granulocytopenia: An abnormal blood condition where there is a decrease in the number of granulocytes, white blood cells with granules in their cytoplasm.

Gynecomastia: An abnormal enlargement of one or two breasts in men.

Half-life ($t_{1/2}$): The time needed to decrease the plasma concentration of a drug by half.

Hematuria: Abnormal presence of blood in the urine.

Hemolysis: The breakdown of red blood cells and the release of hemoglobin.

Hemolytic anemia: An anemia, or loss of hemoglobin, characterized by red blood cell destruction.

Hepatic: Pertaining to the liver.

Hepatic portal system: A vascular bed that runs from the capillary bed surrounding the small intestine and includes the hepatic capillary beds.

Hepatomegaly: Abnormal enlargement of the liver.

Hepatotoxic: Toxic to the liver.

Herxheimer reactions: Also called "die-off reactions," they are a type of toxic reaction due to microbial die-off induced by correct medication.

Hirsutism: Excessive body hair in a masculine distribution.

Histology: The science dealing with the microscopic identification of cells, microbes, and tissues.

Huntington's disease: A genetic disease causing degeneration of the nerves affecting muscle coordination and eventual cognitive decline and psychiatric problems leading to a reduced life span. Chorea is one hallmark sign.

Hydrophilic: Chemicals that prefer to be in an aqueous solution rather than a fat- or oil-based solution.

Hydrophobic: Chemicals that prefer to be in a fat- or oil-based solution rather than an aqueous solution.

Hydroxyapatite: A chemical made of calcium, phosphate, and hydroxide that forms a lattice-like structure that helps bones and teeth become rigid.

Hyperbilirubinemia: A condition of too much of the bile pigment bilirubin in the blood.

Hypercalcemia: Too much calcium in the blood.

Hypercalciuria: Too much calcium in the urine.

Hyperglycemia: Too much glucose in the blood.

Hyperkalemia: Too much potassium in the blood.

Hyperplasia: An increase in the number of cells of a given body part.

Hyperpolarization: The state where a neuron's membrane is more electrically negative than normal, and therefore it is much more difficult to initiate an action potential.

Hyperpyrexia: Very high fever.

Hypersensitivity: An abnormal reaction to a stimulus; an allergy or allergic reaction.

Hypertensive crisis: A sudden, severe, life-threatening increase in blood pressure.

Hypertriglyceridemia: Abnormally high amounts of triglycerides in the blood.

Hyperuricemia: A condition of increased uric acid in the blood; associated with gout.

Hypnotic: A class of drugs that help people sleep.

Hypoglycemia: Too little glucose in the blood.

Hypogonadism: A lack of secretion of sex hormones from the testes or ovaries.

Hypokalemia: Too little potassium in the blood.

Hypokinesia: Decreased movement, a common symptom of Parkinson's disease.

Hypomania: A condition similar to mania but less severe in its symptoms.

Hypomagnesemia: Abnormally low magnesium in the blood.

Hyponatremia: Lower than normal levels of sodium in the blood.

Hypoplasia: An incomplete or underdeveloped organ or tissue usually due to a reduced number of cells.

Hypotension: Lower than normal blood pressure. Can cause light-headedness, dizziness, and fainting.

Hypovolemia: Abnormally low blood volume.

Hypoxia: A state where oxygen levels are below normal.

Iatrogenic: Caused by treatment of diagnostic procedures.

Inducer: A drug that stimulates a process.

Infarction: A sudden stoppage of blood flow that causes tissue death.

Inhibitor: A drug that interferes or prevents a process.

Inhibitory postsynaptic potential: A decrease of voltage that decreases the likelihood of an action potential and a nerve impulse.

Intercellular: Between cells.

Intermittent claudication: A condition of intermittent pain and/or cramping in the leg, especially the calf, during physical activity that most often is a symptom of peripheral arterial disease.

Interstitium: The space between cells that is filled with fluid.

Intracellular: Within the cell.

Intracranial: Within the head.

Intraocular: Within the eye.

Intraventricular administration: Administration of a drug directly into the ventricles of the brain in order to bypass the blood-brain barrier.

Ischemia: Decreased blood flow to an organ or body part, often accompanied by pain and dysfunction.

Isoenzymes: Subtypes of a specific enzyme.

K_e: A rate constant for drug elimination from the total body. In other words, it is a constant, different for each drug, that helps describe how fast a drug is eliminated from the body.

In vitro: Latin for "within glass," means an experiment done in the lab.

In vivo: Latin for "within life," means an experiment occurring in a living organism, usually human.

Junctional arrhythmia: An arrhythmia originating from the junction of the atria and ventricles.

Lennox-Gastaut syndrome: A severe form of epilepsy involving different types of seizures. Most children with this syndrome have some degree of impaired intellectual function, developmental delays, and behavioral disturbances.

Leukocytosis: An abnormal increase in the number of circulating white blood cells.

Leukopenia: A decreased number of white blood cells in the blood; defined as fewer than 5,000 cells per cubic millimeter.

Leukorrhea: White vaginal discharge.

Leukotrienes: Biological compounds that have a role in inflammation and allergic reactions.

Lipodystrophy: A problem with fat metabolism usually involving loss of adipose tissue but can also indicate abnormal accumulations. Examples include fat atrophy or buffalo hump.

Lipolysis: The splitting of a fat molecule.

Lipophilic: The opposite of hydrophobic, these are chemicals that prefer to be in a fat- or oil-based solution rather than an aqueous solution.

Lipopolysaccharides: Chemical compounds consisting of fat and multiple sugars.

Lumen: The opening or channel within an organ or other structure of the body; for example, the lumen of the intestines.

Lysis: Destruction of a cell or molecule through the action of an agent.

Macule: A flat area of skin that is less than 1 cm in diameter that has changed color.

Megaloblastic anemia: A blood disorder characterized by the production and proliferation of immature, large, and dysfunctional red blood cells, usually associated with pernicious anemia and folic acid deficiency.

Merozites: Any organisms resulting from the asexual reproduction phase of the life cycle of certain protozoa known as sporozoans.

Metabolites: Chemicals that are a result of metabolism. They can be either an intermediate product (one that will undergo further transformation) or an end product.

Metaplastic: Pertaining to an abnormal transformation of adult, fully differentiated tissue of one kind into a differentiated tissue of another kind; often cancerous or precancerous.

Methemoglobinemia: The presence in the blood of methemoglobin, a form of hemoglobin that cannot bind and transport oxygen.

Microcytic: "Small cell." Used to describe a smaller than normal cell.

Micrographia: Very small writing, a common symptom of Parkinson's disease.

Mineralocorticoids: Hormones produced by the adrenals in the zona glomerulosa that regulate water and salt metabolism and excretion.

Minimum bactericidal concentration (MBC): The minimal concentration of an agent at which bacteria are killed.

Minimum inhibitory concentration (MIC): The minimum concentration of an agent at which bacterial growth stops.

Miosis: Constriction of the pupil.

Mitosis: A type of cell division that results in two identical daughter cells.

Mobilliform rash: A rash that is measles-like: macular lesions that are red and are usually 2-10 mm in diameter but may be confluent.

Monoamine oxidase (MAO): An enzyme that metabolizes norepinephrine and other catecholamines.

Monoamine oxidase inhibitor (MAOI): A class of antidepressants.

Moon facies: A rounded, puffy face caused by high doses of corticosteroids.

Morbidity: Rate of illness or abnormality.

Morphology: The study of the size and shape of a specimen.

Mortality: Rate of death.

Muscarinic receptor: Acetylcholine receptor subtype primarily located on the postsynaptic membrane of the effector organ in the parasympathetic division of the autonomic nervous system.

Mutagen: An agent (environmental or physical) that causes, induces, or increases the rate of genetic mutation.

Myasthenia gravis: An autoimmune disease where antibodies attack acetylcholine receptors and cause muscle weakness and fatigue.

Mydriasis: Dilation of the pupil.

Myelosuppression: A decrease in blood cell production from the bone marrow.

Myenteric plexus: A plexus of unmyelinated nerve fibers and postganglionic autonomic cell bodies lying within the musculature of the esophagus, stomach, and intestine; it communicates with the enteric plexus.

Myocardial infarction: Necrosis of part of the heart muscle; heart attack.

Myoclonus: A single or series of shock-like contractions of muscle groups.

Myoglobinemia: Abnormal presence of myoglobin in the blood indicating muscle breakdown.

Myoglobinuria: Abnormal presence of myoglobin in the urine.

Myopathy: An abnormal condition of the skeletal muscles that includes wasting and weakness.

Myxedema: The most severe form of hypothyroidism,; may lead to coma or death.

Narcolepsy: A sleep disorder of recurring episodes of sleep during the day.

Nasopharyngitis: Inflammation or infection of the nose and throat.

Necrosis: Localized tissue death.

Negative chronotrope: A drug that reduces the rate of heartbeats.

Negative inotrope: A drug that reduces the force of the heart's contraction.

Nematodes: Elongated roundworms that have a complete digestive system including a mouth and anus unlike any of the other categories of worms.

Neoplasm: Any abnormal growth of new tissue, whether benign or malignant.

Neostriatum: See striatum.

Nephrolithiasis: A disorder of calculi/stones in the kidney.

Nephrotic syndrome: Any of several kidney diseases that involve protein in the urine with low blood protein levels and edema.

Neuritis: Inflammation of a nerve.

Neurogenic: Stemming from or caused by the nervous system.

Neuroleptic drugs: Another name for antipsychotic drugs.

Neuroleptic malignant syndrome: Can occur with the use of any neuroleptic drug and may be fatal. Symptoms include muscle rigidity, fever, stupor, unstable blood pressure, and myoglobinemia.

Neurotransmitter: A chemical released from a neuron that is used to communicate, either excitatory or inhibitory, with a receiving cell such as another neuron, a muscle, or an effector organ.

Neutropenia: A reduction in the number of neutrophils, one type of immune cell, in the blood.

N-methyl-D-aspartate (NMDA): An excitatory neurotransmitter.

Nocturia: Excessive urination at night.

Non-competitive binding: Agents act at sites on the receptor that are different from and do not interfere with active sites for endogenous molecules.

Non-steroidal anti-inflammatory drug (NSAID): Used in pain relief; includes aspirin and acetaminophen.

Norepinephrine: A neurotransmitter that stimulates the sympathetic nervous system.

Neurogenic: Originating from the nervous system.

Nystagmus: Involuntary, rhythmic movements of the eyes; may be horizontal, vertical, rotary, or mixed.

Off label: Once a drug is approved by the Food and Drug Administration, it can be prescribed for any purpose. When this purpose is not the approved use, its use is considered "off label."

Oligohidrosis: Abnormal lessening of perspiration.

Oligosaccharide: A compound made up of a small number of monosaccharides such as glucose.

Onychomycosis: A fungal infection of a nail; plural: onychomycoses.

Orthostatic hypotension: A period of reduced blood pressure due to standing rapidly from a seated or lying position; usually causes light-headedness.

Osteoclast: A cell located in the bone that functions to break down bone during remodeling.

Osteomalacia: An abnormal condition of the bone characterized by loss of calcification resulting in softening of the bone and weakness.

Ototoxic: Having a harmful effect on the ear or Cranial Nerve VIII.

Oxidation: A chemical reaction that either increases oxygen in a molecule or loses an electron from a molecule.

Pancytopenia: A great reduction in the number of red blood cells, white blood cells, and platelets.

Papule: An elevated, firm area on the skin of less than 1 cm diameter.

Parasympathomimetic: Either mimicking or stimulating the parasympathetic nervous system.

Paravertebral: Near the vertebral column.

Parenchyma: The distinguishing or specific cells of a gland or organ supported in a connective tissue framework.

Parenteral: Outside of the intestines; a route of administration of a drug that does not enter the intestinal or digestive tract; for example, injections.

Paresthesias: Numbness and tingling.

Paroxysmal atrial tachycardia: Periods of very rapid (often 160-200 bpms), regular heart beats originating in the atrioventricular node.

Passive diffusion: The movement of small molecules across a cell membrane without the need for energy.

Pericarditis: Inflammation and/or infection of the pericardium.

Peristalsis: The rhythmic contraction of smooth muscle in the gastrointestinal tract, the main purpose of which is to propel food through the digestive tract.

pH: The inverse log of the concentration of hydrogen ions. Used as a measurement of acidic and basic level; 7 is neutral, below that is acidic, and above that is basic. The further away from 7 the more basic or acid the solution is. A acidic pH of 2 is more acidic than a pH of 4.

Phagocytosis: A method where certain cells engulf and dispose of cellular debris and microorganisms.

Phenotype: The complete observable characteristics of an organism regardless of its genetics.

Pheochromocytoma: A tumor of the adrenal medulla that causes excessive release of catecholamines especially epinephrine and norepinephrine.

Phospholipid bilayer: A description of a cell membrane. It comprises lipids or fats and phosphate groups and is arranged in two layers.

Photophobia: An abnormal sensitivity to light, especially by the eyes.

Phototoxic: A substance that causes a rapidly developing, non-immune reaction of the skin when exposed to light.

Pinocytosis: A method of absorption for a cell where it indents and encloses an external area and internalizes it.

pKa: The inverse log of the acid constant. A measure of a drug's interaction with a proton (acid). A low pKa indicates that the drug is more acidic, while a high pKa indicates a more basic drug.

Plaque: A skin condition identified as a large, irregular area of elevated skin.

Poikilothermia: A condition where body temperature fluctuates with the environment.

Polydipsia: Excessive thirst.

Polypeptide: A chain of many amino acids so named because of the peptide bond between any two adjacent amino acids.

Polyuria: Excessive urination.

Porins: Enzymes that allow transmembrane transport of specific compounds.

Porphyria: A group of inherited disorders characterized by accumulation of porphyrins, intermediaries of hemoglobin production.

Postictal: Pertaining to the period after a convulsion.

Postprandial: After a meal.

Postsynaptic neuron: The neuron that is after a synapse; the neuron receiving neurotransmitters from the synaptic cleft.

Potency: How much of the drug is necessary to reach a certain effect. See EC_{50}.

Premature ventricular complex: An abnormal heart rhythm caused by the ventricle initiating depolarization before it is expected.

Presynaptic neuron: The neuron before a synapse; the neuron releasing neurotransmitters into the synaptic cleft.

Priapism: An abnormally prolonged or constant erection of the penis.

Proanalog: A drug or other chemical that after metabolism is similar in structure or constituents to another but differs in effects.

Prodrug: A drug that is not chemically active when administered but is converted in the body to an active drug.

Prostaglandins: A group of bioactive, hormone-like chemicals derived from fatty acids that have a wide variety of biological effects including roles in inflammation, platelet aggregation, vascular smooth muscle dilation and constriction, cell growth, protection from acid in the stomach, and many more.

Proteinuria: The presence of an abnormally large quantity of protein in the urine.

Pruritis: Itching.

Psychosis: A severe emotional and behavioral disorder that includes symptoms of gross distortion of a person's mental capacity, ability to recognize reality, and inability to relate to others or perform ADLs.

Psychotomimetic: "Psychosis mimicking"; a drug or substance that induces psychological and behavioral changes resembling those of psychosis.

Psychotropic: Can affect the mind, emotions, and behavior; pertaining to drug use in the treatment of mental illness.

Pyelonephritis: A fever inducing infection of the kidney.

Raynaud's phenomenon: A disorder that causes pain and discoloration of the extremities.

Rebound: Where the symptoms or condition treated by an agent come back stronger than originally when the agent was ceased.

Refractory period: Referring to the period after an event has occurred and before another can be initiated again.

Renin: An enzyme that converts angiotensinogen to angiotensin I.

Rhabdomyolysis: An acute, potentially fatal disease of destruction of skeletal muscle; signs include myoglobinemia and myoglobinuria.

Rhinitis: Inflammation of the mucous membranes of the nose.

Rhinorrhea: Discharge of thin nasal mucus.

Sedative: See hypnotic.

Selective serotonin reuptake inhibitors (SSRIs): A class of antidepressants.

Sepsis: The presence of pathogenic organisms or their toxins in the blood or tissues.

Septum: A thin wall dividing two cavities or two areas of soft tissue; septa is plural.

Serotonin and norepinephrine reuptake inhibitors (SNRIs): A class of antidepressants.

Sinus arrhythmias: An arrhythmia with its origin in a dysfunction of the sinoatrial (SA) node.

Sinus rhythm: A heart rhythm initiated by the SA node; a normal rhythm.

Sjogren's syndrome: An autoimmune disease whose main symptoms include dry eyes and mouth.

Sporozites: Any cells resulting from the sexual union of spores during the life cycle of certain protozoa known as sporozoans.

Status epilepticus: A condition of a sustained epileptic seizure that can be life threatening.

Steady state: When the dosing of a drug and the elimination of the drug maintain a relatively stable amount of the drug in the body.

Stenosis: Narrowing.

Stent: A device that is designed to anchor skin grafts or support body openings or cavities.

Steven-Johnson syndrome: A serious, often fatal inflammatory disease, potentially caused by an allergic reaction to a drug. Symptoms include fever, skin lesions, and mucous membrane ulcers.

Stomatitis: An inflammation and/or infection of the mouth.

Striatum (also referred to as corpus striatum or neostriatum): The part of the basal ganglia of the brain that includes the caudate nucleus and putamen. Its function is to plan and modulate movement and some higher cognitive functions. Lack of dopamine prevents proper modulating function in Parkinson's disease.

Stricture: A narrowing or stenosis of a tube, duct, or hollow structure usually consisting of a contracture or deposition of abnormal tissue.

Stroke volume: How much blood is pumped by each contraction of the heart. It is determined by heart muscle contractility and the amount of venous blood return.

Sublingual: Below the tongue refers to a method of administration where a drug is held under the tongue until dissolved.

Substrate: The specific chemical that is acted upon by an enzyme.

Superinfection: An infection that develops during antimicrobial treatment of another infection.

Supraventricular tachycardia (SVT): An arrhythmia that originates above the ventricle,either in the SA node, atria, or atrioventricular (AV) junction.

Sympathomimetic: Either mimicking or stimulating the sympathetic nervous system.

Synapse: A junction between 2 nerves or a nerve and an effector organ.

Synaptic cleft (also called synaptic space): The space between the two neurons of a synapse; the space into which the neurotransmitters are released.

Syncope: Momentary loss of consciousness, a faint.

Tachyarrhythmias: Arrhythmias with an overall rate of over 100 bpm.

Tachycardia: A rapid heart rate defined as over 100 bpms.

Tachyphylaxis: When repeated drug use results in a smaller effect.

Tardive dyskinesia: A motor disorder that includes involuntary movements such as lateral jaw movements and "fly-catching" movements of the tongue.

TD_{50}: The drug dose that produces toxic effects in 50% of the population.

Teratogen: A substance that causes congenital defects in fetuses.

Therapeutic index: A measurement of how safe a drug is. It

is the ratio between the therapeutic dose and the toxic dose.

Therapeutic margin: See therapeutic index.

Therapeutic window: See therapeutic index.

Thrombocytopenia: A decreased number of platelets in the blood.

Thrombocytopenic purpura (sometimes referred to as thrombotic thrombocytopenic purpura): A condition of reduced platelets (thrombocytopenia) causing pin-prick bleeding and bruising under the skin (purpura). It runs the gamut from the relatively benign idiopathic thrombocytopenic purpura to the life-threatening emergency of thrombotic thrombocytopenic purpura.

Thromboembolism: Blockage of a blood vessel due to a piece of a clot breaking off from another location and preventing blood flow.

Thrombolytic: A drug that breaks up a thrombus or clot.

Thrombophlebitis: Inflammation of a vein often accompanied by a blood clot.

Thyroid storm: A crisis of uncontrolled hyperthyroidism characterized by high fever, rapid pulse, respiratory distress, apprehension, restlessness, and irritability; can lead to delirium, coma, or fatal heart failure.

Tinnitus: Ringing in the ears.

Tolerance: The need for increasing doses of a substance in order to maintain the same effect or to avoid negative symptoms.

Tonic convulsion: A prolonged generalized contraction of the voluntary muscles.

Torsade de pointes: A specific type of ventricular tachycardia characterized by rapid irregular QRS complexes. It may end spontaneously or degenerate into ventricular fibrillation. It causes significant blood flow compromise and often causes death.

Total peripheral vascular resistance: Degree of resistance to blood flow from systemic blood vessels.

Toxic megacolon: A severe complication of several conditions that involves a large dilation of the colon with possible local bacterial overgrowth. Rupture of the colon is a possibility and has a 50% mortality. Emergency treatment for this condition is necessary and can prevent sepsis, shock, and possibly death.

Trematodes: Flukes that are leaf-shaped flatworms.

Triacylglycerol: A chemical with three fatty acids attached to a glycerol molecule. High levels in the blood have been linked to atherosclerosis and therefore heart disease and stroke.

Triglyceride: See triacylglycerol.

Troche: A small tablet containing a drug and a flavored base that dissolves in the mouth releasing the drug.

Trophozites: Protozoa that are in the active phase of their life cycle, where reproduction and other activities of life are occurring.

Tyrosine: An amino acid.

Urticaria: Skin condition consisting of wheals, usually the result of hypersensitivity; commonly called hives.

Valproate: The ionic form of valproic acid; in vivo they are equivalents.

Valproic acid: The root acid form of the ionic valproate,;in vivo they are equivalents.

Vasculitis: Inflammation of the blood vessels.

Vasoconstriction: A decrease in diameter of a blood vessel.

Vasodilation: An increase in diameter of a blood vessel.

Vasopressin: See antidiuretic hormone.

Ventricular extrasystoles: An extra contraction started in a ventricle.

Ventricular fibrillation: Causes uncoordinated quivering of the ventricle without any useful contractions. Immediate syncope occurs, and death happens within minutes.

Ventricular premature beats(VPB): A single impulse in the ventricle caused by reentry or abnormal automaticity of ventricular cells. VPBs are asymptomatic or can cause palpitations and usually require no intervention.

Vesicle: A storage "bubble" located in the cytoplasm of a cell, it is surrounded with a phospholipid bilayer. Also a skin lesion identified as a small, circumscribed, elevated area of fluid-filled skin.

Vestibular: Pertaining to the inner ear apparati in control of body balance.

Viral load: The level of viral RNA present in the blood plasma.

Virion: A rudimentary viral particle that includes a capsid, a protein sheath, and a central nucleoid.

Volume of distribution (Vd): A measurement of how much drug is in the body versus how much is in the blood. A large Vd indicates wide distribution to the body, while a small Vd indicates a drug that is generally sequestered in the blood.

Wheal: A circumscribed papule or irregular plaque of skin edema.

Withdrawal: The psychological and/or physical syndrome caused by abrupt cessation of the use of a drug in a habituated individual.

Wolff-Parkinson-White (WPW) syndrome: The most common reentrant supraventricular tachycardia. When combined with atrial fibrillation, WPW is a medical emergency.

Xenobiotics: Biological compounds from outside the body a generic way to describe drugs and other compounds.

Xerostomia: A dry mouth.

General Index

Amigesic, 170, 341
Amiloride, 140, 143-144
Aminocaproic acid, 180-181
Aminoglutethimide, 110, 220-221, 328, 366
Aminoglycoside, 146, 270, 272, 275, 372, 425
Aminophylline, 231, 233, 235, 423
Aminopyrine, 101
Aminosalicylic acid, 281-284
Amiodarone, 110, 154, 156, 159, 161-162, 165, 169, 366, 420-421, 430
Amitiza, 261
Amitriptyline, 98-99, 101-102, 423
Amlodipine, 165-166, 168, 190, 420
Amnesia, 44, 46, 84, 87-88, 379-380, 388, 428, 439
Amnesteem, 367
Amobarbital, 83, 85, 92
Amoclan, 267
Amomum, 153, 175, 179
Amoxapine, 98-99, 423
Amoxicillin, 245, 247, 250, 262, 267-270
Amphetamine, 63, 92-95, 121, 378
Amphotericin B, 147, 287, 290
Ampicillin, 267-270
Amprenavir, 310
Ampyra, 72
Amrix, 365
Amturnide, 134, 140, 165
Amyl nitrite, 148, 150
Amyotrophic lateral sclerosis (ALS), 72-73, 433, 439
Anacin, 93, 170, 348
Anacin Advanced Headache Formula, 93, 348
Anadrol, 207
Anaerobic organisms, 266, 268
Anafranil, 98
Analgesic, 89-92, 118-121, 240-241, 341-342, 345-346, 349, 365, 414, 439
Analgesic Creme Rub/Aloe, 341
Anaphylaxis, 266, 346, 439
Anaplasia, 317, 439
Anaplex, 54, 113, 236
Anaplex DM, 54, 113, 236
Anaprox, 341
Anaspaz, 43
Anastrozole, 328-329
Ancobon, 285
Ancylostoma duodenale, 298
Androderm, 207, 215
AndroGel, 207, 215
Androgens, 192, 207, 209-210, 215, 219, 227, 329, 381, 403
Android, 207

Androstenedione, 328
Androxy, 207
Anemarrhena, 204-206
Anemia, 129, 181-182, 202, 280, 284, 290, 297, 311, 319, 330, 336, 346, 351, 353, 356, 400-401, 411-414, 440, 443-444
Anesthetic, 56, 84, 243, 439
Angelica, 152, 173, 178, 216, 350, 426, 428-429
Angelica root, 152, 173, 178
Angelica sinensis, 152, 173, 178, 216, 426, 428-429
Angeliq, 207-208
Angina, 59-61, 95, 140, 149-151, 157, 161, 165-167, 172, 195, 297, 360, 390-392, 398-401
Angina pectoralis, 61, 149, 151, 161
Angioedema, 89, 195, 211, 280, 439
Angiotensin converting enzyme, 133-135, 433, 439
Angiotensin converting enzyme inhibitors, 133, 135
Angiotensin I, 59, 134-135, 439, 447
Angiotensin II, 134-135, 439
Angiotensin-receptor blockers, 135, 433
Anhedonia, 98, 439
Ankylosing spondylitis, 342, 344-346
Anolor, 83
Anolor 300, 83
Anorexia, 71, 95, 161, 301, 319, 323-324, 327, 329, 334, 339, 356, 366, 391-393, 399, 401, 405, 411-412, 439
Anorexiant, 362, 439
Anorgasmia, 105, 394, 395, 439
Antacid, 15, 22, 245, 247-248, 250-251
Antacid Extra Strength, 245
Antagonist, 73, 94, 143, 145, 211, 215, 253-254, 282, 322, 439, 443
Antara, 186
Anterograde amnesia, 84, 88, 439
Anti-Hist, 236
Anti-Hist Allergy, 236
Anti-Itch Maximum Strength, 236
Antiandrogens, 207, 210, 215, 403
Antiarrhythmic, 60, 154, 157-164, 166, 398-399, 439
Antibiotics, 33, 141, 146, 242, 246, 249-250, 263-272, 276-278, 280-281, 284, 286, 323-324, 356, 372, 410, 413, 425, 428-429
Anticancer agents, 315, 319, 323-324, 327, 329, 331, 334-335, 339, 413
Anticholinergic agents, 22, 231, 233, 253, 406-407, 409

Anticoagulant, 151-153, 173-175, 177-180, 347, 427
Anticonvulsant, 85-88, 96, 101, 123-124, 126, 128
Antidepressants, 24, 53, 56, 71-72, 78, 80, 96-99, 101-103, 105-112, 115, 121, 169, 347, 354, 365-366, 394-395, 423, 445, 447
Antidiabetic, 53, 56, 62, 89, 97, 130, 139, 147, 195-198, 202-206, 363, 403
Antidiarrheals, 256, 409
Antidiuresis, 181, 193
Antiemetic, 44, 46, 71, 76, 77, 87, 222, 240, 253-255, 316, 354, 409, 440
Antifungals, 23, 167, 168, 263, 285-287, 290, 355, 366, 411, 433
Antihistamines, 83-84, 138, 237-238, 240, 253, 407, 409
Antihypertensives, 56, 62-63, 89, 97, 130, 134, 136, 139, 147, 165, 168, 195, 204, 363, 400
Antihyperthyroid, 53, 56, 62, 89, 97, 130, 139, 147, 195, 203-204, 206, 363, 364
Antimetabolites, 320, 321, 413
Antimicrobial agents, 245, 263, 265, 267, 269, 271, 273, 275, 277, 279, 281, 283, 285, 287, 289, 291, 293, 295, 297, 299, 301, 303, 305, 307, 309, 311, 313, 408, 410
Antimotility agents, 256, 409
Antimuscarinic agents, 43-45, 66-67, 70, 245-248, 251, 388, 408, 440
Antimycobacterial drugs, 281, 411
Antineoplastic, 315-316, 323, 440
Antiplatelet agents, 151-153, 173-175, 177-180
Antiprogestin, 207, 210-211, 215, 403
Antiprotozoals, 263, 292-293
Antipsychotic agents, 71, 77, 81, 105, 121
Antipsychotic drugs, 67, 71, 74, 347, 396, 445
Antipsychotics, 22, 75, 78, 82, 112, 253, 254, 409, 432
Antipyretic, 171, 342-344, 349, 413-414, 440
Antiretroviral agents, 307
Antirheumatic, 171, 350, 414, 434, 437
Antischizophrenic drugs, 74
Antiseizure, 53, 56, 62, 89, 97, 125, 130, 139, 147, 195, 203-204, 206, 354, 363-364
Antispasmodic agent, 44

Genahist, 237

Generalized anxiety disorder, 84, 103-105, 394, 435

Generess Fe, 208

Generlac, 258

Gengraf, 369

Genie, 380

Genpril, 341

Gentamicin, 272, 274

Gentian violet, 285, 288

Gentiana, 90, 92, 121, 147, 241

Gentiana macrophylla root, 90, 92, 121, 241

Gentle laxative, 258

Geodon, 79

Georgia Home Boy, 379

Geri-Dryl, 237

Geri-kot, 258

Geri-Mucil, 256

Geri-Stool, 258

Geri-Tussin, 242

GHB, 376, 379

GHB/sodium oxybate, 379

GI motility, 21-22, 24, 41, 43, 47, 247

Gianvi, 208

Giardia lamblia, 293-294, 296

Giardiasis, 295-296

Giazo, 356

Gildess FE, 208

Gildess FE 1.5/30, 208

Gildess FE 1/20, 208

Gilenya, 72

Gilotrif, 332

Ginger, 152, 174, 178, 320, 347, 425, 428-429, 432

Ginkgo leaf, 91, 105-106, 148, 153, 167, 175, 180, 347

Ginseng, 30, 46, 53, 72, 109, 151, 163, 164, 173, 177, 179, 203-206, 217, 225, 313, 320, 323, 334, 388, 425-426, 428-431

Glass, 378, 444

Glatiramer, 72, 73

Glaucoma, 40, 46, 59, 71, 96, 101, 125, 130, 142, 144, 225, 436, 443

Gleevec, 332

Gliadel Wafer, 316

Glimepiride, 196-197, 199, 207, 228, 420

Glioblastoma multiforme, 317-319

Gliomas, 317

Glipizide, 196-197, 200, 204, 206-207, 228, 290, 420

Glossitis, 280, 443

Glossy privet herb, 203, 205-206

Glucagon, 61, 161-162, 197, 199, 443

Glucocorticoids, 192, 219-220, 222,

225, 361, 369, 440, 443

Gluconeogenesis, 199, 219, 443

Glucophage, 196

Glucose-6-phosphate dehydrogenase deficiency, 297

Glucotrol, 196, 200

Glucovance, 196

Gluey, 382

Glumetza, 196

Glyburide, 196-197, 200, 204, 206-207, 228, 420

Glycerin, 258-259

Glycerin (adult), 258

Glycerin (pediatric), 258

Glycine, 66, 443

GlycoLax, 258

Glycopyrrolate, 43-45

Glycosuria, 129, 138, 443

Glycyrhizzin, 152, 174, 178

Glynase, 196, 200

Glyset, 196

Go, 1, 23, 29, 31-32, 34, 191, 258, 267, 380, 428, 431

Go-Fast, 378

God's Drug, 377

God's Medicine, 377

Goiter, 193-194, 443

Gold, 9, 297, 350-351

GoLYTELY, 258

Gonadotropin-releasing hormone, 211, 435

Gonal-f, 226

Gonal-f RFF, 226

Gonal-f RFF Pen, 226

Gondola, 377

GoodSense Mucus Relief, 242

GoodSense Senna Laxative, 258

Goody's Extra Strength Headache Powder, 93, 348

Goody's Extra Strength Pain Relief, 93, 348

Goody's PM, 237, 348

Goof Balls, 379

Goop, 379

Gordofilm, 367

Goric, 377

Gou Teng, 96, 152, 174, 178

Gout, 146, 189, 284, 342, 345, 347, 349, 352-353, 414, 443

Gouty arthritis, 342, 345-346, 414

Graft vascular disease, 369

Graft-versus-host reactions, 324, 330, 336, 435

Gralise, 122

Gram stain, 263, 269, 282, 443

Gram-negative cocci, 266, 268

Gram-negative rods, 266, 268

Gram-positive bacilli, 266, 268

Gram-positive cocci, 266, 268

Grand mal siezure, 123-124

Granisetron, 253, 255

Granisol, 253

Granulocytopenia, 280, 297, 327, 443

Grapefruit juice, 12, 24, 151

Grass, 381

Great Tobacco, 377

Green tea, 55, 216, 252

Grievous bodily harm, 379

Grifulvin, 285

Gris-PEG, 285

Griseofulvin, 285-290

Growth factors, 192, 370

GTP, 16, 18, 306, 359, 435

Guaiatussin AC, 113, 242

Guaicon DMS, 114, 242

Guaifenesin, 63-64, 131-132, 242-244, 407

Guan Ye Lian Qiao, 25, 82, 89, 91, 101, 105-106, 112, 121, 163-164, 167, 178, 186, 216, 226, 235, 241, 252, 258, 276, 290, 312-313, 334, 356, 366, 373, 419, 422

Guanabenz, 48, 51, 53, 58, 110, 139, 147, 153, 167, 169

Guanfacine, 48, 51, 53-54, 58, 110, 139, 147, 153, 167, 169

Guanidine, 40

Guanine, 322, 324, 434

Guanosine triphosphate, 18, 359, 435

Gui Ban Jiao, 22

Gui Zhi, 147

Guma, 377

Gynazole, 285

Gynazole-1, 285

Gyne-Lotrimin, 285

Gyne-Lotrimin 3, 285

Gynecomastia, 146, 169, 215, 251, 290, 320, 443

Gynostemma, 89-90, 121, 241

H

H. influenzae, 303

H2-histamine antagonists, 245, 247-248, 251, 408

Hai Ge Fen, 22

Hai Piao Xiao, 22

Halaven, 325

Halcinonide, 218, 223

Halcion, 83

Haldol, 75

Half-life, 13

HalfLytely and Bisacodyl, 258

Halfprin, 170

Hallucinations, 70, 74, 95, 123, 129,

Lovaza, 186
Lover's Speed, 380
Low-Ogestrel, 208-209
Loxapine, 75, 77
Loxitane, 75
LSD, 93, 376, 380, 381, 435
Lu Cha, 55, 216, 252, 419
Lu Han Cao, 276
Lu Hui, 148, 162-164, 203-204, 206, 225
Lu Jiao Jiao, 22
Lubiprostone, 261-262
Ludiomil, 98
Lufyllin, 231
Lumefantrine, 291, 297, 420
Luminal, 141, 144, 292, 294
Lunar Wave, 383
Lunch Money drug, 379
Lunesta, 83, 430
Lupus erythematosus, 225, 293, 295, 437
Lurasidone, 79, 80, 83, 420
Lutera, 208
Lutropin alpha, 226-227
Luvox, 102
Luxiq, 218
Lybrel, 208
Lychee seed, 203-204, 206
Lycium root bark, 203-205
Lycopus, 147
Lysergic acid diethylamide, 93, 376, 380, 435
Lysimachia, 147
Lysodren, 218, 335
Lysteda, 180

M

M-Clear, 113, 242
M-Clear WC, 113, 242
M-END, 236
M-END DM, 236
Ma Huang, 53, 55-56, 62-63, 71, 96-97, 102, 109, 139, 147, 163-164, 225-226, 235, 252, 320, 347, 356, 363, 392, 406, 416, 431
Maalox, 245, 261
Maalox Advanced Maximum Strength, 245, 261
Maalox Advanced Regular Strength, 245, 261
Maalox Children's, 245
Maalox Junior Plus Antigas, 245, 261
Macrobid, 277
Macrodantin, 277
Macrolides, 266, 272, 275, 282
Maculopapular rash, 397
Mag-Al, 245

Mag-Al Ultimate, 245
Magic Bullets, 258
Magic Mushrooms, 380
Magnesium citrate, 258, 259
Magnesium hydroxide, 245, 249, 258, 262
Magnesium oxide, 258, 260
Magnesium salicylate, 341, 345
Magnesium sulfate, 258, 260, 262
Magnesium trisilicate, 262
Magnolia bark, 152, 174, 178
Mai Ya, 203-204, 206
Makena, 208
Malaria, 157, 291-296
Malarone, 291
Male pattern baldness, 213, 382
Malignant hyperthermia, 365
Man Jing Zi, 78, 82, 216-217
Mania, 76, 79-81, 110, 112, 126, 129, 391-392, 394-396, 443
Mannitol, 146
Mao Dong Qing, 152, 174, 179
MAO inhibitors, 55, 68, 71, 72, 89, 96, 108, 109, 111, 202, 240, 356, 363, 366, 436, 445
Mapap, 48, 114, 237, 348
Mapap Arthritis Pain, 348
Mapap Children's, 348
Mapap Extra Strength, 348
Mapap Infant's, 348
Mapap Junior Rapid Tabs, 348
Mapap Multi-Symptom Cold, 48, 114, 348
Mapap PM, 237, 348
Mapap Sinus PE, 48, 348
Mapo bath, 258
Maprotiline, 98, 100
Mar-Cof CG, 113, 242
Maraviroc, 302, 305, 308, 311-313, 422
Margesic, 83, 114, 348
Margesic H, 114, 348
Maria, 377, 383
Maria pastora, 377, 383
Marijuana, 93, 376, 380-381, 437
Marinol, 253
Marlissa, 208
Marplan, 106
Mary Jane, 381
Mast cell stabilizers, 231, 233-234, 237- 238, 406-407
Mast cells, 94, 232-233, 407
Mastocytosis, 233, 332, 334
Matulane, 316
Matzim LA, 165
Mavik, 133
Maxair, 47
Maxalt, 354

Maxichlor, 48, 54, 114, 236
Maxichlor PEH, 48, 114, 236
Maxichlor PEH DM, 114
Maxichlor PSE, 54, 114, 236
Maxichlor PSE DM, 54, 114
Maxidone, 114, 348
Maxifed, 54, 114, 242
Maxifed DM, 54, 114
Maxifed DMX, 54, 114, 242
Maxifed-G, 54
Maxiphen, 48, 114, 242
Maxiphen DM, 48, 114
Maxiphen DMX, 48, 114, 242
Maxzide, 140
MDMA, 380
Mebendazole, 298-302, 420
Mechlorethamine, 316-317, 319
Meclizine, 237, 240, 253
Meclofenamate, 341, 345-347, 420
Medent, 48, 242
Medent-PEI, 48, 242
Medi-First, 48, 285
Medi-First Anti-Fungal, 285
Medi-Meclizine, 237
Medi-Phenyl, 48
Medicone, 48
Mediplast, 367
Mediproxen, 341
Medrol, 218
Medrol Pak, 218
Medroxyprogesterone, 208, 213, 217, 228
Medulloblastoma, 319
Mefenamic acid, 341, 343, 345-346
Mefloquine, 291-295, 297, 420, 422
Megace, 204, 208
Megaloblastic anemia, 129, 280, 444
Megestrol, 208, 210, 213, 328
Meglitinide derivatives, 196, 199, 201-202
Mekinist, 335
Melanoma, 183, 316-318, 326, 330-332, 335-339, 400
Melfiat, 362
Mellow Yellow, 380
Meloxicam, 341-343, 345, 347, 420
Meloxicam Comfort Pac, 341
Melphalan, 316-317, 319
Memantine, 72-73
Menest, 207
Meningitis, 122, 265, 283, 301, 303, 321
Meningococcal Menopur, 226
Menostar, 207
Menotropins, 226-228
Mentax, 285, 288
Meow Meow, 383
Mepenzolate, 43-45, 246

OTHER BOOKS ON CHINESE MEDICINE AVAILABLE FROM:
BLUE POPPY ENTERPRISES, INC.

Oregon: 4804 SE 69th Avenue, Portland, OR 97206
For ordering 1-800-487-9296 PH. 503-650-6077 FAX 503-650-6076
California: 1815 W. 205th Street, Suite 304, Torrance, CA 90501
For ordering 1-800-293-6697 PH. 424-488-2000 FAX 424-488-2024
Email: info@bluepoppy.com Website: www.bluepoppy.com

ACUPOINT POCKET REFERENCE
by Bob Flaws
ISBN 0-936185-93-7
ISBN 978-0-936185-93-4

ACUPUNCTURE, CHINESE MEDICINE & HEALTHY
WEIGHT LOSS   Revised Edition
by Juliette Aiyana, L. Ac.
ISBN 1-891845-61-6
ISBN 978-1-891845-61-1

ACUPUNCTURE & IVF
by Lifang Liang
ISBN 0-891845-24-1
ISBN 978-0-891845-24-6

ACUPUNCTURE FOR STROKE REHABILITATION
Three Decades of Information from China
by Hoy Ping Yee Chan, et al.
ISBN 1-891845-35-7
ISBN 978-1-891845-35-2

ACUPUNCTURE PHYSICAL MEDICINE: An Acupuncture
Touchpoint Approach to the Treatment of Chronic Pain,
Fatigue, and Stress Disorders
by Mark Seem
ISBN 1-891845-13-6
ISBN 978-1-891845-13-0

ACUPUNCTURE MEDICINE: Bodymind Integration for Bodily
Distress and Mental Pain
by Mark Seem
ISBN 1-891845-70-5
ISBN 978-1-891845-70-3

AGING & BLOOD STASIS: A New Approach to TCM Geriatrics
by Yan De-xin
ISBN 0-936185-63-6
ISBN 978-0-936185-63-7

AN ACUPUNCTURISTS GUIDE TO MEDICAL RED FLAGS &
REFERRALS
by Dr. David Anzaldua, MD
ISBN 1-891845-54-3
ISBN 978-1-891845-54-3

BETTER BREAST HEALTH NATURALLY with CHINESE
MEDICINE
by Honora Lee Wolfe & Bob Flaws
ISBN 0-936185-90-2
ISBN 978-0-936185-90-3

BIOMEDICINE: A TEXTBOOK FOR PRACTITIONERS OF
ACUPUNCTURE AND ORIENTAL MEDICINE
by Bruce H. Robinson, MD Second Edition
ISBN 1-891845-62-4
ISBN 978-1-891845-62-8

THE BOOK OF JOOK: Chinese Medicinal Porridges
by Bob Flaws
ISBN 0-936185-60-6
ISBN 978-0-936185-60-0

CHANNEL DIVERGENCES Deeper Pathways of the Web
by Miki Shima and Charles Chase
ISBN 1-891845-15-2
ISBN 978-1-891845-15-4

CHINESE MEDICAL OBSTETRICS
by Bob Flaws
ISBN 1-891845-30-6
ISBN 978-1-891845-30-7

CHINESE MEDICAL PALM IS TRY: Your Health in Your Hand
by Zong Xiao-fan & Gary Liscum
ISBN 0-936185-64-3
ISBN 978-0-936185-64-4

CHINESE MEDICAL PSYCHIATRY: A Textbook and Clinical
Manual
by Bob Flaws and James Lake, MD
ISBN 1-845891-17-9
ISBN 978-1-845891-17-8

CHINESE MEDICINAL TEAS: Simple, Proven, Folk Formulas
for Common Diseases & Promoting Health
by Zong Xiao-fan & Gary Lis cum
ISBN 0-936185-76-7
ISBN 978-0-936185-76-7

CHINESE MEDICINAL WINES & ELIXIRS
by Bob Flaws Revised Edition
ISBN 0-936185-58-9
ISBN 978-0-936185-58-3

CHINESE PEDIATRIC MASSAGE THERAPY: A Parent's &
Practitioner's Guide to the Prevention & Treatment of Childhood
Illness
by Fan Ya-li
ISBN 0-936185-54-6
ISBN 978-0-936185-54-5

CHINESE SCALP ACUPUNCTURE
by Jason Jishun Hao & Linda Lingzhi Hao
ISBN 1-891845-60-8
ISBN 978-1-891845-60-4

CHINESE SELF-MASSAGE THERAPY: The Easy Way to Health
by Fan Ya-li
ISBN 0-936185-74-0
ISBN 978-0-936185-74-3

THE CLASSIC OF DIFFICULTIES: A Translation of the Nan Jing
translation by Bob Flaws
ISBN 1-891845-07-1
ISBN 978-1-891845-07-9

A CLINICIAN'S GUIDE TO USING GRANULE
EXTRACTS
by Eric Brand
ISBN 1-891845-51-9
ISBN 978-1-891845-51-2

A COMPENDIUM OF CHINESE MEDICAL MENSTRUAL
DISEASES
by Bob Flaws
ISBN 1-891845-31-4
ISBN 978-1-891845-31-4

CONCISE CHINESE MATERIA MEDICA
by Eric Brand and Nigel Wiseman
ISBN 0-912111-82-8
ISBN 978-0-912111-82-7

CONTEMPORARY GYNECOLOGY: An Integrated Chinese-
Western Approach
by Lifang Liang
ISBN 1-891845-50-0
ISBN 978-1-891845-50-5

CONTROLLING DIABETES NATURALLY WITH CHINESE
MEDICINE
by Lynn Kuchinski
ISBN 0-936185-06-3
ISBN 978-0-936185-06-2

CURING ARTHRITIS NATURALLY WITH CHINESE
MEDICINE
by Douglas Frank & Bob Flaws
ISBN 0-936185-87-2
ISBN 978-0-936185-87-3

CURING DEPRESSION NATURALLY WITH CHINESE
MEDICINE
by Rosa Schnyer & Bob Flaws
ISBN 0-936185-94-5
ISBN 978-0-936185-94-1

CURING FIBROMYALGIA NATURALLY WITH CHINESE
MEDICINE
by Bob Flaws
ISBN 1-891845-09-8
ISBN 978-1-891845-09-3

CURING HAY FEVER NATURALLY WITH CHINESE
MEDICINE
by Bob Flaws
ISBN 0-936185-91-0
ISBN 978-0-936185-91-0

CURING HEADACHES NATURALLY WITH CHINESE
MEDICINE
by Bob Flaws
ISBN 0-936185-95-3
ISBN 978-0-936185-95-8

CURING IBS NATURALLY WITH CHINESE
MEDICINE
by Jane Bean Oberski
ISBN 1-891845-11-X
ISBN 978-1-891845-11-6

CURING INSOMNIA NATURALLY WITH CHINESE
MEDICINE
by Bob Flaws
ISBN 0-936185-86-4
ISBN 978-0-936185-86-6

CURING PMS NATURALLY WITH CHINESE MEDICINE
by Bob Flaws
ISBN 0-936185-85-6
ISBN 978-0-936185-85-9

DISEASES OF THE KIDNEY & BLADDER
by Hoy Ping Yee Chan, et al.
ISBN 1-891845-37-3
ISBN 978-1-891845-35-6

THE DIVINE FARMER'S MATERIA MEDICA: A Translation of
the Shen Nong Ben Cao
translation by Yang Shouz-zhong
ISBN 0-936185-96-1
ISBN 978-0-936185-96-5

DUI YAO: THE ART OF COMBINING CHINESE HERBAL
MEDICINALS
by Philippe Sionneau
ISBN 0-936185-81-3
ISBN 978-0-936185-81-1

ENDOMETRIOSIS, INFERTILITY AND TRADITIONAL
CHINESE MEDICINE: A Layperson's Guide
by Bob Flaws
ISBN 0-936185-14-7
ISBN 978-0-936185-14-9

THE ESSENCE OF LIU FENG-WU'S GYNECOLOGY
by Liu Feng-wu, translated by Yang Shou-zhong
ISBN 0-936185-88-0
ISBN 978-0-936185-88-0

EXTRA TREATISES BASED ON INVESTIGATION &
INQUIRY: A Translation of Zhu Dan-xi's Ge Zhi Yu Lun
translation by Yang Shou-zhong
ISBN 0-936185-53-8
ISBN 978-0-936185-53-8

FIRE IN THE VALLEY: TCM Diagnosis & Treatment of Vaginal
Diseases
by Bob Flaws
ISBN 0-936185-25-2
ISBN 978-0-936185-25-5

FULFILLING THE ESSENCE:
A Handbook of Traditional & Contemporary Treatments for
Female Infertility
by Bob Flaws
ISBN 0-936185-48-1
ISBN 978-0-936185-48-4

FU QING-ZHU'S GYNECOLOGY
trans. by Yang Shou-zhong and Liu Da-wei
ISBN 0-936185-35-X
ISBN 978-0-936185-35-4

GOLDEN NEEDLE WANG LE-TING: A 20th Century Master's
Approach to Acupuncture
by Yu Hui-chan and Han Fu-ru, trans. by Shuai Xue-zhong
ISBN 0-936185-78-3
ISBN 978-0-936185-78-1

A HANDBOOK OF CHINESE HEMATOLOGY
by Simon Becker
ISBN 1-891845-16-0
ISBN 978-1-891845-16-1

A HANDBOOK OF TCM PATTERNS & THEIR TREATMENTS
Second Edition
by Bob Flaws & Daniel Finney
ISBN 0-936185-70-8
ISBN 978-0-936185-70-5

A HANDBOOK OF TRADITIONAL CHINESE DERMATOLOGY
by Liang Jian-hui, trans. by Zhang Ting-liang
& Bob Flaws
ISBN 0-936185-46-5
ISBN 978-0-936185-46-0

A HANDBOOK OF TRADITIONAL CHINESE GYNECOLOGY
by Zhejiang College of TCM, trans. by Zhang Ting-liang
& Bob Flaws
ISBN 0-936185-06-6 (4th edit.)
ISBN 978-0-936185-06-4

A HANDBOOK of TCM PEDIATRICS
by Bob Flaws
ISBN 0-936185-72-4
ISBN 978-0-936185-72-9

THE HEART & ESSENCE OF DAN-XI'S METHODS OF
TREATMENT
by Xu Dan-xi, trans. by Yang Shou-zhong
ISBN 0-926185-50-3
ISBN 978-0-936185-50-7

HERB TOXICITIES & DRUG INTERACTIONS:
A Formula Approach
by Fred Jennes with Bob Flaws
ISBN 1-891845-26-8
ISBN 978-1-891845-26-0

IMPERIAL SECRETS OF HEALTH & LONGEVITY
by Bob Flaws
ISBN 0-936185-51-1
ISBN 978-0-936185-51-4

INSIGHTS OF A SENIOR ACUPUNCTURIST
by Miriam Lee
ISBN 0-936185-33-3
ISBN 978-0-936185-33-0

INTEGRATED PHARMACOLOGY: Combining Modern
Pharmacology with Chinese Medicine
by Dr. Greg Sperber with Bob Flaws
ISBN 1-891845-41-1
ISBN 978-0-936185-41-3

INTEGRATIVE PHARMACOLOGY: Combining Modern
Pharmacology with Integrative Medicine   Second Edition
by Dr. Greg Sperber with Bob Flaws
ISBN 1-891845-69-1
ISBN 978-0-936185-69-7

INTRODUCTION TO THE USE OF PROCESSED CHINESE
MEDICINALS
by Philippe Sionneau
ISBN 0-936185-62-7
ISBN 978-0-936185-62-0

KEEPING YOUR CHILD HEALTHY WITH CHINESE
MEDICINE
by Bob Flaws
ISBN 0-936185-71-6
ISBN 978-0-936185-71-2

THE LAKESIDE MASTER'S STUDY OF THE PULSE
by Li Shi-zhen, trans. by Bob Flaws
ISBN 1-891845-01-2
ISBN 978-1-891845-01-7

MANAGING MENOPAUSE NATURALLY WITH CHINESE
MEDICINE
by Honora Lee Wolfe
ISBN 0-936185-98-8
ISBN 978-0-936185-98-9

MASTER HUA'S CLASSIC OF THE CENTRAL VISCERA
by Hua Tuo, trans. by Yang Shou-zhong
ISBN 0-936185-43-0
ISBN 978-0-936185-43-9

THE MEDICAL I CHING: Oracle of the Healer Within
by Miki Shima
ISBN 0-936185-38-4
ISBN 978-0-936185-38-5

MENOPAIUSE & CHINESE MEDICINE
by Bob Flaws
ISBN 1-891845-40-3
ISBN 978-1-891845-40-6

MOXIBUSTION: A MODERN CLINICAL HANDBOOK
by Lorraine Wilcox
ISBN 1-891845-49-7
ISBN 978-1-891845-49-9

MOXIBUSTION: THE POWER OF MUGWORT FIRE
by Lorraine Wilcox
ISBN 1-891845-46-2
ISBN 978-1-891845-46-8

A NEW AMERICAN ACUPUNTURE By Mark Seem
ISBN 0-936185-44-9
ISBN 978-0-936185-44-6

PLAYING THE GAME: A Step-by-Step Approach to Accepting
Insurance as an Acupuncturist
by Greg Sperber & Tiffany Anderson-Hefner
ISBN 3-131416-11-7
ISBN 978-3-131416-11-7

POCKET ATLAS OF CHINESE MEDICINE
Edited by Marne and Kevin Ergil
ISBN 1-891-845-59-4
ISBN 978-1-891845-59-8

POINTS FOR PROFIT: The Essential Guide to Practice Success
for Acupuncturists   5th Fully Edited Edition
by Honora Wolfe with Marilyn Allen
ISBN 1-891845-64-0
ISBN 978-1-891845-64-2

PRINCIPLES OF CHINESE MEDICAL ANDROLOGY: An
Integrated Approach to Male Reproductive and Urological
Health by Bob Damone
ISBN 1-891845-45-4
ISBN 978-1-891845-45-1

PRINCE WEN HUI's COOK: Chinese Dietary Therapy
by Bob Flaws & Honora Wolfe
ISBN 0-912111-05-4
ISBN 978-0-912111-05-6

THE PULSE CLASSIC: A Translation of the Mai Jing
by Wang Shu-he, trans. by Yang Shou-zhong
ISBN 0-936185-75-9
ISBN 978-0-936185-75-0

THE SECRET OF CHINESE PULSE DIAGNOSIS by Bob Flaws
ISBN 0-936185-67-8
ISBN 978-0-936185-67-5

SECRET SHAOLIN FORMULAS FOR THE TREATMENT OF
EXTERNAL INJURY
by De Chan, trans. by Zhang Ting-liang & Bob Flaws
ISBN 0-936185-08-2
ISBN 978-0-936185-08-8

STATEMENTS OF FACT IN TRADITIONAL CHINESE MEDICINE
by Bob Flaws   Revised & Expanded
ISBN 0-936185-52-X
ISBN 978-0-936185-52-1

STICKING TO THE POINT: A Step-by-Step Approach to TCM
Acupuncture Therapy
by Bob Flaws & Honora Wolfe 2 Condensed Books
ISBN 1-891845-47-0
ISBN 978-1-891845-47-5

A STUDY OF DAOIST ACUPUNCTURE
by Liu Zheng-cai
ISBN 1-891845-08-X
ISBN 978-1-891845-08-6

THE SUCCESSFUL CHINESE HERBALIST
by Bob Flaws and Honora Lee Wolfe
ISBN 1-891845-29-2
ISBN 978-1-891845-29-1

THE SYSTEMATIC CLASSIC OF ACUPUNCTURE &
MOXIBUSTION: A translation of the Jia Yi Jing
by Huang-fu Mi, trans. by Yang Shou-zhong & Charles Chace
ISBN 0-936185-29-5
ISBN 978-0-936185-29-3

THE TAO OF HEALTHY EATING: DIETARY
WISDOM ACCORDING TO CHINESE MEDICINE
by Bob Flaws Second Edition
ISBN 0-936185-92-9
ISBN 978-0-936185-92-7

TEACH YOURSELF TO READ MODERN MEDICAL CHINESE
by Bob Flaws
ISBN 0-936185-99-6
ISBN 978-0-936185-99-6

TEST PREP WORKBOOK FOR BASIC TCM THEORY
by Zhong Bai-song
ISBN 1-891845-43-8
ISBN 978-1-891845-43-7

TEST PREP WORKBOOK FOR THE NCCAOM BIOMEDICINE
MODULE: Exam Preparation & Study Guide
by Zhong Bai-song
ISBN 1-891845-34-9
ISBN 978-1-891845-34-5

TREATING PEDIATRIC BED-WETTING WITH ACUPUNCTURE
& CHINESE MEDICINE
by Robert Helmer
ISBN 1-891845-33-0
ISBN 978-1-891845-33-8

TREATISE on the SPLEEN & STOMACH: A Translation and
annotation of Li Dong-yuan's Pi Wei Lun
by Bob Flaws
ISBN 0-936185-41-4
ISBN 978-0-936185-41-5

THE TREATMENT OF CARDIOVASCULAR DISEASES WITH
CHINESE MEDICINE
by Simon Becker, Bob Flaws & Robert Casañas, MD
ISBN 1-891845-27-6
ISBN 978-1-891845-27-7

THE TREATMENT OF DIABETES MELLITUS WITH CHINESE
MEDICINE
by Bob Flaws, Lynn Kuchinski & Robert Casañas, M.D.
ISBN 1-891845-21-7
ISBN 978-1-891845-21-5

THE TREATMENT OF DISEASE IN TCM, Vol. 1: Diseases of
the Head & Face, Including Mental & Emotional Disorders New
Edition
by Philippe Sion neau & Lü Gang
ISBN 0-936185-69-4
ISBN 978-0-936185-69-9

THE TREATMENT OF DISEASE IN TCM, Vol. II:
Diseases of the Eyes, Ears, Nose, & Throat
by Sionneau & Lü
ISBN 0-936185-73-2
ISBN 978-0-936185-73-6

THE TREATMENT OF DISEASE IN TCM, Vol. III: Diseases of
the Mouth, Lips, Tongue, Teeth & Gums
by Sionneau & Lü
ISBN 0-936185-79-1
ISBN 978-0-936185-79-8

THE TREATMENT OF DISEASE IN TCM, Vol IV: Diseases of
the Neck, Shoulders, Back, & Limbs
by Phi lippe Sion neau & Lü Gang
ISBN 0-936185-89-9
ISBN 978-0-936185-89-7

THE TREATMENT OF DISEASE IN TCM, Vol V: Diseases of
the Chest & Abdomen
by Philippe Sionneau & Lü Gang
ISBN 1-891845-02-0
ISBN 978-1-891845-02-4

THE TREATMENT OF DISEASE IN TCM, Vol VI: Diseases of
the Urogential System & Proctology
by Phi lippe Sion neau & Lü Gang
ISBN 1-891845-05-5
ISBN 978-1-891845-05-5

THE TREATMENT OF DISEASE IN TCM, Vol VII:
General Symptoms
by Phi lippe Sion neau & Lü Gang
ISBN 1-891845-14-4
ISBN 978-1-891845-14-7

THE TREATMENT OF EXTER NAL DIS EASES WITH
ACUPUNCTURE & MOXIBUSTION
by Yan Cui-lan and Zhu Yun-long, trans. by Yang Shou-zhong
ISBN 0-936185-80-5
ISBN 978-0-936185-80-4

THE TREATMENT OF MODERN WESTERN
MEDICAL DISEASES WITH CHINESE MEDICINE
by Bob Flaws & Philippe Sionneau
ISBN 1-891845-20-9
ISBN 978-1-891845-20-8

UNDERSTANDING THE DIFFICULT PATIENT: A Guide for
Practitioners of Oriental Medicine
by Nancy Bilello, RN, L.ac.
ISBN 1-891845-32-2
ISBN 978-1-891845-32-1

WESTERN PHYSICAL EXAM SKILLS FOR PRACTITIONERS
OF ASIAN MEDICINE
by Bruce H. Robinson & Honora Lee Wolfe
ISBN 1-891845-48-9
ISBN 978-1-891845-48-2

YI LIN GAI CUO (Correcting the Errors in the Forest of
Medicine)
by Wang Qing-ren
ISBN 1-891845-39-X
ISBN 978-1-891845-39-0

70 ESSENTIAL CHINESE HERBAL FORMULAS
by Bob Flaws
ISBN 0-936185-59-7
ISBN 978-0-936185-59-0

160 ESSENTIAL CHINESE READY-MADE MEDICINES
by Bob Flaws
ISBN 1-891945-12-8
ISBN 978-1-891945-12-3

630 QUESTIONS & ANSWERS ABOUT CHINESE HERBAL
MEDICINE:
A Work book & Study Guide
by Bob Flaws
ISBN 1-891845-04-7
ISBN 978-1-891845-04-8

260 ESSENTIAL CHINESE MEDICINALS
by Bob Flaws
ISBN 1-891845-03-9
ISBN 978-1-891845-03-1

750 QUESTIONS & ANSWERS ABOUT ACUPUNCTURE
Exam Preparation & Study Guide
by Fred Jennes
ISBN 1-891845-22-5
ISBN 978-1-891845-22-2